Principles of EXPERIMENTAL PHONETICS

Principles of
EXPERIMENTAL
PHONETICS

Edited by

Norman J. Lass, Ph.D.

Professor
Department of Speech Pathology and Audiology
West Virginia University
Morgantown, West Virginia

with 22 contributors
with 300 illustrations

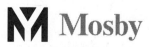 Mosby

St. Louis Baltimore Boston Carlsbad Chicago Naples New York Philadelphia Portland
London Madrid Mexico City Singapore Sydney Tokyo Toronto Wiesbaden

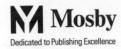
Mosby
Dedicated to Publishing Excellence

A Times Mirror
Company

P
95
P75
1996

Editor: Martha Sasser
Associate Developmental Editor: Kellie White
Project Manager: John Rogers
Editing and Production: Graphic World Publishing Services
Manufacturing Supervisor: Betty Richmond
Cover Design: Jeanne Wolfgeher

Printed in the United States of America
Composition by Graphic World, Inc.
Printing/binding by Maple Vail-York

Mosby–Year Book, Inc.
11830 Westline Industrial Drive
St. Louis, Missouri 63146

Library of Congress Cataloging in Publication Data

Principles of experimental phonetics / edited by Norman J. Lass.
     p.   cm.
  Includes bibliographical references and index.
  ISBN 0-8016-7975-3
  1. Speech. 2. Phonetics, Experimental. I. Lass, Norman J.
P95.P75 1995
302.2'242--dc20   95-15515
                                CIP

95 96 97 98 99 / 9 8 7 6 5 4 3 2 1

Contributors

James H. Abbs, Ph.D.
Departments of Neurology and
    Neurophysiology
University of Wisconsin Medical School
Madison, Wisconsin

Scott G. Adams, Ph.D.
Department of Communicative Disorders
Elborn College
University of Western Ontario
London, Ontario
Canada

Jared Bernstein, Ph.D.
Entropic Research Laboratory, Inc.
Menlo Park, California

James Dembowski, Ph.D.
Waisman Center on Mental Retardation and
    Human Development and
Department of Communicative Disorders
University of Wisconsin-Madison
Madison, Wisconsin

Horacio Franco, M.S.
SRI International
Menlo Park, California

Stephen D. Goldinger, Ph.D.
Department of Psychology
Arizona State University
Tempe, Arizona

Steven Greenberg, Ph.D.
Department of Linguistics
University of California, Berkeley
Berkeley, California and
International Computer Science Institute
Berkeley, California

Hector R. Javkin, Ph.D.
Speech Technology Laboratory
Panasonic Technologies, Inc.
Santa Barbara, California and
Department of Linguistics
University of California, Santa Barbara
Santa Barbara, California

Peter W. Jusczyk, Ph.D.
Department of Psychology and
Center for Cognitive Sciences
State University of New York at Buffalo
Buffalo, New York

Joel C. Kahane, Ph.D.
Department of Audiology and Speech
    Pathology
University of Memphis
Memphis, Tennessee

Ray D. Kent, Ph.D.
Waisman Center on Mental Retardation and
    Human Development and
Department of Communicative Disorders
University of Wisconsin-Madison
Madison, Wisconsin

Norman J. Lass, Ph.D.
Department of Speech Pathology and
    Audiology
West Virginia University
Morgantown, West Virginia

Ilse Lehiste, Ph.D.
Department of Linguistics
The Ohio State University
Columbus, Ohio

Paul A. Luce, Ph.D.
Department of Psychology and
Center for Cognitive Sciences
State University of New York at Buffalo
Buffalo, New York

Robert F. Orlikoff, Ph.D.
Laryngology Laboratory
Department of Surgery
Head and Neck Service
Memorial Sloan-Kettering Cancer Center
New York, New York

David B. Pisoni, Ph.D.
Speech Research Laboratory
Department of Psychology
Indiana University
Bloomington, Indiana

James R. Sawusch, Ph.D.
Department of Psychology and
Center for Cognitive Sciences
State University of New York at Buffalo
Buffalo, New York

Maureen Stone, Ph.D.
Speech and Voice Pathology Program
Division of Otolaryngology
University of Maryland Medical School
Baltimore, Maryland

Greg S. Turner, Ph.D.
Waisman Center on Mental Retardation and
  Human Development and
Department of Communicative Disorders
University of Wisconsin-Madison
Madison, Wisconsin

Hisashi J. Wakita, Ph.D.
Panasonic Technologies, Inc.
Santa Barbara, California

Donald W. Warren, D.D.S., Ph.D.
University of North Carolina
Craniofacial Center
Schools of Dentistry and Medicine
University of North Carolina at Chapel Hill
Chapel Hill, North Carolina

Richard M. Warren, Ph.D.
Department of Psychology
University of Wisconsin-Milwaukee
Milwaukee, Wisconsin

In Loving Memory of My Parents:

Fay Lerner Lass
and
Louis Lass

"Hear, my son, the instruction of thy father,
And forsake not the teaching of thy mother . . . "

—Proverbs 1:8

Acknowledgments

I am very grateful to the 22 authors who have contributed to this book. In addition to their highly skillful writing, they have shown an exceptional amount of cooperation and patience. My appreciation is also extended to the staff at Mosby, including Martha Sasser, Kellie White, and Amy Dubin, for their invaluable assistance throughout the various stages of development of this volume.

The efforts of Anne Gassett of Graphic World Publishing Services are acknowledged for her assistance with the editing and production of the book, and Kelly Johnson of the Department of Speech Pathology and Audiology at West Virginia University for her contribution to the preparation of the glossary.

I also wish to express my very sincere gratitude to my former mentors, particularly Professors J. Douglas Noll, Kenneth W. Burk, Ralph L. Shelton, and John F. Michel, who have had a profound influence on my education and career. I will always be indebted to them.

And finally, to my wife, Martha, whose never-ending patience and understanding were most helpful to me throughout the duration of this project, my deepest gratitude and appreciation.

Norman J. Lass

Preface

Principles of Experimental Phonetics provides comprehensive coverage of relevant contemporary topics of importance to graduate students and professionals in speech-language pathology, audiology, speech, language, and hearing sciences, psychology, the cognitive sciences, and linguistics. This volume will also prove valuable to those involved in research on the speech production and speech perception processes.

The book contains features that make it very user friendly, including (1) a chapter outline and key terms at the beginning of each chapter, (2) all key terms presented in boldface type when first mentioned in a chapter and defined in a glossary at the end of the volume, (3) review questions presented at the end of each chapter, and (4) a listing of suggested readings on the subtopics discussed within each chapter.

The authors are experienced researchers and writers who have presented a thorough discussion of their topics, including a comprehensive review of the pertinent literature as well as a delineation of the unresolved issues on each topic. In addition, they have provided specific suggestions for further inquiry and/or general directions for future research.

The book contains 15 chapters in four major sections. The Speech Production section includes four chapters. The first addresses models of speech production (feedback, feedforward, motor program, dynamic systems, gestural patterning, connectionist, subsystem, and composite) and the critical issues concerning these models. The second chapter discusses the aerodynamic principles of speech production, including the mechanics of breathing and speech, upper airway dynamics, the regulation of speech aerodynamics, experimental evidence of a speech regulating system, and the instrumentation employed in the study of speech aerodynamics. The third chapter is concerned with the mechanisms of speech motor execution and control, including passive and active peripheral mechanical properties of the speech production system; motor-sensory programming, execution, and control; sensorimotor contributions to speech motor control; multiple roles for speech motor-sensory mechanisms; and time-varying contributions of motor-sensory processes. Laryngeal structure and function is the topic of the fourth and final chapter in this section, which includes a detailed discussion of the structure, neurology, and phonatory function of the larynx as well as theories of phonation, the modification of phonation, and phonatory behavior involved in speech.

The Speech Signal section has three chapters. The first is concerned with the acoustic characteristics of American English, including the defining acoustic features of consonants, vowels, and diphthongs as well as the acoustic manifestations of the suprasegmental features of intonation, stress, and quantity. The second chapter addresses in detail the physiological, acoustic, and perceptual aspects of the prosodic features of duration and quantity, tone and intonation, as well as stress and emphasis. Also included are comparative analyses of these suprasegmental features across languages. Speech analysis and speech synthesis are discussed in the third chapter in this section, including Fourier analysis, spectrographic analysis, visual analysis of the time waveform of speech, time analysis of the glottal waveform, cascade and parallel formant synthesizers, synthesis based on linear predictive coding, as well as synthesis by rule and text-to-speech.

There are five chapters in the Speech Perception section. The first is concerned with issues in speech perception and spoken word recognition, including linearity, lack of acoustic-phonetic invariance, the segmentation problem, the specialization of speech perception, and normalization problems in speech perception. Also addressed are theories of speech perception (motor, direct-realist, information-processing, as well as LAFS and fuzzy logical models) and theories of spoken word recognition (logogen, cohort, autonomous search, neighborhood activation, as well as TRACE and other connectionist models). The second chapter discusses developmental speech perception, including the capacities of infants to recognize native and nonnative language contrasts, the nature of the underlying speech perception mechanisms in infants, and the relationship of speech perception and language acquisition in children. The third chapter addresses auditory processing of speech, including the relevance of auditory physiology to speech processing, anatomy and physiology of the auditory pathway, spectral representations of the auditory periphery, central auditory mechanisms, and information coding. In addition, the author discusses clinical implications and implications for models of speech recognition, general models of speech perception, and the sound patterns of language. The fourth chapter describes speech recognition by computer, including a technical overview and design of speech recognition systems, evaluation of speech recognizers, as well as commercial and educational applications of speech recognition devices. The fifth and final chapter in this section deals with auditory illusions and perceptual processing of speech, including the illusory presence of obliterated sounds (phonemic restorations and auditory induction), perception and confusions of temporal order, illusory organization of loud and clear vowel sequences, and illusory changes in repeated words (the verbal transformation effect).

The final section of the book, Research Techniques, contains three chapters. The first deals with digital speech analysis techniques for the study of speech acoustics, including the cepstrum method, linear prediction method, methods for computing vocal tract area functions, and perceptually based analysis. The second chapter addresses instrumentation for the study of speech physiology, including three types: point-tracking techniques (electromagnetic midsagittal articulometer, x-ray microbeam, strain gauges, and Optotrak), imaging techniques (x-ray, xeroradiography, tomography, computed tomography, magnetic resonance imaging, and ultrasound), and measures of complex behaviors (electropalatography, electromyography, electroglottography, and inductance plethysmography). The third and final chapter in this section is concerned with instrumentation and methodology for the study of speech perception. This chapter includes psychophysical methods (adjustment, limits, and constant stimuli), signal detection theory, experimental tasks and converging operations (reaction time, categorical perception, speech mode, and selective adaptation), methods for nonadult listeners, as well as audio reproduction, listener participation, and on-line system instrumentation.

It is our intention that the contents of this volume will result in the reader's understanding of relevant contemporary topics and important issues in experimental phonetics. It is also our hope that this understanding will lead to increased clinical application of normative data as well as further investigation of unresolved issues that will ultimately result in their resolution.

Norman J. Lass

Contents

Principles of EXPERIMENTAL PHONETICS

Part I

SPEECH PRODUCTION

Chapter 1

Models of Speech Production

Ray D. Kent, Scott G. Adams, Greg S. Turner

INTRODUCTION

What is a **model?** It is difficult to give an answer that fits everything that has been called a model in the literature on speech production. One source of difficulty is that the words *model* and *theory* are not used consistently, so that one person's theory may be another person's model. Rather than impose a vocabulary on the various proposals considered in this review, this chapter usually retains the terminology used by the various authors. However, there are reasons to distinguish between theory and model. A model is a simplified description of a complex system or process. A model is always an abstraction or simplification. Modeling helps the scientist to identify the important parameters or elements of a system or process that is too complicated to be comprehended in its complete, natural form. A model may be related to a theory, as in the case of implementing a theory, and may be used to test a theory directly or indirectly.

A theory is an overall conception that encompasses the known facts in a (preferably) parsimonious way and typically includes a set of assumptions and a number of principles from which predictions (hypotheses) can be derived. Another way of viewing the distinction between theory and model is that a model often is used as an analogy to the theory, especially as a way of visualizing the theory. Schmidt (1988) gives an example from atomic theory. When this theory was developed in the 1930s, electrons and protons were imaginary constructs. A common model used to describe these constructs was a system of little balls, with neutrons and protons clustered in a central nucleus and with electrons orbiting the nucleus. Most of the ideas to be discussed in this chapter are better described as models than theories. They help us to visualize the processes and structures thought to be involved in speech production.

Because speech is a complex phenomenon, it can be modeled in various ways for different purposes. The box on p. 5 summarizes some major directions in the modeling of speech production. The variability in content and purpose of these models can make it difficult to compare or evaluate them because they are not necessarily intended to do exactly the same thing. For example, a **neural model** of speech production is an account of the nervous system processes that control speaking. Such a model typically is couched in terms of neural regulatory loops, brain centers, or some other conception of neural organization. An **articulatory model** is concerned primarily with **articulation,** or the movements of the speech structures (e.g., the tongue, jaw, lips, and velum). This kind of model usually describes articulatory positions, movements, and configurations. It may neglect neural processes altogether or treat them only indirectly. It also may neglect the muscles that make up the articulators and refer only to gross structural movements, such as a closing movement of the jaw or an alveolar closure of the tongue tip.

Another kind of model, the **vocal tract model,** focuses on the shaping of the vocal tract (the pharyngeal, oral, and nasal cavities). The vocal tract may be considered as an acoustic tube or combination of tubes that is adjusted in its cross-sectional dimensions and length for different speech sounds. Although human speech accomplishes these adjustments by means of articulatory actions that give shape to the vocal tract, a vocal tract model can neglect the underlying articulations and refer to the vocal tract only as an acoustic tube that undergoes changes in its overall length and its cross-sectional area as a function of length. A vocal tract model might refer to a constriction in the palatal region without explaining how such a constriction comes about.

Other models of speech production are functional. For example, an information-processing model attempts to account for the ways various types of information regulate speaking. An example is a **servosystem model,** in which feedback control is a major feature. An error signal derived from the feedback is used to generate the desired movement. Still other models are developed at the level of motor control. These **motor control models** are concerned with the activation patterns of muscles or muscle groups and therefore may be explicitly defined in terms of motoric processes. It would be a very ambitious undertaking to develop a comprehensive model that incorporated all of these models. Most scientists work on a narrower set of issues, so it is important to recognize the type of model under discussion.

All of these are models of speech production. They all represent important knowledge about the act of speaking and guide research on speech production. Given the diversity among these theories and models and the limited space available to discuss them, this chapter summarizes major directions of theorizing and model-

Some general types of models of speech production

Model Type	Purpose
Neural	Accounts for nervous system processes that control speaking; may specify neural structures, control circuits, information flow, other neural variables.
Articulatory	Describes articulatory positions, movements, or configurations; typically specifies individual articulators, such as tongue, lips, jaw, velum.
Vocal tract	Focuses on the shaping of the vocal tract for the production of speech; does not necessarily specify actions of individual articulators; may be concerned with overall descriptions of vocal tract configuration.
Functional	Accounts for the ways in which various types of information regulate speech production; variables may be linguistic (syllables, phonemes, etc.), control signals (feedforward or feedback signals) or generally defined in terms of movement sequence.
Motor control	Describes the motor processes of the activation of muscles for the production of speech; usually expressed in motoric terms, such as specification of muscle synergies or kinematic descriptions of movement.

ing rather than exhaustively reviewing individual proposals. The various theories and models of speech production can be put into relief by asking of each: What is being modeled? What is the purpose of the theory or model? These two questions are important not only to understand the proposals themselves but also to identify the kinds of evidence against which they can be tested.

The following definitions will apply in this chapter: *A theory of speech production accounts for the conversion of a linguistic representation of a message to the actions of the speech production system. A model of speech production is a simplified representation of speech production or some aspect of speech production.* The linguistic representation typically is viewed as a symbolic string, for example, a string of phonemes. The speech production system includes the respiratory subsystem, the laryngeal subsystem, and the supraglottal subsystem (the latter corresponding to the vocal tract). This definition can accommodate several types of theories, including those mentioned earlier in this chapter. It also announces the fundamental problem that all such theories face: how to relate the output of language formulation to the working of a speech production model. Although some proposals ig-

nore this problem, it must be faced if the theories and models are to account for speech as a language modality.

Carre and Mrayati (1990) proposed some general criteria by which models of vocal tract function (particularly articulatory-acoustic-phonetic relations) can be evaluated. The same criteria, given here in slightly modified form, are useful in evaluating the models to be discussed in this chapter:

1. The model should closely describe natural phenomena, such as coarticulation, vowel and consonant production, declination of fundamental frequency, speech breathing, and adjustment to speaking rate. Naturally, the more of these phenomena the model addresses, the better.
2. The parameters of the model should be based on observations of the system to be modeled. Ideally, the parameters should be orthogonal (independent of one another, so as to be maximally efficient) and capable of producing all possible states or functions of the modeled system.
3. The number of model parameters should be as small as possible (*parsimony*), and the command strategies should be simple yet significant (*economy with power*).

4. The model should enable simple interpretations across domains (e.g., neural to articulatory, articulatory to acoustic, acoustic to phonetic).
5. The model should exhibit nonlinear phenomena characteristic of speech production. That is, some aspects of speech cannot be described as linear operations. A purely linear model would not account for these aspects.
6. The model should account for relevant scientific facts.

CONCEPTUALIZING SPEECH QUA LANGUAGE: LEVELS OF ORGANIZATION

Theorizing about speech production is complicated by several factors. One is the relationship between speech and language. Because speech is a modality of language, it cannot be separated from its role as language expression. Speech is derived from intent to communicate and formulation of a linguistic message. If some articulatory or acoustic pattern is to be called speech, then the implicit assumption is that the pattern expresses an underlying linguistic message known to the speaker. There are a few exceptions to this general assumption, including speaking in tongues as practiced in some churches, deliberate attempts of a talker to produce gibberish, and neologistic jargon produced by some individuals with aphasia.

Knowing where to draw the line between language and speech helps in constructing and evaluating theories of speech production. Consider sequencing errors in speech, such as when a speaker says "food the peech" instead of "feed the pooch" (example from Fromkin, 1989). If these errors are thought to arise in speech production processes, they become a source of information about speech production. On the other hand, if they are thought to arise in processes that precede speech (such as a system for phonological assembly), they need not be accounted for in a speech production model and in fact may be irrelevant to such a model. Recent evidence indicates that speech errors are pertinent to speech production models and may have to be considered at the motoric level (Mowrey and MacKay, 1990).

This is the fundamental question about the relationship of speech to language: What is the input to the model of speech production? In other words, what output of the language system drives the production of speech? Figure 1-1 is a general diagram of the components commonly described in accounts of language formulation and speech production. A brief description of each component follows:

Cognition—prelinguistic formulation; ideas not yet cast as language; may take the form of schema, notions, general plans.

Affect—emotional accompaniments of cognition and language.

Syntax—the rules governing the arrangements of words in an utterance; pertains to the linear order of words in sentences, the categorization of words into parts of speech, and the grouping of words into structural constituents.

Semantics—the meaning of words and of groups of words.

Phonology—the principles and patterns by which sounds are used in a language.

Lexicon—the vocabulary of a language user; may specify morphologic, phonologic, orthographic, syntactic, semantic, and pragmatic information for words and the morphemes of which words are composed.

Phonetics—the specification of ways phonologic units are produced; output is presumably the input to the motor processes of speech production. The more elaborate the output of the phonetic component, the fewer are the problems to be resolved at the level of motor control. An output that

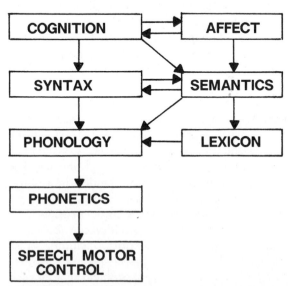

FIGURE 1-1 A general diagram of the processes of spoken language, including language formulation and speech production.

specifies allophonic variations (detailed considerations of sound pattern) provides more information than a phonemic output. For example, a phonetic output of the form [s p⁼ ū n] is more detailed than the phonemic representation /s p u n/. The former specifies certain features, such as lack of aspiration for /p/ following /s/ and nasalization of the vowel /u/ preceding the nasal consonant.

Motor control system — the structures and processes that regulate the muscular actions of the speech production system; composed of muscles and other tissues within the head, neck, thorax and abdomen.

An important feature of this diagram is that the processes of language formulation must relate to the processes of speech production. Exactly how this relation takes place is a matter of much speculation. To say that the phonological component of language accomplishes the relation is not satisfactory unless this component is clearly defined with respect to language processes on the one hand and to the motoric events in speech production on the other hand. Modern phonological theory may hold some interesting answers, and those who would understand speech should be aware of developments in phonology. These developments can have important implications for the study of the production and perception of speech.

Meyer and Gordon (1985) observed that conceptualizations of speech organization generally recognize three levels (box). Basically, this table is an elaboration of the motor control component. The first level in the box is a multiunit representation based on networks or sequences of some kind, typically extending over several segments or syllables. For example, Kozhevnikov and Chistovich (1965) proposed the **syntagma,** a rhythmic grouping of syllables tending toward seven constituent syllables. Another perspective, after Chomsky (1965), is that surface-structure sequences of words are the highest level of organization.

The second level is the basic unit of phonetic or articulatory representation. Candidates at this level include the syllable, phoneme, allophone, and feature. Possibly more than one unit is involved, as would be the case if units were nested into a hierarchical structure, such as features within phonemes and phonemes within syllables.

The third level is motor control, or the direct regulation of the musculature. Here possibilities include an abstract articulatory target or goal (e.g., a kind of snapshot of the intended vocal tract configuration), a motor command (a specific neural instruction to a muscle or set of muscles), an acoustic template (an acoustic goal to be achieved by articulation), and a **coordinative structure** (a synergy or linkage among a group of muscles to accomplish a particular task).

These terms will be considered in more detail later in this chapter. The central point of this discussion is that speech organization can be modeled with different units selected from different levels of control or representation. In-

Hypothesized levels of speech organization with candidate units at each level

Several models of speech production propose a multilevel organization, often reflecting the levels and units shown here. The usual strategy is to select one or more units from each level to formulate a hierarchical control system of the form: sequence of units — prearticulatory representation — motor realization.

SEQUENCE OR NETWORK OF UNITS (MULTI-UNIT ASSEMBLY OR PATTERN)

Conceptual dependency networks
Surface structure word sequences
Syntagma
Breath group
Articulatory phrase

PREARTICULATORY REPRESENTATION

Syllables
Demisyllables
Phonemes
Allophones
Phonetic features
Gesture bundles

MOTOR REALIZATION (VOCAL TRACT CONTROL)

Spatial targets
Motor commands
Acoustic templates
Coordinative structures
Vocal tract and articulatory model variables
Motor or gestural score

deed, models of speech production often reflect different levels of organization, and furthermore, different units or constructs have been proposed for each level. The possible permutations are impressive. But this feature also complicates the empirical test of these models. For example, if a multilevel model misses the mark in accounting for a phenomenon or predicting an experimental outcome, which stage should be revised?

The principal reason that different levels have been proposed for speech organization is the belief that different phenomena seem to be explained more effectively at different levels. However, it is difficult to test a multilayered theory because processes or events at one level usually depend on processes or events at other levels. Therefore, a conceptual error at one level can affect the rest of the model.

A proper study of speech production models rests on a careful reading of this entire book. A useful theory draws from several sources of knowledge and accounts for a large number of facts with reasonable parsimony (simplicity). Beginning students may find it difficult to appreciate the parsimony of a theory until they have digested a volume of facts about speech production. But a theory can also help to guide and integrate the facts on speech production. Always remember, any given theory may very well be wrong, if not in its major concepts, at least in its details. But an incorrect theory is not a bad theory if it clearly directs research efforts to disprove it.

CRITICAL ISSUES FACING SPEECH PRODUCTION MODELS

Why has it been difficult to model speech production? After all, if speech is regulated by a string of linguistic units, such as phonemes, then should it not be possible simply to define for each phoneme a set of muscle commands (or vocal tract adjustments) and execute them in the order specified by the linguistic string, much as one might type the consecutive letters that make up a word? By this reasoning, a word like *soon* would be produced by sequentially executing the stored motor instructions for the phonemes [s], [u] and [n]. This has appealing simplicity: The language production system generates a string of phonemes (or segments of some kind), and the speech production system then gives

physical realization to each phoneme in turn.

However, this simple idea does not survive empirical tests. The actual articulations in speech are not easily reconciled with a linear string of control units. Beyond the general issue of how linguistic units relate to the control of the speech production system, there are three major problems from a motor control perspective.

The Serial Order Problem

The problem of serial order in behavior, classically formulated by Lashley (1951), remains a challenge to contemporary speech research. Speech is a string or sequence that evolves in time. A fundamental issue in its regulation is the determination of how its elements are strung together. What are the elements of control? Several units have been proposed, including the extrinsic allophone, the phoneme, the syllable, the demisyllable, and so on. And even when two scientists agree on the choice of the element, they may differ on how serial ordering is accomplished. For example, one might maintain that the elements cohere in a larger structure, such as a stress grouping. The other might argue that peripheral feedback mechanisms are sufficient to control the temporal ordering of speech events, so that feedback that verifies the completion of one event is sufficient to trigger the next. The simple word *soon* can be conceptualized in several ways; for example, as a string of phonemes, a string of allophones, a consonant-vowel-consonant (CVC) syllable structure, or a syllable combination of consonant-vowel (CV), ([s] + [u]) followed by CV ([n] + null element).

The Degrees of Freedom Problem

The speech production system has potential for a large number of degrees of freedom. Gracco (1990) cites (but does not necessarily concur with) the frequent observation that there are more than 70 different muscular degrees of freedom in the production of speech. The tongue, lips, jaw, velum, larynx, and respiratory system all possess several possible types of movement with respect to range, direction, speed, and temporal combinations with one another. Moreover, they can combine in various ways; for example, the lower lip and jaw can move in phase and in the same direction, out of phase but in the same direction, or in phase but in opposite directions. The **degrees of freedom problem** is general to action and not unique to speech (Jordan and Rosenbaum, 1989). On the one hand, excessive degrees of freedom allow a great degree of behavioral flexibility. But on the other hand, many degrees of freedom also present a challenge: How does the control system contend with so many degrees of freedom to achieve a desired action? The system must either expend a great deal of computational effort to manage a large number of degrees of freedom or somehow reduce the degrees of freedom. Production of even the simple word *soon* involves the respiratory system (which itself is multistructural, containing the abdominal muscles, the diaphragm, and the rib cage), the larynx (also a multistructural assembly of cartilage, muscles, and other tissues), the velopharynx, the tongue body, the tongue tip, and the lips. The magnitude of the problem can be appreciated by attempting to list the sequence of articulations and other actions needed to utter this single monosyllabic word. The challenge grows considerably if we attempt such a listing for a longer utterance, such as "Soon the snow began to melt and the grass began to grow." How does the speech production system manage the movements of so many structures?

The Context-Sensitivity Problem

Another problem is that the production of a given sound varies with the context in which it is produced. Just as the degrees of freedom problem is not unique to speech, neither is the context-sensitive aspect of action unique to speech; it is true of motor behavior in general. In fact, any given sound of speech has a large number of physical instantiations. If speech were produced by a simple library of motor commands retrieved as needed for individual phonemes, how would the control system regulate action in the face of a tremendous number of degrees of freedom, and how would it permit extensive adjustments to context?

Many of these effects are subsumed under the term **coarticulation,** which means that at any one time the speech system shows adjustments for more than one segment (see Kent and Minifie [1977] for a general discussion). Some examples of coarticulatory patterns are shown in Figure 1-2. Figure 1-2, *A* shows how the tongue position for the velar consonants /k/ and /g/ varies with the tongue carriage for the following vowel. When the vowel is produced with a relatively front position of the tongue (as in *key*),

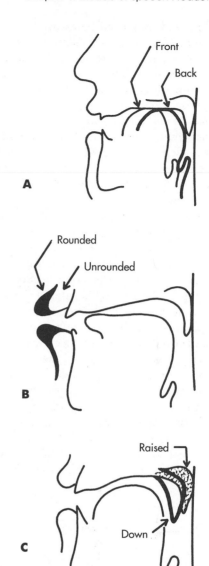

FIGURE 1-2 Examples of coarticulation: *A,* Variation in place of constriction for a velar consonant. *B,* Variation in lip configuration for the fricative /s/. *C,* Variation in velar position for a vowel. (From Nielson, M. D., & Neilson, P. D. [1987]. Speech motor control and stuttering: A computational model of adaptive sensory-motor processing. *Speech Communication, 6,* 325-333.)

the constriction for the velar consonant is also relatively front. But when the vowel has a relatively back tongue position, the constriction for the velar consonant also is made with a back articulation. As shown in Figure 1-2, *B,* careful observations of the lips during production of word pairs such as *soup* and *seep* show that the [s] in *soup* is produced with rounding of the lips, whereas the [s] in *seep* is not produced with such rounding and may even be associated with lip retraction. The labial articulation for the [s] sound apparently is affected by an upcoming sound in the string. The [s] in *soup* is rounded in anticipation of the rounded vowel [u]. However, the [s] in *seep* is not rounded because [i] is not a rounded vowel. Finally, Figure 1-2, C illustrates that the velum may be raised or lowered during a vowel, depending on whether the following segment is a nasal or oral sound. Vowels in English are typically nasalized when they occur before nasal consonants.

For the sample word *soon,* coarticulation is manifest in several ways, including these: (1) during the production of the initial [s], the body of the tongue, to some degree, anticipates the retracted and elevated position needed for the upcoming high-back vowel [u]; (2) the lips are rounded during the production of the initial [s] as preparation for the following rounded vowel [u]; and (3) the velopharynx opens during production of the vowel [u] because of the influence of the following nasal consonant [n].

Coarticulation has come to subsume a number of phenomena, not all of which necessarily involve the same level of explanation. Some coarticulatory effects may result from anticipation of forthcoming phonetic requirements in a string of segments; other effects may be deter-mined by biomechanical constraints; and still others may be determined by variations in the timing of articulatory movements within different sequences. These explanations can have profound implications for linguistic theory as well as speech production. Fujimura (1990) noted that some contextual variations traditionally classified as allophones may be interpreted as the expressions of variably timed characteristic gestures of different articulators. Browman and Goldstein (in press) described how variations in interarticulator timing could account for phenomena such as deletions, insertions, and feature alterations. Similar ideas have been used by Saltzman and Munhall (1989) and Lofqvist (1990) to explain the motor patterns of speech. Figure 1-3 illustrates how the articulatory movements can be variably timed during the production of a phonetic sequence. One way of understanding these complex patterns is to recognize that control of the vocal tract is determined by the strength or dominance of a given articular at a given time. At point a in Figure 1-3, the jaw and tongue have the greatest influence on shaping the vocal tract.

Lofqvist (1990) viewed the segment as a bundle of gestures characterized by an internal stability of patterns of muscle activation, movement, or both. The gestural coherence, or

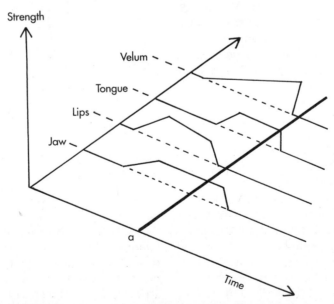

FIGURE 1-3 **Diagram showing complex temporal relationships among the movements in a phonetic sequence; a is the point where the jaw and tongue have the greatest influence on shaping the vocal tract.** (From Kent, R. D. [1981]. Sensorimotor aspects of speech development. In Aslin, R. N., Alberts, J.R., & Petersen, M. R. [Eds.], *Development of Perception: Psychobiological Perspectives* [Vol. 1, pp. 162-185]. New York: Academic Press.)

togetherness, can be defined at three levels: (1) spatial, meaning activation of the same set of muscles, (2) temporal, meaning that the gestures should be related by synchronicity, fixed temporal order, or fixed phase, and (3) scaling, meaning that a scaling or parameter change is distributed over all activated gestures. An example of scaling is the effect of placing stress on a syllable. When a syllable is given increased stress, several different articulations in the syllable tend to have a greater range of movement and greater movement velocities (Kent and Netsell, 1972).

These issues speak directly to the question of input to a speech production model. One model might take allophones as the input segment, thereby referring the assignment of allophonic variations to a phonological stage that precedes speech production per se. Another model might assume that phonemes (or a similar unit) are the input and that the so-called allophonic variations are a result of variably timed relationships among the articulators. However, *the form of a speech production model depends critically on the assumptions of its formation; one such assumption is the nature of the input to the model.*

Many models implicitly or explicitly assume that the phoneme or a similar segment is a major form of input to the speech production system. The phoneme is a convenient unit for the conversion from a phonological domain to an articulatory system, although the phoneme itself does not necessarily explain all of the details in this conversion. However, some interpretations of *segment* are highly restrictive. The eminent phonetician Kenneth L. Pike (1959) spoke of language in terms of particles, waves, and fields, much as modern physics views light as having both a particle and wave nature. Meyer (1987) emphasized that Pike's idea extends to the phoneme as well as to language more generally. That is, he argued that the phoneme has some properties of the particle, other properties of the wave, and still other properties of the field. The phoneme has a unitary property insofar as listeners can hear segments, that is, identify successive units in the speech stream. But the identification of phonemes also is subject to contextual influences, such that a given acoustic segment may be identified quite differently depending on the sound stream that surrounds it. Although this formulation makes it difficult to define the phoneme, it is an alternative to the more traditional conceptualizations, which tend to emphasize the phoneme as unit.

SCHOOLS OF THOUGHT IN THE MODELING OF SPEECH

Theories proposed to account for these problems fall into several general notions of the control of speech production. Some license has been taken in placing individual models within the following categories. A given model may in fact fall under more than one heading, depending on the emphasis given to its properties.

The box below offers a comparison of selected models with respect to primary modeling strategy, advantages, disadvantages, and current directions. This summary is highly selective and is intended to point out only a few major properties of the models. It may be helpful to refer to it during the discussion of each model. For a thorough discussion of each model, see the papers cited in this review.

Summary of major classes of speech production models

MOTOR PROGRAM MODELS

Basic Strategy: Goals or targets used to construct a plan of motor action; feedback no role or limited role.

Advantages: Account for predictable (learned) variations in motor performance; movement control can continue despite interruptions or distortions of feedback or despite changes in peripheral status.

Disadvantages: Contain highly detailed information on spatial and temporal features of movement (hence, a risk of being top-heavy in high-level control responsibilities); may neglect peripheral and environmental variables that affect motor performance.

Current Directions: Based on (1) motor schema that take into account initial conditions, intended action, previous experience, etc.; (2) stages of program construction, such as

---

Continued.

retrieval and unpacking; or (3) multilevel operations defined at various levels, with particular objectives handled at each level.

GESTURAL PATTERNING MODELS

Basic Strategy: Families of functionally equivalent movement patterns regulated to achieve speech goals.

Advantages: Movement goals specifically defined in terms of movement patterns that permit goal to be reached in a flexible, biomechanically appropriate manner; has been used with good results in an articulatory synthesis system.

Disadvantages: Leave unresolved some questions regarding serial order; strategy may have a table-lookup character in which functionally equivalent patterns specified ad hoc.

Current Directions: Strategy supplemented with aspects of connectionist theory to resolve serial order problem; system readily modified to reflect new data on speech motor properties.

FEEDBACK MODELS

Basic Strategy: Feedback from periphery used to ensure that movement goals are reached; feedback signal allows correction of movements to reach desired goals.

Advantages: Accounts for spatial accuracy of movements in the face of peripheral disturbances or variations in load.

Disadvantages: Feedback loops sometimes too slow to account for the precision of speech movements; little or no use of prediction based on knowledge of system-task interactions.

Current Directions: Feedforward and feedback control combined so that predictive and/or adaptive control features are possible; adaptive sensorimotor control accomplished by noncontinuous monitoring of movements with amendment as needed for intended actions.

CONNECTIONIST MODELS

Basic Strategy: Establishes (learns) weighted connections in a large network of interconnected units.

Advantages: General success in modeling various aspects of speech behavior, including sequencing errors, coarticulation, and serial order.

Disadvantages: Generally do not reveal the working of the natural system (e.g., invariants or control processes); difficult to choose among alternative architectures.

Current Directions: State units and hidden units incorporated to model speech behaviors; biological or psychological constraints may be applied to networks.

ACTION THEORY (DYNAMIC SYSTEM) MODELS

Basic Strategy: Action responses based on task-determined synergies (coordinative structures) with few degrees of freedom and well-defined control parameters.

Advantages: Minimizes degrees of freedom and recognizes biomechanical properties of system in relation to tasks; control strategy flexible but parsimonious.

Disadvantages: Responses not clearly linked with phonological input to speech production; some predictions based on phase relations not confirmed; neglects acoustic and language-specific timing factors.

Current Directions: Implementation of some basic features into articulatory models, e.g., gestural patterning theory (families of functionally equivalent movement patterns regulated to achieve speech goals).

FEEDBACK AND FEEDFORWARD MODELS

The first set of solutions consists of feedback and feedforward models. The components of a *feedback model* are shown in Figure 1-4, *A*. The strategy is to use characteristics of the output of the system to modify the controlling process. The reference signal is the *actuating signal,* which causes the system to act or respond in some way. For example, if we take the tongue as a speech structure to be controlled, the reference signal is a motor command (a neural instruction to the tongue muscles), and the output signal is a movement of the tongue. Information about the movement is sent to the brain via the feedback loop, which contains a feedback controller. The loop for the tongue might include feedback from sensory receptors for touch, position, or movement. The controller has various purposes, typically to generate an error signal from the feedback. For example, if the tongue fails to move far enough to reach a specified target, the error signal is used to correct the deficiency. The error and reference signals are summed in the feedback operation.

The **feedback system** can work very well if the feedback loop is fast enough to regulate the movement. However, for many human movements, the response to feedback is too slow to keep up with precise movements. Hence, a limiting condition for a feedback model is the latency of the feedback signal. If the latency is too great for the time within which control must be exercised, the feedback model loses credibility.

A particular type of feedback model applied to speech is a servosystem model. In control theory a servomechanism is a power-amplifying control system in which the controlled variable is a mechanical position or one of its time derivatives (velocity or acceleration). A familiar servomechanism is the power-steering system of an automobile. When the driver turns the steering wheel, the small rotational torque that the driver applies is amplified hydraulically so that the front wheels of the car move as desired. When the intended angular position of the front wheels is reached, negative feedback is used to decrease the torque from the hydraulic amplifier to zero. The essential feature of the control system is the use of a feedback path that allows

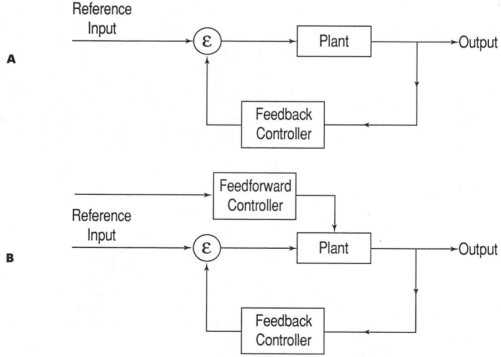

FIGURE 1-4 *A,* General diagram for a feedback system, in which information from the system (plant) output is fed back to the controller. *B,* General diagram for a system combining feedback and feedforward signals; ε is the summation operator. (From Perkell, J. S. [1980]. Phonetic features and the physiology of speech production. In Butterworth, B. [Ed.], *Language Production* [Vol. 1, pp. 337-372]. New York: Academic Press.)

the output (the angular position of the front wheels) to affect the actuating signal (the signal that drives the hydraulic apparatus). To understand how this idea is applied to speech, consider the angular movements of the jaw around the temporomandibular joint. Just as the servosystem ensures that the wheels of the car reach the desired position, it can ensure that the jaw reaches the intended amount of opening.

One of the early theories of speech production was the servosystem theory of Fairbanks (1954), who proposed that speech relied on feedback to generate an error signal, which was the means by which the desired output could be achieved. Feedback control is one way to reduce the degrees of freedom in a system. The feedback loop allows for the correction of errors during the operation of the system. This kind of approach is still used today, often for subsystems of speech production, considered later in the chapter. The general application of feedback for the regulation of speech movements was discussed by MacNeilage (1970), who considered how various receptors, particularly the muscle spindle, could participate in a feedback (closed loop) control system. The term *closed loop* implies that once the command to move has been issued, no further action of the command center is needed because feedback loops control the outcome.

As noted earlier, the application of the feedback model to speech regulation is limited by the slowness of many important feedback signals. There is another important issue to consider. If speech is under feedback control, disruption of feedback channels should greatly disturb the production of speech. A number of experiments have tested this prediction. Although the results are mixed, the most persistent conclusion is that attempts to eliminate or distort sensory feedback usually have, at most, slight effects on speech production. Kent, Martin, and Sufit (1990) concluded that speech regulation, at least in the mature speaker, does not appear to require *continuous* feedback information. Speakers often seem to compensate quite well for a variety of disruptions, including trigeminal nerve block, topical anesthesia, and noise masking. Although delayed auditory feedback can produce disruptive effects on speech, some speakers learn to speak fluently despite the delayed feedback.

In view of the difficulties with feedback models, several writers have proposed **feedforward systems** (possibly combined with feedback mechanisms) as a more appropriate model. Figure 1-4, *B*, shows a system with both feedback and feedforward information. Feedforward signals make adjustments at the periphery so that the system can respond efficiently to forthcoming instructions. Sometimes the signals bias the operational status of the system, giving it a status suited to the movement about to be performed. Feedforward is particularly useful for systems for planning or prediction. This capability lets the system adjust for rapid movements and various disturbances or restrictions on motor performance and its sensory feedback. Gracco (1990) summarizes research indicating that sensory information plays two major roles in speech motor control. They are (1) to allow comparison of feedback from the periphery with the intended speech goal, and (2) to set parameters or adjust predictively for forthcoming control actions.

One example of contemporary use of feedback control is the adaptive model theory (Figure 1-5), which uses feedback adaptively to control speech (Neilson and Neilson, 1987). This theory does not assume that a highly practiced motor skill like speech requires continuous sensory feedback. Instead, movements are monitored to determine *whether* the regulatory process needs to be modified. Afference, or feedback, is the means by which errors are corrected if they are detected. The essence of adaptive model theory is an adaptable store of information based on sensory feedback. This substrate, accomplished over time as feedback derived from motor sequences, generates new actions. A planned sensory trajectory (which prescribes the intended action) is transformed into a corresponding set of motor commands. Feedback is used to monitor the relationship between the motor commands and their multimodal sensory consequences. If necessary, the relationship is modified. In this way the system performs intended movements and gains expertise in planning movements. This model allows for the capability for continual updating of the strategies that relate movement to its sensory outcomes. According to this model, continuous feedback is not essential to speech regulation, but feedback signals can be incorporated into speech production on a provisional and discontinuous basis.

MOTOR PROGRAM MODELS

The second set of solutions is a **motor program** perspective. A motor program is a plan or prescription of movement. The word *preplan-*

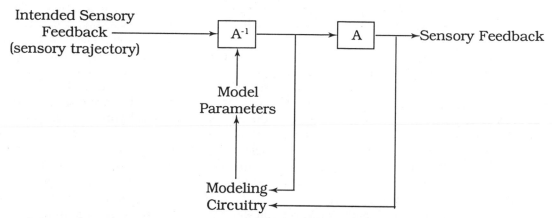

FIGURE 1-5   The adaptive sensory-motor control model of Neilson and Neilson (1987). Intended sensory feedback is compared with actual feedback through a modeling circuitry. A^{-1} and A are inverse operations. (From Nielson, M. D., & Neilson, P. D. [1987]. Speech motor control and stuttering: A computational model of adaptive sensory-motor processing. *Speech Communication, 6,* 325-333.)

ning is sometimes used, apparently to emphasize that the movement plan is prepared in advance of its execution and therefore can be said to reside somewhere in the control system even before movements are performed. The ready-made plan is executed by the speech system, much as a computer executes a computer program. Different conceptualizations of motor programs have been described. The extreme version makes no use of peripheral feedback; the commands contained in the program are sufficient. Other versions of motor program theory make allowances for feedback participation in some aspects of regulation (e.g., Abbs, Gracco, and Cole, 1984; Gracco, 1990). Various terms have been introduced to convey the concept of motor program, including *motor score, motor goal score, motor plan,* and *movement sequence*. At the heart of these concepts is the idea that speech movements are available in a preassembled form that directs the actual muscular regulation of the production system.

The concept of motor programming for speech has been criticized on several grounds, including its excessive rigidity, failure to account for corrections in the ongoing movement, and inability to assess the status of the periphery and take proper advantage of these initial conditions. These and other criticisms of motor program theory are discussed at length in Reed (1982). Some critics find it untenable

to assume that the action sequences of speech are contained in the brain before the actions of speech are evident.

The concept of a program has not been abandoned by all speech scientists. Its proponents believe that it accounts for some types of data that are not easily explained by other models. As one example, motor programs can address latency data in the production of utterances of varying length. When subjects read aloud words or digits, the voice-onset latency, or the interval from the onset of the stimulus (a visual display) to the beginning of voicing for the response, increases with the number of syllables to be uttered (Eriksen, Pollack, and Montague, 1970; Klapp, Anderson, and Berrian, 1973). In other words, the more complex the utterance, the longer it takes to produce it. However, if the speaker is given time to prepare the response before a signal to speak is given, the syllable latency effect disappears (Klapp, Anderson, and Berrian, 1973). Therefore, the latency is not simply an initiation effect in which more time is needed to initiate long utterances than short ones. One interpretation is that the utterance to be produced is represented in a motor program. The execution of this program depends on its content, especially the number of syllables it contains.

Latency effects occur even for simple tasks such as rapid repetition of the same utterance (MacKay, 1974). It appears that latency depends on the motoric complexity of the utterance, not just on the length of the utterance in segments. For example, monosyllables containing the same number of phonetic segments are associated with different latencies. A sequence composed of CV (consonant + vowel) syllables has shorter syllable durations *and* shorter intersyllable pauses than a sequence composed of VC (vowel + consonant) syllables (MacKay, 1974). One interpretation of this observation is that the intersyllable pause reflects programming time.

Using latency data from behavioral responses, Sternberg et al. (1978) proposed a three-stage process in the control of motor sequences such as those required for typing and speech:

1. *Retrieval stage.* A search is made for a unit in a preplanned buffer. The search continues until the unit is found, but the unit remains in the buffer after the search is complete.
2. *Unpacking stage.* The constituents of a retrieved unit are separated to make them available for motor execution.
3. *Execution stage.* The motor commands are sent for production of the utterance.

Each stage might contribute to latencies in a speech response. Levelt (1989) suggested that retrieval delay varies with the number of units in the buffer, that unpacking delay varies with the complexity of a motor unit, and that during actual production, a speaker can lengthen syllables to absorb latencies in retrieval.

More recently, Sternberg et al. (1988) described a two-process model for the control of rapid action sequences in speech production. The first process is subprogram selection, the duration of which varies directly with sequence length. The second process is command, whose duration depends on the type of unit. Sternberg et al. (1988) also proposed that the stress group or metrical foot is the fundamental action unit of speech production. The model can be summarized as a series of two-process connections as follows:

[UNIT 1 SELECTION + UNIT 1 COMMAND] + [UNIT 2 SELECTION + UNIT 2 COMMAND] + . . .

Mulder (1983) has commented on certain limitations of the additive-factor method inherent to the motor program model of Sternberg et al. (1978). First, this method does not directly show the duration or order of the various stages. Second, it does not yield a substantive interpretation of the proposed stages. Third, if an experimental variable affects both the duration and output of a stage, then the effect of one stage is carried over to subsequent stages. These limitations complicate the experimental test of additive-factor stage models. The newer model (Sternberg et al., 1988) is conceptually simpler than its predecessor and is therefore not so seriously challenged by Mulder's objections. An appealing simplicity is the distinction between the two processes of subprogram selection and command and the way each relates to measurable properties of response timing.

An approach that may avoid some of the objections to the concept of motor programs is a *generalized motor program* (or **schema theory**), in which motor programs are composed of *schemata* (Schmidt, 1975). Schemata are learned relationships among movement outcomes, control signals, and boundary conditions. For example, a schema may be based on the relationships among initial conditions (e.g., the momentary positions of the articulators), the intended outcome (desired goal of movement), expected sensory consequences (the predicted sensory feedback), and the actual sensory consequences (the actual feedback resulting from movement). These relationships allow execution of responses, including ones not previously performed, based on a variety of experiences. An important feature of schema theory is that it can account for the learning of novel responses (ones not previously encountered). The schema represents learned relationships and the use of these learned patterns to prepare motor programs for a response that has not been performed before. The schemata are enhanced and strengthened by experience; therefore, practice with variable motoric requirements is a route to the development of effective schemata.

An example of schema theory applied to speech production is shown in Figure 1-6. The inputs are the desired outcome (e.g., a spatial target for a phonetic unit) and the initial conditions (the current state of the speech system, including the positions of the articulators). These inputs are needed for response recognition as a motor response schema. Past outcomes (earlier speech) and their response specifications determine the response specifications for any desired outcome, even if it has never been produced before. This strategy applies to any motor skill, including athletic skills such as golf, tennis, and archery. In each case it is often necessary to perform a movement slightly different from earlier movements. Per-

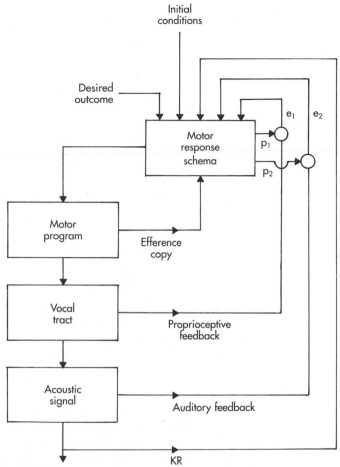

FIGURE 1-6 A version of schema theory applied to speech production. The motor response schema generates a motor program based on the desired outcome and initial conditions. Feedback signals are generated in the form of efference copy, proprioceptive feedback (e_1), and auditory feedback (e_2). The actual feedback signals are compared with expected feedback (p_1, and p_2), and discrepancies between actual and expected feedback are used to adjust the motor response schema. In this way, the motor response schema can be adapted to deal with novel responses. (KR = Knowledge of results). (From Kent, R. D. [1981]. Sensorimotor aspects of speech development. In Aslin, R. N., Alberts, J. R., & Petersen, M. R. [Eds.], *Development of perception: Psychobiological perspectives* [Vol. 1, pp. 162-185]. New York: Academic Press.)

formance is based on experience represented in the motor schema, and motor program is executed from this information. The expected sensory consequences are also generated. For the sake of simplicity, only three examples of such feedback are shown in the figure, but a plurimodal feedback system is more likely. The expected feedback is compared with the actual feedback to derive error information (e1 and e2), which is used to adjust the motor response schema. A motivating feature of the schema approach is that it tries to account for motor learning. Kent (1981) discusses the possible relevance of this model to the learning of speech by children.

MODELS THAT COMBINE MOTOR PROGRAMS AND FEEDBACK CONTROL

Another way of viewing the regulation of speech movements is in terms of combined processes of programming and feedback control. One model that uses such an approach is Perkell's (1980) conceptual model of the physiology of speech production (Figure 1-7). This example of a functional model attempts to identify general processes and types of information used in speech production. It is "physiological" in the sense that it refers to classes of physiological information, such as sensory or motor goals. It is also an example of a common approach to

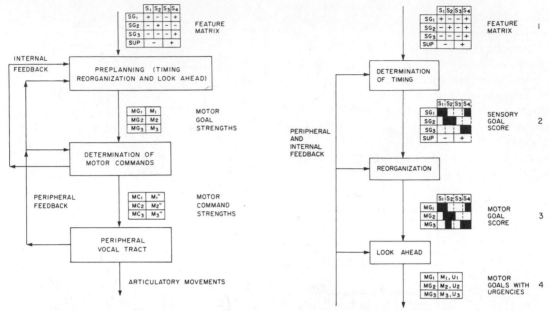

FIGURE 1-7 Perkell's (1980) physiological model of speech production. The three major components of the conceptual model are preplanning, motor command generation, and the peripheral vocal tract. Preplanning is elaborated at the right to show three subcomponents: determination of timing, reorganization, and look-ahead. (From Perkell, J. S. [1980]. Phonetic features and the physiology of speech production. In Butterworth, B. [Ed.], *Language production* [Vol. 1, pp. 337-372]. New York: Academic Press.)

model building in speech production, to endow the model with various levels of regulation and allow selective feedback to operate across the levels.

Perkell's model has three major components. The input is a matrix in which sensory goals are specified for phonetic segments. The sensory goals are regarded as correlates of phonetic features and may refer to patterns of articulatory contact, levels of intraoral air pressure, or articulatory configurations. Accompanying suprasegmental information also is represented in the input matrix. Situated under the input matrix are three blocks arranged in descending order. These blocks determine the following:

Block 1. Timing, reorganization, and coarticulation
Block 2. Motor commands
Block 3. Peripheral (vocal tract) events

Figure 1-7 shows block 1's different functions, *timing, reorganization,* and *look-ahead.* Block 1 timing is thought to fulfill its role by assigning temporal specifications for sensory goals, such as a specified duration for an articulatory contact. Block 1 reorganization works by reconciling and integrating the sensory goals for different features and suprasegmental factors. The result is a temporal sequence of

motor goal specifications, or a motor goal score. This can be thought of as a set of assigned times for individual articulatory actions. Finally, block 1 look-ahead accounts for anticipatory coarticulation by scanning the input motor goal score (with a window size of about six segments). As it does so, it assigns urgency to each motor goal to reflect the immediacy of the need for achievement. The components of block 1 incorporate aspects of motor programming, including assignment of timing, preparation of a motor score, and forward scan of the score to make adjustments for coarticulation.

Perkell's model separates the biomechanical properties of the speech system from the major components of control. The input matrix and the three functions of block 1 are not immediately constrained by the physical characteristics of the periphery. For example, the timing specifications for the sensory and motor goals are set at early levels in the process. Furthermore, it is not clear that these need to take into account the articulatory biomechanics.

DYNAMIC SYSTEMS MODELS

Another set of solutions to speech production fall in the category of **dynamic systems** (also known as *task dynamics* or *action theory*), in which motor behavior is viewed in terms of the interactions between biomechanical and environmental variables. Concepts from dynamic systems theory have been applied to many fields of science, including speech and virtually all other human motor activities. A fundamental idea is to emphasize the interactions of living systems (which are considered nonlinear) with the physical world on which these living systems operate. These interactions define a nonlinear dynamic model that has several stable operational regions with relatively simple control features. That is, the interactions give rise to conditions that afford a comparatively simple and powerful description. Identification of these regions of stability is an important step toward understanding the control of behavior. The interactions between any living system and the physical world occur in a number of regions of stable performance, each having relatively few degrees of freedom. These stable regions can be controlled quite easily because there are few degrees of freedom in their regulation. In this way, a system that appears highly complex when its individual components are described can be considered much simpler when the components are functionally linked.

In dynamic systems theory (and in related theories known by other names), the degrees of freedom problem is resolved by recognizing functional groupings, or **synergies**, among the muscles that comprise a system. This view avoids the implication that each degree of freedom in a system is controlled individually and continuously. Rather, muscles are grouped together to act as a unit in accord with shared afferent and efferent signals. An analogy sometimes used to explain this notion is the control of an airplane. Suppose that an airplane has five movable parts: the two ailerons on the trailing edge of the wings, the two elevators on the horizontal piece of the tail section, and the rudder on the vertical tail fin. The student pilot initially contends with a control system having five degrees of freedom. (Of course, the degrees of freedom increase as other factors, such as speed of flight, are added.) The pilot soon learns that banking and turning are accomplished with a combination of aileron and rudder movements. This combined action can be defined by an equation of constraint, or a mathematical expression that defines their relative motions for the purpose of banking and turning. Similarly, the elevators have a combined

action to change the elevation of the plane. Smooth and effective control of the plane can be described by appropriate combinations of control actions. These combinations are analogies of coordinative systems in motor control. The essential point is that combined or coordinated control of a system can achieve the intended action of that system. *Coordination* and *intended action* are the key words.

In the study of motor control, functional groupings have been called *linkages* (Boylls, 1975), *synergies* (Gurfinkel et al., 1971), *collectives* (Gel'fand, et al., 1971), and *coordinative structures* (Easton, 1972; Kelso, Southard, and Goodman, 1979; Saltzman, 1979). These terms may be regarded as essentially synonymous. The term *synergies* will be used in this chapter. Movements come about when synergies are selected for a given action. The synergies are by their nature task specific, context sensitive, and adaptive.

The synergies possess both essential and nonessential parameters, and these two types of parameters are important for their description. *Essential parameters* are qualitative aspects of a movement's structure (e.g., lip closure for the bilabial stop [b]). *Nonessential parameters* are quantitative, scalar variations (e.g., differing displacements of the lower lip in reaching bilabial closure when variations are introduced in phonetic context, stress, or speaking rate). The combination can be economically powerful in accounting for speech movements because essential parameters can account for the phonetically distinctive (characteristic) aspects of movement, and the nonessential ones can account for the effects of stress, rate, and other scalar variables that operate within the phonetic requirements of the movements.

The following account describes how the fundamental ideas of task dynamics may be used to produce the syllable *bat* ([b æ t]). The phonological prescription for the syllable does not contain detailed production instructions but only a general form of the intended action. That is, there is no motor program to direct the details of performance. The details of the motor events are determined by the coordinate grouping, or synergies, among the many possible active elements. The relationships between the components of a synergetic group and the motor consequence of that synergy are determined by *equations of constraint* that specify how the members of the group can interact within the limits of a particular action and its environmental circumstances. The equations allow a principled variation in the actions of the group members. A given member may vary somewhat in its participation, depending on the actions of other members in the group. For example, the consonant [b] can be instantiated (a term often used by action theorists to denote a particular motor action) by various combinations of jaw, lower lip, and upper lip movements (Figure 1-8). But the relative contributions of the mandibular and labial musculature to the final articulation are constrained by the equations that define their performance within the motor objective or goal. The goal is bilabial closure, so the jaw and lip are controlled to reach that goal. The equation of constraint specifies the ways jaw and lower lip may covary while accomplishing the closure of the two lips.

An important concept in dynamic systems is the *emergent property,* a function or action

created through preexisting functions. The idea is not to create something out of nothing but rather to create a new thing out of things that already exist. This possibility often rests on the combination of the preexisting functions into coalitions, or cooperative sets. As synergies combine within a nested or coalitional organization, particular combinations of synergies can bring about properties that were not fully defined in any one synergy acting alone. An emergent property arises naturally through the dynamics of the system. Whereas a motor program account may specify in detail how components are arranged to accomplish a certain pattern of movement, action theory proposes that the pattern of movement is a natural and predictable consequence of the system's dynamics.

It has been proposed that coordination of movements is an emergent property in the sense that coordination is enabled by the dynamics of cooperating synergies. In this view, coordination is not preassigned, as by a motor program, but rather follows directly from the system dynamics. How can this be? One possibility is that the dynamics of the different synergies are formed into a superordinate organization that is defined by the interactions of the various participating synergies. Consider the simple motor act of reaching to grasp a pencil that someone has handed to you. A smooth and successful accomplishment of this act requires that the muscles of the shoulder, arm, wrist, and fingers be properly timed. Obviously, it will not suffice to close the fingers in a grasp before the arm is fully extended to bring the fingers close to the pencil. The dynamics of the grasping motions performed by the fingers must be properly timed with respect to the extension of the arm. Coordination therefore is a blending of the dynamics of the participating synergies.

Von Holst (1973) and Haken (1975, 1983) describe general principles by which the degrees of freedom problem can be solved in a number of physical and biological systems. The central idea is to compress system complexity to a small number of degrees of freedom, sometimes called *order parameters.* These parameters have equations of motion (dynamics) that are low-dimensional and nonlinear. A first step in reducing the number of degrees of freedom in a system is to define the task or pattern of action. Take again the bilabial closure for a [b]. The task, closure of the lips, can be accomplished through various movement combinations of the jaw,

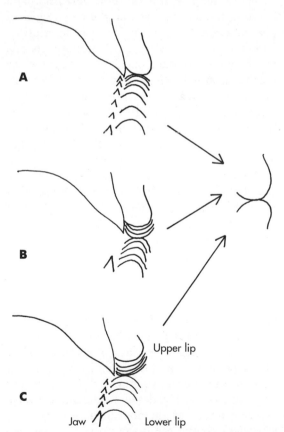

FIGURE 1-8   **Examples of different combinations of lip and jaw movement associated with the goal of bilabial closure.** *A*—jaw movement predominates; *B*—jaw is fixed so that bilabial closure is affected by upper and lower lip movements; *C*—jaw and upper lip movements predominate.

upper lip, and lower lip. The degrees of freedom can be precisely determined by examining this behavior for **phase transitions,** or circumstances that introduce a qualitative change in the system's behavior. For example, a horse demonstrates phase transitions as it changes from a trot to a gallop. Phase transitions are studied to determine the order parameter that characterizes the pattern and the control parameters within which patterns occur. One way to search for phase transitions in speech is to study articulatory movements under changing conditions, such as rate of speech or stress pattern.

The equations of motion can be used to identify **attractors,** or stable solutions. Attractors are a very interesting feature of dynamic systems theory. An especially important aspect of an attractor is that it represents a point of convergence for a system that may have had different initial conditions, or starting points. That is, regardless of where the system might have been at the start, it can settle into certain regions of stability in its field of dynamic potential.

Several types of attractors may define stable motor solutions. These include the *point attractor,* the *limit cycle,* and the *strange attractor.* A point attractor can be illustrated with a pan of water. Shake the pan vigorously so that the water is set into motion. Place the pan on a table and observe the water. Eventually the water ceases its motion until it seems placid. This settled state is a point attractor. No matter how you shook the pan (clockwise rotation, up and down movements, rocking from side to side), the water will return to this stable state given time for the motions to dissipate. Finger-pointing tasks often are described as having a point attractor. The final goal of pointing is the attractor. An example in speech production is the contact of the tip of the tongue against the alveolar ridge. The tongue may have had very different initial conditions (different positions), but eventually it must reach the desired point of contact.

The limit cycle is a stable state of oscillatory systems such as the pendulum of a large clock. The pendulum settles into a highly repeatable movement. That is, it reaches a stable state defined by a cycle of limiting action. Do our bodies have limit cycles? Observe a person walking briskly. What happens to the person's arms? Are they held rigidly against the body? No, they usually swing like the pendulum. Swinging is a stable oscillatory state. Limit cycles in speech conceivably could take the form of syllable sequences, stress groupings, or some other rhythmic pattern.

The strange attractor is so named because it is not easily explained. The system under examination has certain stable states, including some that occur only infrequently. Stability can be demonstrated by showing that if the right initial conditions are replicated, the system reaches the same condition. Flowing water is an interesting example because many people think that the detailed motions of falling water have no predictable pattern; that is, the motion seems random. A person sitting close to a small waterfall may sit safely by the churning water for some time without feeling anything more than a weak spray or mist, but suddenly the action of the water changes and a cold splash arouses our complacent observer. Why did this abrupt change occur? Explanation by strange attractor holds that under certain conditions the overall pattern of the water flow changes and assumes a new form. The event is not random because this occasional form recurs *if the right conditions are repeated.* The person may have to sit by the waterfall for several hours before such patience is rewarded with another splash.

Much literature has accumulated on dynamic systems applied to speech. A special issue of the *Journal of Phonetics* (1986) was devoted to the theory of dynamic systems applied to speech production. Nolan (1982) and Wilson and Morton (1990) evaluated action theory as it relates to normal linguistic behavior and pathologies of linguistic behavior.

A primary argument used to support dynamic-system or action-theory approaches to speech production is that they overcome the inherent limitations of translation theories. Translation theory is based on the idea that information is passed through various levels of control of speech production. One problem with translation theories is that the degrees of freedom can quickly become very large, necessitating a complex control operation. Moreover, many studies of movement, both of speech and other systems, have shown that the control and coordination of motor actions are not necessarily determined in a rigid top-down process in which the topmost level has all of the information needed to control the motor events. To the contrary, lower-level systems may account for various aspects of control and coordination that are not specifically addressed at some higher level.

Proponents of dynamic systems also have asserted several advantages in the temporal features of motor regulation. Kelso, Saltzman, and Tuller (1986) described a model of movement control in which timing is not an absolute, independent property but rather a feature intrinsic to a more basic description in terms of stable phase relationships between events in various task-coupled articulators. In *phase stability* two or more movements have an invariant phase relationship. Task-coupled articulators cooperate in the performance of a specific task. Consider the lower lip and jaw (coupled articulators) participating in the formation of bilabial closure (the task). Movement regulation based on absolute time may take a form such as this: The lower lip begins to close 14 ms after the jaw begins to elevate. Figure 1-9 describes a stable phase relationship, an invariant pattern of movement in a phase portrait. This approach specifies the interarticulator patterns not in clock time but in phase relationships.

Kelso, Saltzman, and Tuller (1986) interpreted their data to support their hypothesis of stable phase relationships between lip and jaw articulations in a speaking task. However, this conclusion has been criticized on several grounds, including failure of replication (Lubker, 1986; Keller, 1987; Nittrauer et al., 1988), possible statistical artifacts (Barry, 1983; Munhall, 1985; Benoit, 1986), and dependence of the data on speech rates, which may fully explain the apparent phase stability (Munhall, 1985; Keller, 1987). Moreover, Gentner (1987), in a review of literature on rate variations in movement, concluded that the movements performed at different rates are quite variable and that relative timing measures do not describe the data well.

Another timing advantage was ascribed to dynamic systems theory by Fowler (1980), who contrasts the dynamic systems approach with what she calls extrinsic timing models. She describes dynamic systems as having features of intrinsic timing to explain movement patterns. The extrinsic timing models must in some way impose time on a movement plan. Fowler sees

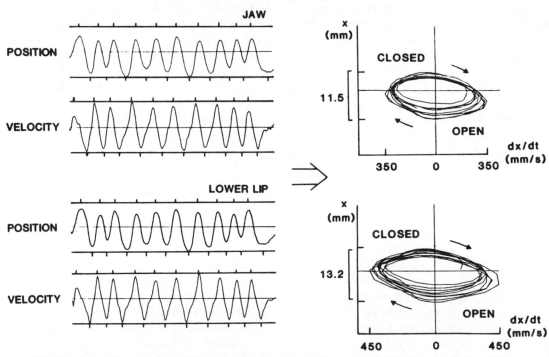

FIGURE 1-9 Phase portrait of jaw and lip movements for a repetitive series of /ba/ syllables. *Left,* position-time and velocity-time profiles of jaw and lower lip (plus jaw) during reiterant speech (in which the syllable /ba/ replaces the real syllables in a sentence). *Right,* phase portraits corresponding to the articulatory profiles shown on the left. The phase portraits are plotted as position-velocity relationships. *Closed* refers to articulatory trajectory into and out of bilabial closure; *open* refers to the vocalic part of the syllable. (From Kelso, J. A. S., & Tuller, B. [1984]. Conveying evidence in support of common dynamical principles for speech and movement coordination. *American Journal of Physiology,* 1984, 246, p. R933.)

particular advantage in proposing **coproduction** of consonants and vowels, that is, production in parallel, coordinated systems. Coproduction is a possible explanation for coarticulation in that vowel and consonant movements can be performed in parallel to yield combined effects in articulation at a given time. (Coarticulation of consonants is not explained by this formulation.) Fowler also uses coproduction to account for the fact that variations in stress and speaking rate affect the relative timing of vowel and consonant movements. However, Shaffer (1982) argues that the explanation does not work because it predicts one of two outcomes, both wrong: (1) only one stream of segments (vowels or consonants) should change because they are parallel, or (2) both streams of segments should change proportionately because they are coordinated. Whether temporal features are determined intrinsically, extrinsically, or both remains a fundamental question in the regulation of speech.

Interestingly, Gracco (1990, p. 10) argues that coordinative structures (synergies) are *synonymous* with motor programs. He writes, "Coordinative structures may be more rigidly specified than previously thought and the distinction between a flexible coordinative structure and a hard-wired motor program algorithm may be more rhetorical than real."

Gracco proposes that speech relies on sensorimotor specifications that determine the relative contribution of the articulators to the overall configuration of the vocal tract. These fixed neuromuscular specifications are compatible with either a motor program or coordinative structure hypothesis. As evidence of the rigidity of these specifications, Gracco points to studies showing that when the mandible is fixed with a block clenched between the teeth, the jaw-closing muscles are nonetheless active (Folkins and Zimmerman, 1981). In addition, experiments involving jaw perturbation demonstrated both functionally specific responses and nonfunctional responses (Kelso et al., 1984; Shaiman, 1989). Some of the key ideas in task dynamics have been incorporated in other models of speech production that are discussed in the following section.

MODELS OF GESTURAL PATTERNING

One recent development is the **gestural patterning model**. The term *gesture* in these models refers to a family of functionally equivalent movement patterns that are actively regulated to achieve a goal relevant to speech. Again, bilabial closure for [b] may include various combinations of jaw, lower lip, and upper lip movements. A gesture includes many aspects of speech production that have been discussed under categories such as context sensitivity and motor equivalence. Concepts of gestural patterning have been proposed by Browman and Goldstein (1986), Saltzman and Munhall (1989), Boyce, Krakow, Bell-Berti and Gelfer (1990), Lofqvist (1990).

Saltzman and Munhall (1989) assumed that the invariant units of speech are gestures that relate to context-independent sets of parameters in a dynamical system. The spatiotemporal patterns of speech are considered to be the product of a dynamical system that has two interacting levels: (a) an *intergestural level,* defined by a set of activation coordinates, and (b) an *interarticulator level,* defined by both model articulator and tract-variable coordinates. The activation coordinate associated with a particular gestural unit gauges the strength of that gesture in effecting the vocal tract movements at a particular instant. Gestures may compete in terms of their activation coordinates. Each gestural unit is associated with model articulator variables that specify articulatory movements

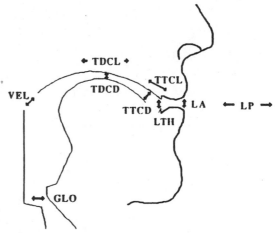

FIGURE 1-10 **Part of Saltzman and Munhall's model for articulatory synthesis, showing tract variables labeled as follows: LP, lip protrusion; LA, lip aperture; TTCL, tongue tip constriction location; LTH, lower tooth height; TTCD, tongue tip constriction degree; TDCL, tongue dorsum constriction location; TDCD, tongue dorsum constriction degree; VEL, velic constriction; and GLO, glottal constriction. (From Saltzman, E. L., & Munhall, K. G. [1989]. A dynamical approach to gestural patterning in speech production. *Ecological Psychology, 1,* 333-382.)**

and tract variables, hence vocal tract configurations. Figure 1-10 shows the tract variable coordinates, and the box below lists the relationships between these coordinates and the model articulator variables. The tract variable coordinates pertain to *context-independent* gestural goals (e.g., bilabial closure). The model articulator coordinates pertain to *context-dependent* performances of a gesture. Therefore, a given vocal tract configuration can have various articulatory implementations, depending on the tract-articulator relationships that apply.

Activation of gestural units at the intergestural level accounts for patterns of relative timing and cohesion for a particular utterance. This level defines an active set of gestures that in turn are related to events at the interarticulator level, where the coordination among articulators is determined. Each gesture is related to a tract-variable dynamical system. In the computer implementation of the model, the dynami-

cal systems are defined as tract-variable point attractors (or stable equilibrium points). The attractors are modeled as damped second-order linear differential equations that permit the model to generate articulatory motions in an articulatory synthesizer. Early results are promising; the articulatory patterns are consistent with certain effects in natural speech, including articulatory compensation (motor equivalence) and coarticulation.

Saltzman and Munhall (1989, p. 355) succinctly state the essence of their model: "It defines, in effect, a selective pattern of coupling among the articulators that is specific to the set of currently active gestures." In so doing, it gives an intrinsically dynamical account of multiarticulator coordination for gestural activation intervals. However, it does not provide a comparable intrinsically dynamical account of the *intergestural* timing patterns. That is, it lacks serial dynamics. Saltzman and Munhall point

---

Relationships between tract variables and model articulatory variables

Each tract variable* can be implemented in terms of the model articulatory variables listed in parentheses. For example, LA, lip aperture, is related to some combination of jaw angle, upper lip vertical position and lower lip vertical position.

Tract Variable	Model Articulator Variables
LP, lip protrusion	(Horizontal lip movement)
LA, lip aperture	(Jaw angle) (Upper lip vertical position) (Lower lip vertical position)
TDCL, tongue dorsum constriction location	(Jaw angle) (Tongue body radial position) (Tongue body angular position)
TDCD, tongue dorsum constriction degree	(Jaw angle) (Tongue body radial position) (Tongue body angular position)
LTH, lower tooth height	(Jaw angle)
TTCL, tongue tip constriction location	(Jaw angle) (Tongue body radial position) (Tongue body angular position) (Tongue tip radial position) (Tongue tip angular position)
TTCD, tongue tip constriction	(Jaw angle) (Tongue body radial position) (Tongue body angular position) (Tongue tip radial position) (Tongue tip angular position)
VEL, velic constriction	(Velar position)
GLO, glottic constriction	(Glottal configuration)

* See Figure 1-10.
(From Saltzman, E. L., & Munhall, K. G. [1989]. A dynamical approach to gestural patterning in speech production. *Ecological Psychology, 1,* 333-382.)

to connectionist approaches as a solution, and this recommendation brings us to the next class of models.

CONNECTIONIST AND SPREADING ACTIVATION MODELS

Connectionist models, also called parallel-distributed processing (PDP), have recently had great influence in a number of disciplines. Not surprisingly, these models have been applied to both speech production and speech perception. The common property of connectionist models, which differ in several particulars, is that they have networks of densely interconnected units. Figure 1-11 shows a simple example of units connected by lines. Depending on the particular connectionist model, the units can be arranged in various configurations, or layers. The input lines to any given unit carry excitatory or inhibitory signals, often called activity, which in most models are simply summed by the unit to determine its state. The state usually is evaluated with respect to a threshold. The activity carried by a given connection can be modulated by a property called weight. The weights assigned to individual connections constitute a kind of memory and can be modified by experience. The overall behavior of the network depends on the initial state of activation of its units and on the weights of the connections between units. The network can "learn" by using feedback to change the weights of its connections or its threshold values. The network as a whole is a computing device whose configuration of connections is an analog to a computer program.

PDP is the use of cooperative and parallel processing elements, as opposed to the use of strictly serial steps. Parallel processing allows a great increase in the speed of operation, particularly when individual units have significant processing times. Massively parallel systems can work much faster than serial systems, in which delays (serial bottlenecks) build up with the sequence of computations. As a crude analogy, imagine five statistics students, each of whom has a statistical calculation to solve. Only one calculator is available to the group of five. If each waits for his or her turn, some time will pass before the solutions to all five problems are in hand. But if five calculators are available, they can work in parallel and arrive at the full set of solutions in short order.

The network in Figure 1-11 includes input units, hidden units, and output units. The input units are the information given to the system. The output units are the product of the model. The input units are connected to the output units by hidden units. The hidden units allow the network to create an internal representation as it works to generate an output. Without hidden units, the network simply links input to output units and may not be appropriate for complex tasks. Hidden units are a powerful addition to the network, particularly since they enable the network to construct an internal representation.

Connectionist models have been implemented on computers and have been used to

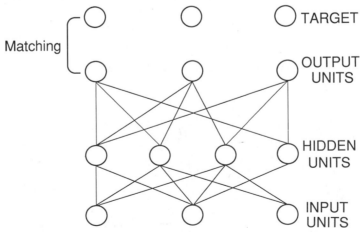

FIGURE 1-11 Example of a connectionist network in which the units (circles) are connected by lines carrying activation signals. The activation signals are weighted so that the inputs to a particular unit are the sum of its weighted activation signals. The units shown are input units, hidden units, and output units.

recognize patterns (such as those of speech), to demonstrate rulelike behaviors (such as the rules of language), and to map the relationships between patterns of input and patterns of output. These models are considered by some to have another attractive feature—they are thought to work much as the brain works. Substitute "neuron" for "unit" and "synaptic connectivity" for "weighted connection," and the analogy comes clear. The term *neural networks* sometimes is used to refer to connectionist systems. However, the analogy to the brain is not universally accepted.

Dell (1986) developed a connectionist model for speech production errors, or slips of the tongue. He defined these errors as unintended, nonhabitual deviations from a speech plan. His goal was to determine whether a connectionist network could produce errors like those reported for natural speech. Dell's model was based on two intersecting systems of interconnected nodes, one for linguistic representation (with levels for words, syllables, phonemes, and phonological features), and another for output sequencing (with levels for rimes and clusters, which are constituents of syllables). The network is illustrated in Figure 1-12.

Dell's model works by *spreading activation,* or the selective radiation of activation along its connections. Both the linguistic subsystem and the sequencing subsystem provide activation input to a phoneme. As a phoneme is activated, it activates in turn all of the features and syllables to which it is connected. The activated features and syllables (and words) then activate other phonemes. When applied under certain conditions, this spreading activation allows errors to occur. When they do, they are constrained by some of the same factors that seem to constrain errors in natural speech. For example, syllable position of a sound is a potent factor in accounting for sequencing errors. A general assumption of the spreading activation theory is that representations of an utterance are constructed simultaneously at various levels, but within the limits of coordinated information that operates across levels. For example, a lexical selection must precede assignment of phonological structure. Activation is modeled as a real variable with the properties of spreading (distributing nonzero levels of activation to all connected nodes), summation (integration or addition of activation at each node), and decay (a temporal, passive loss of activation at each node).

A major attraction of PDP models is that they can permit context sensitivity without increasing the number of degrees of freedom. Rumelhart and Norman (1982) developed a PDP model for

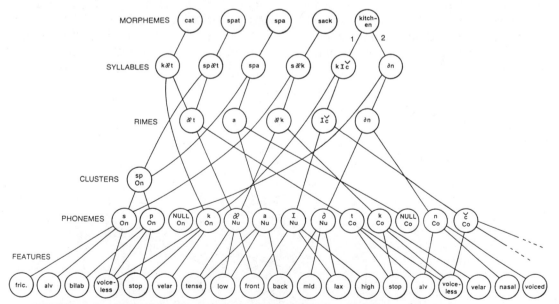

FIGURE 1-12 Part of the network from Dell's spreading activation model developed to account for sequencing errors in speech. The network shown accounts for phonological coding. The nodes for phonemes, clusters, and null elements are labeled to indicate whether they are potential onsets, nuclei, or codas. (From Dell, G. S. [1986]. A spreading-activation theory of retrieval in sentence production. *Psychological Review, 93,* 283-321.)

typing, a task that has interesting similarities to speech, particularly in regard to the goal of a serially ordered output—alphabet letters for typing and phonetic segments for speech.

Jordan and Rosenbaum (1989) and Jordan (1990) propose a parallel approach to account for serial order that has special relevance to speech production. Jordan's (1990) connectionist sequential machine is illustrated in Figure 1-13. It operates as follows: An action is a pattern of activation across the output units. Sequences of actions are generated by changing weights in the network. The network receives an external input in the form of a constant *plan* vector, which specifies the sequence to be executed. The network also receives input from a *state* vector, a time function changing in response to recurrent connections affecting the state units. The model works by decomposing the serial order problem into two subproblems. The first is how to change the state vector in time; the second is how to map the states to actions. The only requirement of the recurrent connections is that they produce discriminable

state patterns at each time step. Additional discriminability comes from the plan. The other parts of the network learn to map the state patterns to target output patterns at each time step. The single output vector means that all actions are a function of one set of tunable weights. As a particular learned action affects the weights, other actions in the sequence are also affected. That is, context sensitivity arises naturally from the operation of the network.

Connectionist systems have become popular in many fields. The many issues surrounding connectionist systems are discussed further by Massaro (1988), Pinker and Meher (1988), and Hanson and Burr (1990). Some hints of the controversy can be offered here. Fant (1989, p. 5) expresses one of the major sources of uneasiness about the connectionist solution for speech production: "It may prove fruitful, but at the same time it implies a failure. We leave it to the computer to learn what we have failed to understand. The computer might do the job but can it tell us how?" Fant explains that the connectionist approach reveals neither the sys-

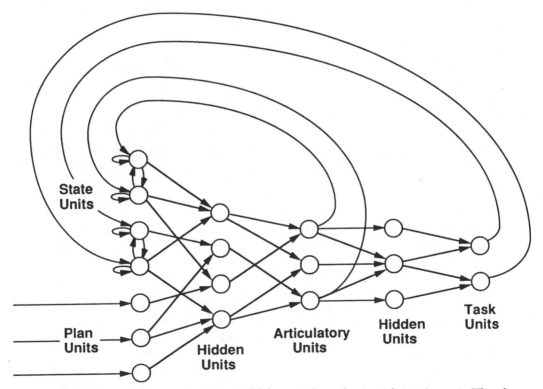

FIGURE 1-13 Jordan's connectionist model for speech production (shown in part). The plan and state units together constitute the input units for the network. The articulatory units are the output units of the network. (From Jordan, M. I. [1990]. Motor learning and the degrees of freedom problem. In Jeannerod, M. [Ed.], *Attention and performance XIII* [pp. 796-836]. Hillsdale, NJ: Erlbaum.)

tem at hand nor invariance criteria. It yields "... only a complex pattern of joint probabilities set by a large number of weighting factors within complex layers of neuron-like units trained for the specific task."

Some proponents of connectionist systems have admitted that features such as hidden units may have little or no bearing on the behavioral or cognitive phenomena of interest (Hanson and Burr, 1990). Commenting on this issue, Lamberts and d'Ydewalle (1990, p. 500) observed that hidden-unit nets will be of greater psychological relevance if their features are constrained by knowledge gained from psychological research. They assert that "Hidden-unit nets can be used as tools for generating candidate psychological theories, but unless network features are constrained in a psychologically plausible way, a principled choice among these candidates is impossible."

SUBSYSTEM MODELS AND COMPOSITE MODELS OF SPEECH PRODUCTION

The models addressed to this point have intended to explain how speech movements are regulated to accomplish phonetic objectives. Many modeling efforts have been made at subsystem levels. This section addresses models for individual subsystems such as the larynx or vocal tract. It also considers attempts to model the overall system of speech production by taking together various subsystem models into a model of the complete system. Such endeavors have particular value as models for the articulatory synthesis of speech.

The term **composite model** here refers to models that incorporate several submodels or concepts to arrive at an overall model of the speech production system, or at least several of its components. A great deal of modeling has focused on the vocal tract, that subsystem of the speech production system that extends from the vocal folds to the lips. Many of these models neglect the contributions of the larynx and the pulmonary system. Other models are devoted exclusively to the laryngeal or pulmonary subsystem. Putting these subsystems into a reasonably complete model of the speech production system is an ambitious task. It is best to begin with a brief assessment of each subsystem — respiratory, laryngeal, and supraglottal. This assessment is aimed at a characterization of each subsystem and a very brief introduction to subsystem models.

A number of models attempt to characterize the operation of specific components of speech production. In recent years separate models have been advanced for the respiratory, laryngeal, and supralaryngeal subsystems. A brief discussion of some of these models will illustrate the complexity of behaviors considered in any complete model of speech production.

Respiratory Subsystem

During speech, one of the main goals of the respiratory system is to maintain an adequate and fairly constant subglottal pressure over the course of an utterance by the coordination of active muscular forces and passive elastic forces. The passive forces are produced by the elastic properties of the respiratory tissues (e.g. lungs, muscles, and tendons of the rib cage), which attempt to return an inflated or deflated respiratory system to its resting position. These recoil forces are analogous to the force that causes an inflated balloon to deflate. The muscular forces correspond to the active contraction of various respiratory muscles such as those of the rib cage, diaphragm, and abdomen. These act to modulate the passive recoil forces and to produce the ongoing adjustments in subglottal pressure required for speech.

In some early models of speech breathing, the active muscular forces were thought to be turned off whenever the passive recoil forces were sufficient to produce the desired subglottal pressures (Draper, Ladefoged, and Whitteridge, 1959). However, more recent research has demonstrated that the muscular forces are active throughout the speech breathing cycle (Hixon, Goldman, and Mead, 1973; Hixon, Mead, and Goldman, 1976). The continuous muscular activity associated with speech breathing may represent a more efficient control strategy than one in which muscular forces are turned on and off. Hixon et al. (1987) suggest that this control strategy involves setting the muscles of the respiratory system into a configuration that is optimal for generating rapid pressure changes without requiring major changes in the shape of the system. In other words, the respiratory system may be tuned to a posture optimally suited to the rapid and fine-grained changes in subglottal pressure required for speech breathing.

For a number of years the muscular forces used during the expiratory phase of speech breathing were thought to be caused primarily by the contraction of the muscles of the rib cage (e.g., internal intercostals). The muscles of the abdomen were thought to contribute to the muscular forces only during loud speech or possibly toward the end of the expiratory phases of speech breathing (Draper, Ladefoged, and Whitteridge, 1959). However, recent kinematic and dynamic studies of respiration conducted by Hixon and his coworkers have reinterpreted this traditional view, showing that the abdominal muscles are generally quite active throughout the expiratory phase of speech breathing and thus appear to play an important role in speech production (Hixon, Goldman, and Mead, 1973; Hixon, Mead, and Goldman, 1976). Weismer (1985) has argued that this relatively continuous abdominal activity during speech represents a biologically efficient mode of action. First, the continuous contractions of the abdominal muscles appear to provide a platform that optimizes the expiratory actions of the rib cage during speech. Without such a platform, the expiratory actions of the rib cage would expand the abdomen, reducing the force available for the expiration of air from the lungs. It is further argued that the ongoing contractions of the abdomen may maintain the muscles of the diaphragm at an optimal length for rapid inspiration. In a sense this may reflect the abdomen's contribution to what was described earlier as the speaker's attempt to maintain a preferred respiratory posture that is most efficient for the demands of speech production.

The foregoing describes in a very general way certain characteristics of chest wall behavior during speech breathing. However, when speech breathing patterns are examined in more detail, a great deal of variability is observed across subjects and speaking tasks. For example, speech breathing patterns have been found to vary with the subject's age, gender, and body type (Hodge, Putnam, and Weismer, 1986; Hixon et al., 1987). The nature of the spoken material (e.g., conversation versus prolonged vowels), the subject's body position (e.g., standing versus supine), and loudness of speech can also influence chest wall configurations (Hixon et al., 1987). Furthermore, a certain amount of variability has been noted in an individual subject's breathing pattern across repeated productions of the same utterance (Hunker and Abbs, 1982). This may reflect a form of motor equivalence whereby the speaker uses a variety of chest wall configurations to accomplish similar respiratory goals during speech.

These are just a few of the sources of variation that must be explained in any model of speech breathing. Both Hixon et al. (1987) and Weismer (1988) emphasize the need for research to describe the influence of various linguistic factors in speech breathing. Hixon et al. (1987) call for studies to quantify the relatively minute chest wall adjustments observed during utterances of varying linguistic content. In addition, Weismer (1988) points out the paucity of studies on the organization of speech breathing during connected discourse. He suggests that an in-depth analysis of the effects of grammatical structure or passage content on chest wall behavior is necessary.

Laryngeal Subsystem

Attempts to model laryngeal behavior during speech production have been approached from a number of perspectives. First, because the vocal folds play such an important role in the generation of sound for speech production, attention has been focused on the mechanisms responsible for vocal fold vibration. Models of vocal fold vibration attempt to explain the biomechanical and aerodynamic forces responsible for different patterns of vibration. For example, Ishizaka and Matsudaira (1972a,b) developed a *two-mass model* of vocal fold vibration in which the upper and lower portions of each vocal fold are characterized as two separate masses connected by elastic components (Figure 1-14). This model describes how aerodynamic forces due to subglottal pressure and the flow of air through the glottis (Bernoulli forces) are sequenced with the elastic forces of the vocal fold tissues to produce

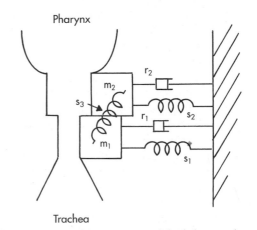

FIGURE 1-14   **Two-mass model of the vocal folds. The terms m, s, and r represent the equivalent mass, stiffness, and viscous resistance, respectively.**

the continuous vibrations of the vocal folds. The two-mass model also helps to explain certain microaspects of laryngeal kinematics such as the vertical wave in vocal fold vibration, which is characterized by the bottom edge of the vocal fold moving in advance of the top edge throughout the vibratory cycle. Some theorists have further refined the two-mass model by adding more components (e.g., the 16-mass model by Titze [1973]) with the result that additional microaspects of laryngeal vibration can be explained. (See Broad [1979] for a comprehensive review of theories of vocal fold vibration.)

Anatomical and histological studies of the vocal folds have led to the development of theories to explain some of the prosodic and qualitative aspects of vocal behavior. For example, the cover-body theory (Hirano and Kakita, 1985) posits that certain aspects of vocal behavior result from the speaker's explicit control of the mechanical properties of different layers of tissue in the vocal folds. As a first approximation, the vocal fold is seen to be composed of two separate layers, a cover layer near the surface of the fold and a body layer lying deeper in the vocal fold. Contraction of different laryngeal muscles alters the relative stiffness of these two layers, and this causes different patterns of vocal fold vibration. For example, Hirano (1974) suggests that weak contractions of the vocalis and cricothyroid muscles produce both a slack cover and body layer, resulting in a soft phonatory pattern produced at a low fundamental frequency. In contrast, if the strength of contraction in the vocalis muscle is increased while that of the cricothyroid remains relatively weak, the body layer will become stiffer than the cover layer. According to the theory, this will result in a louder phonatory pattern at a medium fundamental frequency. Thus, through graduated changes in the relative stiffness of the vocal fold layers, it is hypothesized, the speaker can make a variety of prosodic changes during speech.

Vocal fold vibration and its timing relative to supralaryngeal movements are also seen to be critical for certain segmental aspects of speech production. For example, the coordination of voice onset with lingual and labial releasing gestures has a major contribution to the voicing contrast in obstruent consonants (e.g., [p] versus [b]). In the case of voiceless obstruents (e.g., [p t s k]), vocal fold vibration is interrupted briefly by what Weismer (1980) called the "laryngeal devoicing gesture." This gesture appears to have an immutable and fairly stereotypical topology across a variety of contexts. A very tight temporal relationship exists between this laryngeal gesture and other oral gestures. For example, the sound /p/ is produced with a laryngeal devoicing gesture whose peak in laryngeal abduction coincides with the onset of the bilabial opening gesture (Lofqvist and Yoshioka, 1981). Attempts to explain the mechanisms by which the speaker achieves such precise control in the timing of multiple gestures has been a central issue in the development of many recent models of speech production (Fowler et al., 1980; Kelso, Saltzman, and Tuller, 1986; Saltzman and Munhall, 1989). This issue will be treated in more detail in subsequent sections.

Supralaryngeal Subsystem

Attempts to characterize the supralaryngeal subsystem form the basis of much theoretical work in speech production. The models discussed here are those that attempt to describe the principles for controlling a single speech articulator or a restricted portion of the supralaryngeal system.

The major task of the supralaryngeal system in speech is to shape and constrict the vocal tract in ways that accomplish specific patterns of acoustic output. For many speech sounds these constrictions are due in large part to the movements of a single supralaryngeal articulator. For example, the production of an alveolar lingual plosive (e.g., [t]) is due primarily to movements of the front of the tongue. Other parts of the tongue and other articulators (e.g., the jaw) are also involved, but they have a relatively minor or indirect role in the production of this sound.

To a large extent, models of single-articulator movements and of subsystems have intended to explain the variability of speech movements. For example, the **quantal theory** of articulation (Stevens, 1972, 1989) explains the variability in speech production in terms of acoustic and perceptual constraints. Drawing on the acoustic theories of speech production (Stevens and House, 1955; Fant, 1960), the quantal theory holds that in critical regions of the vocal tract, small articulatory adjustments can have relatively large acoustic consequences. The sensitivity in these critical regions is seen as a problem for articulatory control because these regions demand a high degree of articulatory precision to produce a specific result. The quantal theory posits that the speech production system employs a control strategy that avoids these critical regions as places of articulation for speech sounds. The quantal theory accounts for certain articulatory-acoustic relations in speech production, but it is not a complete theory for the regulation of speech sounds. For further discussion, see the theme issue on quantal theory in *Journal of Phonetics, 17* (1), 1989.

Wood (1979) and Perkell and Nelson (1985) support the basic conceptions of quantal theory by showing that during vowel productions the articulations of the tongue are least variable in dimensions that are the most critical for acoustic output (e.g., the degree of vocal tract constriction). Thus, in the supralaryngeal system, there may be acoustically driven constraints operating to control the amount of variation in articulatory positions. Examples of variation in cross-sectional area for different classes of vowels are

shown in Figure 1-15. For each diagram, there is a region of conspicuous narrowing.

Other models describe the variability of movements from one articulatory position to another. For example, Fujimura (1986) and Kent (1986) have observed that vowel-to-consonant and consonant-to-vowel articulatory transitions are produced in a fairly standard manner. Fujimura (1986) emphasizes the importance of these stable transitional movements in his *iceberg model* of articulatory invariance. In this model, the transitions are seen as fixed elementary gestures that are free to vary with respect to one another in time. The metaphor of icebergs continuously shifting their relative positions in currents of water emphasizes the concept of these stable transitional movements in speech production. Kent (1986) argues that stereotypical transitional segments may reflect optimized movement patterns for speech produced under normal conditions. He suggests

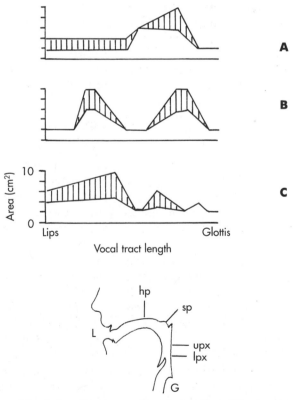

FIGURE 1-15 **Examples of variation in cross-sectional area for different classes of vowels:** *(A)* **high-front vowels,** *(B)* **high-back vowels, and** *(C)* **low vowels. The vocal tract sketch at the bottom of the illustration identifies regions where the vocal tract is narrowly constricted for vowel production, specifically, the hard palate (hp), soft palate (sp), upper pharynx (upx), and lower pharynx (lpx) (L = lips, G = glottis).** (Adapted from Wood, S. [1979]. A radiographic analysis of constriction locations for vowels. *Journal of Phonetics, 7,* 25–43.)

that under certain abnormal circumstances such as neuropathology or possibly during certain prosodic changes (e.g., slow speaking rate), the form of these transitional movements may change. Presumably this results from some change in the underlying movement variables being controlled or optimized.

Many studies of supralaryngeal articulation describe the variations of specific movement parameters such as the amplitude of a movement, the average or maximum velocity of a movement, and the duration of a movement (see Weismer [1988] for a review). Some researchers have modeled the mechanisms of motor control responsible for changes in these variables. Ostry and Munhall (1985) model the control of specific movement variables associated with transitional movements produced at various speaking rates. They found systematic changes in certain movement variables (e.g., peak velocity and movement amplitude) as speakers increased their rates of speech. They interpret their data in the context of a **mass-spring model** of articulation, in which the transitional movements in speech are likened to the movements of a mass attached to a spring. The speed of movement of the mass can be increased if the stiffness of the spring is increased. Similarly, the mass-spring model suggests that changes in the speed of transitional movements are accomplished by explicit control of the stiffness of the speech articulators.

Ostry, Keller, and Parush (1983) and Ostry, Cooke, and Munhall (1987) have also applied the mass-spring model to other oral nonspeech transitional movements and transitional movements of the limbs. Thus, it appears that controlling articulatory stiffness to change the rate of movement may reflect a general strategy of motor control that has been incorporated into the speech production system. It seems likely that in a behavior as complex as speech, there may be a nesting of numerous motor control strategies, some specific to speech and others related to more global aspects of movement control. Determination of the physical economies of movement (Nelson, 1983) should underlie an understanding of movement control.

Many models focus on simplifying notions of vocal tract configurations. The work on vowels is illustrative. Stevens and House (1955) and Fant (1960) developed a three-parameter model of the vocal tract shape for vowels based on (1)

location of the constriction, (2) size of the constriction, and (3) the ratio of mouth opening to length. Liljencrants (1971), Harshman, Ladefoged, and Goldstein (1977), Kiritani (1977), and Maeda (1990) have taken statistical approaches, especially factor analysis. Generally, the factor analytical studies agree that vowel articulation can be described with two tongue factors, a lip factor, and perhaps a jaw factor. Still another direction in modeling is to identify independently controllable functional blocks, or solid articulatory structures, by which the articulatory organs can be represented (Lindblom and Sundberg, 1971; Mermelstein, 1972; Coker, 1976; Rubin, Baer, and Mermelstein, 1981). Rubin, Baer, and Mermelstein incorporated their model in the gestural patterning model of Saltzman and Munhall (1989). A basic goal in this work is to reduce the number of degrees of freedom compared with that required for an acoustic tube model of the vocal tract divided into sections 0.5 to 1 cm long. As Scully (1990) points out, ideally the number of degrees of freedom in an articulatory model should be identical to that defined by the physiological constraints of the actual articulatory system. We thus return to the fundamental issue of degrees of freedom.

Composite Models

The foregoing illustrates that the speech production system can be viewed as a complex arrangement of multiple subsystems operating in parallel or in series and that each one is fairly complicated. Unfortunately, most models of speech production address only individual subsystems or single levels within a subsystem. One of the great challenges of modeling is to explain the way these subsystems are integrated together in the production of speech.

Allwood and Scully (1982) and Scully (1986, 1987, 1990) have produced a composite model of the speech production process (Figure 1-16). The model identifies parameters at the pulmonary, laryngeal, and supralaryngeal levels. The parameters are divided into three major categories: articulatory, aerodynamic and mechanical. Computer implementation requires three major programs, one for timing and articulation, another for aerodynamics with acoustic sources, and a third for filtering the acoustic sources by the vocal tract and radiating the sound pressure wave of speech. Scully (1990) describes the application of this model to the study of differences between speakers, with the intent of developing rules to identify types of speakers. Figure 1-16 may be deceptively simple if it leaves the impression that the modeling of speech production is a matter of turning parameters on and off. In fact, the parameters must be precisely regulated and coordinated. The accuracy of the

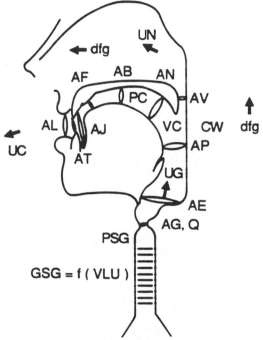

$$GSG = f (VLU)$$

FIGURE 1-16   Scully's model of speech production. The parameters are as follows. *Articulatory:* PLU (not shown in figure; air pressure in the lungs, reflecting subglottal control of lung walls); Q (effective mass and stiffness of the vocal folds); AG (articulatory component of glottal area); AE, EP (not shown), AN, AB, AC (not shown), and AF (defining shape of the tongue); AJ (jaw); AT (teeth); AL (lips); AV (velum); AP (pharynx). *Aerodynamic:* VLU (lung volume); PSG (subglottal air pressure); PC (oral air pressure behind the vocal tract constriction of area AF); UG, UC and UN (volume flow rate of air through the glottis, oral constriction and velopharyngeal port, respectively); VC (volume enclosed behind the vocal tract constriction), CW (compliance of the walls of the vocal tract); GSG (subglottal airflow conductance, which increases with lung volume). The distance from the glottis along the length of the vocal tract is indicated by dfg. (From Scully, C. [1990]. In Hardcastle, W. J., & Marchal, A. [Eds.], *Speech production and speech modelling* (pp. 151-186.) Dordrecht, Netherlands: Kluwer Academic Publishers.)

model depends on the availability of data on the various subsystems of speech production. Therefore, the actual implementation of Figure 1-16 is a highly involved set of computer programs that reflect much accumulated knowledge about speech production.

SPEECH PRODUCTION MODELS AND LANGUAGE BEHAVIOR

Although one could become completely occupied in the study of speech as a motor behavior or a conversion of articulation to sound pattern, speech is, after all, of greatest interest because of its primacy as a language modality. One of the most exciting facets of a speech production model is what it can tell us about language. The study of language generally may also direct research and theory on speech production. That is, speech is constrained not only by the task dynamics of its production system and the articulatory-acoustic relations of the vocal tract, but also by its service to language. Unfortunately, only a few brave scientists have directly attacked the formidable question of how speech production relates to a more general model or theory of language formulation. A particularly comprehensive source of information on this topic is Levelt (1989), who considers speech from "intention to articulation" (the subtitle of his book). Another valuable source is Bock's 1982 presentation of a model for utterance formulation. Gee and Grosjean (1983) have done related work on prosodic patterns as performance structures of language, and Martin (1972) has studied the rhythmic structure of spoken language. Eventually speech must be integrated into a fuller understanding of human language and its social utility. One aspect of speech is often taken as an important attribute but is neglected in speech production models. This aspect, **rhythm**, may hold particular significance in relating speech to language behavior.

Speech has a rhythmic quality, as is most evident in the recitation of verse. Simply, rhythm is the distribution of various levels of stress across a chain of syllables. The implementation of rhythm involves a complex interaction beginning at the sentence or phrase level and going down to the actuation of individual phonemes (Fourakis and Monahan, 1988). Rhythm also plays a key role in the understanding of speech. It is thought to provide a listener with the means to anticipate future elements in the speech stream for more efficient perceptual processing (Martin, 1972).

To give credence to the concept of rhythm, researchers have attempted to uncover consistent aspects of stress patterning. Temporal measures, such as the interval between two stressed syllables and the duration of metrical feet (a foot consists of a combination of stressed and unstressed syllables), have been analyzed for consistency (Bolinger, 1965; Nakatani, O'Connor, and Aston, 1981; Hoequist, 1983). The only positive durational finding was a tendency for constancy (isochronicity) in some types of metrical feet. This difficulty in uncovering the rhythmic units of speech has led some researchers to speculate that the perceptual phenomena of rhythm may be based on some other acoustical aspect of stress besides duration (Allen, 1975; Nakatani, O'Connor, and Aston, 1981).

More recently, metric phonology has set forth a different view of rhythmic organization (Selkirk, 1984). To establish rhythmic constancy, individuals manipulate the placement of stress by avoiding strings of adjoining stressed syllables or adjoining unstressed syllables. That is, speakers alternate strong and weak stress. One means of testing this hypothesis is to observe whether individuals shift syllable stress in phrases where stress clashing (two adjacent strong stress syllables) occurs. If Selkirk's hypothesis holds true, there is a tendency for a speaker to adjust the metrical pattern of the second stressed syllable. Perceptually, the stressed syllable may provide the beat for which anticipatory perceptual processing can be undertaken. The perceptual salience of the stressed syllable is enhanced by the adjacent unstressed syllable.

Cooper and Eady (1986) and Kelly and Bock (1988) undertook relevant studies. Cooper and Eady measured the duration and pitch change associated with the stress clash. They did not find an acoustic reduction in stress (reduced duration and pitch) for either syllable of the stress clash pair. Kelly and Bock chose a perceptual means to test for changes in the metrical feet. Their findings indicated that speakers did tend to change the metrical feet so as to impose alternating stress rhythm. These mixed but promising results provide a slightly clearer picture of the rhythmic characteristics of speech, which need to be accounted for in a model of speech.

Rhythm has not been addressed with much satisfaction in the majority of models discussed in this chapter. Indeed, many models ignore it altogether. It will be interesting to observe in the development of speech production models whether rhythm will be a clarifying and organizing influence on models or simply an add-on feature. Edelman (1989, pp. 178-179), writing on the *theory of neuronal group selection,* gives particular emphasis to rhythm as a potent factor in the evolution of language:

> In the evolution of speech systems, the linkage of the means of sound production to the breath period and to the rhythm of speech was probably particularly important. This temporal aspect of the production of speech sounds was, in all likelihood, correlated with the phasic reentrant signaling of cortical systems yielding correlations among various memory systems.

A concept of speech organization with implications for rhythm and other aspects of prosody is known as *slots and fillers* (Shattuck-Hufnagel, 1983) or *frames and contents* (MacNeilage, Studdert-Kennedy, and Lindblom, 1984). Slots (or frames) are syllable markers embodying information such as speaking rate and stress. Fillers (or contents) are the phonetic segments assigned to slots (or frames). In this view, speech is organized in two channels, one representing syllable markers and the other representing the phonetic content associated with syllables.

Lindblom (1990) introduced the *H & H theory,* which has a number of implications for understanding speech behavior in its communicative function. Basically, this theory holds that speech is controlled along a continuum of *hyperspeech* to *hypospeech* (hence H & H). Hyperspeech is described as output-oriented because this kind of control is purposive and prospectively organized. Speakers use hyperspeech to ensure that speech sound discriminations can be made by a listener. Hypospeech is system-oriented in the sense that it seeks a low-cost form of regulation. Speakers tend to use hypospeech to minimize the energy costs of speech production. Especially when other factors, such as context and topic familiarity, can be relied on to facilitate transmission of the message, speakers are inclined to use hypospeech. The output-oriented aspects of hyperspeech (insure speech sound discriminability) are in conflict with the system-oriented aspects of hypospeech (save energy), which is to say that both sets of aspects cannot be completely satisfied at the same time. The theory holds that a speaker selects for a given situation the degree to which hyperspeech or hypospeech will prevail. In other words, speech production is not undertaken with an invariant regulatory process but rather with a regulatory process that is adjusted to the demands of the situation.

It has been suggested that when speakers make adjustments along a certain hypo-hyper continuum, such as intended clarity, there may be an active reorganization of phonetic gestures (Lindblom and Moon, 1988; Moon, 1991). Results from an acoustic study of duration-dependent formant undershoot during clear speech have been offered as support for this reorganization hypothesis (Moon, 1991). (*Formant undershoot* is a formant pattern that falls short of the formant-frequency values observed in an isolated or context-free production of the sound in question; in other words, the speaker falls short of the full movement for a sound.) Moon's results indicate that while clear speech is associated with a certain degree of formant undershoot at shorter vowel durations, the amount of undershoot is much less than that observed during a more casual citation-form of speech. Thus, for equivalent vowel durations, clear speech appears to show less formant undershoot than more casual styles of speech.

A parallel finding was obtained in a kinematic analysis of clear and casual speech (Adams, 1990). Tongue movements produced during clear speech were found to have larger movement amplitudes and greater peak velocities than movements produced at equivalent durations during a more casual style of speech. However, these kinematic differences were not associated with any fundamental changes in the relationship between peak velocity and movement amplitude or the topology of movements, as measured by the velocity profiles, during clear speech. This led Adams to conclude that although clear speech may be associated with slightly larger movement amplitudes in some speakers, there is little evidence that variations in clarity are associated with a basic reorganization of motor control processes.

NEURAL MODELS OF SPEECH PRODUCTION

The challenges of modeling loom even larger with the neural regulation of human speech. This chapter does not present detailed models of

the neural control of speech or discuss putative differences between the cerebral hemispheres in the processing of various kinds of information for speech and language. Netsell (1986) and Kuehn, Lemme, and Baumgartner (1989) offer general coverage of neural bases of speech and language. Instead this brief section considers some general models for the neural control of speech as a voluntary motor behavior.

One of the most frequently reproduced diagrams to represent the motor control of speech is one adapted from Allen and Tsukahara (1974), as shown in Figure 1-17. This diagram, in the original or a modified form, has been presented as a model for speech regulation by Hirose (1982), Netsell (1986), and Barlow and Farley (1989), among others. The pathways for the planning, programming, and execution of movement are depicted. Obviously, this is a very general conception of the neural control of voluntary movement. The brain structures and pathways are not specific to speech. The model serves primarily to identify parts of the nervous system that control various aspects of movement. The parietal, frontal, and temporal cortices are thought to be involved in the initial planning for action (or *intent*). In addition, movement is programmed in a system composed of the premotor cortex, supplementary motor area, thalamus, lateral cerebellum, and motor cortex. The medial cerebellum monitors the motor instructions from the motor cortex and may revise them as needed to accomplish the goal. Somatosensory afference is the primary feedback channel and the feedback is probably plurimodal, involving taction, movement, position, aerodynamic, and other signals (Kent, Martin, and Sufit, 1990).

Certain observations on the control of voluntary movement suggest some changes in the picture of Figure 1-17. The effect of these changes is illustrated in Figure 1-18. First, Eccles (1982) has reviewed evidence that the initial neuronal event in all voluntary movements is in the supplementary motor areas of both hemispheres. Another possible change is motivated by the work summarized by De Long and Alexander (1987) showing that the basal ganglia-thalamocortical circuit (shown as a unitary circuit in Figure 1-17) may consist of segmental circuits, with at least a motor loop and an association loop, if not several such loops. Alexander, De Long and Strick (1986) and Miller and De Long (1988) have proposed a

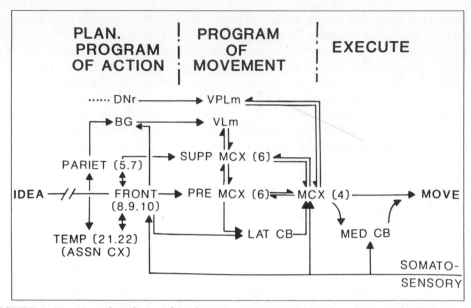

FIGURE 1-17 Neural pathways for planning, programming and execution of voluntary movement. BG, basal ganglia; DNr, dentate nucleus of cerebellum; FRONT, frontal cortex (areas 8, 9, 10); LAT CB, lateral cerebellum; MED CB, medial cerebellum; MCX, motor cortex (area 4); PARIET, parietal cortex (areas 5, 7); PRE MCX, premotor cortex (area 6); SUPP MCX, supplementary motor cortex (area 6); TEMP, temporal association cortex (areas 21, 22); VLm, medial part of ventral lateral thalamic nucleus; VPLm, medial part of the ventral posterior lateral thalamic nucleus. (From Kuehn, D. P., Lemme, M. L., & Baumgartner, J. M. [Eds.], [1989]. *Neural bases of speech, hearing, and language*, Austin, Texas: Pro-Ed Publishing.)

parallel organization of several such segmental circuits, in which a portion of the striatum, principally the putatem, receives partially overlapping projections from the motor cortex, premotor cortex, supplementary motor area, primary somatosensory cortex, and superior parietal lobule. The somatopically organized projections are thought to be maintained from putamen to globus pallidus and substantia nigra. The putamen thus represents a convergence of segmental circuits from various cortical regions. The basal ganglia are thought by many neuroscientists to be involved somehow in the programming of movement, one major aspect of which may be the coupling of sensory and motor responses (Lidsky, Manetto, and Schneider, 1985; Edelman, 1989). One possibility of such coupling for speech is the preparation of sensorimotor trajectories that guide the performance of movement (Kent, 1990). Edelman (1989) wrote that the basal ganglia, by virtue of their connections to prefrontal, premotor, and motor areas, may play an important role in linking motor programs to behavioral plans.

Another feature that may require modification, or at least essential elaboration, is the interconnections among various cortical and subcortical sites. Edelman (1989, p. 116) proposed that serially-ordered behavior is based on interconnections among neuronal groups in various regions "that are responsive to moment-to-moment sensory input." The importance of these interconnections is that they enable cortical neuronal groups to anticipate the consequences of their own activity and thereby prepare for the next action in a series. Cortical regions may be particularly responsible for longer intervals in the preparation and planning of action. Edelman wrote of "organs of succession," meaning brain structures that participate in the regulation of successive actions. He ascribed time constants to various structures in the following manner: neocortex—short, medium, and long; basal ganglia—short; and cerebellum—short. With respect to the control of voluntary movements like speech, these time constants can be interpreted to mean that the neocortex maintains the long-term pattern of an action series, while the basal ganglia and cerebellum are responsible for relatively short spans

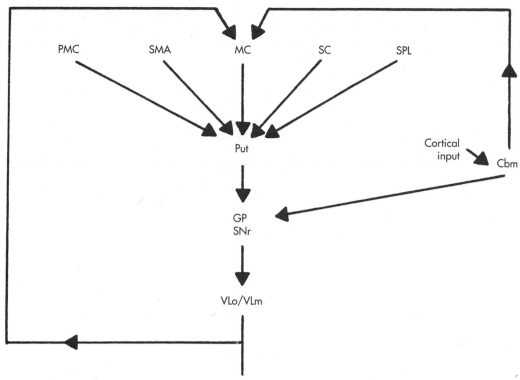

FIGURE 1-18   Neural pathways for the control of voluntary movement, a revised version. PMC, premotor cortex; SMA, supplementary motor area; MC, motor cortex; SC, somatosensory cortex; SPL, superior parietal lobule; Put, putamen; Cbm, cerebellum; GP, globus pallidus; SNr, substantia nigra pars reticularis; VLo, pars oralis of ventrolateral thalamus; VLm, pars medialis of ventrolateral thalamus. (From Kent, R. D. [1990]. In Hardcastle, W. J., & Marchal, A. [Eds.], *Speech production and speech modelling* (p. 388.) Dordrecht, Netherlands: Kluwer Academic Publishers.)

of time. The basal ganglia participate in aspects of programming and sensorimotor coordination, and the cerebellum engages primarily in the control of timing and synchronization of movements. In this conceptualization, the control of succession is distributed among various parts of the brain according to time constants of activity.

The extension of this idea to language as well as speech may provide some useful hypotheses for the governance of syntactic relationships, semantic associations, and morphologic units. Ideas about the neural control of language are changing rapidly. New data from brain imaging are providing new insights into patterns of brain activity associated with language. In addition, new hypotheses are being formulated about brain structures that have not been clearly represented in extant theories of neural bases of language. For example, recent speculations attribute important cognitive and language functions to the cerebellum (Leiner, Leiner, and

Dow, 1990), a structure conspicuously lacking in classical accounts of brain systems in language. Research on neural function in oral and vocal behavior of animals also is a rich source of hypotheses about the neural bases of language. Although humans may be unique in possessing language, some mechanisms related to language may be shared by humans and animals (Larson, 1988; Jurgens, 1992).

This section only touches the surface of possibilities in the neural modeling of speech production. Additional information on neural models of vocal communication is available in Larson (1988), Jurgens (1992), Kent and Tjaden (in press), and Square and Martin (in press).

CONCLUSION

A complete, valid and accurate model of speech production awaits the answers to all of the questions raised in this and other chapters in this book. Each area of investigation contributes to an understanding of speech and therefore to a better sense of how speech can be modeled. Although much remains to be done (is it not ever so?), progress in modeling speech production has been substantial. Interesting possibilities have been proposed, and the stage is set for studies to test the models. Speech has been modeled in different ways for different purposes. Much progress has been made in articulatory and vocal tract models, in connectionist models, and in task dynamic models. Rather less has been accomplished in neural models. But even here, the prospects are very good, particularly as brain imaging systems are used to study brain activity associated with speech.

An especially exciting prospect is the convergence or combination of various models. For example, Saltzman and Munhall (1989) combine aspects of task dynamics, articulatory phonology, and connectionism in their model of gestural patterning. Similarly, Scully (1990) draws from a large body of work to develop a composite model of speech production. This is not to say that all models are compatible (far from it), but rather that at least some of them may fit together in a comprehensive theory of speech production. At present, that may be the closest approach to a theory with general applicability. The combination of models may have another happy consequence—a kind of emerging property in which a suitable interaction of models generates theoretical notions not defined in any model working alone. Many speech production models virtually ignore perception of the acoustic signal as a determining influence. Indeed, some of them neglect audition to the degree that we might suppose that speech is produced in a world of silence.

A better understanding of speech production might be generated by an attempt to fit together complementary aspects of different theories. Because the conversion of articulatory configuration to acoustic output is an essential aspect of speech, careful evaluations are needed of theories such as Stevens's (1989) quantal theory and similar theories (Badin et al., 1990; Carre and Mryati, 1990) that propose powerful parsimonies in the articulatory-acoustic relationship. Characteristics of this relationship may define important constraints within which motor control of the articulators can be described. Additional steps in specifying motor control require study of the articulatory kinematics to determine invariant properties. Such invariances can characterize the gestures associated with particular acoustic-phonetic goals. If kinematic invariants exist, they may become the language for the higher order problem of serial order, or the temporal assembly of movements to form a phonetic string.

Theories of speech production also may be extended to include considerations of speech development in children, speech disorders, and bilingualism. A theory of speech production can hold implications for many aspects of speech behavior. In addition, knowledge gained from the study of speech development, speech disorders, and bilingualism may help to shape a general theory of speech production.

Acknowledgments
This work was supported in part by research grants DC00319 and DC00820 from the National Institute on Deafness and Other Communication Disorders, National Institutes of Health.

Review Questions

(The word *theory* is used here to designate the various theories and models discussed in this chapter.)

1. Describe three major issues to be accounted for in a theory of speech production. How have different theories attempted to resolve these issues?

2. Choose five theories discussed in this chapter and describe the following for each: What is being modeled or represented in the theory?

What is the purpose or goal of the theory? What kinds of evidence might be used to test the theory?

3. Choose any theory discussed in this chapter and develop an experiment to test some aspect of it. You may want to test a prediction that is generated by the theory.

4. What kind of information might be contained in a motor program for speech production? Take the simple sentence "There is much

to be considered." List the various kinds of information that a motor program conceivably would have to contain to represent the motoric events associated with this sentence.

5. What are some of the reasons for adopting a dynamic systems approach to understand speech production?

6. What are the strengths and weaknesses of a connectionist theory in accounting for speech production?

7. What difficulties arise in the development of a composite model (that is, a complete model) of speech production?

References

Abbs, J. H., Gracco, V. L., & Cole, K. J. (1984). Control of multimovement coordination: Sensorimotor mechanisms in speech motor programming. *Journal of Motor Behavior, 16*, 195-231.

Adams, S. G. (1990). *Rate and clarity of speech: An x-ray microbeam study.* Unpublished doctoral dissertation, University of Wisconsin, Madison.

Alexander, G. E., De Long, M. R., & Strick, P. L. (1986). Parallel organization of functionally segregated circuits linking basal ganglia and cortex. *Annual Review of Neuroscience, 9*, 357-381.

Allen, G. D. (1975). Speech rhythm: its relation to performance universals and articulatory timing. *Journal of Phonetics, 3*, 75-86.

Allen, G. I., & Tsukahara, N. (1974). Cerebrocerebellar communication system. *Physiological Review, 54*, 957-1006.

Allwood, E., & Scully, C. (1982). A composite model of speech production. *Proceedings of International Congress on Acoustics, Speech and Signal Processing*, IEEE, ICASSP 82, 2, 932-935.

Badin, P., Perrier, P., Boe, L.J., & Abry, C. (1990). Vocalic nomograms: Acoustic and articulatory considerations upon formant convergences. *Journal of the Acoustical Society of America, 87*, 1290-1300.

Barlow, S. M., & Farley, G. R. (1989). Neurophysiology of speech. In Kuehn, D. P., Lemme, M. L., & Baumgartner, J. M. (Eds.), *Neural bases of speech, hearing, and language.* Boston: College-Hill (pp. 146-200).

Barry, W. J. (1983). Some problems of interarticulator phasing as an index of temporal regularity in speech. *Journal of Experimental Psychology: Human Perception and Performance, 9*, 826-828.

Benoit, C. (1986). Note on the use of correlations in speech timing. *Journal of the Acoustical Society of America, 80*, 1846-1848.

Bock, C. (1982). Toward a cognitive psychology of syntax: Information processing contributions to sentence formulation. *Psychological Review, 89*, 1-47.

Bolinger, D. L. (1965). Pitch accent and sentence rhythm. In Abe, I., & Kanekiyo, T. (Eds.), *Forms of English.* Cambridge, MA: Harvard Press (pp. 123-141).

Boyce, S. E., Krakow, R. A., Bell-Berti, F., & Gelfer, C. E. (1990). Converging sources of evidence for dissecting articulatory movements into core gestures. *Journal of Phonetics, 18*, 173-188.

Boylls, C. C. (1975). A theory of cerebellar function with applications to locomotion: 2. The relation of anterior lobe climbing fiber function to locomotor behavior in the cat. *COINS Technical Report 76-1*, Department of Computer and Information Science, University of Massachusetts, Amherst.

Broad, D. (1979). The new theories of vocal fold vibration. In Lass, N. J. (Ed.), *Speech and language: Advances in basic research and practice* (Vol. 2). New York: Academic Press (pp. 203-256).

Browman, C., & Goldstein, L. (1986). Towards an articulatory phonology. *Phonology Yearbook, 3*, 219-252.

Browman, C. P., & Goldstein, L. (1990). Tiers in articulatory phonology, with some implications for casual speech. In Kingston, J. & Beckwith, M. (Eds.), *Papers in laboratory phonology I: Between the grammar and the physics of speech.* Cambridge, UK: Cambridge University Press (pp. 219-252).

Carre, R., & Mrayati, M. (1990). Articulatory-acoustic-phonetic relations and modelling, regions and modes. In Hardcastle, W. J., & Marchal, A. (Eds.), *Speech production and speech modelling* (pp. 211-240). Dordrecht, Netherlands: Kluwer Academic Publishers.

Chomsky, N. (1965). *Aspects of the Theory of Syntax.* Cambridge, MA: MIT Press.

Coker, C. (1976). A model of articulatory dynamics and control. *Proceedings of IEEE, 64*, 452-460.

Cooper, W. E., & Eady, S. J. (1986). Metrical phonology in speech production. *Journal of Memory and Language, 25*, 369-384.

Dell, G. S. (1986). A spreading-activation theory of retrieval in sentence production. *Psychological Review, 93*, 283-321.

De Long, M. R., & Alexander, G. E. (1987). The basal ganglia and sensorimotor function. In Struppler, A., & Weindl, A. (Eds.), *Clinical aspects of sensory motor integration.* Berlin: Springer-Verlag (pp. 203-211).

Draper, M. H., Ladefoged, P., & Whitteridge, D. (1959). Respiratory muscles in speech. *Journal of Speech and Hearing Research, 2,* 16-27.

Easton, T. (1972). On the normal use of reflexes. *American Scientist, 60,* 591-599.

Eccles, J. C. (1982). The initiation of voluntary movements by the supplementary motor area. *Archiv fur Psychiatrie und Nervenkrankheiten, 231,* 423-441.

Edelman, G. M. (1989). *The remembered present.* New York: Basic Books.

Eriksen, C. W., Pollack, M. D., & Montague, W. E. (1970). Implicit speech: Mechanisms in perceptual coding? *Journal of Experimental Psychology, 84,* 502-507.

Fairbanks, G. (1954). Systematic research in experimental phonetics: 1. A theory of the speech mechanism as a servosystem. *Journal of Speech and Hearing Disorders, 19,* 133-139.

Fant, G. (1960). *Acoustic theory of speech production.* The Hague: Mouton.

Fant, G. (1989). Speech research in perspective. Speech Transmission Laboratories, Royal Institute of Technology, *Quarterly Progress and Status Reports, STL-QPSR 4,* 1-8.

Folkins, J. W., & Zimmerman, G. N. (1981). Jaw-muscle activity during speech with the mandible fixed. *Journal of the Acoustical Society of America, 69,* 1441-1445.

Fourakis, M., & Monahan, C. B. (1988). Effects of metrical foot structure on syllable timing. *Language and Speech, 31,* 283-306.

Fowler, C. A. (1980). Coarticulation and theories of extrinsic timing. *Journal of Phonetics, 8,* 113-133.

Fowler, C., Rubin, P., Remez, R. E., & Turvey, M. T. (1980). Implications for speech production of a general theory of action. In Butterworth, B. (Ed.), *Speech production* (Vol. 1). New York: Academic Press (pp. 373-420).

Fromkin, V. A. (1989). Grammatical aspects of speech errors. In F. J. Newmeyer (Ed.), *Linguistics: The Cambridge survey. I. Linguistic theory: Extensions and implications.* Cambridge, UK: Cambridge University Press (pp. 117-138).

Fujimura, O. (1986). Relative invariance of articulatory movements: An iceberg model. In Perkell, J. S., & Klatt, D. H. (Eds.), *Invariance and variability in speech processes.* Hillsdale, NJ: Erlbaum (pp. 226-242).

Fujimura, O. (1990). Articulatory perspectives of speech organization. In Hardcastle, W. J., & Marchal, M. (Eds.), *Speech production and speech modelling.* Dordrecht, Netherlands: Kluwer Academic Press (pp. 323-342).

Gee, J. P., & Grosjean, F. (1983). Performance structures: A psycholinguistic and linguistic appraisal. *Cognitive Psychology, 15,* 411-458.

Gel'fand, I. M., Gurfinkel, V. S., Tsetlin, M. L., &

Shik, M. L. (1971). Some problems in the analysis of movement. In Gel'fand, I. M., Gurfinkel, V. S., Fomin, S. V., & Tsetlin, M. L. (Eds.), *Models of the structural-functional organization of certain biological systems.* Cambridge, MA: MIT Press (pp. 329-345).

Gentner, D. R. (1987). Timing of skilled motor performance: Tests of the proportional duration model. *Psychological Review, 94,* 255-276.

Gracco, V. L. (1990). Characteristics of speech as a motor control system. In Hammond, G. E. (Ed.), *Cerebral control of speech and limb movements.* Amsterdam: North Holland (pp. 3-28).

Gurfinkel, V. S., Kots, Y. A., Paltsev, E. I., & Feldman, A. G. (1971). The compensation of respiratory disturbances of the erect posture of man as an example of the organization of interarticular interaction. In Gel'fand, I. M., Gurfinkel, V. S., Fomin, S. V., & Tsetlin, M. L. (Eds.), *Models of the structural-functional organization of certain biological systems.* Cambridge, MA: MIT Press (pp. 382-395).

Haken, H. (1975). Cooperative phenomena in systems far from thermal equilibrium and in nonphysical systems. *Review of Modern Physics, 47,* 67-121.

Haken, H. (1983). *Advanced synergetics.* Heidelberg: Springer-Verlag.

Hanson, S. J., & Burr, D. J. (1990). What connectionist models learn: Learning and representation in connectionist networks. *Behavioral and Brain Sciences, 13,* 471-518.

Harshman, R., Ladefoged, P., & Goldstein, L. (1977). Factor analysis of tongue shapes. *Journal of the Acoustical Society of America, 62,*693-707.

Hirano, M. (1974). Morphological structure of the vocal cord as a vibrator and its variations. *Folia Phoniatrica* (Basel), *26,* 89-94.

Hirano, M., & Kakita, Y. (1985). Cover-body theory of vocal fold vibration. In Daniloff, R. G. (Ed.), *Speech science.* San Diego: College Hill Press.

Hirose, H. (1982). Pathophysiology of motor speech disorders. *Folia Phoniatrica (Basel), 38,* 61-88.

Hixon, T. J., and collaborators (1987). *Respiratory function in speech and song.* Boston: College-Hill Press.

Hixon, T. J., Goldman, M., & Mead, J. (1973). Kinematics of the chest wall during speech production: Volume displacements of the rib cage, abdomen, and lung. *Journal of Speech and Hearing Research, 16,* 78-115.

Hixon, T. J., Mead, J., & Goldman, M. (1976). Dynamics of the chest wall during speech production: Function of the thorax, rib cage, diaphragm and abdomen. *Journal of Speech and Hearing Research, 19,* 297-356.

Hodge, M., Putnam, A. H. B., & Weismer, G. (1986).

Respiratory kinematics in adult female speakers. Paper presented at the Annual Convention of the American Speech-Language-Hearing Association, Detroit, MI.

Holst, E. von (1973). *The Behavioral Physiology of Animal and Man: The Collected Papers of Erich von Holst.* (Vol. 1) (R. Martin, trans.). London: Methven.

Hoequist, C. (1983). Syllable duration in stress-syllable- and mora-timed languages. *Phonetica, 40,* 203-237.

Hunker, C. J., & Abbs, J. H. (1982). Respiratory movement control during speech: Evidence for motor equivalence. *Society for Neuroscience, 8,* 946 (Abstract).

Ishizaka, K., & Matsudaira, M. (1972a). Fluid mechanical considerations of vocal cord vibration (SCRL Monograph No. 8). Santa Barbara: Speech Communication Research Laboratory.

Ishizaka, K., & Matsudaira, M. (1972b). Theory of vocal cord vibration. *Reports of the University of Electro-Communications, 23,* 107-136.

Jordan, M. I. (1990). Motor learning and the degrees of freedom problem. In Jeannerod, M. (Ed.), *Attention and performance XIII.* Hillsdale, NJ: Erlbaum (pp. 796-836).

Jordan, M. I. (1991). Serial order: A parallel distributed processing approach. In Elman, J. L., & Rumelhard, D. E. (Eds.), *Advances in connectionist theory: Speech.* Hillsdale, NJ: Erlbaum (pp. 214-249).

Jordan, M. I., & Rosenbaum, D. A. (1989). Action. In Posner, M. I. (Ed.), *Foundations of cognitive science.* Cambridge, MA: MIT Press (pp. 184-202).

Jurgens, U. (1992). On the neurobiology of vocal communication. In Papousek, H., Jurgens, U., & Papousek, M. (Eds.), *Nonverbal vocal communication.* Cambridge, UK: Cambridge University Press (pp. 31-42).

Keller, E. (1987). The variation of absolute and relative measures of speech activity. *Journal of Phonetics, 15,* 225-247.

Kelly, M. H., & Bock, J. K. (1988). Stress in time. *Journal of Experimental Psychology: Human Perception and Performance, 14,* 389-403.

Kelso, J. A. S., Saltzman, E. L., & Tuller, B. (1986). The dynamical perspective on speech production: data and theory. *Journal of Phonetics, 14,* 29-59.

Kelso, J. A. S., Southard, D., & Goodman, B. (1979). On the nature of interlimb coordination. *Science, 203,* 1029-1031.

Kelso, J. A. S., & Tuller, B. (1984). Conveying evidence in support of common dynamical principles for speech and movement coordination. *American Journal of Physiology, 246,* R928-R935.

Kelso, J. A. S., Tuller, B., Vatikiotis-Bateson, E., & Fowler, C. A. (1984). Functionally specific articulatory cooperation following jaw perturbations during speech: Evidence for coordinative structures. *Journal of Experimental Psychology: Human Perception and Performance, 10,* 812-832.

Kent, R. D. (1981). Sensorimotor aspects of speech development. In Aslin, R. N., Alberts, J. R., & Petersen, M. R. (Eds.), *Development of perception: Psychobiological perspectives* (Vol. 1). New York: Academic Press (pp. 162-185).

Kent, R. D. (1986). The iceberg hypothesis: The temporal assembly of speech movements. In Perkell, J. S., & Klatt, D. H. (Eds.), *Invariance and variability in speech processes.* Hillsdale, NJ: Erlbaum (pp. 234-242).

Kent, R. D. (1990). The acoustic and physiological characteristics of neurologically impaired speech movements. In Hardcastle, W. J., & Marchal, A. (Eds.), *Speech production and speech modelling.* Dordrecht, Netherlands: Kluwer Academic Publishers (pp. 365-402).

Kent, R. D., Martin, R. E., & Sufit, R. L. (1990). Oral sensation: A review and clinical prospective. In Winitz, H. (Ed.), *Human communication disorders* (Vol. 3). Norwood, NJ: Ablex (pp. 135-191).

Kent, R. D., & Minifie, F. D. (1977). Coarticulation in recent speech production models. *Journal of Phonetics, 5,* 115-133.

Kent, R.D., & Netsell, R. (1972). Effects of stress contrasts on certain articulatory parameters. *Phonetica, 24,* 23-44.

Kent, R. D., & Tjaden, K. (in press). Brain functions underlying speech. In Hardcastle, W. J., & Laver, J. (Eds.), *Manual of phonetics.* London: Blackwell.

Kiritani, S. (1977). Articulatory studies by the X-ray microbeam system. In Sawashima, M., & Cooper, F. S. (Eds.), *Dynamic aspects of speech production.* Tokyo: University of Tokyo Press (pp. 171-190).

Klapp, S. T., Anderson, W. G., & Berrian, R. W. (1973). Implicit speech in reading, reconsideration. *Journal of Experimental Psychology, 100,* 368-374.

Kozhevnikov, A. A., & Chistovich, L. A. (1965). *Speech: Articulation and Perception.* Moscow-Leningrad, English Translation in Joint Publications Research Service, 30, 543, Clearinghouse for Federal Scientific and Technical Information, U.S. Department of Commerce.

Kuehn, D. P., Lemme, M. L., & Baumgartner, J. M. (Eds.), (1989). *Neural bases of speech, hearing, and language.* Boston, MA: College-Hill.

Lamberts, K., & d'Ydewalle, G. (1990). What can psychologists learn from hidden-unit nets? Open peer commentary on S. J. Hanson and D. J. Burr: What connectionist models learn: Learning and representation in connectionist networks. *Behavioral and Brain Sciences, 13,* 499-500.

Larson, C. R. (1988). Brain mechanisms involved in the control of vocalization. *Journal of Voice, 2,* 301-311.

Lashley, K. (1951). The problem of serial order in behavior. In Jeffress, L. A. (Ed.), *Cerebral mechanisms in behavior.* New York: Wiley (pp. 506-528).

Leiner, H. C., Leiner, A. L., & Dow, R.S. (1990). The human cerebro-cerebellar system: Its computing, cognitive and language skills. *Behavioral and Brain Research, 44,* 113-128.

Levelt, W. J. M. (1989). *Speaking: From intention to articulation.* Cambridge, MA: MIT Press.

Lidsky, T. I., Manetto, C., & Schneider, J. S. (1985). A consideration of sensory factors involved in motor functions of the basal ganglia. *Brain Research Review, 7,* 1-19.

Liljencrants, J. (1971). Fourier series description of the tongue profile. *Speech Transmission Laboratory,* Royal Institute of Technology, Stockholm, Sweden, *QPSR* 9-18.

Lindblom, B. (1990). Explaining phonetic variation: A sketch of the H and H theory. In Hardcastle, W. J., & Marchal, A. (Eds.), *Speech production and speech modelling.* Dordrecht, Netherlands: Kluwer Academic Publishers (pp. 403-439).

Lindblom, B., & Moon, S. (1988). Formant undershoot in clear and citation form speech. Paper presented at the Conference on Distinctive Features, Stockholm University, Stockholm, Sweden.

Lindblom, B. E. F., & Sundberg, J. E. F. (1971). Acoustical consequences of lip, tongue, jaw and larynx movement. *Journal of the Acoustical Society of America, 4,* 1166-1179.

Lofqvist, A. (1990). Speech as audible gestures. In Hardcastle, W. J., & Marchal, A. (Eds.), *Speech production and speech modelling.* Dordrecht, Netherlands: Kluwer Academic Publishers (pp. 289-322).

Lofqvist, A., & Yoshioka, H. (1981). Interarticulator programming in obstruent production. *Phonetica, 38,* 21-34.

Lubker, J. (1986). Articulatory timing and the conception of phase. *Journal of Phonetics, 14,* 133-137.

MacKay, D. G. (1974). Aspects of the symbol of behavior: Serial structure and speech rate. *Quarterly Journal of Experimental Psychology, 26,* 642-657.

MacNeilage, P. (1970). Motor control of serial ordering of speech. *Psychological Review, 77,* 182-196.

MacNeilage, P. F., Studdert-Kennedy, M. G., & Lindblom, B. (1984). Functional precursors to language and its lateralization. *American Journal of Physiology, 246 (Regulatory, Integrative and Comparative Physiology, 15),* R912-R914.

Maeda, S. (1990). Compensatory articulation during speech: evidence from the analysis and synthesis of vocal-tract shapes using an articulatory model. In Hardcastle, W. J., & Marchal, A. (Eds.), *Speech production and speech modelling.* Dordrecht, Netherlands: Kluwer Academic Publishers (pp. 131-150).

Martin, J. G. (1972). Rhythmic (hierarchical) versus serial structure in speech and other behavior. *Psychological Review, 79,* 487-509.

Massaro, D. W. (1988). Some criticisms of connectionist models of human performance. *Journal of Memory and Language, 27,* 213-234.

Mermelstein, P. (1972). Speech synthesis with the aid of a recursive filter approximating the transfer function of the nasalized vocal tract. *Proceedings of the International Conference on Speech Communication and Processing,* Boston: 152-155.

Meyer, D. E., & Gordon, P. C. (1985). Speech production: Motor programming of phonetic features. *Journal of Memory and Language, 24,* 3-26.

Meyer, J. (1987). Contrastive phonology: Particle, wave and field. *International Review of Applied Linguistics in Language Teaching, 25,* 213-219.

Miller, W. C., & De Long, M. R. (1988). Parkinsonian symptomatology: An anatomical and physiological analysis. In Joseph, J. J. (Ed.), *Central Determinants of Age-Related Declines in Motor Function. Annals of the New York Academy of Sciences, 515,* 287-302.

Moon, S. (1991). An acoustic and perceptual study of undershoot in clear and citation-form speech. Unpublished doctoral dissertation, University of Texas at Austin.

Mowrey, R. A., & MacKay, I. R. A. (1990). Phonological primitives: Electromyographic speech error evidence. *Journal of the Acoustical Society of America, 88,* 1299-1312.

Mulder, G. (1983). The information processing paradigm: Concepts, methods and limitations. *Journal of Child Psychology and Psychiatry, 24,* 19-35.

Munhall, K. (1985). An examination of intra-articulatory relative timing. *Journal of the Acoustical Society of America, 78,* 1548-1553.

Nakatani, L. H., O'Connor, K. D., & Aston, C. H. (1981). Prosodic aspects of American English speech rhythm. *Phonetica, 38,* 84-106.

Neilson, M. D., & Neilson, P. D. (1987). Speech motor control and stuttering: A computational model of adaptive sensory-motor processing. *Speech communication, 6,* 325-333.

Nelson, W. L. (1983). Physical principles for economies of skilled movements. *Biological cybernetics, 46,* 135-147.

Netsell, R. (1986). *A neurobiologic view of speech production in the dysarthrias.* San Diego: College-Hill.

Nittrauer, S., Munhall, K., Kelso, J. A. S., Tuller, B.,

& Harris, K. S. (1988). Patterns of interarticulatory phasing and their relation to linguistic structure. *Haskins Laboratories Status and Progress Report, SR-95*, 1-15.

Nolan, F. J. (1982). The role of action theory in the description of speech production. *Linguistics, 20*, 287-308.

Ostry, D. J., Cooke, J. D., & Munhall, K. G. (1987). Velocity curves of human arm and speech movements. *Experimental Brain Research, 68*, 37-46.

Ostry, D. J., Keller, E., & Parush, A. (1983). Similarities in the control of the speech articulators and the limbs: kinematics of tongue dorsum movement in speech. *Journal of Experimental Psychology (Human Perception), 9*, 622-636.

Ostry, D. J., & Munhall, K. G. (1985). Control of rate and duration of speech movements. *Journal of the Acoustical Society of America, 77*, 640-648.

Perkell, J. S. (1980). Phonetic features and the physiology of speech production. In Butterworth, B. (Ed.), *Language production* (Vol. 1). New York: Academic Press (pp. 337-372).

Perkell, J. S., & Nelson, W. L. (1985). Variability in the production of vowels /i/ and /æ/. *Journal of the Acoustical Society of America, 77*, 1889-1895.

Pike, K. L. (1959). Language as particle, wave and field. *The Texas Quarterly, 2*, 37-54.

Pinker, S., & Meher, J. (1988). *Connections and symbols*. Cambridge, MA: MIT Press.

Reed, E. S. (1982). An outline of a theory of action systems. *Journal of Motor Behavior, 14*, 98-134.

Rubin P. E., Baer, T., & Mermelstein, P. (1981). An articulatory synthesizer for perceptual research. *Journal of the Acoustical Society of America, 70*, 321-328.

Rumelhart, D. E., & Norman, D. A. (1982). Simulating a skilled typist: A study of skilled cognitive-motor performance. *Cognitive Science, 6*, 1-36.

Saltzman, E. L. (1979). Levels of sensorimotor representation. *Journal of Mathematical Psychology, 20*, 91-163.

Saltzman, E. L., & Munhall, K. G. (1989). A dynamical approach to gestural patterning in speech production. *Ecological Psychology, 1*, 333-382.

Schmidt, R. A. (1975). A schema theory of discrete motor learning. *Psychological Review, 82*, 255-260.

Schmidt, R. A. (1988). *Motor Control and Learning* (2nd ed.). Champaign, IL: Human Kinetics Publishers.

Scully, C. (1986). Speech production simulated with a functional model of the larynx and the vocal tract. *Journal of Phonetics, 14*, 407-414.

Scully, C. (1987). Linguistic units and units of speech production. *Speech Communication, 6*, 77-142.

Scully, C. (1990). Articulatory synthesis. In Hard-castle, W. J., & Marchal, A. (Eds.), *Speech production and speech modelling*. Dordrecht, Netherlands: Kluwer Academic Publishers (pp. 151-186).

Selkirk, E. (1984). *Phonology and syntax: The relation between sound and structure*. Cambridge, MA: MIT Press.

Shaffer, L. H. (1982). Rhythm and timing in skill. *Psychological Review, 89*, 109-122.

Shaiman, S. (1989). Kinematic and electromyographic responses to perturbation of the jaw. *Journal of the Acoustical Society of America, 86*, 78-87.

Shattuck-Hufnagel, S. (1979). Speech errors as evidence for a serial-ordering mechanism in sentence production. In Cooper, W., & Walker, E. (Eds.), *Sentence processing*. Hillsdale, NJ: Erlbaum.

Shattuck-Hufnagel, S. (1983). Sublexical units and suprasegmental structure in speech production planning. In MacNeilage, P. F. (Ed.), *The production of speech*. New York: Springer-Verlag (pp. 109-136).

Square, P. A., & Martin, R. E. (in press). The nature and treatment of neuromotor speech disorders in aphasia. In Chapey, R. (Ed.), *Language intervention strategies in adult aphasia* (Vol. 3). Baltimore: Williams & Wilkins.

Sternberg, S., Knoll, R. L., Monsell, S., & Wright, C. E. (1988). Motor programs and hierarchical organization in the control of rapid speech. *Phonetica, 45*, 172-197.

Sternberg, S., Monsell, S., Knoll, R. L., & Wright, C. E. (1978). The latency and duration of rapid movement sequences: Comparison of speech and typewriting. In Stelmach, G. E. (Ed.), *Information processing in motor control and learning*. New York: Academic Press (pp. 117-152).

Stevens, K. N. (1972). The quantal nature of speech: evidence from articulatory-acoustic data. In Denes, P. B., & Davis, E. E. (Eds.), *Human communication: A unified view*. New York: McGraw-Hill (pp. 51-66).

Stevens, K. N. (1989). On the quantal nature of speech. *Journal of Phonetics, 17*, 3-46.

Stevens, K. N., & House, A. S. (1955). Development of a quantitative description of vowel articulation. *Journal of the Acoustical Society of America, 27*, 484-493.

Titze, I. (1973). The human vocal cords: A mathematical model. *Phonetica, 28*, 129-170.

Weismer, G. (1980). Control of the voicing distinction for intervocalic stops and fricatives: Some data and theoretical considerations. *Journal of Phonetics, 8*, 417-428.

Weismer, G. (1985). Speech breathing. In Daniloff,

R. G. (Ed.), *Speech science*. San Diego: College-Hill Press (pp. 46-72).

Weismer, G. (1988). Speech production. In Lass, N. J., McReynolds, L. V., Northern, J. L., & Yoder, D. E. (Eds.), *Handbook of speech-language pathology and audiology*. St. Louis: Mosby.

Wilson, W. R., & Morton, K. (1990). Reconsidera-

tion of the action-theory perspective on speech motor control. *Clinical Linguistics and Phonetics, 4*, 341-362.

Wood, S. (1979). A radiographic analysis of constriction locations for vowels. *Journal of Phonetics, 7*, 25-43.

Suggested Readings
General Discussion of Theorizing and Modeling

Fujimura, O. (1990). Articulatory perspectives of speech organization. In Hardcastle, W. J., & Marchal, M. (Eds.), *Speech production and speech modelling*. Dordrecht, Netherlands: Kluwer Academic Press (pp. 323-342).

Hardcastle, W. J., & Marchal, A. (Eds.), *Speech production and speech modelling*. Dordrecht, Netherlands: Kluwer Academic Press (pp. 365-402).

Schmidt, R. A. (1988). *Motor control and learning* (2nd ed.). Champaign, IL: Human Kinetics Publishers.

Feedback and Feedforward Models

Kent, R. D., Martin, R. E., & Sufit, R. L. (1990). Oral sensation: A review and clinical prospective. In Winitz, H. (Ed.), *Human communication disorders* (Vol. 3). Norwood, NJ: Ablex (pp. 135-191).

MacNeilage, P. (1970). Motor control of serial ordering of speech. *Psychological Review, 77*, 182-196.

Neilson, M. D., & Neilson, P. D. (1987). Speech motor control and stuttering: A computational model of adaptive sensory-motor processing. *Speech Communication, 6*, 325-333.

Motor Programs

Gracco, V.L. (1990). Characteristics of speech as a motor control system. In Hammond, G. E. (Ed.), *Cerebral control of speech and limb movements*. Amsterdam: North Holland (pp. 3-28).

Schmidt, R. A. (1975). A schema theory of discrete motor learning. *Psychological Review, 82*, 255-260.

Sternberg, S., Knoll, R. L., Monsell, S., & Wright, C. E. (1988). Motor programs and hierarchical organization in the control of rapid speech. *Phonetica, 45*, 172-197.

Dynamic Systems (Action) Models

Keller, E. (1987). The variation of absolute and relative measures of speech activity. *Journal of Phonetics, 15*, 225-347.

Kelso, J. A. S., Saltzman, E. L., & Tuller, B. (1986). The dynamical perspective on speech produc-

tion: data and theory. *Journal of Phonetics, 14*, 29-59.

Nolan, F. J. (1982). The role of action theory in the description of speech production. *Linguistics, 20*, 287-308.

Models of Gestural Patterning

Saltzman, E. L., & Munhall, K. G. (1989). A dynamical approach to gestural patterning in speech production. *Ecological Psychology, 1*, 333-382.

Connectionist and Spreading Activation Models

Dell, G. S. (1986). A spreading-activitation theory of retrieval in sentence production. *Psychological Review, 93*, 283-321.

Hanson, S. J., & Burr, D. J. (1990). What connectionist models learn: Learning and representation in connectionist networks. *Behavioral and Brain Sciences, 13*, 471-518.

Subsystem and Composite Models

Broad, D. (1979). The new theories of vocal fold vibration. In Lass, N. J. (Ed.), *Speech and language: Advances in basic research and practice.* (Vol. 2), New York: Academic Press (pp. 203-256).

Fant, G. (1960). *Acoustic theory of speech production.* The Hague: Mouton.

Fujimura, O. (1986). Relative invariance of articulatory movements: An iceberg model. In Perkell, J. S., & Klatt, D. H. (Eds.), *Invariance and variability in speech processes.* Hillsdale, NJ: Erlbaum (pp. 226-242).

Hirano, M., & Kakita, Y. (1985). Cover-body theory of vocal fold vibration. In Daniloff, R. G. (Ed.), *Speech science*. San Diego: College-Hill Press.

Hixon, T.J., & collaborators (1987). *Respiratory function in speech and song*. Boston: College-Hill Press.

Ostry, D. J., & Munhall, K. G. (1985). Control of rate and duration of speech movements. *Journal of the Acoustical Society of America, 77*, 640-648.

Stevens, K. N. (1989). On the quantal nature of speech. *Journal of Phonetics, 17*, 3-46.

Weismer, G. (1985). Speech breathing. In Daniloff, R. G. (Ed.), *Speech science*. San Diego: College-Hill Press (pp. 46-72).

Speech Production Models and Language Formulation

Levelt, W. J. M. (1989). *Speaking: From intention to articulation.* Cambridge, MA: MIT Press.

Neural Models

Edelman, G. M. (1989). *The remembered present.* New York: Basic Books.

Jurgens, U. (1992). On the neurobiology of vocal communication. In Papousek, H., Jurgens, U., & Papousek, M. (Eds.), *Nonverval vocal communication.* Cambridge, UK: Cambridge University Press (pp. 31-42).

Kent, R. D., & Tjaden, K. (in press). Brain functions underlying speech. In Hardcastle, W. J., & Laver, J. (Eds.), *Manual of the phonetic sciences.* London: Blackwell.

Kuehn, D. P., Lemme, M. L., & Baumgartner, J. M. (Eds.), (1989). *Neural bases of speech, hearing, and language.* Boston, MA: College-Hill.

Chapter 2

Regulation of Speech Aerodynamics

Donald W. Warren

Chapter Outline

Key Terms

INTRODUCTION

The movement of air through the respiratory tract is governed by physical forces and controlled by neural and chemical events. Changes in the shape and size of the airway affect airflow significantly, especially when the system is used for speech. Since breathing and speech are so closely related, a description of the mechanical factors of breathing aids understanding of the **regulation** and **control** of speech aerodynamics.

MECHANICS OF BREATHING AND SPEECH

Generation of Driving Pressures

Air flows from a region of higher pressure to one of lower pressure. For phonation to occur, pressure in the lung must be greater than atmospheric pressure. The movement of air into and out of the lung is controlled by the respiratory muscles, which change the volume of the chest cage (Comroe, 1965) (Figure 2-1). The muscles have no inherent rhythm, and they contract only when they receive nerve impulses from the respiratory centers. The increase in lung volume during inspiration occurs in three dimensions: anteroposterior, transverse, and longitudinal, through elevation of the ribs and descent of the diaphragm (Cherniack and Cherniack, 1961). Ordinarily, the muscles used for inspiration include the diaphragm, the external and intercartilaginous segment of the internal intercostals, and the scalene (Campbell, 1968). They are active throughout inspiration as well as during the first part of expiration. During forceful voluntary inspiration, the sternomastoids, trapezius, and pectorals are used as accessory muscles. The diaphragm is the principal muscle of inspiration and in quiet breathing may be the only active inspiratory muscle.

While inspiration is an active process, normal expiration is primarily a passive event (Figure 2-2). The elasticity of stretched tissues and gravitational forces tend to return the thorax to

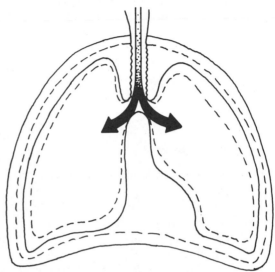

FIGURE 2-1 Lung volume increases during inspiration, and the resulting drop in pressure causes air to flow in.

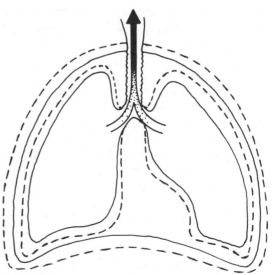

FIGURE 2-2 Recoil of the lungs and chest cage during expiration compresses the air in the lungs, and the resulting increase in pressure causes air to flow out.

its resting position without any further expenditure of energy.

Contraction of the inspiratory muscles enlarges the lung because the outer surface of the lung (**visceral pleura**) is in intimate contact with the inner surface of the thoracic cavity (**parietal pleura**). The two pleural layers are in apposition, separated only by a thin film of fluid. Thus, the lung tends to follow the bony thorax during the expansion that accompanies inspiration. The breathing mechanism can be characterized as a bellows pump having two connective parts, the lung and the chest wall (Agostini and Mead, 1964). The lung is specialized to disperse the gas, and the chest wall is specialized to power the pump.

Elastic Resistance

The forces required to overcome elastic resistance are stored during inspiration, and after muscle action ceases, recoil returns the stretched fibers to their resting position. Resting level is actually a balance between elastic forces pulling in opposite directions (Figure 2-3). That is, the lung would collapse if it were not held in apposition to the thorax, and similarly, the thoracic cavity would enlarge if it were not constrained by the elastic properties of the lung.

The elasticity of the respiratory system may be described in terms of its pressure-volume relationship, exemplified by the relaxation pressure curve (Figure 2-4). The elastic forces of the lung and chest wall vary with lung volume (Agostini and Mead, 1964). At resting level, pulmonary pressure is atmospheric because the lung and chest wall pull in equal but opposite directions. At 60% of **total lung capacity,** the chest wall is at its natural size; its elastic fibers offer no recoil pressure. On the other hand, the elastic fibers in the lung are stretched, so that at that volume lung recoil pressure equals relaxation pressure. As inspiration continues, both lung and chest wall recoil when the muscles relax, and the pressures are additive.

During expiration, when the muscles are relaxed and the lung is deflated below resting level, negative pressure develops. This negative pressure indicates the effort previously exerted to overcome the elastic resistance of the chest wall and lung. Although the lung would exert a positive pressure until it completely collapsed, the lung's pressure is more than counterbalanced by the chest wall, which exerts a greater negative

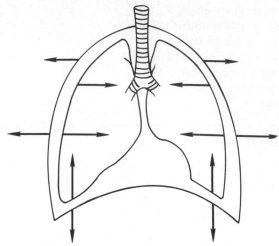

FIGURE 2-3 At resting level elastic forces are balanced as the lung and chest wall pull in opposite directions. (From Warren, D. W. [1976]. Aerodynamics of speech production. In Lass, N. J. [Ed.], *Contemporary issues in experimental phonetics.* New York: Academic Press [105-137].)

pressure when it is smaller than its natural size.

Most of the work of filling the lung is to overcome elastic recoil, and the energy required is stored during inspiration and used during expiration. The compliance of the respiratory system, or the degree of distensibility that occurs with the application of pressure, is an important factor in determining the amount of energy required to move air into and out of the lung.

Nonelastic Resistances

For speech or breathing, the respiratory muscles must overcome not only the elastic forces of the lung and chest wall but also certain nonelastic resistances. There are essentially two types of nonelastic resistances. The more important one, **airway resistance,** is produced by friction (Dubois, 1964). Mechanical energy is dissipated as heat as air moves through the tracheobronchial tree and upper airway. Several physical factors determine the magnitude of resistance encountered in the airway. When airflow is laminar (Figure 2-5), the pressure required to maintain streamline movement is directly proportional to the viscosity of the fluid, or

$$P = k_1 \dot{V}$$

where:
  P = pressure

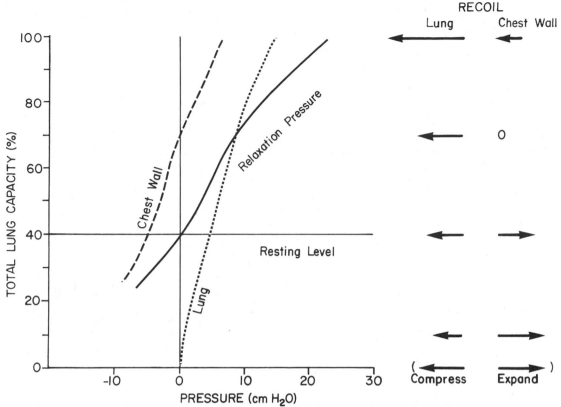

FIGURE 2-4   The relaxation pressure curve. The pressure at any lung volume is the result of elastic forces of the lung and chest wall. The curve is obtained by stopping airflow at various points of inspiration and expiration. (Modified from Rahn, H., Otis, A. B., Chadwick, L. E., & Fenn, O. W. [1946]. The pressure-volume diagram of the thorax and lung. *American Journal of Physiology, 146,* 161-178.)

k_1 = constant including such factors as viscosity, length, and radius

$\dot{V}$ = airflow.

This equation, known as *Poiseuille's law,* can also be written as

$$R = \frac{8\,\mu\,l}{\pi r^4}$$

where:

R   = resistance
μ   = viscosity
l   = length
r   = radius
π   = 3.1416.

Thus, the pressure difference between two points in the airway is proportional to the length of the airway and the coefficient of viscosity and is indirectly proportional to the fourth power of the radius.

Because of the branching, irregular shape of

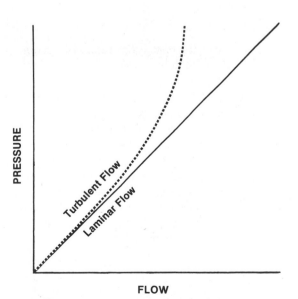

FIGURE 2-5   The relationship between pressure and airflow is linear when airflow is laminar and quadratic when airflow is turbulent.

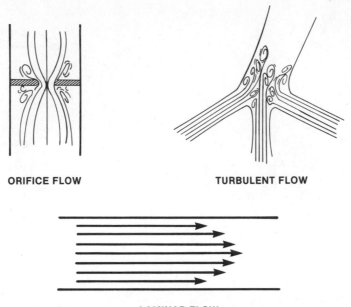

ORIFICE FLOW   **TURBULENT FLOW**

LAMINAR FLOW

FIGURE 2-6 When airflow is turbulent, eddying occurs and pressure is quadratically related to airflow (top right). Constrictions along the vocal tract produce an orifice type of airflow (top left). When airflow is laminar, the lines of flow are smooth and pressure is linearly proportional to airflow (bottom).

the respiratory tract, flow is not always **laminar.** Eddying occurs at bifurcations and when the surface is rough or constricted, producing **turbulent flow.** When airflow is turbulent (Figure 2-5), the pressure necessary to produce a given amount of airflow varies with the square of the flow, or

$$P = k_2 \dot{V}^2$$

Density of the gas, rather than viscosity, becomes important. Turbulence occurs when the relationship of density × velocity × diameter ÷ viscosity, which is known as the **Reynolds number,** exceeds 2000 (Comroe, 1965).

One of the main differences between the airflow patterns in breathing and those in speech results from an **orifice** type of airflow which develops as constrictions form within the vocal tract during phonation. This type of airflow may occur at the glottis, the velopharyngeal orifice, and at various points along the oral airway. The resulting pressure drop is expressed as

$$\Delta P = \frac{d}{2k^2} \left(\frac{\dot{V}}{A} \right)^2$$

where d is the density of air and A is the area of the orifice. The discharge coefficient (k) depends on the sharpness of the edge of the orifice and on the Reynolds number. It has a value of 0.6 to 0.7 in the speech and breathing range of flow (Dubois, 1964). Figure 2-6 illustrates the types of airflow that occur along the vocal tract during speech.

In addition to airway resistance, which must be overcome for airflow to occur, there is **tissue viscous resistance** (Cherniack and Cherniak, 1961). This resistance is due to friction from the peribronchial tissues, lung parenchyma, and vascular structures sliding over one another during movement of the lung. However, tissue viscous resistance is only a small part of the total nonelastic resistance and usually becomes important only in certain disease states.

Lower Airway Dynamics

Airflow in the lower airway is influenced by the shape of the alveolar sacs, the bronchi, and the trachea (Jaeger and Matthys, 1970). The bronchi branch dichotomously, each giving rise to two more bronchi. The length and diameter of the bronchi decrease with each generation in a regular fashion, and their total cross-sectional area increases with each generation. The area of the peripheral bronchi is about 1,000 times that of the trachea. Since the mean velocity of the

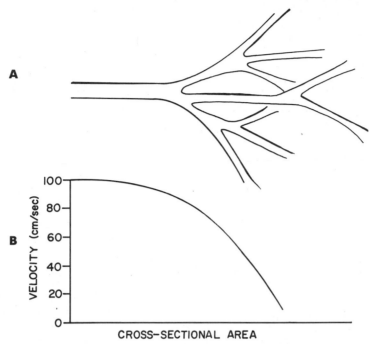

FIGURE 2-7   As cross-sectional area increases, velocity of airflow decreases. *A,* Branching in
the respiratory tract. *B,* Velocity decreases as cross-sectional area increases. (From Warren,
D. W. [1976]. Aerodynamics of speech production. In Lass, N. J. [Ed.], *Contemporary issues
in experimental phonetics.* New York: Academic Press [105-137].)

airstream varies inversely with the cross-
sectional area, the velocity of airflow increases as
it moves from the periphery upward (Figure
2-7). Thus, airflow may increase in velocity from
less than 0.1 cm per second in the small bronchi
to 100 cm per second in the trachea.

Airway Pressures During Speech

A constant **pressure head** must be maintained to
power speech. In spite of the complex interplay
between muscular and nonmuscular forces, the
actual generation of pressure in the lower airway
and the air movement that results appear to be
well controlled. Since speech occurs during the
expiratory phase of breathing, normal expiratory pressure must be modified to some extent.
The subglottal pressure head during normal
expiratory breathing fluctuates between 10 cm
H_2O and atmospheric, depending upon the
phase of expiration (Figure 2-8). However, the
subglottal pressure head for speech is maintained at approximately 6 to 10 cm H_2O. Thus,
expiratory forces must be modified so that an
appropriate and consistent magnitude of subglottal pressure is generated during speech. That
is, to maintain a constant subglottal pressure,

relaxation pressure resulting from the recoil of
elastic fibers in the lung and chest wall must be
checked initially by active contraction of the
inspiratory muscle (Hixon, 1973). Similarly, as
lung volume decreases, relaxation pressure falls,
and activation of the expiratory muscles is
necessary at some stage to maintain the subglottal pressure head, which appears to remain fairly
stable throughout the production of speech
(Ladefoged, 1962, 1968; Mead, Bouhuys, and
Procter, 1968; Netsell, 1969). Pressure is maintained by the respiratory muscles, which check
elastic recoil and prevent overpressure or compress the chest cage further to prevent under-
pressure as speech is produced (Figure 2-9).

The flow of air is also modulated by the glottis
and the supraglottal constrictors (i.e., tongue,
palate, nose, lips, and teeth) so that pressure is
maintained over time. The increase in subglottic
pressure that occurs with increased loudness or
stress apparently is mainly due to changes in
activity of the respiratory muscles (Ladefoged,
1968). There is less external intercostal muscle
suppression of elastic recoil at high lung volumes
and greater internal intercostal augmentation at
lower lung volumes. The result is higher subglottal pressure during stress or loud utterances.

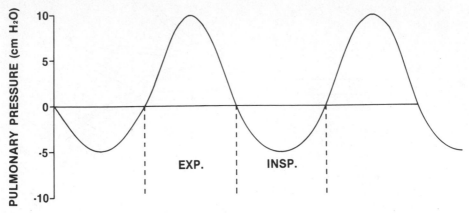

FIGURE 2-8 Pulmonary pressures during breathing. During inspiration pulmonary pressure is below atmospheric, and during expiration it is above atmospheric.

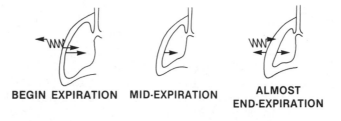

BEGIN EXPIRATION   MID-EXPIRATION   ALMOST END-EXPIRATION

⟵ᴟᴟᴟ BRAKING ACTION BY INSPIRATORY MUSCLES
ᴟᴟᴟ➤ CONTRACTION OF EXPIRATORY MUSCLES
⇌ RECOIL FORCE OF LUNG OR CHEST CAGE

FIGURE 2-9 Subglottal pressure is maintained by checking elastic recoil at the beginning of expiration and contraction of expiratory muscles near the end of expiration.

Normal conversational speech occurs at a mid-range of total lung capacity (Mead, Bouhuys, and Proctor, 1968). The breathing cycle is modified by increasing the depth of inspiration and prolonging the expiration. Approximately 25% of the total lung capacity is used and about 1.2 to 1.5 L of air is involved (Figure 2-10) (Hixon, Goldman, and Mead, 1973). In comparison, during quiet breathing approximately 0.5 L of air is moved with each inspiration or expiration, and this breathing uses only 10% to 15% of the total lung capacity (Cherniack and Cherniack, 1961). Larger lung volumes, perhaps as great as 4 to 5 L, are used when loudness is increased; similarly, **respiratory effort** is lower when the utterance is softer than normal (Ladefoged and McKinney, 1963; Lieberman, 1967; Hixon, 1973).

Hixon (1982) observed that speakers usually initiate conversational speech at approximately 60% of vital capacity and continue speaking until about 35% of vital capacity. As shown in Figure 2-11, relaxation pressures in the 60% to 35% range of vital capacity are not too far above or below the usual magnitude of subglottal pressure. Thus, only little respiratory muscle effort is required to maintain appropriate subglottal pressures.

Russell and Stathopoulos (1988) compared respiratory behaviors of children and adults as a function of articulatory and intensity factors. They observed that children and adults used similar percentages of **vital lung capacity** during comfortable vocal intensity but that adults used a significantly greater percentage of vital capacity during loud vocal intensity.

There is also evidence that small changes in respiratory muscle activity influence the intensity of the sound produced by the vocal folds. Voice intensity is approximately proportional to the third or fourth power of the subglottal pressure (van den Berg, 1956; Isshiki, 1964; Cavagna and Margaria, 1965). Moreover, an increase in subglottal pressure also tends to raise the fundamental frequency (Isshiki, 1964). Fundamental frequency is a dominant parameter

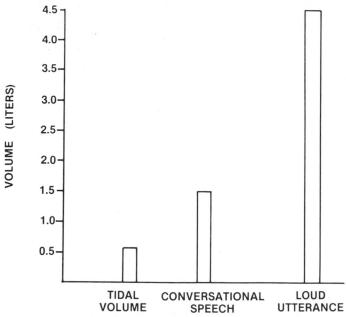

FIGURE 2-10   Comparison of lung volumes used during breathing, conversational speech, and loud utterances.

used to denote stress, although other parameters, such as manner of production and duration, also have an effect (Fry, 1955; Lieberman, 1960; Brown and McGlone, 1974).

Laryngeal Activity

The glottis is the first major constrictor used in forming speech. Air passing through the glottis produces sounds when the vocal folds are properly adducted. During voicing the folds open and close, producing quasiperiodic airflow. The vibration-like movement of the folds results from a complex set of aerodynamic, muscular, and elastic tissue forces. The aerodynamic forces exerted on the vocal folds include subglottal air pressure, the **Bernoulli force** produced by negative pressure created transglottally by high velocity airflow, and supraglottal pressure produced by articulatory constrictions in the upper airway. The Bernoulli force is essentially the work-energy theorem for fluid flow. Although the effect of opening and closing the vocal folds is complex, the aerodynamic events that produce glottal movements can be described in the oversimplified terms of Bernoulli's principle (Lieberman, 1968). Consider that airflow through the glottal constriction is steady, nonviscous, and incompressible (Figure 2-12). The volume velocity of airflow across A_1 is equal to

A_1v_1d, where d is the density of air, A_1 is the cross-sectional area of the trachea, and v_1 is the velocity of airflow. Assuming that airflow is uniform, the same mass of air must travel per unit of time through the constricted vocal folds so that $A_1v_1d = A_2v_2d$ where A_2 is the cross-sectional area of the vocal folds and v_2 is the velocity of airflow at the glottis. Since the density (d) is constant ($A_1v_1 = A_2v_2$), the velocity of airflow at the vocal folds is greater than the velocity of airflow in the pharynx because

$$v_2 = \frac{A_1v_1}{A_2}$$

The net work done on the system by pressure must equal the net gain in mechanical energy. The kinetic energy of the airflow

$$\tfrac{1}{2}d\,\frac{A_1v_1^2}{A_2}$$

is higher in the constriction and therefore the potential energy must decrease. Bernoulli's equation demonstrates that pressure falls at the site of a constriction when the velocity of airflow increases (Lieberman, 1968). That is,

$$\tfrac{1}{2}dv^2 + P = \text{constant.}$$

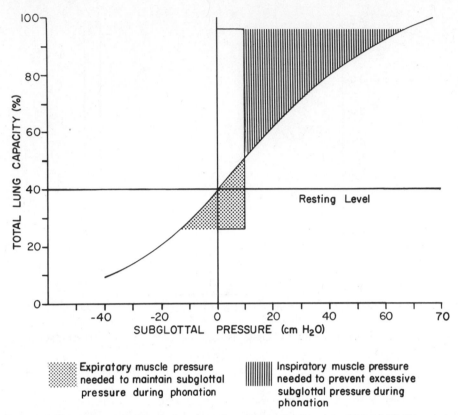

FIGURE 2-11 **Lung volume and pressure relationships during speech. At high lung volumes inspiratory muscle action is required to check recoil pressure and prevent excessive subglottal pressure. At low lung volumes expiratory muscle activity is required to maintain subglottal pressure for speech.** (Modified from Hixon, T., [1973]. Respiratory function in speech. In Minifie, F., Hixon, T., & Williams, F. [Eds.], *Normal aspects of speech, hearing and language,* Englewood Cliffs, NJ: Prentice-Hall.)

The pressure at the glottal constriction may fall below atmospheric pressure, drawing the folds together. Glottal tissue resistance then increases as the area of the constriction decreases, allowing the Bernoulli force to increase only up to a certain point (van den Berg, Zantema, and Doornenbal, 1957). This interaction of aerodynamic forces with muscle and elastic activity produces vocal fold vibrations which, in turn, provide the acoustic source of voicing.

This discussion is an idealized and simplified approximation of voicing. It assumes laminar and incompressible airflow. However, although flow is probably incompressible, it is not always laminar or uniform. Similarly, the folds may not act symmetrically, and the static forces provided by the muscles and ligaments may not behave as idealized springs. Ishizaka and Matsudaira (1972) present a more complex model of vocal fold activity that to some extent accounts for vertical phase differences between the upper and lower parts of the folds. They have shown that different pressures acting on the upper and lower parts of the folds cause a drag and the slight lag of the upper part of the folds behind the lower part.

Titze (1984) presented a configurational model that depicted the vocal folds in three dimensions. His model describes the relation between structure and vibration of the vocal fold more completely than the Ishizaka and Matsudaira (1972) two-mass model. Scherer, Curtis, and Titze (1980), using such models, suggest that existing pressure-flow equations for the larynx may be adequate approximations, but because they lack sensitivity to glottal shape and geometry, they are not applicable to a range of conditions associated with phonation.

Although models of laryngeal function can be made complex, the outcome of tissue and aerodynamic coupling is still the same: the rapid

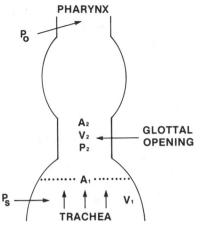

FIGURE 2-12 Schematic view of the vocal folds. A_2, Cross-sectional area of the glottal constriction. V_2 and P_2, Particle velocity and air pressure, respectively, at the glottal constriction. A_1, Cross-sectional area of the trachea. V_1 and P_s, Particle velocity and pressure in the trachea. P_o, Pressure in the mouth. (From Lieberman, P. [1968]. Vocal cord motion in man. In Bouhuys, A. [Ed.], *Sound production in man. Annals of the New York Academy of Science, 155*, 28-38.)

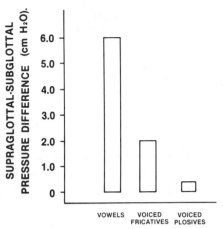

FIGURE 2-13 The supraglottal-subglottal pressure difference is influenced by the oral airway opening. Airway opening is largest for vowels, and supraglottal pressure is nearly atmospheric under these circumstances. A closed oral airway for voiced plosives results in a small pressure drop. Voiced fricatives fall between vowels and plosives as the slight opening of the oral port helps to maintain airway pressure.

closing and opening of the vocal folds mold airflow into a modulated stream that is the basic source of speech.

The Effects of Glottal Activity on Air Pressure and Airflow

The vocal folds, like other articulatory structures, have a significant effect on pressure and airflow during speech (Klatt, Stevens, and Mead, 1968). The size of the glottal constriction affects the transglottal pressure loss, although changes above the glottis also influence pressure at the folds. For example, opening the airway for vowels reduces supraglottal pressure almost to atmospheric pressure, while glottal constriction maintains subglottal pressure (Figure 2-13). In comparison, the small oral port opening for fricatives raises intraoral pressure, and glottal constriction causes only a slight transglottal pressure drop. Plosives prior to voicing have approximately equal supraglottal and subglottal pressures.

Voicing requires airflow across the vocal folds. This airflow in the closed system of stop consonants requires a difference in pressure between the subglottal and supraglottal cavities. Although in many instances voicing occurs on release of the plosive, sometimes it occurs during the stop phase of the consonant. Rothenberg

(1968) has proposed three mechanisms for producing transglottal airflow during voiced stop productions: (1) a passive, pressure-activated expansion of one or more walls of the supraglottal cavity, (2) a muscularly activated enlargement of the supraglottal cavity, and (3) nasal airflow through a slightly open palatal sphincter. Lubker (1973) discounts nasal airflow and favors the active-expansion mechanism. Kent and Moll (1969) and Perkell (1969) have demonstrated that voiced stops are produced with larger supraglottal volumes than their voiceless cognates. Further, the Kent and Moll data reveal that pharyngeal expansion is simultaneous with the depression of the hyoid bone, which is an active process.

Rothenberg (1968) indicates that considering the range of supraglottal cavity compliance, in many instances the voiced interval of voiced alveolar plosives is too long and/or the voicing too strong to be maintained by passive expansion alone. Similarly, if passive expansion did result from greater respiratory muscle activity during voicing, cognate differences in supraglottal pressure should occur, but they apparently do not (Netsell, 1969). Bell-Berti (1975) has proposed two modes of expanding the pharynx for voiced stops, each applying to a different group of muscles. She presents evidence for an active mode requiring increased muscle activity and a passive mode requiring suppression of muscle activity to expand the pharynx.

Glottal Resistance

Glottal resistance is the ratio of transglottal pressure to airflow through the glottis (Figures 2-14, 2-15). The fact that glottal resistance is much lower for voiced fricatives than for vowels indicates that the vocal folds do not adduct as much for fricatives as for vowels (Klatt, Stevens, and Mead, 1968). An estimate of glottal opening for vowels is about 0.05 cm^2, and for fricatives, about 0.1 to 0.15 cm^2. When the opening is larger than 0.5 cm^2, resistance is negligible. The volume rate of airflow used during sound production also affects glottal resistance (Figure 2-16). Increased effort results in a higher resistance for a given amount of glottal opening. Similarly, adduction of the vocal folds has a considerable effect on respiratory volumes and the volume velocity of airflow (Warren and Hall, 1973). Figure 2-17 suggests that greater respiratory effort is required for voiceless consonant production. Figure 2-18 compares volumes. It is not known whether the differences arise simply

as a result of glottal resistance or because greater respiratory effort is required to provide additional acoustic cues in the absence of a glottal sound voice or both.

UPPER AIRWAY DYNAMICS

Structures in the upper airway play an essential role in speech by modulating the airstream into precise patterns. The direction and velocity of air movement are controlled primarily by changes in airway size. These changes occur well in advance of the sounds to be produced and so influence the preceding segments of speech as well (Warren, 1964).

Most speech is directed through the oral airway, and the resistance to airflow varies from less than 1 cm H_2O/L/s for low vowels to an infinite resistance or complete obstruction in the case of plosives. Air actually flows more readily through the oral cavity than the nasal cavity because resistance is approximately one-half, provided the tongue is not elevated to any great extent. That is, for low vowels, most airflow passes through the oral cavity even if the velopharyngeal orifice is open. Whether air exits from the mouth or nose under these circumstances depends upon the relative amounts of resistance. Ordinarily, nasal airway resistance is between 1 and 3.5 cm H_2O/L/s (Warren, Duany, and Fischer, 1969). However, lip, tongue, and soft palate movement can modify resistance considerably and shunt airflow through the nose, as in nasal sounds.

Figure 2-19 illustrates the effect of oral port opening on velopharyngeal sphincter resistance at different degrees of velopharyngeal opening. It is evident that despite an open velopharyngeal orifice, the nasal chamber, with its smaller cross-sectional area and higher resistance, receives substantial amounts of airflow only when the oral airway is constricted. This relationship between oral and nasal airway resistance is very important in individuals with a cleft palate (Warren and Ryon, 1967).

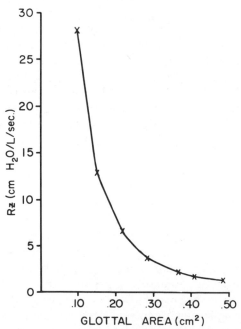

FIGURE 2-14 **The relationship between glottal area and glottal resistance.** (From Warren, D. W. [1976]. Aerodynamics of speech production. In Lass, N. J. [Ed.], *Contemporary issues in experimental phonetics.* New York: Academic Press [105-137].)

Voiceless Plosives

During production of a voiceless plosive (Figure 2-20), the rise in intraoral pressure is determined by speech effort. This is usually 3 to 7 cm H_2O (Malécot, 1955). Supraglottal pressure usually equals subglottal pressure, but it can be slightly less. If after initial release of air into the oral

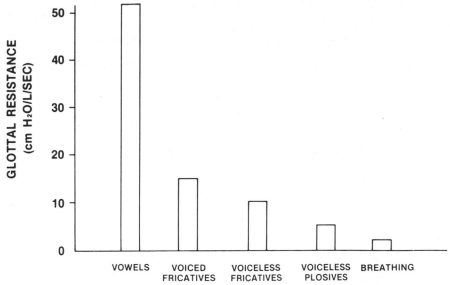

FIGURE 2-15   Approximate glottal resistances for vowels and consonants compared with breathing.

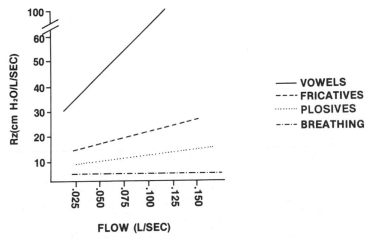

FIGURE 2-16   The relationship between glottal resistance and airflow rate for vowels, fricatives, plosives, and breathing. Resistance increases as effort increases. Glottal resistance is also influenced by the size of the oral airway opening.

cavity the vocal folds close until release of oral air pressure, a small pressure difference between the supraglottal and subglottal cavities can occur, especially if the oral cavity enlarges slightly. The approximate volume of air used for voiceless plosives is 80 ml, and pressure is impounded for approximately 125 ms. When the oral port opens, pressure falls rapidly.

Voiced Plosives

The pressure profile of a voiced plosive depends to a great extent on when voicing begins. As

noted earlier, voicing can occur only if a transglottal pressure drop is created. This is presumed to result from active enlargement of the supraglottal cavity during the stop phase. This increase in size causes supraglottal pressure to drop slightly below subglottal pressure, and the resulting airflow through the glottis initiates voicing. As shown in Figure 2-21, when voicing begins at the onset of the pressure rise, the shape and magnitude of the pressure pulse are altered. The pressure magnitude of voiced sounds is between 3 and 5 cm H_2O, which is slightly lower than its voiceless counterpart (Arkebauer,

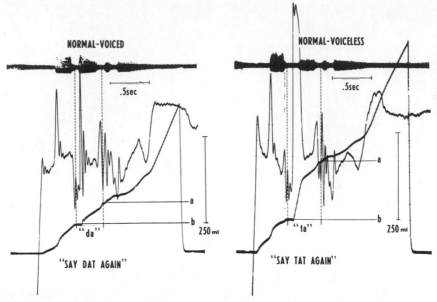

FIGURE 2-17 Typical sound, volume rate of airflow, and volume patterns for voiced and voiceless plosives. A higher rate of airflow and greater respiratory air volume for voiceless sounds are apparent. The distance between *a* and *b* represents the volume of air for the consonant-vowel.

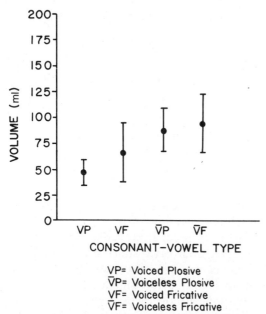

VP= Voiced Plosive
V̄P= Voiceless Plosive
VF= Voiced Fricative
V̄F= Voiceless Fricative

FIGURE 2-18 Means and standard deviations of respiratory air volume. (From Warren, D. W. [1976]. Aerodynamics of speech production. In Lass, N. J. [Ed.], *Contemporary issues in experimental phonetics.* New York: Academic Press [105-137].)

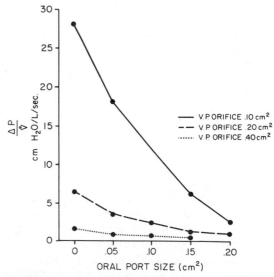

FIGURE 2-19 The relationship between velopharyngeal orifice resistance and oral port size at varying degrees of velopharyngeal closure. (From Warren, D. W. [1976]. Aerodynamics of speech production. In Lass, N. J. [Ed.], *Contemporary issues in experimental phonetics.* New York: Academic Press [105-137].)

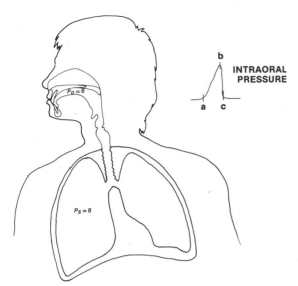

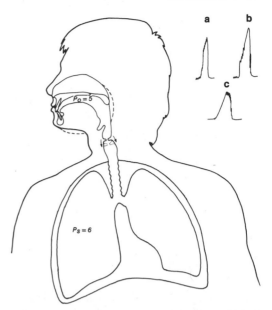

FIGURE 2-20   Aerodynamics of the voiceless plosive /p/. The lips close at *a,* and pressure rises until *b,* when the lips part. Voicing of the vowel begins at *c.* There is no airflow until the lips part. Subglottal pressure (P_s) is usually equal to intraoral pressure (P_o) during the impounding phase (*a* to *b*).

FIGURE 2-21   Aerodynamics of the voiced plosive /b/. The shape of the pressure pulse is determined by when voicing begins. In *a* voicing occurred throughout the pressure-rise phase. This usually lowers pressures to some degree. In *b* voicing occurred only during a portion of the pressure-rise interval. Usually pressure is higher. In *c* voicing occurred at pressure release. Whenever voicing occurs, a slight supraglottal-subglottal pressure difference is present. For voicing to occur during the stop phase, intraoral volume must increase to create this pressure difference (broken lines). P_s, Subglottal pressure. P_o, Intraoral pressure.

Hixon, and Hardy, 1967). Similarly, the airflow rate is lower for voiced plosives (Isshiki and Ringel, 1964). Usually about 50 ml of air is used, and air is impounded for approximately 125 ms. If voicing begins after pressure release, the peak pressure of voiced plosives may equal the peak pressure of voiceless plosives.

Voiceless Fricatives

Figure 2-22 illustrates the pressure and airflow profiles of voiceless fricatives. Respiratory effort is greater for voiceless fricatives than for other consonants because of the need to maintain a pressure head behind an air leak (Warren and Wood, 1969). The oral port opens slightly (about 0.05 cm^2), and a pressure head of approximately 3 to 8 cm H_2O forces airflow through this constriction at a high velocity (Klechak, Bradley, and Warren, 1976). The turbulence created by this high-velocity airflow makes the sound (Hixon, 1966). The volume of air used for a typical voiceless fricative is approximately 100 ml, a larger volume than for other consonants. The two peaks characteristic of fricatives may be due to adjustments in airflow rate to maintain intraoral pressure over an adequate period.

Warren, Hall, and Davis (1981) believe that the larger the opening, the greater the rate of airflow. This would maintain fairly consistent magnitude intraoral pressure. Brown and McGlone (1969) reported such a consistency on consonant repetitions. Thus, the dip in the airflow record may relate to reaching the maximum constriction of the oral port. However, pressure magnitude is reached prior to that point through increased airflow (first peak) and maintained during the initial reopening of the oral port (second peak) by increasing the rate of airflow. Flow rate then declines for the vowel.

Voiceless fricatives also have longer duration times (150 ms) than voiced fricatives or plosives (Warren and Mackler, 1968). This fact may reflect a need to generate sufficient acoustic cues for the listener. In addition, the oral constriction is usually larger for voiceless fricatives than for

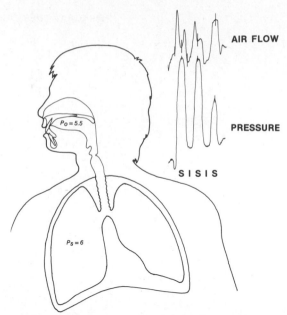

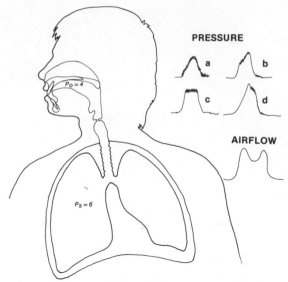

FIGURE 2-22 Aerodynamics of the voiceless fricative /s/. The airflow profile demonstrates two peaks with the dip corresponding to the pressure peak. The increased airflow rate during the pressure-rise phase and the increased airflow rate at the pressure-fall phase may maintain pressure magnitude duration during the closing and opening of the oral constriction. The pressure difference between the supraglottal and subglottal cavities is small. P_s, Subglottal pressure. P_o, Intraoral pressure.

FIGURE 2-23 Aerodynamics of the voiced fricative /z/. The pressure gradient between subglottal (P_s) and supraglottal (P_o) pressure is larger because of vocal fold resistance. The shape and size of the pressure pulse depends upon when voicing begins. Voicing occurred throughout (*a*), in the middle of the pressure-rise phase (*b*), at the peak (*c*), and the release phase (*d*). Airflow demonstrates the twin peak phenomenon.

their voiced counterparts (Smith et al., 1978). Bilabial fricatives differ aerodynamically from linguoalveolar fricatives; as with stop consonants, there is almost no airflow at one point as a result of momentary but complete lip closure against the teeth.

Voiced Fricatives

Figure 2-23 illustrates the pressure and airflow profiles of voiced fricatives. Respiratory effort is less for these sounds than for their voiceless counterparts, possibly owing to less reliance on airflow turbulence for acoustic cues, since sound is generated at the vocal folds. The shape and magnitude of the pressure pulse are influenced by the timing of voicing. Moreover, airflow rate is lower than for voiceless sounds, and the air volume used (about 75 ml) is less (Isshiki and Ringel, 1964; Warren and Wood, 1969). Oral port constriction is about 0.05 cm² but can range from 0.01 to about 0.15 cm². The duration of

constriction for impounding air is approximately 125 ms.

Vowels

Figure 2-24 illustrates the pressure and airflow profiles for vowels. Intraoral pressure is almost atmospheric for vowels, since the oral airway is open. Approximately 50 to 70 ml of air is used. Airflow rate is low, since the vocal folds impede it to provide voicing as well as to maintain the subglottal pressure head. Glottal resistance is much greater for vowels than for voiced fricatives; this may serve an aerodynamic need as well as an acoustic one. That is, the glottis is the only valve protecting the subglottal pressure head during vowel production, whereas for voiced fricatives the oral port is constricted to about 0.05 cm². Thus, aerodynamically, the glottis does not have to close as much to maintain subglottal pressure.

REGULATION OF SPEECH AERODYNAMICS

Physiologists have long observed that the human body maintains a degree of constancy, or ho-

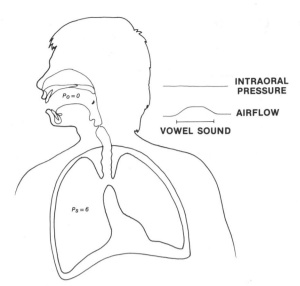

FIGURE 2-24 Aerodynamics of vowel production. Intraoral pressure (P_o) is atmospheric because the mouth is open. Airflow is fairly constant and does not peak at release of the sound. P_s, Subglottal pressure.

meostasis, for its many systems. Circulation, respiration, acid-base balance, body temperature, and food intake are bodily functions operating under rules that tend to preserve physiologic balance (Figure 2-25). These systems have common features that are fundamental to homeostasis: (1) regulation for the purpose of stability and (2) control mechanisms to achieve relatively stable conditions (Brobeck, 1965).

For example, in the cardiovascular system, blood pressure is regulated, and heart rate, stroke volume, and blood flow are controlled (Figure 2-26). A system is said to be regulated if its structures respond to change and preserve or attempt to preserve constancy. That is, the purpose of a regulating system is to maintain a parameter at an acceptable level. Control is the means by which this is accomplished. The term *control* is sometimes used interchangeably with *regulation,* but there are valid reasons for distinguishing between the two. Control describes the process of management. Thus, in cardiovascular regulation, control of heart rate, stroke volume, and peripheral blood flow is necessary to maintain an appropriate amount of blood within the arterial system and thereby regulate blood pressure. The terms *control mechanism, response, behavior,* and *strategy* all imply that the brain receives information,

processes it, and then directs the control activity.

Supporting Evidence

A physiologic parameter is said to be regulated if it remains relatively stable under varying conditions. Response mechanisms, or controls, tend to moderate change. When change does occur, it is detected by receptors that send information to a control center, which determines the response necessary to bring the system back into balance. For example, mean blood pressure may be 100 mm Hg for a supine individual but drop slightly when the individual stands. Before the person stands up, the vasomotor control center programs the vascular system to initiate compensatory maneuvers to prevent a precipitous drop in pressure. Adjustments in peripheral vascular resistance, blood flow volume, and other responses stabilize pressure. In addition, constant monitoring of the system results in minimal change in pressure.

There is evidence that the mechanics of breathing also follow the rules of a regulating system (Remmers and Bartlett, 1977; Warren, 1986b). That is, respiratory performance is guided by the need to preserve physiologic balance, or homeostasis. Apparently, respiratory maneuvers are controlled to ensure adequate gas exchange and a stable chemical environment or blood chemistry. Among the prerequisites of a balanced system is maintenance of optimal upper airway resistance.

Control of respiratory activity, specifically airway resistance, is fairly precise. For example, airway resistance is greater during expiration than inspiration. This increase in resistance provides a longer duration for alveolar gas exchange. Gautier, Remmers, and Bartlett (1973) noted that the vocal folds adduct more strongly during expiration. Similarly, Hairfield et al. (1987) observed that the nasal valve is approximately 10% smaller during expiratory rest breathing.

The drop in pressure that results from air moving across a structure is proportional to the reciprocal of the fourth power of the radius. Reducing the radius of an airway by half increases the pressure drop sixteenfold (van den Berg, 1956; Isshiki, 1964; Cavagna and Margaria, 1965). The pressure drop is also proportional to volume rate of airflow. Thus, airway resistance is an important control factor for

REGULATING SYSTEMS - HOMEOSTASIS

System	Regulated Parameter
Respiratory (Chemical Mechanics)	CO$_2$ Airway Resistance? Airway Pressure? or some correlate
Cardiovascular	Blood Pressure
Temperature	Core Body Temperature
Feeding	Food Intake
Acid-Base	pH
Body Fluids	Fluid Volume
Speech Aerodynamics	Consonant Pressure head

FIGURE 2-25   Homeostatic systems regulate for stability and use control mechanisms to maintain relatively steady conditions.

EXAMPLES OF REGULATION/CONTROL ACTIVITY

System	Regulated Parameter	Control Responses
Cardiovascular	Blood Pressure	Peripheral Vascular Resistance Heart Rate Cardiac Output Contractility Neural Endocrine Local Reflexes

FIGURE 2-26   Blood pressure is regulated through heart rate, stroke volume, blood flow, and contractility.

maintaining stable upper airway breathing pressures, and its magnitude is determined primarily by the smallest cross-sectional area of the airway.

There is evidence that muscles in the upper airway help control airflow to compensate for changes in airway resistance during breathing. Remmers and Bartlett (1977) observed that extrathoracic tracheal stretch receptors monitor changes in upper airway resistance and suggested that responses of the respiratory muscles compensate for differences in resistance. This was confirmed by Warren, Hairfield, and Dalston (1991), who investigated the effects of high nasal resistance on oral posture among adult subjects with documented nasal airway impairment. As expected, all subjects were oral breathers to some extent because of the associated high nasal airway resistance.

The most intriguing finding was how the oral response to nasal airway impairment controlled upper airway resistance. Normally, nasal airway resistance in healthy adults is in the range of 1 to

3.5 cm H$_2$O/L/s (Warren, Duany, and Fischer, 1969). Mean resistance of the subjects in the study was 8.7 cm H$_2$O/L/s, corresponding to a mean nasal cross-sectional area of .17 cm^2. A model of the upper airway was used to simulate the human subject findings. The authors found that a resistance of 8.7 cm H$_2$O/L/s was reduced to 3.2 cm H$_2$O/L/s when the model's mouth was opened to 0.5 cm^2 (Figure 2-27). Some 80% of the air was shunted orally under those conditions. Since about 80% of the air was also shunted orally in the human subjects, this suggested that the degree of mouth opening in response to nasal airway impairment and high nasal resistance is determined by the amount of air that must be shunted orally to reduce upper airway resistance to an acceptable level. Thus, the study supports the concept that postural responses are fairly well controlled to maintain an appropriate level of respiratory tract resistance. Cole (1985) observed similar responses in normal subjects. He occluded the nasal airway and found that oral respiratory resistance as-

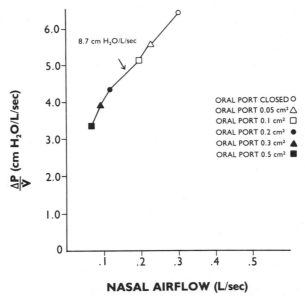

FIGURE 2-27   Data for the model showed that as mouth opening increases, more air is shunted through the oral port and upper airway resistance falls from 8.7 cm $H_2O/L/s$ to about 3.2 cm $H_2O/L/s$. (From Warren, D. W., Hairfield, W. M., & Dalston, E. T. [1991]. Nasal airway impairment: The oral response in cleft palate patients. *American Journal of Orthodontics, 99,* 346-353.)

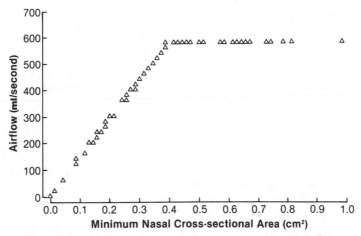

FIGURE 2-28   The relationship between nasal airway size and nasal airflow rate. The data reflect statistical treatment using correlational cutpoints.

sumed a value similar to when the nasal airway was open.

The literature also reveals at what dimension an aperture controls volume rate of airflow. Warren et al. (1987) demonstrated that airflow rate is highly correlated with airway size when the cross-sectional area is less than 0.4 cm^2. Figure 2-28 illustrates the statistically treated data. Correlation coefficients were computed at various cutpoints and, as illustrated, the correlation is very high below 0.4 cm^2 (Pearson

$r = 0.82$) and very low above that point (Pearson $r = 0.23$). Airflow rate becomes independent of cross-sectional area at 0.4 cm^2. Further analysis of the data revealed that airflow is severely limited when constriction size is less than 0.18 cm^2. Thus, while the flow of air appeared to be controlled by constriction sizes less than 0.4 cm^2, dimensions about half that size actually limit flow.

The flow-resistance characteristics of an airway during breathing are shown in Figure 2-29.

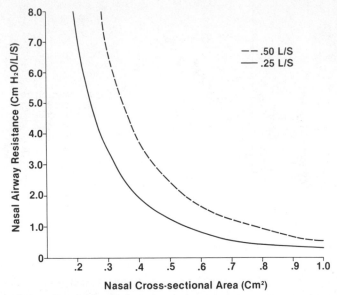

FIGURE 2-29   Relationship between nasal cross-sectional size and nasal airway resistance.

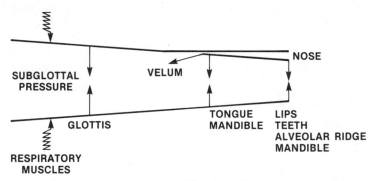

FIGURE 2-30   Vocal tract structures are capable of producing a variety of constrictions.

Resistance increases dramatically at airway sizes less than 0.2 cm^2. This is the same dimension that was shown to be flow-limiting during breathing. In comparison, studies of speakers with velopharyngeal inadequacy indicate that when the velopharyngeal orifice is greater than 0.1 cm^2, individuals have some difficulty impounding air for pressure consonants. As Figure 2-29 illustrates, resistance falls dramatically as cross-sectional size increases. Thus, it is not surprising that individuals with velopharyngeal inadequacy develop structural adjustments such as increased respiratory effort in the attempt to maintain adequate pressures for speech.

Certain responses of the speech articulators are similar to those of the respiratory structures, and there appears to be control of resistances along the vocal tract during speech, somewhat paralleling the controls within the respiratory tract during breathing. The vocal tract is a tube containing oral, pharyngeal, and glottal structures capable of producing a variety of constrictions (Figure 2-30). These constrictions provide the resistances necessary to maintain adequate levels of subglottal and supraglottal pressures for speech. Subglottal pressure, which is the primary energy source for speech, is kept relatively constant at a specific loudness level (Ladefoged, 1962, 1968; Mead, Bouhuys, and Proctor, 1968; Netsell, 1969).

Maintenance of the subglottal pressure head requires more than the checking or enhancement of elastic recoil forces. The sudden changes in respiratory load that occur when the upper airway closes or opens must be compensated for almost instantaneously if pressure is to be nearly constant. Otherwise, sound intensity and fundamental frequency would be unstable. This poses

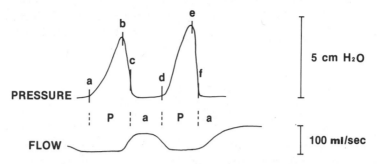

FIGURE 2-31   The constant subglottal pressure head is modulated into discrete patterns by movement of upper airway structures. For example, in the word /papa/, the lips close (*a*) and intraoral pressure builds (*b*). At that point the lips part and pressure falls. Voicing for the vowel begins at (*c*). The lips close again and pressure rises (*d*) until the lips part (*e*). Voicing begins again at *f.* Airflow occurs during vowel production.

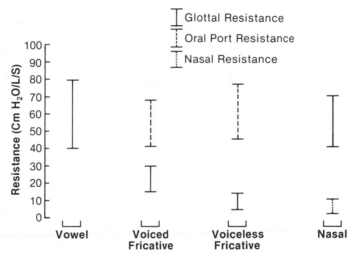

FIGURE 2-32   Approximate ranges of resistance across the vocal tract, controlled to maintain pressures across consonant types.

a considerable control problem not encountered in breathing. For example, phonation of the word /papa/ involves abrupt closure of the lips and impounding of air (Figure 2-31). The subglottal pressure head is maintained by labial closure. The lips open for the vowel, and the vocal folds adduct to maintain the pressure head. The flow of air from the lungs does not appreciably affect pulmonary pressure because the respiratory muscles adjust recoil forces. The lips close again for /p/, and the glottis opens. Once again the pressure head is sustained by closure of the oral port.

Although the position of an articulatory structure varies according to phonetic context, overall resistance across the vocal tract remains fairly stable (Figure 2-32). In normal speech, glottal resistance for a vowel is approximately 40 to 80 cm H_2O/L/s (Smitheran and Hixon, 1981; Warren, 1982), but for voiced fricatives, only 25 cm H_2O/L/s. However, oral port resistance for fricatives, at approximately 75 cm H_2O/L/s, provides an overall resistance within the airway similar to that observed for vowels (Warren, 1982).

Another example of stable resistance is glottal resistance for voiceless fricatives and plosives. The resistance for voiceless fricatives is approximately 10 cm H_2O/L/s, compared with about 6 cm H_2O/L/s for voiceless plosives. On the other hand, resistance is infinite for plosives at the oral port and about 75 cm H_2O/L/s for fricatives. Such relationships suggest that resistances of the speech structures may be synchronously controlled in a manner analogous to respiratory control (Warren, 1982).

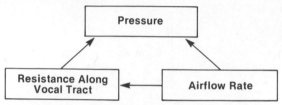

FIGURE 2-33 Pressure is regulated through the movements of articulatory structures and the airflow rate. Control over movements provides the resistance necessary to maintain pressures.

Supraglottal pressures are much more variable than subglottal pressures. For example, peak intraoral pressures during consonant productions usually range from 3 to 8 cm H_2O (Warren, 1988). These pressures vary somewhat as a function of the speaker's age (Bernthal and Beukelman, 1978; Stathopoulos and Weismer, 1985) and gender (Subtelny, Worth, and Sakuda, 1966; Bernthal and Beukelman, 1978; Lotz and Netsell, 1986). In addition, they have been found to vary by word position (Malécot, 1955; Arkebauer, Hixon, and Hardy, 1967; Malécot, 1968; Brown et al., 1970), voicing characteristics (Black, 1950; Malécot, 1966; Netsell, 1969; Lubker and Parris, 1970; Lisker, 1971; Warren and Hall, 1973; Weismer and Longstreth, 1980; Stathopoulos, 1986), vowel context (Brown, McGlone, and Proffit, 1973; Karnell and Willis, 1982; Klich, 1982), utterance length (Brown and McGlone, 1969; Prosek and House, 1975; Flege, 1983), and syllable stress (Malécot, 1970; Flege, 1983). Intraoral pressures for vowels are close to zero. Obviously, if pressure is regulated in the speech system, it is subglottal pressure that is maintained nearly constant. A speech regulating system prevents a rapid fall in subglottal pressure across phonetic contexts but provides flexible local energy sources throughout the vocal tract. The structures that modify airway resistance during breathing are also used as articulatory structures during speech. These structures modulate upper airway resistance to produce the necessary local energy source, such as peak intraoral pressures for plosives and fricatives. Figure 2-33 illustrates the probable relationship among the speech pressure head, speech airflow rate, and vocal tract resistance.

EXPERIMENTAL EVIDENCE OF A SPEECH REGULATING SYSTEM

Systematic study of a regulating system requires experiments that identify and describe the

mechanisms of **control.** Evidence of a regulating system has been obtained by studies that perturb the airway and introduce an "error" such as a change in vocal tract resistance.

Bite-Block and Bleed-Valve Studies

Bite blocks have been used to produce unnatural jaw openings as a means to assess aerodynamic responses to sudden changes in the vocal tract. Insertion of a bite block forces a speaker into compensatory maneuvers that can be evaluated quantitatively (Warren, Nelson, and Allen, 1980; Warren, Hall, and Davis, 1981; Warren, Allen, and King, 1984). These studies clearly show the remarkable adaptive behaviors of the speech structures. When the vertical dimension was dramatically increased, oral port cross-sectional opening for fricatives showed little or no change. Whenever port size did increase slightly, airflow rate also increased, and as a result, intraoral pressure was maintained. On the other hand, frequency of misarticulations increased with vertical dimension, in spite of the fact that port size did not change significantly (Warren, Nelson, and Allen, 1980). These studies indicated that structural responses to sudden change successfully maintain a normal aerodynamic environment for speech, but the speech outcome, as judged by listeners, may be compromised.

Warren, Allen, and King (1984) found that auditory information appears to decrease the frequency of speech distortions. In this bite-block study, vertical dimension was increased from 0 to 6 mm in four increments under three conditions: normal, auditory masking, and unmasked. As Figure 2-34 illustrates, the frequency of /s/ distortions increased with vertical opening as judged by trained and untrained listeners. However, the effect of masking with quasi-white noise presented binaurally through headphones on the frequency of /s/ distortions across different vertical openings differed significantly from the other two unmasked conditions (Figure 2-35). Furthermore, the total number of distortions decreased in time under the two unmasked conditions but did not change in the masked condition. Presumably, subsequent auditory feedback after articulation reveals /s/ distortions, and over time lingual adjustments decrease the frequency of distortions.

Putnam, Shelton, and Kastner (1986) used bite-block and **bleed-valve** maneuvers to assess aerodynamic compensations. When bite blocks

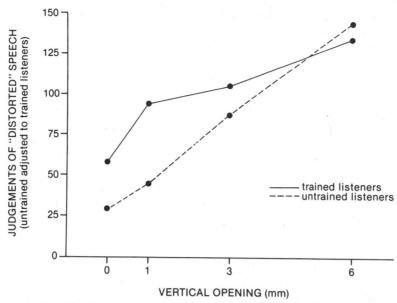

FIGURE 2-34 Combined frequency of /s/ distortions under all conditions. Comparison of judgments by trained and untrained listeners. (From Warren, D. W., Allen, G., & King, H. A. [1984]. Physiologic and perceptual effects of induced anterior open bite. *Folia Phoniatrica, 36,* 164-173.)

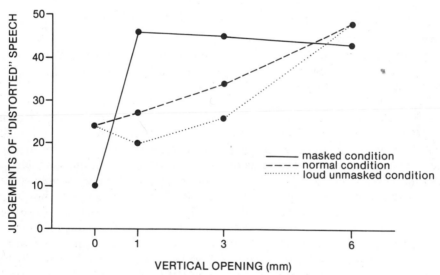

FIGURE 2-35 Frequency of /s/ distortions under masked, normal, and loud conditions as judged by trained listeners. (From Warren, D. W., Allen, G., & King, H. A. [1984]. Physiologic and perceptual effects of induced anterior open bite. *Folia Phoniatrica, 36,* 164-173.)

were inserted, appropriate intraoral pressures were maintained and airflow rate increased. Presumably, as in other bite-block studies, the tongue was manipulated to close the induced open bite, and these maneuvers resulted in maintenance of adequate oral port resistance. The increased airflow observed in their study also would have augmented port resistance.

Another segment of this study used bleed tubes of different diameters during production of plosive consonants. The bleed device prevented lingual maneuvers as a compensatory response. The investigators found that airflow rate increased in a linear fashion as the size of the bleed tubes increased. Although pressure fell with increased opening, it was always maintained above 4 cm H_2O.

Putnam, Shelton, and Kastner (1986, p. 47) observed another characteristic of aeromechanical integrity. Airflow in the postconsonantal vowels exhibited remarkably stable patterns across bleed and block conditions. The investigators reported that

> . . .this implies some accommodating adjustments in laryngeal airway resistance to normalize vowel flow in spite of the aeromechanical perturbations introduced during the preceding /p/ and /s/ segments. . . . Such data lend credence to the attractive but inherently elusive hypothesis that vocal tract pressures are somehow monitored. . .

Studies of Velopharyngeal Inadequacy

Individuals with **velopharyngeal inadequacy** present a unique opportunity to study the dynamics of a pressure-regulating system. Velar inadequacy causes diminished vocal tract resistance, or an "error" that requires a response if the speech pressure head is to be maintained. Dalston et al. (1988) and Warren (1985a) have reported that even at inadequacies greater than 0.20 cm^2, many individuals with cleft palates can maintain speech pressures above 3 cm H$_2$O during nonnasal consonant productions. Several compensatory strategies may be involved. Some such speakers attempt to regulate intraoral pressure by increasing respiratory effort (Warren, 1967; Warren, Wood, and Bradley, 1969). Others use articulatory compensations to maintain intraoral pressure (Warren, 1986a). Some may not have to employ compensatory strategies because their nasal airway resistance is high (Warren, 1985b, 1986a, 1986b).

Recently, Warren et al. (1985) reported that the timing of articulatory movements was also influenced by regulation and control strategies. In a follow-up study Warren et al. (1989) provided additional evidence of aerodynamic regulation of speech pressures. Temporal and respiratory responses to a loss of velar resistance were measured in subjects demonstrating varying degrees of velopharyngeal inadequacy. The subject data were then compared with data generated by a mechanical model that represented a passive system.

The subjects were asked to produce a series of the bilabial plosive consonant /p/ within the carrier word "hamper". The nasal-plosive blend /mp/ was used to stress the palatal mechanism, since it involves an open-to-close movement. Mean nasal airflow rate, mean intraoral pressure,

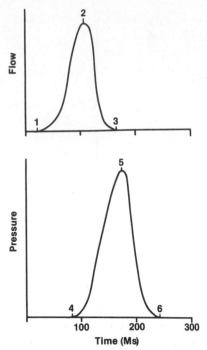

FIGURE 2-36   Timing variables for "hamper". They include (*1*) begin airflow, (*2*) peak airflow, (*3*) end airflow, (*4*) begin pressure, (*5*) peak pressure, and (*6*) end pressure.

and mean area of the **velopharyngeal orifice** during the production of /p/ were calculated from a series of utterances.

The subjects were then divided into four groups according to the size of their velopharyngeal orifice. These groups represented different degrees of "error" to be managed by the control system. The groups included cleft palate subjects with adequate **velopharyngeal closure** ($\leq$ 0.04 cm^2), adequate to borderline closure (0.05-0.09 cm^2), borderline to inadequate closure (0.10-0.19 cm^2), and inadequate closure ($\geq$ 0.20 cm^2). Those criteria are in part perceptually based and in part aerodynamically based (Warren, 1964, 1979, 1982). That is, velopharyngeal areas less than 0.05 cm^2 were considered adequate because normal, noncleft speakers do not manifest areas greater than this value (Warren, 1964). Conversely, the definition of inadequate closure was based on aerodynamic data demonstrating that oral-nasal differential pressure during speech is very low at areas equal to or greater than 0.2 cm^2 (Warren and DuBois, 1964). In addition, unpublished clinical observations lead to the conclusion that speakers with velopharyngeal areas in the inadequate range invariably manifest **hypernasality** and/or **nasal emission**.

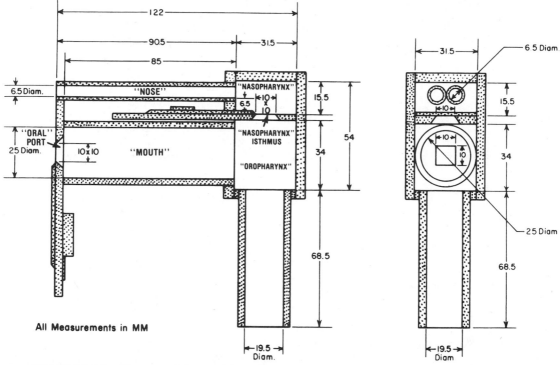

FIGURE 2-37 Diagram of the model used to simulate a passive system. The model was designed to replicate the upper airway, and its dimensions were based on radiographic and physiological data. (From Warren, D. W., & Devereux, J. L. [1966]. An analog study of cleft palate speech. *Cleft Palate Journal, 3,* 103-114.)

The categories of adequate to borderline closure (0.05-0.09 cm^2) and borderline to inadequate closure (0.10-0.19 cm^2) are somewhat more arbitrary. However, aerodynamic and perceptual evidence suggests these groupings (Warren, 1979). Again, the categories represent different degrees of velopharyngeal resistance, or "errors" in the regulating system.

Timing parameters measured are shown in Figure 2-36. The timing changes are associated with aerodynamic events that occurred during repeated productions of the /mp/ blend in "hamper". Figure 2-37 illustrates the mechanical model used in this study. Respiratory activity was simulated by a pump that produced airflow in the form of sine waves. The airflow was adjusted to generate a pressure comparable to that of speakers. Oral cavity pressure was measured at several velopharyngeal apertures to define the relationship between velopharyngeal aperture size and pressure in this passive system. The apertures were set at 0.03, 0.09, 0.13, and 0.45 cm^2.

A normal pressure and airflow relationship for the /mp/ blend in the word "hamper" is illustrated in Figure 2-38, and a pattern typical of velar inadequacy is shown in Figure 2-39. The obvious difference is shifting of the airflow pulse for /m/ to the right with overlap of the pressure pulse for /p/. In the case of adequate closure, peak airflow (2) and end airflow (3) occur before peak pressure (5). By contrast, in the case of velopharyngeal inadequacy, peak airflow (2) occurs almost in unison with peak pressure (5) and end airflow (3) occurs after peak pressure (5). Table 2-1 lists the mean durations of the airflow pulse in milliseconds across groups. The duration increased with increased degree of inadequacy, and the difference for each group was statistically significant. However, the data for duration of the pressure pulse (4-6) were very different. Duration of pressure did not change across groups; no differences among any of the groups were identified.

Table 2-2 lists mean peak intraoral pressure across groups for the model and the human subjects. As expected, peak intraoral pressure fell as inadequacy increased. The differences between the model and human data reflect the active responses of human subjects. Peak intraoral pressure in the model dropped dramatically across groups, but the decrease was much

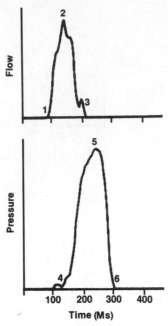

FIGURE 2-38   Typical normal airflow-pressure relationship for /hamper/. (See text for more information.)

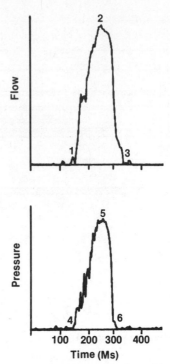

FIGURE 2-39   Typical record of a subject with velopharyngeal inadequacy. The airflow pulse has shifted to the right. (See text for more information.)

TABLE 2-1   Means for durations of the airflow and pressure pulses in milliseconds

	Category			
Variable	Adequate	Adequate to Borderline	Borderline to Inadequate	Inadequate
Airflow	136.4	178.8	198.8	226.5
Pressure	175.9	174.0	174.4	182.5

less among the human subjects. Moreover, the mean pressure never dropped below 3 cm H_2O.

Table 2-3 better indicates the difference between the model and the human subjects. If the ratio of peak intraoral pressure in the adequate group to peak intraoral pressure in the adequate to borderline group is calculated, a value of 4.3 is obtained for the model compared with a value of 1.2 in the subjects. This reflects a more than fourfold drop in pressure in the passive system compared with only a slight drop in the active human system. The ratio comparison of the adequate group and the inadequate group is more dramatic, namely 9.6 for the model and only 1.4 for the subjects. These differences clearly demonstrate that the subjects can compensate for the loss in resistance imposed by velopharyngeal impairment.

Measurements of peak intraoral pressure do not account for any temporal adjustments within the pressure pulse. Therefore, the pressure was integrated and the area under the pressure curve (cm H_2O/s) was calculated. These data are listed in Table 2-4, which shows no differences across groups.

Mean peak volume rate of airflow, mean average volume rate of airflow, mean volume rate of nasal airflow measured at the pressure peak, and mean air volume values are listed in Table 2-5. As expected, all variables related to airflow increased across groups. Comparison of two of the airflow variables, namely peak volume rate and nasal volume rate measured at the pressure peak, is especially revealing (Table 2-5). Both variables increased significantly across groups, but as the airflow pulse shifted to the right, the data points almost coincide in the inadequate group. This finding indicates that respiratory effort shifted from the nasal consonant to the plosive consonant. Normally, the airflow peak coincides with the nasal consonant and occurs before the pressure peak. Instead, it moved closer to the pressure peak as velar resistance fell.

TABLE 2-2   Mean peak intraoral pressures (cm H_2O)

Category	Model	Human
Adequate	8.6	5.0
Adequate to borderline	2.0	4.3
Borderline to inadequate	1.6	4.2
Inadequate	0.9	3.6

TABLE 2-3   Ratios of peak intraoral pressure across groups in the model and human subjects

Category	Ratios of Peak Intraoral Pressures	
	Model	Human
Adequate	4.3	1.2
Adequate to borderline		
Borderline to inadequate	5.4	1.2
Inadequate	9.6	1.4

These data illustrate that both temporal adjustments and respiratory responses are used to maintain the speech pressure head. When pressure was integrated over time, the area under the pressure curve remained nearly constant across groups. When airflow rate was integrated, volume increased significantly across groups (Figure 2-40). The constancy of the integrated pressure pulse compared with changing volume is characteristic of an operational regulation-control system.

One may argue that the increase in airflow rate across groups is merely a function of lowered velar resistance rather than an active response. That is, airflow rate increases because the velopharyngeal orifice is larger and therefore offers less resistance to airflow. However, that does not explain the increase in duration of the airflow pulse (Table 2-1) that raises air volume.

Similarly, the movement of the airflow pulse from the nasal consonant to the plosive consonant cannot be construed as passive (Figure 2-41). In the adequate group, peak airflow is the

TABLE 2-4   Integration of the pressure pulse or area under the curve for the subjects studied (cm H_2O/s)

Category			
Adequate	Adequate to Borderline	Borderline to Inadequate	Inadequate
.53	.46	.46	.45

TABLE 2-5   Mean standard deviation for peak volume rate of airflow (ml/sec), average volume rate of airflow (ml/sec), volume rate of nasal airflow at pressure peak (cc/sec), and air volume (ml) by degree of inadequacy

Category	Peak Volume Rate (ml/sec)	Average Volume Rate (ml/sec)	Nasal Airflow at Pressure Peak (ml/sec)	Volume (ml)
Adequate	140 ± 59	78 ± 25	32 ± 25	11 ± 5
Adequate to borderline	178 ± 59	94 ± 25	102 ± 34	17 ± 8
Borderline to inadequate	256 ± 148	118 ± 57	149 ± 51	24 ± 12
Inadequate	320 ± 180	184 ± 23	313 ± 188	43 ± 26

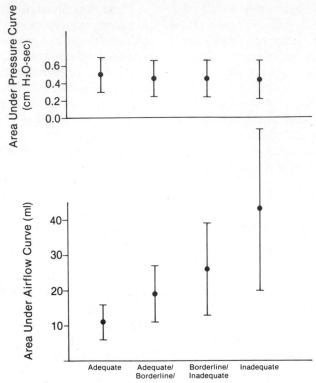

FIGURE 2-40   An illustration of regulation and control. The pressure pulse is regulated and remains constant across groups. The airflow pulse is controlled and responds so as to produce a constant pressure pulse. (From Warren, D. W., Dalston, R. M., Morr, K. E., Hairfield, W. M., & Smith, L. R. [1989]. The speech regulating system: Temporal and aerodynamic responses to velopharyngeal inadequacy. *Journal of Speech and Hearing Research, 32,* 566-575.)

maximum for the nasal consonant. Airflow at peak pressure occurs at the plosive consonant. Both airflow variables increased across groups. However, the increase at the airflow peak represents an active increase in respiratory effort, whereas the increase in airflow at the pressure peak represents the effect of decreased velar resistance as well as increased respiratory effort.

Additional evidence of a regulating system lies in the remarkable parallelism between the loss of pressure in the model and gain in airflow in subjects. Figure 2-42 compares the ratio of change in model peak pressure across groups with the inverse ratio of change in airflow in the subjects. The drop in pressure when adequacy is compared with inadequacy in the model is paralleled by the increase in airflow rate when the inadequate group is compared with the adequate group in the human subjects. The fact that the clinical research data are inversely proportional to the modeling data indicates that the subjects adopted active responses to main-

tain pressure. Moreover, the subject data (Table 2-3) reveal that the strategies were fairly successful in regulating pressure. The extent to which the pressures observed in this study exceed those measured in the passive system may be considered a rough estimate of success of that effort. The extent to which those pressures were not held constant across the groups may simply reflect the physiologic limits of this compensatory response. However, when time responses were included in the measurements, regulation of the pressure pulse was very successful.

Acquired Velopharyngeal Inadequacy

Individuals with velopharyngeal inadequacy resulting from cleft palate represent a group with long-term structural deficits. However, compensations for a congenital defect may differ from those for a defect acquired after speech patterns have matured. Minsley et al. (1988)

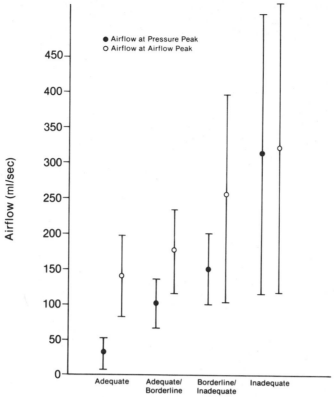

FIGURE 2-41 Peak airflow rate and airflow rate measured at the pressure peak increase across groups. The data points coincide at the inadequate group, indicating a shift in airflow to the right with loss of velar resistance. (From Warren, D. W., Dalston, R. M., Morr, K. E., Hairfield, W. M., & Smith, L. R. [1989]. The speech regulating system: Temporal and aerodynamic responses to velopharyngeal inadequacy. *Journal of Speech and Hearing Research, 32,* 566-575.)

studied four subjects who had a normal speech mechanism until treatment of a malignancy produced a large oronasal defect. An **obturator** fabricated for each subject prior to surgery was to be worn immediately after surgery to prevent long-term adaptation to the defect. Thus, any responses in speaking without the prosthesis could be considered fairly immediate. The structural defect introduced a significant loss of upper airway resistance, and a rather large drop in intraoral pressure would be expected if no compensation occurred. Figure 2-43 illustrates that while intraoral pressures did drop without the obturator in place, the mean pressure remained above 3 cm H_2O. Respiratory volumes increased fourfold (Fig. 2-44). However, voiced-voiceless distinctions among consonants (Warren and Wood, 1969) were maintained even when respiratory volumes quadrupled. This finding may reflect the speaker's desire to maintain the acoustic contrast, not to alter the associated laryngeal articulations, or both.

Simulation Studies

Warren et al. (1989) had normal subjects simulate velopharyngeal inadequacy and measured the effects of reduced vocal tract resistance on respiratory effort and intraoral pressure. Subjects were asked to say the word "papa" in a series of five repetitions produced in a single breath. The subject then perturbed the velopharyngeal mechanism, lowering the soft palate, or "talking through the nose," while performing the same task. The pressure-flow contrasts between normal and perturbed productions are shown in Figure 2-45.

Table 2-6 lists average peak intraoral pressures and average expiratory speech volumes for each subject during normal and perturbed conditions. For all but one subject (GM), pressure fell

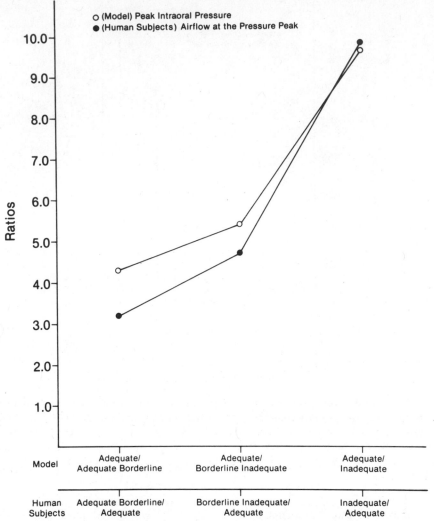

FIGURE 2-42   A tenfold drop in intraoral pressure in the model represents the passive relationship between velopharyngeal size and intraoral pressure. The tenfold increase in airflow rate
reflects the active respiratory response of subjects to loss of velar resistance. (From Warren,
D. W., Dalston, R. M., Morr, K. E., Hairfield, W. M., & Smith, L. R. [1989]. The speech
regulating system: Temporal and aerodynamic responses to velopharyngeal inadequacy. *Journal of Speech and Hearing Research, 32,* 566-575.)

during the perturbed speech task, and for two
speakers (HF and JW), pressure fell below 3 cm
H_2O. Despite this decrease, comparing the normal condition with the experimental condition
revealed no statistically significant difference.
On the other hand, speech expiratory volumes
increased significantly across conditions. In most
instances, speech volumes doubled under the
perturbed condition. However, in the case of
one subject, who had increased intraoral pressure, speech volume almost quadrupled.

Table 2-7 compares mean inspiratory and
expiratory volumes across conditions. Statistical

analysis revealed no significant difference between the inspiratory and expiratory phases of
normal speech but a significant difference between these phases during perturbed speech.
Five of the eight subjects had higher inspiratory
than expiratory volumes during normal speech,
while all eight subjects had higher expiratory
than inspiratory volumes during perturbed
speech.

Comparisons of inspiratory and expiratory
volumes during normal and perturbed speech
produced similar results. No difference was
noted for inspiratory breathing, and a highly

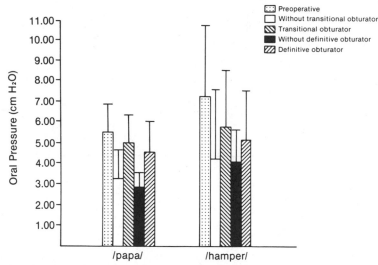

FIGURE 2-43   Mean oral pressures during /p/ production for all subjects. (From Minsley, G. E., Warren, D. W., & Hinton, V. A. [1987]. Physiologic responses to maxillary resection and subsequent obturation. *Journal of Prosthetic Dentistry, 57,* 338-344.)

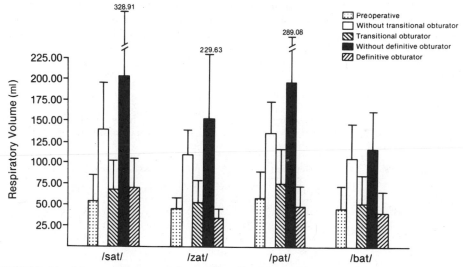

FIGURE 2-44   Mean respiratory volumes for all subjects. (From Minsley, G. E., Warren, D. W., & Hinton, V. A. [1987]. Physiologic responses to maxillary resection and subsequent obturation. *Journal of Prosthetic Dentistry, 57,* 338-344.)

significant difference was noted for expiratory speech breathing.

Since changes in utterance duration could affect respiratory volume, the duration of the single expiratory breath during production of a series of five "papa"s was measured. Table 2-8 compares the mean durations across conditions. Each series was measured at the onset of the intraoral pressure pulse of the first /p/ in the first "papa" to the offset of the /a/ at the end of the fifth "papa". No significant difference was noted.

A mechanical model was then used to estimate the effect of decreased velopharyngeal resistance on intraoral pressure in a passive system. The orifice was set at an opening of 0.5 cm^2, corresponding to the mean velopharyngeal opening in the human sample under the perturbed condition. The pump was set at a pulse volume of 100 ml to simulate a normal /pa/

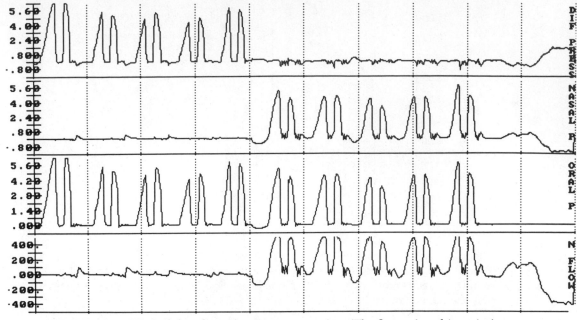

FIGURE 2-45 Typical data from the computer monitor. The first series of /papa/ s is a normal sequence. The second series is produced with the velum lowered. Note the large difference in airflow rate and the negligible orifice differential pressure when the velum is lowered, indicating successful completion of the task. (From Warren, D. W., Morr, K. E., Rochet, A. P., & Dalston, R. M. [1989]. Respiratory response to a decrease in velopharyngeal resistance. *Journal of the Acoustical Society of America, 86,* 917-924.)

TABLE 2-6 Average peak intraoral pressure and expiratory speech volumes for normal and simulated velopharyngeal inadequacy. Speech volumes include the entire expiratory volume during the string of utterances.

Subject	Pressure (cm H_2O)		Speech Volume (ml)	
	Normal	VPI	Normal	VPI
JB	5.1	5.0	390	780
TL	5.4	3.1	338	613
PP	5.3	4.9	713	1267
HF	4.7	2.6	563	775
JW	5.0	2.6	608	1225
GS	4.7	3.7	904	1646
GM	4.4	6.8	537	2316
BJ	4.5	3.8	399	758
Mean	4.9	4.1	557	1173
s.d.	0.37	1.4	188	578

(Warren and Wood, 1969). The resulting intraoral pressure at this setting was 1.8 cm H_2O. Volume was then increased to 200 ml to approximate the doubling in expiratory volume observed under the perturbed condition (Table 2-6). Pressure rose to 6.3 cm H_2O. This is a fourfold difference in intraoral pressure across conditions and is in marked contrast to the minimal pressure change of 0.8 cm H_2O observed among the subjects studied here.

These findings indicate that responses to voluntary lowering of the velum in normal subjects

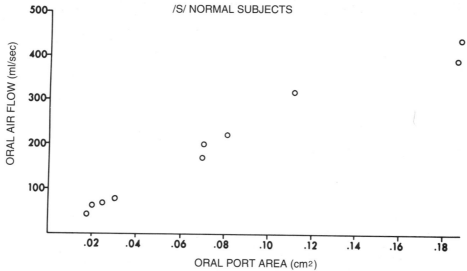

FIGURE 2-46 The relationship between oral port area and rate of airflow is linear. The data presented are averaged for each subject and the middle /s/ in "say /sasas/ again" was used. (From Warren, D. W., Hall, D. J., & Davis, J. [1981]. Oral port constriction and pressure airflow relationships during sibilant productions. *Folia Phoniatrica, 33,* 380-394.)

TABLE 2-7 Mean inspiratory and expiratory volumes (ml) and standard deviation for normal and perturbed speech

Paired t-test *p* values are shown within and across conditions.

	Inspiratory	Expiratory	*p* value
Normal	787 ± 420	557 ± 188	n.s.
Perturbed	747 ± 287	1173 ± 578	<0.03
p value	N.S.	<0.01	

TABLE 2-8 Duration of five utterances

Subject	Duration(s)	
	Normal	VPI
JB	3.23	3.27
TL	2.95	3.00
PP	3.03	3.00
HF	3.23	3.23
JW	3.03	3.08
GS	3.59	3.72
GM	2.77	3.08
BJ	2.50	2.47
Mean	3.04	3.11
Standard deviation	0.33	0.35

are similar to the compensatory responses observed in cleft palate subjects with velopharyngeal impairment. Approximately 75% of the subjects in this study were able to maintain intraoral pressure above 3 cm H_2O during plosive consonant productions, while approximately 70% of cleft subjects with velopharyngeal impairment were able to maintain such pressures (Dalston et al., 1988). Both populations responded to decreased velopharyngeal resistance by actively increasing respiratory effort.

Pressure Regulation during Production of Sibilants

Warren, Hall, and Davis (1981) demonstrated that the relationship between intraoral pressure and respiratory airflow is similar for sibilant sounds. Differences in constriction size at the oral port (i.e., the space between tongue, alveolar ridge, and teeth) have little effect on intraoral pressures during production of sibilants because airflow rate covaries with port size. That is, larger port openings are associated with larger flow rates. Figure 2-46 illustrates the relationship between port area and airflow rate at openings between 0.02 and .18 cm², and Figure 2-47 demonstrates that pressures are maintained above 3 cm H_2O across those port dimensions. Rochet, Morr, and Warren (1989) measured respiratory effort in response to manipulation of

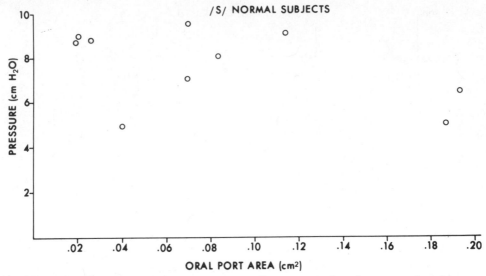

FIGURE 2-47   The relationship between intraoral pressure and oral port area is stable over the normal range of openings. However, there does appear to be a slight drop in pressure at the largest openings. (From Warren, D. W., Hall, D. J., & Davis, J. [1981]. Oral port constriction and pressure airflow relationships during sibilant productions. *Folia Phoniatrica, 33,* 380-394.)

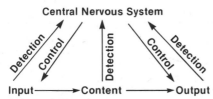

FIGURE 2-48   Relationships among input, content, and output, with outline of how physiologic mechanisms detect and control rates of change. (From Brobeck, J. R. [1965]. Exchange, control, and regulation. In Yamamoto, W. S., & Brobeck, J. R. (Eds.), *Physiological controls and regulations.* Philadelphia: W. B. Saunders, pp 1-13.)

port size during sibilant production and found that the increase in airflow reflects an active increase in respiratory effort rather than a passive increase in airflow through a larger anterior opening.

Sensory Information

In any regulating system, there must be a relationship among input, processing, and output (Fig. 2-48). Mechanisms to identify change are necessary for control factors to operate. The presence of sensory receptors must be established, their location identified, and their sensitivity determined. However, the physiologic detection system does not have to respond to the variable being regulated; it can respond to some correlate or function related to it (Brobeck, 1965).

Respiratory receptors have been found in the trachea (Sant'Ambrogio, 1982), larynx (Sant'-Ambrogio et al., 1983), nasopharynx (McBride and Whitelaw, 1981) and oral cavity (Furusawa et al., 1992) of man. Intrathoracic receptors signal both volume and flow; extrathoracic receptors signal flow and upper airway resistance (Sant'Ambrogio, 1982). Similarly, laryngeal receptors sensing pressure, airflow, and contraction of muscles have also been described (Sant'Ambrogio, 1982). Muscles in the upper airway may also play a functional role in instantaneous control of airflow and compensation for changes in airway resistance during breathing (Cohen, 1975; Brouillette and Thach, 1980). Remmers and Bartlett (1977) observed tracking behavior involving extrathoracic tracheal stretch receptors in which the respiratory muscles responded to changes in upper airway resistance. The expiratory discharge of the receptors was determined by the relationship between upper airway resistance and instantaneous flow. This information is useful for coordinating the activity of expiratory flow controllers. If this afferent information were compared centrally with that derived from intrathoracic pulmonary receptors, the relative magnitude of upper airway resistance could be estimated. Such information might allow adjustment of laryngeal resistance in response to changes in supralaryngeal pressures. Studies by England and Bartlett (1982) demonstrate that the laryngeal activity controls respiratory flow in man by varying the degree of glottal adduction. Thus, the detection system for breathing may in some fashion operate in speech as well.

Several early studies addressed somatosensory feedback mechanisms in speech using nerve block approaches (Ringel and Steer, 1963; Gammon et al., 1970; Scott and Ringel, 1971; Putnam and Ringel, 1972). Although Smith (1992) has argued that changes in motor performance after a nerve block may be the result of other factors than reduced afferent input, the importance of somatosensory information is unequivocal. For example, Gracco and Abbs (1985) demonstrated that afferent information from the perioral region is used to control lip movements during speech.

Malécot (1966, 1970) and Williams, Brown, and Turner (1987) provide evidence of such a system. However, whether the detection system actually senses pressure or some correlate of pressure remains to be seen. Malécot (1966, 1970), Müller and Brown (1980), Wyke (1981), Williams, Brown, and Turner (1987) and McClevan and Furusawa et al. (1992) have indicated that aerodynamic monitoring may direct the activity of speech structures. Indeed, several investigators have shown that trigeminal mucosal and cutaneous mechanoreceptors are responsive to the application of external stimuli and to minute degrees of lateral stretch, and encode information about the magnitude of these events affecting their receptive fields (Johansson et al., 1988 a and b; Nordin and Thomander, 1989; Nordin and Hagbarth, 1989; Furusawa et al., 1992). They also signal the velocity and direction of stresses and strains similar to those likely produced by changes in vocal tract air pressures (Essick, Edin and Trulsson, unpublished findings).

Elice (1990) reported that a 30% change in resistance can be detected during breathing. Subjects were able to detect an increase or decrease of about 0.7 cm H_2O/L/s of resistance. Interestingly, subjects in the Elice study responded to increases in applied resistance load by decreasing airflow rate. Similarly, when resistance load was decreased stepwise, airflow

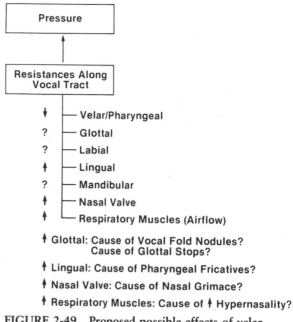

FIGURE 2-49   Proposed possible effects of velar resistance deficit resulting from velopharyngeal inadequacy.

rate was increased to minimize the change in intraoral pressure.

IMPLICATIONS OF A SPEECH-REGULATING SYSTEM

If speech aerodynamics does conform to the principles of a regulating system, new explanations for certain maladaptive articulatory behaviors are possible. Aerodynamic performance would receive some priority in the speech-motor control program. In fact, in many studies compensatory responses to errors in the system usually met the criteria for aerodynamic stability, sometimes at the expense of speech performance. Since almost all clinical studies that have tested the regulating system hypothesis involved patients with velopharyngeal deficits, the following discussion will be limited to that population. However, one should easily see the relevance to other populations having deficits that affect the speech structures. Figure 2-49 suggests possible responses to a decrease in velopharyngeal resistance associated with cleft palate. Greater respiratory muscle activity increases airflow rate. Since resistance is flow dependent, velar resistance increases, and so intraoral pressure rises. Individuals with high nasal resistance require less airflow to maintain intraoral pressure. Additionally, nasal resistance

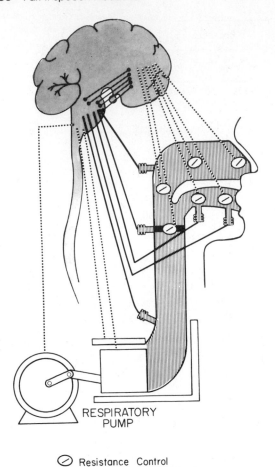

○ Resistance Control
▨ Possible Sensing Mechanisms
······ Motor
—— Sensory

FIGURE 2-50 A possible feedback system to regulate speech pressures. According to this theory, sensors send error messages to resistance controllers via the brain.

can be increased by constricting the nasal valve. This physiologic manifestation of the **nasal grimace** can increase nasal resistance by 10% to 30%. As discussed earlier, the nasal valve normally constricts more during expiration than during inspiration, and this reflex associated with breathing is also available for speech function.

High tongue carriage and the pharyngeal fricatives also increase vocal tract resistance in the presence of a velar deficit. Similarly, the glottis normally serves as an expiratory brake during breathing and adducts more during expiration than during inspiration. The glottal stop may be a more forceful manifestation of this reflex. The well-known **Passavant's pad** activity of the posterior pharyngeal wall may also be an airway response to a loss of resistance. The anterior movement of the muscle decreases

cross-sectional size of the airway and therefore increases airway resistance. The point is that a speech-regulating system would be dedicated to maintaining speech pressures, and many of the compensatory behaviors in cleft palate appear to fit the description of control responses.

Although the hypothesis that speech aerodynamics follows regulation and control principles may be novel, it is very much in line with modern theories of speech-motor control as described by Kelso, Tuller, and Harris (1983) and Kelso and Tuller (1984). Speech-motor control theory is framed in such terms as *motor equivalence* and *coordinative structures*. In terms of segmental speech activities, the postulate is that functionally and anatomically distinct parts of the speech system are constrained to act together toward a common goal. Within this framework the respiratory and articulatory systems are hypothesized to form a coordinative structure whose goal is to regulate speech patterns.

Figure 2-50 illustrates a possible feedback system for regulating speech pressures. Although pressure would vary somewhat according to consonant type, the system would be driven to maintain an adequate level of pressure for consonant productions. The system proposed is very similar to pressure regulation in cardiovascular dynamics. It is purposefully cryptic to convey the uncertainty of many of the components of this "black box" arrangement.

INSTRUMENTATION FOR AERODYNAMIC STUDIES

Manometry

Various devices have been used to measure intraoral pressures during breathing and maximum expiratory efforts (Warren, 1975). Most of these instruments are modifications of the U-tube **manometer**. Their use has been limited because nonspeech tasks, such as maximum expiratory effort, may not reflect the capability of the speech mechanism. However, in some instances oral manometers provide a gross measure of the efficiency of the velopharyngeal mechanism during blowing.

Aerodynamic Devices

Instruments that precisely measure respiratory parameters associated with speech include flow-

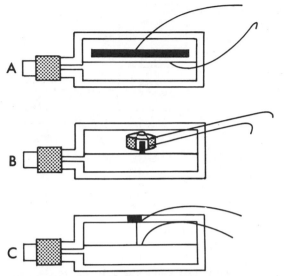

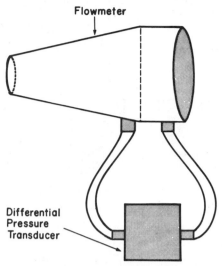

FIGURE 2-51   Types of transducers used to measure air pressure: *A*, variable capacitance; *B*, variable inductance; *C*, variable resistance.

FIGURE 2-52   The pneumotachograph consists of a flowmeter and a differential pressure transducer. As air flows across the mesh screen in the flowmeter, pressure drops and is recorded by the transducer. The pressure drop is proportional to the rate of airflow.

meters, which record volume rates of airflow, and pressure transducers, which record airway pressures within the vocal tract (Lubker, 1970).

Air Pressure Devices

Strain gauge transducers are the most common devices for measuring pressure. The pressure-transducing element activates whenever pressure is applied to a diaphragm in the unit. Displacement of the diaphragm is transmitted to a Wheatstone bridge, and these changes in resistance unbalance the bridge in proportion to the applied pressure (Figure 2-51).

It is common practice to amplify the signal from transducers to provide power to drive galvanometers. However, the mechanical inertia of some direct-writing galvanometers is so great that the frequency response is limited, and amplification is required to provide any measurable response. Usually a carrier amplifier is used with a strain gauge transducer. An oscillator supplies an alternating current, and the amplitude is continuously affected by the varying resistance of the Wheatstone bridge. The output of the transducer enters a capacitance-coupled amplifier, which amplifies the modulated carrier wave. Then the signals are rectified and the carrier wave is filtered out, leaving a direct current voltage that powers the recording in-

strument. Usually a small catheter is used to transmit the pressure to the transducer (Warren, 1982).

Airflow Devices

The most widely accepted instrument for measuring the volume rate of airflow is the heated **pneumotachograph**, which consists of a flowmeter and a differential pressure transducer (Figure 2-52). It uses the principle that as air flows across a resistance, the resulting pressure drop is linearly related to the volume rate of airflow. In most cases, the resistance is a wire mesh screen that is heated to prevent condensation. Pressure taps on each side of the screen are connected to a sensitive differential pressure transducer. The pressure drop is converted to a voltage that is amplified and recorded either on tape or on a direct-writing instrument. Both ingressive and egressive airflow can be measured (Warren, 1982).

APPLICATION OF AERODYNAMIC TECHNIQUES

Pressure and airflow devices have been used in a variety of ways to measure the aerodynamics of speech production (Warren, 1975). Intraoral

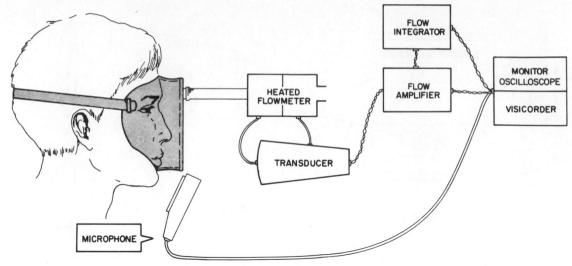

FIGURE 2-53   Airflow is measured by means of a face mask, pneumotachograph, and recorder.

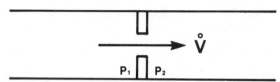

FIGURE 2-54   The area of a constriction of pipes can be calculated from measurements of airflow through the constriction (V̊) and the pressure drop (P_1 to P_2) across the constriction.

pressure can be recorded by a small catheter placed in the mouth and attached to a pressure transducer, amplifier, and recorder. Similarly, subglottal pressure can be measured by insertion of a needle attached to a catheter into the trachea below the glottis. Pressures can be measured anywhere along the vocal tract as long as access can be provided.

Airflow along the vocal tract can be recorded with a pneumotachograph appropriately attached by tubing or a mask to the mouth, nose, or both (Figure 2-53). Integration of airflow values over time provides a measure of air volumes used in speech.

Aerodynamic techniques provide important information about normal and abnormal speech production. The techniques usually involve the application of hydraulic principles (Warren, 1976). Upper airway structures such as the tongue, teeth, lips, and palate form numerous constrictions that affect airflow and pressure. Hydraulic equations are used to estimate the size of these constrictions. The basis for such mea-

surements can be explained by the analogy of air flowing through simple pipes (Figure 2-54). The size of the constriction in a pipe can be calculated by measuring the airflow through the pipe (V̊) and the pressure drop across the pipe (ΔP). The area of the constriction is then calculated by

$$A = \frac{\overset{\circ}{V}}{k\sqrt{\dfrac{2\Delta P}{d}}}$$

where k = 0.65 and d = density of air.

As Figure 2-55 illustrates, the size of articulatory constriction can also be estimated in this manner (Warren, 1976). Thus, to measure the size of the velopharyngeal orifice, record the pressure difference between the nose and the mouth and the volume rate of airflow through the nose during speech. This measurement is especially important in people with cleft palates. Similarly, the size of the oral opening during fricative productions can be estimated by the placement of catheters and a face mask in the positions illustrated in Figure 2-56 (Warren, 1975; Smith et al., 1978).

Upper airway structures also constrain airflow. The equation

$$R = \frac{\Delta P}{\overset{\circ}{V}}$$

where R = resistance, can be used to estimate

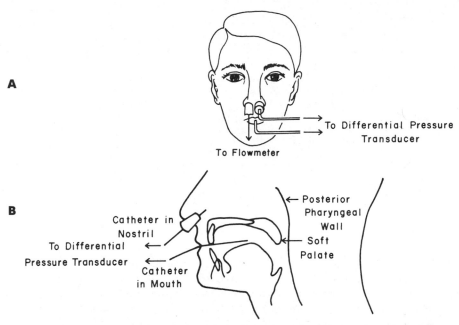

FIGURE 2-55   Catheters are placed above and below the orifice to measure the differential pressure. *A,* The catheter placed in the left nostril is secured by a cork, which plugs the nostril and creates a stagnant air column above the orifice. *B,* The second catheter is placed in the mouth. Both catheters are connected to a differential pressure transducer. The pneumotachograph is connected to the right nostril and collects orifice airflow through the nose. (From Warren, D. W. [1976]. Aerodynamics of speech production. In Lass, N. J. [Ed.], *Contemporary issues in experimental phonetics.* New York: Academic Press [105-137].)

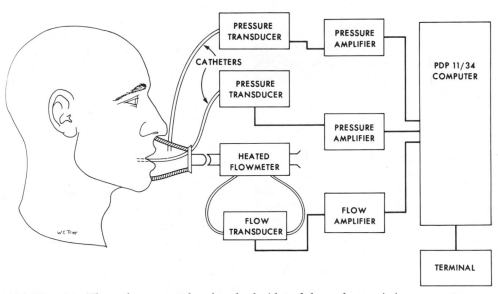

FIGURE 2-56   The catheters are placed on both sides of the oral constriction to measure oral port opening for fricatives. Airflow is collected in a face mask and goes to the pneumotachograph. (From Smith, H. Z., Allen, G. D., Warren, D. W., & Hall, D. J. [1978]. The consistency of the pressure-flow technique for assessing oral port size. *Journal of the Acoustical Society of America, 64,* 1203-1206.)

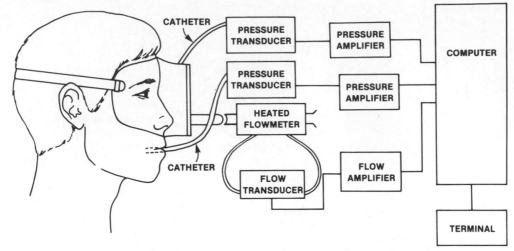

FIGURE 2-57 Nasal airway resistance is measured by recording the pressure drop across the structure and the airflow through it. A face mask is used to collect airflow from the nose. Closing the lips around the pressure catheter provides a measure of pressure across the nasal airway. (From Warren, D. W., Duany, L. F., & Fischer, N. D. [1969]. Nasal pathway resistance in normal and cleft lip and palate subjects. *Cleft Palate Journal, 6,* 134-140.)

these resistances during speech (Warren, Duany, and Fischer, 1969). For example, to calculate nasal resistance, measure the pressure drop across the nose and airflow through the nose, as in Figure 2-57. The same technique can be used to measure lingual, palatal, or oral port resistance during speech. A self-contained software and related hardware package (PERCI-PC, Microtronics Corporation, Chapel Hill, NC) does aerodynamic assessment of speech and breathing. This system is used to collect pressure-flow data, and the software provides analysis modes for measuring the pressure, airflow, volume, constriction areas, resistance, conductance, and timing associated with speech. The system also uses the Smitheran and Hixon (1981) method for estimating laryngeal resistance during vowel production.

Resistance measurements can also be generated from area measurements. The actual relationship between nasal airway size and nasal resistance can be described in mathematical terms by means of an empirical conversion equation, as follows:

$$R = 1.9 + \left(\frac{0.03 + 0.0009 \times \text{flow}}{A^2} \right)$$

Figure 2-58 illustrates inspiratory and expiratory breathing data from which measurements of resistance and area are generated.

DIRECTIONS FOR FUTURE RESEARCH

Although evidence in this chapter shows that the aerodynamics of speech conforms to patterns typical of a physiologic regulating system, many questions remain. Netsell (1990), for example, suggests an **acoustic regulation hypothesis** as an alternative to the pressure regulation hypothesis. He proposes that a speaker's attempt to maintain an appropriate level of pressure is for acoustic consequences rather than for pressure regulation per se. Similarly, Dalston et al. (1988) observed that regardless of how adjustments are made to maintain pressure, it is reasonable to ask why these pressures are maintained. Is their maintenance a primary goal, a secondary goal, or merely a by-product of some other system activity?

Although speakers maintain intraoral pressures in the face of transient and persistent system disturbances, it may be argued that the maintenance of pressure in such circumstances is required merely for the acoustic power necessary to generate perceptually acceptable pressure consonants. In that case, pressure maintenance would not necessarily indicate that speech aerodynamics is subject to regulation and control. It would merely reflect the fact that pressure is requisite to the primary goal of impounding air for pressure-consonant productions. However, the fact that listeners perceived a deterioration in speech during induced ante-

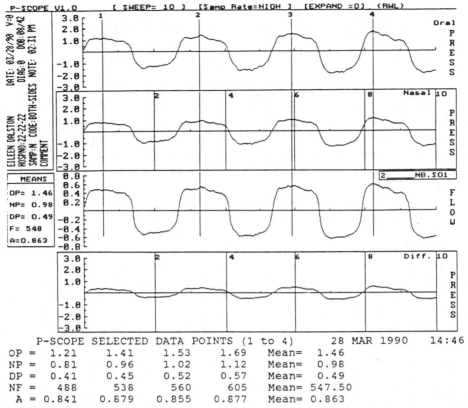

FIGURE 2-58 Resistance and area measurements can be generated from pressure-airflow data. Bottom to top, the records are differential pressure, nasal airflow, nasal pressure, and oral pressure. Data for pressures, airflow, area, and resistance are at the bottom. Numbers on records denote where measurements were obtained.

rior open-bite conditions suggests one or more of the following:

1. Pressure maintenance took precedence over perceptual accuracy.
2. Pressure maintenance does not have a one-to-one relationship with perceived speech normality.
3. Pressure maintenance was necessary but not sufficient for accurate speech, and speakers could maintain pressure but not produce all the requisites for acceptable speech.
4. Speakers may adopt a minimum competency strategy leading to adjustments that do not fully compensate for imposed perturbations.
5. The speakers perceived that their own speech remained acceptable under the various experimental conditions.

None of the studies cited here addressed the speakers' perceptions of their own speech. This would be the easiest of the five alternatives to test experimentally.

It would be interesting to compare performance under varying conditions of anterior open bite and auditory masking. If speakers maintain equivalent pressures and perceive themselves as having comparable speech proficiency with and without auditory masking under identical open-bite conditions, it might suggest that pressure maintenance is a primary goal of the speaking mechanism and not secondary to acoustic and perceptual accuracy. The relative importance of auditory feedback in the maintenance of acceptable speech might be reflected in the extent to which accuracy deteriorates under masking. The study by Warren, Allen, and King (1984) comes closest to examining this question.

That study reported the speech of normal individuals under auditory masking and varying conditions of imposed anterior open bite. The researchers found that these subjects tended to maintain oral port sizes appropriate for the production of fricative consonants even though the perceptual quality of these phonemes deteriorated noticeably. Although intraoral pressure measurements were not reported, unpublished data from that investigation do show that these pressures were consistently maintained above 3 cm H_2O.

Moon and Folkins (1991) assessed the relative importance of auditory feedback in the regulation of intraoral pressure and reported some preliminary findings. Subjects who spoke normally were forced into a choice between aerodynamic and auditory feedback. Manipulation of the acoustic signal often resulted in adjustments of peak pressure and/or duration of pressure. However, the changes in pressure were not of the magnitude expected for the large adjustment in the acoustic signal. They found that the system is somewhat resistant to changes in speech pressures.

Moon, Folkins, and Smith (1993) indicate that sensory information may not always be necessary to drive the respiratory system reflexively. They suggest that the inherent physiological properties of the human respiratory system provide pressure stability. However, because they cannot explain certain compensatory processes, such as changes in airflow duration, passavant pad activity, nasal valve constrictions, among others, in response to changes in vocal tract resistance (see Warren, Wood, and Bradley, 1969; Warren, 1986 a and b; Warren et al., 1989; Liu, Warren, and Dalston, 1991), they believe that maintaining pressure during speech may also require some active responses as well.

It should also be noted that a subject who monitors or attempts to regulate pressure during speech may be doing so because of associations established much earlier between pressure and other perhaps more fundamental variables such as perceived speech quality or acoustics. It is quite possible that such associations are formed and strengthened during the very early stages of speech development. Therefore, the fact that a given variable (e.g., pressure) may be regulated after speech development is complete does not rule out the original and primary importance of some other associated variable. The speech of the congenitally deaf clearly exemplifies the consequences of inadequate acoustic feedback.

An assessment of the aerodynamic patterns of deaf speakers is a direction that should yield important new information on aerodynamic and acoustic interaction. Cain, Seaver, Jackson, and Sandridge (1989) found that deaf speakers have basically normal pressure patterns despite articulatory errors related to their auditory defi-

cits. Seaver and his associates are using bite blocks and bleed valves to perturb speech aerodynamics in deaf speakers to determine whether compensatory responses are similar to those in the normal population.

Physiologic regulating systems often are multifactorial, and responses to change reflect the need to maintain more than one parameter at an optimal level. For example, in respiration the system is managed so that CO_2 concentrations, pH, and peak upper airway breathing pressures are kept within a certain limited range despite changes in the environment or in level of activity. Information concerning the chemical environment of the blood, the status of the airway, and other factors is integrated by the brain and appropriate control responses made. Thus, some interaction of the acoustic and aerodynamic systems may well occur. Whether the one receives a higher priority than the other has particular relevance to speech-motor control theory.

There are still many gaps in our understanding of a regulating system as it pertains to speech. The detection system, an essential component to identify errors, is only now beginning to receive some attention, although Malécot (1966) presented some data on sensitivity of receptors. However, the specific variable being detected is not entirely clear. The regulated parameter is not necessarily the same variable that is detected (Brobeck, 1965). The system may respond to some correlate or function related to the variable. Furthermore, the minimal level of pressure required for adequate consonant production remains unknown. For example, a pressure value of 3 cm H_2O has been routinely adopted as an operational definition of adequate consonant pressure. The validity of this definition has not been tested rigorously, although it is based upon long-term observations of data generated from aerodynamic studies. The relationship between consonant pressure and the perceptual acceptability of its acoustic analog also must be investigated.

Finally, as Netsell (1990) indicates, intraoral pressure reflects subglottal pressure as well as articulatory movements of the larynx and upper airway. Studies of the speech regulation system have limited the speech sample to pressure consonants in which intraoral pressure is expected to reflect subglottal pressure. Vowels have not been used. Thus, a major test of the regulating system hypothesis would be to determine whether subglottal pressures rather than intra-oral pressures remain fairly constant when the system is perturbed during continuous speech.

SUMMARY

The chemical and neural control of respiration is quite complex, and an even more precise and delicate regulatory mechanism is required for speech. The sudden changes in respiratory load that occur when the upper airway closes or opens during phonation must be compensated almost instantaneously if subglottal pressure is to be kept nearly constant. Otherwise, sound intensity and fundamental frequency would be unstable. This poses a considerable error control problem that is not encountered in breathing. Undoubtedly a complicated feedback system regulating pressure and controlling airflow and articulatory movements is involved. Although there is some general information available, current models are still highly speculative.

The system presumably consists of a controller unit or computer coordinating center, sensors or receptors to transmit information, and effectors to power the system and produce articulatory movements. The controller most certainly is in the brain, and higher centers such as the medulla are involved. Sensors are located in the lung and along the vocal tract. The effectors are the respiratory muscles that power the system, and the articulatory structures are the variable resistances that modulate the airstream. The resulting aerodynamic patterns generate the sounds that are perceived by the listener as speech.

Review Questions

1. What is the principal muscle of inspiration?

2. What two main factors determine the amount of energy required to move air into and out of the lung?

3. Explain the hydraulic principle upon which pressure-flow measurements of the size of a constriction are based.

4. What is the difference between regulation and control?

5. Expiration is generally an active event. T   F

6. The aerodynamics of sound production is a biomechanical process.   T   F

7. Airflow through the respiratory tract is always laminar.   T   F

8. The subglottal pressure head remains relatively stable during speech production. T   F

9. To achieve voicing during a stop consonant, a difference in pressure between the subglottal and supraglottal cavities must occur. T   F

10. Respiratory effort is less when a speech utterance is softer than normal.   T   F

11. Smaller lung volumes of air are used during stressed speech.   T   F

12. Air flows more readily through an open oral cavity than it does through the nose.   T   F

13. When loudness is increased, lung volumes as great as 5 L are used.   T   F

14. The rapid adduction and abduction of the vocal folds provide the basic sound source of speech.   T   F

15. During voiceless consonant production, supraglottal and subglottal pressures are about the same.   T   F

16. Oral resistance during vowel production is well above zero.   T   F

17. Subglottal pressures tend to be more variable than supraglottal pressures.   T   F

18. Enlargement of the oropharyngeal cavity during /p/ production is probably a passive event.   T   F

19. The term *homeostasis* refers to bodily functions that operate under rules tending to preserve physiologic balance.   T   F

20. The acoustic regulator hypothesis is a possible alternative to the pressure regulation hypothesis.   T   F

21. Which of the following is *not* a supraglottal constrictor?
a. velum
b. nasal valve
c. tongue
d. lips
e. alveolus
f. teeth

22. For phonation to occur, pressure in the lung must be (greater/lesser) than atmospheric pressure.

23. Glottal resistance is (higher/lower) for voiceless fricatives than for vowels.

24. (Larger/smaller) lung volumes of air are used with increased loudness during speech.

25. During speech peak intraoral pressures range from _____cm H_2O to _____cm H_2O.

26. During normal conversational speech approximately_____% of lung capacity is used, with_____to_____liters of air involved.

27. During quiet breathing, approximately _____% to_____% of lung capacity is used, with_____liters of air involved.

28. During conversational speech approximately_____% to_____% of vital capacity is used.

References

Agostini, E., & Mead, J. (1964). Statics of the respiratory system. In Fenn, W. (Ed.), *Handbook of Physiology, Respiration I.* Washington, DC: American Physiological Society (pp. 387-409).

Arkebauer, H., Hixon, T. J., & Hardy, J. (1967). Peak intraoral air pressure during speech. *Journal of Speech and Hearing Research, 10,* 196-208.

Bell-Berti, F. (1975). Control of pharyngeal cavity size for English voiced and voiceless stops. *Journal of the Acoustical Society of America, 57,* 456-461.

Bernthal, J. E., & Beukelman, D. R. (1978). Intraoral air pressure during the production of /p/ and /b/ by children, youths, and adults. *Journal of Speech and Hearing Research, 21,* 361-371.

Black, J. (1950). The pressure component in the production of consonants. *Journal of Speech and Hearing Research, 15,* 207-210.

Brobeck, J. R. (1965). Exchange, control, and regulation. In Yamamoto, W. S., & Brobeck, J. R. (Eds.), *Physiological controls and regulations.* Philadelphia: W.B. Saunders (pp. 1-13).

Brouillette, R. 1., & Thach, B. T. (1980). Control of genioglossus muscle inspiratory activity. *Journal of Applied Physiology, 49,* 801-808.

Brown, W., & McGlone, R. (1969). Constancy of intraoral air pressure. *Folia Phoniatrica, 21,* 332-339.

Brown, W., & McGlone, R. (1974). Aerodynamic and acoustic study of stress in sentence productions. *Journal of the Acoustical Society of America, 56,* 971-974.

Brown, W., McGlone, R., & Proffit, W. (1973). Relationship of lingual and intraoral air pressure during syllable production. *Journal of Speech and Hearing Research, 16,* 141-151.

Brown, W., McGlone, R., Tarlow, A., & Shipp, T. (1970). Intraoral air pressure associated with specific phonetic positions. *Phonetica, 22,* 202-212.

Cain, M., Seaver, E., Jackson, P., & Sandridge, S. (1989). Aerodynamic and nasometric assessment of velopharyngeal functioning in hearing-impaired speakers. *Asha, 31,* 158 (Abstract).

Campbell, E. J. M. (1968). The respiratory muscles. In Bouhuys, A. (Ed.), *Sound production in man.*

New York: Annals of the New York Academy of Science (pp. 135-139).

Cavagna, G. A., & Margaria, R. (1965). An analysis of the mechanics of phonation. *Journal of Applied Physiology, 20,* 301-307.

Cherniack, R. M., & Cherniack, L. (1961). *Respiration in health and disease.* Philadelphia: W. B. Saunders.

Cohen, M. I. (1975). Phrenic and recurrent laryngeal discharge patterns and the Hering-Breuer reflex. *American Journal of Physiology, 228,* 1489-1496.

Cole, P. (1985). Upper respiratory airflow. In Proctor, D. F. (Ed.), *The nose-upper airway physiology and the atmospheric environment.* The Netherlands: Elsevier (pp. 163-189).

Comroe, J. H. (1965). *Physiology of respiration.* Chicago: Year Book Medical Publishers.

Dalston, R. M., Warren, D. W., Morr, K. E., & Smith, L. R. (1988). Intraoral pressure and its relationship to velopharyngeal inadequacy. *Cleft Palate Journal, 25,* 210-219.

DuBois, A. B. (1964). Resistance to breathing. In Fenn, W. (Ed.), *Handbook of physiology, respiration I.* Washington, DC: American Physiological Society (pp. 451-462).

Elice, C. (1990). Sensitivity to changes in nasal resistance. Unpublished master's thesis, University of North Carolina, Chapel Hill.

England, S. J., & Bartlett, D. (1982). Changes in respiratory movements of human vocal cords during hyperpnea. *Journal of Applied Physiology, 52,* 780-785.

Flege, J. E. (1983). The influence of stress, position, and utterance length on the pressure characteristics of English /p/ and /b/. *Journal of Speech and Hearing Research, 26,* 111-118.

Fry, D. B. (1955). Duration and intensity as physical correlates of linguistic stress. *Journal of the Acoustical Society of America, 27,* 765-768.

Furusawa K., Yamaoka M., Ichikawa N., & Kumai T. (1992). Airflow receptors in the lip and buccal mucosa. *Brain Research Bulletin, 29,* 69-74.

Gammon S. A., Smith P. J., Daniloff R. G., & Kim C. W. (1971). Articulation and stress/juncture production under oral anesthetization and masking. *Journal of Speech and Hearing Research, 14,* 271-281.

Gautier, H., Remmers, J. E., & Bartlett, D. (1973). Control of the duration of expiration. *Respiratory Physiology, 18,* 205-221.

Gracco V. A., & Abbs J. H. (1985). Dynamic control of the perioral system during speech: Kinematic analyses of autogenic and nonautogenic sensorimotor processes. *Journal of Neurophysiology, 54,* 418-432.

Hairfield, W. M., Warren, D. W., Hinton, V. A., & Seaton, D. L. (1987). Inspiratory and expiratory effects of nasal breathing. *Cleft Palate Journal, 24,* 183-189.

Hixon, T. J. (1966). Turbulent noise source for speech. *Folia Phoniatrica, 18,* 168-182.

Hixon, T. J. (1973). Respiratory function in speech. In Minifie, F. D., Hixon, T. J. & Williams, F. (Eds.), *Normal aspects of speech, hearing, and language.* Englewood Cliffs, NJ: Prentice-Hall (pp. 73-125).

Hixon, T. J. (1982). Speech breathing kinematics and mechanism inferences therefrom. In Grillner, S. (Ed.), *Speech motor control.* New York: Pergamon Press (pp. 75-93).

Hixon, T. J., Goldman, M. D., & Mead, J. (1973). Kinematics of chest wall during speech production: Volume displacements of the rib cage, abdomen, and lung. *Journal of Speech and Hearing Research, 16,* 78-115.

Ishizaka, K., & Matsudaira, M. (1972). *Fluid mechanical consideration of vocal cord vibration.* Santa Barbara: Speech Communication Research Laboratory.

Isshiki, N. (1964). Regulatory mechanism of voice intensity variation. *Journal of Speech and Hearing Research, 7,* 17-29.

Isshiki, N., & Ringel, R. (1964). Airflow during the production of selected consonants. *Journal of Speech and Hearing Research, 7,* 233-244.

Jaeger, M., & Matthys, H. (1970). The pressure flow characteristics of the human airways. In Bouhuys, A. (Ed.), *Airway dynamics.* Springfield, IL: CC Thomas (pp. 21-32).

Johansson R. S., Trulsson J., Olsson K. A., Westbery K-G. (1988a). Mechanoreceptor activity from the human face and oral mucosa. *Experimental Brain Research, 72,* 204-208.

Johansson R. S., Trulsson M., Olsson K. A., Abbs J. H. (1988b). Mechanoreceptive afferent activity in the infraorbital nerve in man during speech and chewing movements. *Experimental Brain Research 72,* 209-214.

Karnell, M., & Willis, C. (1982). The effect of vowel context on consonantal intraoral air pressure. *Folia Phoniatrica, 34,* 1-8.

Kelso, J. A. S., & Tuller, B. (1984). Converging evidence in support of common dynamic prin-

ciples for speech and movement. *American Journal of Physiology, 246,* 928-935.

Kelso, J. A. S., Tuller, B., & Harris, K. S. (1983). A "dynamic pattern" perspective on the control and coordination of movement. In MacNeilage, P. (Ed.), *The production of speech.* New York: Springer-Verlag (pp. 137-173).

Kent, R. D., & Moll, K. L. (1969). Vocal-tract characteristics of the stop cognates. *Journal of the Acoustical Society of America, 46,* 1549-1555.

Klatt, D. H., Stevens, K. N., & Mead, J. (1968). Studies of articulatory activity and airflow during speech. In Bouhuys, A. (Ed.), *Sound production in man.* New York: Annals of the New York Academy of Science (pp. 42-55).

Klechak, T. L., Bradley, D. P., & Warren, D. W. (1976). Anterior open bite and oral port constriction. *Angle Orthodontist, 46,* 232-242.

Klich, R. J. (1982). Effects of speech level and vowel context on intraoral air pressure in vocal and whispered speech. *Folia Phoniatrica, 34,* 33-40.

Ladefoged, P. (1962). Subglottal activity during speech. In *Proceedings of the fourth international congress on phonetic sciences.* The Hague: Mouton (pp. 73-91).

Ladefoged, P. (1968). Linguistic aspects of respiratory phenomena. In Bouhuys, A. (Ed.), *Sound production in man.* New York: Annals of the New York Academy of Science (pp. 141-151).

Ladefoged, P., & McKinney, N. P. (1963). Loudness, sound pressure and subglottal pressure in speech. *Journal of the Acoustical Society of America, 35,* 454-460.

Lieberman, P. (1960). Some acoustic correlates of word stress in American English. *Journal of the Acoustical Society of America, 32,* 451-454.

Lieberman, P. (1967). *Intonation, perception, and language.* Cambridge: MIT Press.

Lieberman, P. (1968). Vocal cord motion in man. In Bouhuys, A. (Ed.), *Sound production in man.* New York: Annals of the New York Academy of Science (pp. 28-38).

Lisker, L. (1971). Supraglottal air pressure in the production of English stops. *Language and Speech, 13,* 215-230.

Liu, H., Warren D. W., & Dalston, R. M. (1991). Increased nasal resistance induced by the pressure-flow technique and its effect on pressure and air flow during speech. *Cleft Palate Journal, 28,* 261-265.

Lotz, W. K., & Netsell, R. (1986). *Developmental patterns of laryngeal aerodynamics for speech.* Paper presented at the midwinter meeting of the Association for Research in Otolaryngology.

Lubker, J. F. (1970). Aerodynamic and ultrasonic assessment techniques in speech-dentofacial research. *Asha Reports, 5,* 207-223.

Lubker, J. F. (1973). A consideration of transglottal airflow during stop consonant production. *Jour-*

nal of the Acoustical Society of America, 53, 212-215.

Lubker, J., & Parris, P. (1970). Simultaneous measurements of intraoral air pressure, force of labial contact, and labial electromyographic activity during production of the stop cognates /p/ and /b/. Journal of the Acoustical Society of America, 47, 625-633.

Malécot, A. (1955). An experimental study of force of articulation. Studia Linguistica, 9, 35-44.

Malécot, A. (1966). The effectiveness of intraoral air pressure pulse parameters in distinguishing between stop cognates. Phonetica, 14, 65-81.

Malécot, A. (1968). The force of articulation of American stops and fricatives as a function of position. Phonetica, 19, 95-102.

Malécot, A. (1970). The lenis-fortis opposition: Its physiological parameters. Journal of the Acoustical Society of America, 47, 1588-1592.

McBride, B., & Whitelaw, W. A. (1981). A physiological stimulus to upper airway receptors in humans. Journal of Applied Physiology, 51, 1179-1189.

Mead, J., Bouhuys, A., & Proctor, D. F. (1968). Mechanisms generating subglottic pressure. In Bouhuys, A. (Ed.), Sound production in man. New York: Annals of the Academy of Science (pp. 177-181).

Minsley, G., Warren, D. W., Dalston, R. M., & Hinton, V. A. (1988). Maintenance of intraoral pressure during speech after maxillary resection. Journal of the Acoustical Society of America, 83, 820-824.

Minsley, G., Warren, D. W., & Hinton, V. A. (1987). Physiologic responses to maxillary resection and subsequent obturation. Journal of Prosthetic Dentistry, 57, 338-344.

Moon, J. B., & Folkins, J. W. (1991). The effects of auditory feedback on the regulation of intra-oral air pressure during speech. Journal of the Acoustical Society of America, 90, 2992-2999.

Moon, J. B., Folkins, J. W., & Smith, A. (1993). Air pressure regulation during speech production. Journal of the Acoustical Society of America, 94, 54-63.

Müller, E. M., & Brown, W. S. (1980). Variations in the supraglottal air pressure waveform and their articulatory interpretation. In Lass, N. J. (Ed.), Speech and language: advances in basic research and practice. New York: Academic Press (pp. 317-389).

Netsell, R. (1969). Subglottal and intraoral air pressure during intervocalic contrast of /t/ and /d/. Phonetica, 20, 68-73.

Netsell, R. (1990). An acoustic regulation hypothesis. Cleft Palate Journal, 27, 59-60.

Nordin M., & Hagbarth, K-E. (1989). Mechanoreceptive unity in the human infraorbital nerve. Acta Physiologica Scandinavica, 135, 149-161.

Nordin M., & Thomander L. (1989). Intrafascicular multi-unit recordings from the human infraorbital nerve. Acta Physiologica Scandinavica, 135, 139-148.

Perkell, J. A. (1969). Physiology of speech production: Results and implications of a quantitative cineradiographic study. Cambridge: MIT Press.

Prosek, R. A., & House, A. (1975). Intraoral air pressure as a feedback cue in consonant production. Journal of Speech and Hearing Research, 18, 133-147.

Putnam A. H. B., & Ringel R. L. (1972). Some observations of articulation during labial sensory deprivation. Journal of Speech and Hearing Research, 15, 529-542.

Putnam, A. H. B., Shelton, R. L., & Kastner, C. V. (1986). Intraoral air pressure and oral airflow under different bleed and bite-block conditions. Journal of Speech and Hearing Research, 29, 37-49.

Remmers, J. E., & Bartlett, D. (1977). Reflex control of expiratory airflow and duration. Journal of Applied Physiology, 42, 80-87.

Ringel R. L., & Steer, M. D. (1963). Some effects of tactile and auditory alterations on speech output. Journal of Speech and Hearing Research, 6, 369-378.

Rochet, A. H. B., Morr, K. E., & Warren, D. W. (1989). Respiratory response to oral airflow perturbations during speech. Journal of the Acoustical Society of America, 85, 554 (Abstract).

Rothenberg, M. (1968). The breath-stream dynamics of simple-released-plosive production. Phonetica, 6, 1-117.

Russell, N. K., & Stathopoulos, E. (1988). Lung volume changes in children and adults during speech production. Journal of Speech and Hearing Research, 31, 146-155.

Sant'Ambrogio, G. (1982). Information arising from the tracheobronchial tree in mammals. Physiology Review, 62, 531-569.

Sant'Ambrogio, G., Matthew, O. P., Fisher, J. T., & Sant'Ambrogio, F. B. (1983). Laryngeal receptors responding to transmural pressure, airflow and local muscle activity. Respiratory Physiology, 54, 317-330.

Scherer, R. C., Curtis, J. F., & Titze, I. R. (1980). Pressure-flow relationships within static models of the larynx. Journal of the Acoustical Society of America, 68, 101 (Abstract).

Scott, C. M., & Ringel, R. L. (1971). Articulation without oral sensory control. Journal of Speech and Hearing Research, 14, 804-818.

Smith, A. (1992). The control of orofacial movements in speech. Critical Reviews In Oral Biology and Medicine, 3, 233-267.

Smith, H. Z., Allen, G. D., Warren, D. W., & Hall, D. J. (1978). The consistency of the pressure-flow technique for assessing oral port size. Journal of the Acoustical Society of America, 64, 1203-1206.

Smitheran, R., & Hixon, T. J. (1981). A clinical method for estimating laryngeal airway resistance during vowel production. *Journal of Speech and Hearing Disorders, 46,* 138-147.

Stathopoulos, E. T. (1986). Relationship between intraoral air pressure and vocal intensity in children and adults. *Journal of Speech and Hearing Research, 29,* 71-74.

Stathopoulos, E. T., & Weismer, G. (1985). Oral airflow and intraoral air pressure: A comparative study of children, youths and adults. *Folia Phoniatrica, 37,* 152-159.

Subtelny, J., Worth, J., & Sakuda, M. (1966). Intraoral pressure and rate of flow during speech. *Journal of Speech and Hearing Research, 9,* 498-518.

Titze, I. R. (1984). Parameterization of the glottal area, glottal flow, and vocal fold contact area. *Journal of the Acoustical Society of America, 75,* 570-580.

van den Berg, J. W. (1956). Direct and indirect determination of mean subglottic pressure. *Folia Phoniatrica, 8,* 1-24.

van den Berg, J. W., Zantema, J. T., & Doornenbal, P. (1957). On the air resistance and the Bernoulli effect of the human larynx. *Journal of the Acoustical Society of America, 29,* 626-631.

Warren, D. W. (1964). Velopharyngeal orifice size and upper pharyngeal pressure-flow patterns in cleft palate speech: A preliminary study. *Journal of Plastic and Reconstructive Surgery, 34,* 15-26.

Warren, D. W. (1967). Nasal emission of air and velopharyngeal function. *Cleft Palate Journal, 4,* 148-156.

Warren, D. W. (1975). The determination of velopharyngeal incompetence by aerodynamic and acoustical techniques. *Clinics in Plastic Surgery, 2,* 299-304.

Warren, D. W. (1976). Aerodynamics of speech production. In Lass, N. J. (Ed.), *Contemporary Issues in Experimental Phonetics.* New York: Academic Press (105-137).

Warren, D. W. (1979). Perci: a method for rating palatal efficiency. *Cleft Palate Journal, 16,* 279-285.

Warren, D. W. (1982). Aerodynamics of speech. In Lass, N. J., McReynolds, L. V., Northern, J. L., & Yoder, D. E., (Eds.), *Speech, language and hearing* (vol. I Normal Processes). Philadelphia: W. B. Saunders (pp. 219-245).

Warren, D. W. (1985a). Regulation/control of speech aerodynamics in cleft palate. *Asha, 27,* 111 (Abstract).

Warren, D. W. (1985b). Respiratory significance of the nasal grimace. *Asha, 27,* 82 (Abstract).

Warren, D. W. (1986a). Compensatory speech behaviors in individuals with cleft palate: A regulation/control phenomenon? *Cleft Palate Journal, 23,* 251-260.

Warren, D. W. (1986b). Regulation/control of speech aerodynamics. *Folia Phoniatrica, 38,* 368 (Abstract).

Warren, D. W. (1988). Aerodynamics of speech. In Lass, N. J., McReynolds, L. V., Northern, J. L., &

Yoder, D. E. (Eds), *Handbook of speech-language pathology and audiology.* St. Louis: Mosby (pp. 191-214).

Warren, D. W., Allen, G., & King, H. A. (1984). Physiologic and perceptual effects of induced anterior open bite. *Folia Phoniatrica, 36,* 164-173.

Warren, D. W., Dalston, R. M., Morr, K. E., Hairfield, W. M., & Smith, L. R. (1989). The speech regulating system: Temporal and aerodynamic responses to velopharyngeal inadequacy. *Journal of Speech and Hearing Research, 32,* 566-575.

Warren, D. W., Dalston, R. M., Trier, W. C., & Holder, M. B. (1985). A pressure-flow technique for quantifying temporal patterns of palatopharyngeal closure. *Cleft Palate Journal, 22,* 11-19.

Warren, D. W., & Devereux, J. L. (1966). An analog study of cleft palate speech. *Cleft Palate Journal, 3,* 103-114.

Warren, D. W., Duany, L. F., & Fischer, N. D. (1969). Nasal pathway resistance in normal and cleft lip and palate subjects. *Cleft Palate Journal, 6,* 134-140.

Warren, D. W., & DuBois, A. B. (1964). A pressure-flow technique for measuring velopharyngeal orifice area during continuous speech. *Cleft Palate Journal, 1,* 52-71.

Warren, D. W., Hairfield, W. M., & Dalston, E. T. (1991). Nasal airway impairment: The oral response in cleft palate patients. *American Journal of Orthodontics, 99,* 346-353.

Warren, D. W., & Hall, D. J. (1973). Glottal activity and intraoral pressure during stop consonant productions. *Folia Phoniatrica, 25,* 121-129.

Warren, D. W., Hall, D. J., & Davis, J. (1981). Oral port constriction and pressure airflow relationships during sibilant productions. *Folia Phoniatrica, 33,* 380-394.

Warren, D. W., Hinton, V. A., Pillsbury, H. C., & Hairfield, W. M. (1987). Effects of size of the nasal airway on nasal airflow rate. *Archives of Otolaryngology, 113,* 405-408.

Warren, D. W., & Mackler, S. B. (1968). Duration of oral port constriction in normal and cleft palate speech. *Journal of Speech and Hearing Research, 11,* 391-401.

Warren, D. W., Morr, K. E., Rochet, A. P., & Dalston, R. M. (1989). Respiratory response to a decrease in velopharyngeal resistance. *Journal of the Acoustical Society of America, 86,* 917-924.

Warren, D. W., Nelson, G., & Allen, G. D. (1980). Effects of increased vertical dimension on oral port size and fricative intelligibility. *Journal of the Acoustical Society of America, 67,* 1828-1831.

Warren, D. W., & Ryon, W. E. (1967). Oral port constriction, nasal resistance, and respiratory aspects of cleft palate speech: An analog study. *Cleft Palate Journal, 4,* 38-46.

Warren, D. W., & Wood, M. T. (1969). Respiratory volumes in normal speech: A possible reason for intraoral pressure differences among voiced and voiceless consonants. *Journal of the Acoustical Society of America, 45,* 466-469.

Warren, D. W., Wood, M. T., & Bradley, D. F. (1969). Respiratory volume in normal and cleft palate speech. *Cleft Palate Journal, 6,* 449-469.

Weismer, G., & Longstreth, D. (1980). Segmental gestures at the laryngeal level in whispered speech: Evidence from an aerodynamic study. *Journal of Speech and Hearing Research, 23,* 383-392.

Williams, W. N., Brown, W. S., & Turner, G. E. (1987). Intraoral air pressure discrimination by normal-speaking subjects. *Folia Phoniatrica, 39,* 196-203.

Wyke, B. (1981). Neuromuscular control systems in voice production. In Bless, D. (Ed.), *Vocal fold physiology: Contemporary research and clinical issues.* San Diego: College-Hill Press (pp. 71-76).

Suggested Readings

Mechanics of Breathing and Speech

Hixon, T. J. (1981). Respiratory function in speech. In Hixon, T. J. (Ed.), *Respiratory Function in Speech and Song.* Boston: College Hill Press (pp. 1-54).

Otis, A. B. (1988). Two functions of breathing: Respiration and sound production. In Mathew, O. P. (Ed.), *Respiratory Function of the Upper Airway.* New York: Marcel Dekker (pp. 519-532).

Proctor, D. F. (1980). Structure of breathing and phonatory mechanisms. In Proctor, D. F. (Ed.), *Breathing, Speech, and Song.* New York: Springer-Verlag (pp. 1-13).

Upper Airway Dynamics

Brancatisano, A., & Engel, L. A. (1988). Role of the upper airway in the control of respiratory flow and lung volume in humans. In Mathew, O. P. (Ed.), *Respiratory Function of the Upper Airway.* New York: Marcel Dekker (pp. 447-505).

Brobeck, J. R. (1965). Exchange, control and regulation. In Brobeck, J. R. (Ed.), *Physiological Controls and Regulation.* Philadelphia: W. B. Saunders (pp. 1-13).

Perkell, J. S. (1976). Responses to an unexpected suddenly induced change in the state of the vocal tract. Progress Report #117, Research Laboratory of Electronics, MIT (pp. 273-281).

Proctor, D. F. (1980). Breathing mechanics and phonation. In Proctor, D. F. (Ed.), *Breathing, Speech, and Song.* New York: Springer-Verlag (pp. 67-86).

Warren, D. W. (1986). Compensatory speech behaviors in individuals with cleft palate: a regulation/control phenomenon? *Cleft Palate Journal, 23,* 251-260.

Warren, D. W., Dalston, R. M., Morr, K. E., Hairfield, W. M., & Smith, L. R. (1989). The speech regulating system: Temporal and aerodynamic responses to velopharyngeal inadequacy. *Journal of Speech and Hearing Research, 32,* 566-575.

Application of Aerodynamic Techniques

Warren, D. W. (1975). The determination of velopharyngeal incompetency by aerodynamic and acoustical techniques. *Clinics in Plastic Surgery, 2,* 299-304.

Warren, D. W. (1979). Perci: A method for rating palatal efficiency. *Cleft Palate Journal, 16,* 279-285.

Warren, D. W. (1984). A quantitative technique for assessing nasal airway impairment. *American Journal of Orthodontics, 86,* 306-314.

Warren, D. W., Dalston, R. M., Trier, W. C., & Holder, M. B. (1985). A pressure-flow technique for quantifying temporal patterns of palatopharyngeal closure. *Cleft Palate Journal, 22,* 11-19.

Warren, D. W., & DuBois, A. B. (1964). A pressure-flow technique for measuring velopharyngeal orifice area during continuous speech. *Cleft Palate Journal, 1,* 52-71.

Chapter 3

Mechanisms of Speech Motor Execution and Control

James H. Abbs

INTRODUCTION

Over 15 years ago, in an introduction to a chapter on this same topic, I commented that the physiological mechanisms underlying the oral communication process represented a scientific challenge of major proportion. A very sizable part of that challenge remains. However, distinct gains have been made, and this chapter will examine some of the same issues in the light of those gains and with the benefit of 15 years of hindsight.

To provide a perspective on the importance of understanding speech motor execution and control, let me first restate that primary challenge. Specifically, the current understanding of speech production and its disorders is restricted primarily by comprehension of underlying motor-sensory systems. All of the processes theorized to be carried out by the central nervous system for speech generation (linguistic operations, element selection, movement sequencing and planning, coordination and regulation, and so on) are shaped, implemented, and manifested through motor programming and execution actions. The motor-sensory system thus acts as a filter that prevents one from using speech output as a direct reflection of presumed underlying organization. For this reason, when dealing with biologically based problems of speech, it is not particularly useful to focus on many of the easily measured and popular parameters borrowed, often unimaginatively, from experimental phonetics.

Figure 3-1 clarifies this point. It is a schematic block diagram of the speech motor control system, with specific reference to the accessibility of speech neural mechanisms. As noted, output components of the speech control mechanism are in large part directly observable. At a minimum the motor system functions that are immediately upstream from the speech output include (1) the obvious peripheral structures and their not-so-obvious mechanical response properties and (2) the multiple contributions of on-line sensorimotor control mechanisms, including but not restricted to the cerebellum, basal ganglia, red nucleus, and multiple areas of the cerebral neocortex (i.e., areas classically defined as primary motor, somatic sensory, premotor and supplementary motor, posterior parietal, and others). The nature of these sensorimotor contributions has been presented previously (Abbs, Gracco, and Cole, 1984; Abbs and Welt, 1985; Abbs and Winstein, 1990).

In principle, the mechanical response properties could be approximated through the use of quantitative analyses and modeling techniques. By contrast, however, the higher-level neural processes are simply inaccessible, especially in relation to their specific functional contributions to speech motor control. The only serious means to overcome this difficulty is through more explicit consideration of actual physiological mechanisms. This latter requirement is particularly important if one is to consider such knowledge as a basis for assessment and treatment of speech disorders associated with neurological problems, orofacial anomalies, or other yet-unspecified problems in speech motor coordination, learning, etc. The lack of information and the inaccessibility of the central neural mechanisms underlying speech and language have led to an empty kind of black box

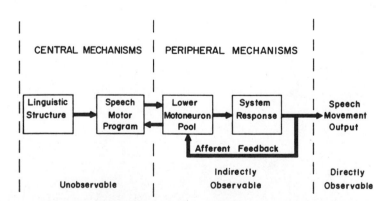

FIGURE 3-1   A highly schematic diagram of accessibility to various central and peripheral processes of speech motor control.

empiricism in speech and language models. The substance of these models is generally a series of consistent but abstract and nonexclusive assertions regarding the presumed central organization of hypothesized elements underlying speech system output. While such models are intellectually stimulating, they are hardly useful as a basis for understanding the physical and physiological functions of speech motor control.

The critical aspects of speech production cannot be appreciated because one cannot discern from an observation of speech output activity which aspects of that output reflect central control or an underlying linguistic code, and which components represent motor output contributions (sensorimotor control mechanisms and/or mechanical properties). In cases of speech disorders the weakness of black box empirical models is most apparent. For example, if we are to appreciate and aid an individual with parkinsonian speech movement control deficits, amyotrophic lateral sclerosis, or cleft palate, it is of little value to know that the acoustic formant transitions of this patient or another are somehow changed. Of course they are changed; but what about their problems in control of muscle contraction and movement? With respect to better understanding speech motor processes, some developments, such as those discussed in other chapters in this volume, facilitate direct observation of speech movements, speech muscle activity, and/or associated aerodynamic events. However, it seems at times that technique development and data gathering without purpose may have distracted from the key issue of underlying processes and mechanisms— analogous to trying to understand the genius of a painter by studying the directions of the brush strokes.

In this challenging context the purpose of this chapter is to synthesize some of what we know about the underlying physiology of speech production, particularly (1) mechanical properties of muscle contraction and movement and (2) motorsensory control mechanisms. As will be apparent, even a detailed account of the data, arguments, and hypotheses provides only a fragmented view of speech motor control. Progress in science is, after all, a series of discontinuous steps and blind alleys. The need for continued programs of research is obvious.

We have arbitrarily divided the speech production process into the peripheral mechanical properties and the mechanisms of sensorimotor

programming, control, and execution. An ideal representation must specify the interdependence of these divisions. However, to make our task manageable, we must evaluate these elements theoretically isolated from the total mechanism. In this vein there are certain dangers inherent in studying the speech motor-sensory system independent of upstream linguistic and planning functions. Breaking down this very complicated process into component parts is the essence of scientific advancement; if we insist that we can only learn from the whole, advances will be limited. Fortunately, over the past decade the long-held superstition that we could not learn from studies of nonspeech sensorimotor functions in humans or from the physiological and anatomical investigations in animals has subsided, at least in most circles. In fact, it is irrefutable that almost all of the major advances in understanding brain function and dysfunction have been based to some, if not a major, degree on basic biomedical research in more than one species. Furthermore, there are distinct advantages in exploring the peripheral orofacial motor system isolated from any single swallowing, deglutition, mastication, or communication function.

PERIPHERAL MECHANICAL PROPERTIES

The speech production system is not simply the bones, muscles, tendons, and ligaments of the respiratory, laryngeal, and orofacial mechanisms. A functional description must include lower motoneurons, somatic sensory receptors, their afferent projections, and the many primary and secondary cortical, cerebellar, and basal ganglia representations of these systems. Imagine if you will the conceptual emptiness of a model of the tongue or larynx without the elegance of a nervous system to control it! On the other hand, the greatest advantage of focusing on the peripheral processes and systems is that analyses of these more peripheral components may make it possible to discern how they operate as part of the whole, including the central nervous system.

The importance of biomechanical factors has for some time been recognized in most models of speech motor control. While some effort has been made to incorporate these factors, sufficiently detailed models specific to the tongue, lips, jaw, or even respiratory system, particularly in their functions for speech, are not available. Basically, in large part, these properties have not been measured, simulated, or synthesized into a functional model; this has not changed significantly over the past two decades. Some workers have labored on these problems, but far too few investigators with the combined backgrounds in physics, biology, and mathematics have focused their efforts on the speech production system. Therefore, there has been little progress in quantitative evaluation of these properties in relation to their actual physical influence on speech movements, particularly in the articulatory system. Nevertheless, they must be considered.

The inherent mechanics of speech are quite complex. The critical movements of the ribs, diaphragm, larynx, tongue, lips, jaw, and velopharyx are much more than a simple consequence of muscle contractions. Muscle-generated forces exert nonlinear, multidimensional and changing pulling actions upon the body parts to be moved, and those body parts each have different resistances to those pulls. The respiratory system is mostly elastic or stiff, while the jaw and tongue have more **inertia** and are more sluggish, given the pulling forces and movement speeds required. The degree to which **stiffness** and inertia must be overcome is not constant but varies with distances and speed of movement; consider pulling a spring a short or long distance or slowly lifting versus throwing a large rock. These features are a critical part of why speech actions are what they are, and determine that the nervous system perform in a certain manner. Interestingly, in our speech-centric view of biology and motor functions, we once thought that stiffness and inertia posed limitations to speech movements. In actuality, of course, inertia and elasticity most appropriately are considered energy storage mechanisms, and although they may absorb energy generated during one interval of time, they can release that energy for later contributions to the system's output. Mechanically stored elastic energy is known to facilitate, not limit, the control of respiratory maneuvers for generation of speech air pressures.

Another example closely related to rapid movement is found in the biomechanics of the frog's jump. The frog's gastrocnemius muscle (the jumping muscle) has a rather long tendon. In this motor phenomenon the energy stored in a stretched tendon allows the frog to move his hind limb much faster than the gastrocnemius muscle contraction alone can provide. Mechanical facilitation of this sort is widespread in motor systems. It is reasonable to expect that in highly evolved systems like those for respiration, swallowing, chewing, and communication, similar mechanical facilitation is operating to assist the generation of speech movements. Research on the biomechanics of the lip muscles also indicates the operation of such phenomena (Müller, Abbs, and Kennedy, 1985).

While the peripheral biomechanical properties of motor systems in their full biophysical complexity are beyond the scope of this chapter, a brief history helps put them in perspective. It is useful to separate biomechanical characteristics into three major categories: (1) the active muscle properties, (2) distribution or translation of muscle forces to create movements and muscle tension, and (3) passive mechanical contributions. The nature of these factors and their hypothetical interaction are illustrated schematically in Fig. 3-2. The interaction of these three factors as illustrated varies considerably, depending on the speech muscle group under study and the desired level of model sophistication.

Active Muscle Properties

The output of the nervous system is a series of motoneuron discharges that activate the several muscles involved. The deceptively simple process by which motoneuron discharge causes muscle fibers to shorten and to produce pulling forces (i.e., the active properties of muscle) has been the subject of a considerable research effort in physiology and biomechanics. For example, the most recent semicomprehensive review on muscle properties (Partridge and Benton, 1981) had 532 references, and Partridge reports that this was but a fraction of the total (personal communication, 1983). The reason for the size of this effort is that the relationship between motoneuron firing as an input to a muscle and force as an output is easily as complex as the generation and manipulation of acoustic signals by the vocal tract. The critical complication lies in the mapping between motoneuron firing and muscle force, or motoneuron firing and muscle shortening. Specifically, a number of intervening variables, such as muscle length, rate of muscle shortening or lengthening, the load against which the muscle is pulling (elastic, inertial, or viscous), the degree of fatigue, and the type of muscle fiber (to name a few), influence how a nervous system input acts upon muscle. For example, even in the simplest case (isometric contraction) without changes in the rate or number of motoneurons firing, the amount of

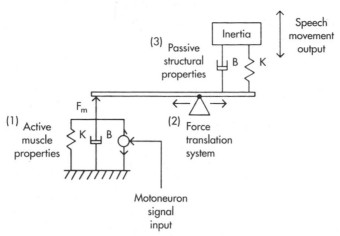

FIGURE 3-2   Schematic illustration of the multiple factors intervening between motoneuron discharge and speech movement. F_m, K, and B are the mechanical properties of force, elasticity, and viscosity, respectively.

force produced by a contracting muscle varies with muscle length. We know this inherently; lifting a heavy object with your arm flexed is easier than lifting the same object with your arm extended because the biceps produce more force for the same activation with the muscle at the length associated with elbow flexion. Similarly, how fast a given muscle will produce the movement depends on the load being lifted; as the load gets heavier, the rate of shortening becomes less, even with the same pattern of motoneuron activation.

One way to illustrate the transfer between motoneuron discharge activity and muscle contraction force is to represent muscle contraction as a mechanical rather than a biological process. Such representations, as shown in Figure 3-3, can be made by thinking about muscles in terms used for mechanical systems with elastic and viscous elements. Muscle models developed in this way have been shown to characterize a large variety of forces and movements. Early efforts to model the mechanical properties of muscle concentrated on developing precise descriptions of isometric and isotonic contractile states and responses of isolated muscle to twitch and tetanus electrical stimuli.

Many such muscle models were activated by an ideal contractile element (Fig. 3-3, C) in parallel or in series with constant viscous and elastic elements. These viscoelastic components are linear approximations to empirically derived curves (Fig. 3-3, *curves a, b, c*). The goal of these models was to provide a means of incorporating active muscle properties into larger neural control models, a purpose not inconsistent with the present chapter. Hence, in these models the

muscle output force, F_m, is not a simple function of the level of neural input but depends, as it must, also on the mechanical parameters associated with the active state. In the model defined here muscle activity is represented on four different levels: (1) bioelectrical level (electromyogram, or EMG, measured in volts); (2) biomechanical contractile force (C, measured in dynes); (3) the biomechanical parameters of elasticity (K, measured in dynes per centimeter) and **viscosity** (B, measured in dynes per centimeter per second); and (4) the muscle length (measured in centimeters), the associated movement variables (velocity and acceleration measured in centimeter per second and centimeter per second^2), and the muscle output force F_m (measured in dynes). The relationship among these levels is not simple. For example, the electromechanical transfer function (Fig. 3-3) would vary with the assumed relationship between EMG and motor unit firing rate.

Because speech movements involve rapid transitions by the articulatory musculature between the active and passive states, the constant linear models described here and shown in Fig. 3-3 may not provide the best means for simulating speech movements. In a parametrically forced model (Milhorn, 1966) where the state variables (K_p and B, in Fig. 3-3) are directly influenced by neural input, the change from a compliant to a stiff elastic viscous body (and the implicit dynamics) is accomplished in an explicit manner (unlike a linear model). In an interesting review (Greene, 1969) it was shown that a three-element model, if parametrically forced, could accurately predict isometric tension as a function of time for twitch and tetanus, and was

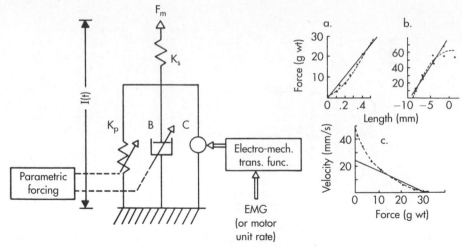

FIGURE 3-3 Basic mechanical features of muscle contraction. Two competing theories for muscle activation are represented (ideal contractile [C] and parametric; refer to text). K_p, K_s, and B are the parallel and series muscle elasticity and apparent viscosity, respectively. The muscle output force, F_m, drives the speech articulator as depicted in Figure 3-2. The curves shown in the right half of the figure (after Green, 1969) are adaptations of earlier results (Abbott and Wilkie, 1953; Jewell and Wilkie, 1958). They illustrate muscle data that the model attempts to encompass: (a) the load—extension curve of the series elastic element in the frog sartorius muscle, (b) the tension—length curve of contracting frog sartorius muscle, and (c) force—velocity curve of isometrically contracting sartorius muscle. The solid lines are linear approximations to the various corresponding data curves.

superior to the ideal contractile model in its prediction of isometric peak tension as a function of stimulus rate. In a parametrically forced model, the ideal contractile element, C, is no longer required to activate the model, since force is produced by changes in K_p.

Because of the necessity to incorporate mechanical properties that are influenced by the activity level of the neuromuscular system, such properties must be considered in the development of speech models. One **active mechanical property** is related to the rate of muscle shortening and is referred to as **apparent viscosity** (Fig. 3-3, *B*) (Fenn and Marsh, 1935; Hill, 1938). The rate at which a muscle can convert chemical energy to mechanical energy is limited. Apparent viscosity is manifested in the observation that the maximum force a muscle can apply is reduced as its rate of shortening increases, as indicated in Fig. 3-3, *curve C*. One would expect this active viscosity to be an important consideration in many of the speech muscles, especially in view of the rather high-velocity transient movements that are required for speech.

In addition to active viscosity, the inherent parallel elasticity (Fig. 3-3 K_p) of a muscle is known to vary directly with the level of active contraction; that is, the greater the contraction,

the greater the internal muscle elasticity. Wilkie (1956, p. 177) suggests that "resting muscle is soft and freely extensible. On stimulation the muscle passes into a new physical state—it becomes hard, develops tension, resists stretching, lifts loads." This statement illustrates a unique role of muscle contraction in speech production. Active elasticity appears to be a particularly significant element, since many of the moving parts in the speech system, such as the tongue, soft palate, and throat walls, are composed primarily of muscle tissue. It is conceivable that the mechanical properties of these structures are actively tuned to optimize particular patterns of movement. An active tuning mechanism is associated with contractions of the vocalis muscle in the control of vocal fold vibration.

Much of the mass of the lips, tongue, velopharynx, and pharynx is muscle tissue. In this respect the role of muscle stiffness in speech actions becomes important. For example, the orbicularis oris muscle acts as a sphincter that closes the oral cavity and provides interlabial contact forces for bilabial occlusion. However, since the orbicularis oris makes up much of the mass of the lips, as the level of contraction increases, the lips appear to become stiffer. In

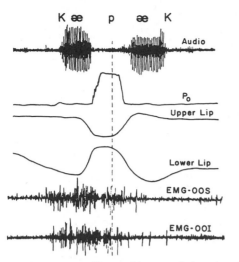

FIGURE 3-4 An oscillographic record showing the speech acoustic signal (Audio), intraoral air pressure (P_o) for upper and lower lips, and electromyographic tracing (EMG) from lip muscles: orbicularis oris superior (OOS) and orbicularis oris inferior (OOI). The record illustrates the momentary *inhibition* of the orbicularis oris muscle in synchrony with the release of the bilabial stop [p]. The time of release is indicated by the vertical dashed line.

the relaxed state, the lips have an average elasticity of 200 dynes per centimeter. At a level of contraction equivalent to that observed for bilabial closure, the value increased to 200 dynes per centimeter. It appears that without the active muscle stiffening, the lips would not maintain an appropriate seal for the impoundment of intraoral air pressure. Likewise, sudden relaxation of the orbicularis oris would result in reduced elasticity of the lips, making them distensible. This observation suggests that muscle elasticity of the orbicularis oris is part of the mechanism of bilabial stop release.

To illustrate the operation of this phenomenon, Figure 3-4 shows an oscillographic record of orbicularis oris EMG, along with the speech acoustic signal, intraoral air pressure, and upper and lower lip movement (inferior-superior dimension only). Just prior to the instant of bilabial release (as indicated on the record), there is a momentary shutdown in orbicularis oris EMG activity. These observations suggest that the release of the bilabial stop is implemented via control of inherent orbicularis oris elasticity. That is, the release event appears to be implemented, at least in part, by a pulse of inhibition to the orbicularis oris muscle. This example illustrates the importance of active muscle prop-

erties in understanding even some of the basic features of speech. Without this perspective, one might assume that labial stop release is generated exclusively by a positive separating force from the depressor labii inferior or levator labii superior muscles. It is obvious from the present example that to generate such interpretations one must appreciate fully peripheral mechanical properties and particularly the central levels of speech motor control. Observation of speech movement and/or speech EMG without considering active muscle elasticity may well lead to simplistic conclusions. The widespread analyses of EMG without movement that were so popular in the 1970s and early 1980s were in this respect seriously flawed.

Variations in the Muscle Force Translation System

While the level of muscle force, F_m, can be viewed as resulting from electromechanical processing of motoneuron activation, the contribution of this force to movement in various speech and nonspeech tasks depends on its geometry in relation to what is being moved. Most motor acts, including speech, result from many muscles acting in three dimensions to create a net force or torque that generates movement. As structures are changed in their position and a muscle shortens or lengthens, the effective muscle force provided will change, even though the activation level of that muscle may not. One common example of variations in the muscle force translated to a structure is the lever type of biomechanical mechanism found in skeletal muscle systems. Most investigators find it necessary to take into account changes in effective muscle force that occur as a result of such structure position changes (Penrod, Davy, and Singh, 1972; Alexander, 1981).

A hypothetical example of this phenomenon in the orofacial system is the change in effective muscle force generated by the anterior belly of the digastric (ABD) for jaw lowering movements. As illustrated in Figure 3-5,*A*, the ABD has its origin in the diagastric fossa of the mandible and inserts into the hyoid bone via a tendinous loop. If it can be assumed that (1) the mandible rotates around an axis at the condyle and (2) during jaw lowering the hyoid bone and skull remain fixed, the variation in the effective muscle force provided by the ABD as a function of jaw position can be specified. As illustrated

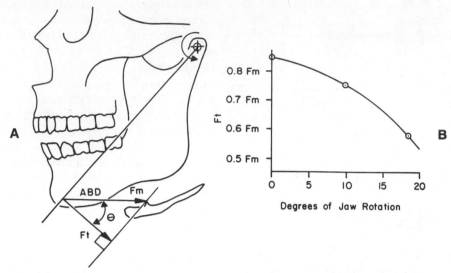

FIGURE 3-5 Influence of variations in moment arm (mechanical advantage) for contraction forces of the anterior belly of the diagastric muscle (ABD) with changes in jaw position. *A,* A schematic representation of the force generated by ABD (Fm) and the vector of that force that is tangent to the arc of rotation θ of the jaw (Ft), and *B,* Calculated variation in Ft as a function of degrees of jaw rotation from rest (0 degrees) to approximately 2 cm of inter incisor separation (18.5 degrees).

in Figure 3-5, *A,* of the total muscle force provided by the ABD (F_m), only the component tangent to the arc of mandibular rotation (Ft) produces mandibular rotation. It is also apparent from Figure 3-5, *A,* that the magnitude of the *Ft* vector is proportional to the cosine of the angle θ. Thus, as the jaw is lowered, θ becomes increasingly large and the effective force available to rotate the jaw, *Ft,* is reduced in proportion to the cosine of this angle. The curve shown in Figure 3-5, *B,* is an illustration of the hypothetical change in the effective ABD jaw lowering force *(Ft)* as a function of the position of the jaw. This example is not to be taken literally but merely illustrates the fact that the contribution of a muscle contraction with a constact muscle contraction force varies with position of the joint across which that muscle acts.*

The variations in effective ABD force illustrate the limitations in interpreting measures from these systems. Specifically, if one were to observe EMG in the ABD during jaw movement, the relative amplitude changes for various speech tasks could only be understood in relation to the effective jaw-lowering force of that muscle, which appears to depend on jaw position. In other words, the EMG levels would be expected to correspond to the force generated by the ABD (F_m), not the force available to generate movement *(Ft).* In respect to speech movements and muscles, this kind of variation is seemingly ubiquitous. For example, a related and even more complicated example of this same phenomenon is that of the effective lip closing force provided by the orbicularis oris inferior *(OOI)* muscle. When the lower lip is depressed, the muscle force provided by the OOI has a distinct superiorly directed component that acts to raise the lip toward closure. However, when the lip is at rest, the primary vector of muscle force of this OOI is horizontal and appears to act primarily to draw the corners of the mouth medially; the ability of the OOI to elevate the lip from rest is practically nil. At any position between lip depression and rest, the effective superiorly directed force provided by the OOI thus varies as a function of the sine of the angle between the fibers of this muscle and the horizontal plane. Thus, as with the ABD, it is obvious that EMG from the orbicularis oris can be interpreted only with a knowledge of the position of the lip itself. This kind of variation is especially significant for researchers who are

*I am aware that the mandible does not rotate around a constant center of rotation; the first research on jaw rotation and translation was conducted in my laboratory (Eilenberg and Abbs, 1974).

attempting to relate relative levels of EMG activity to certain speech production tasks.

While variations in muscle force translation are additional complications in our attempt at understanding the motor execution of speech production, such phenomena in turn highlight the elegance of the neural control mechanisms, which must take into account such variations to generate proper speech movements.

Passive Mechanical Properties

Often when speech researchers speak of system mechanical properties, they refer to passive properties. These components can be thought of as (1) the bone, skin, tendons, ligaments, and fatty tissue, which do not receive neural input, and (2) muscle in a nonactivated state. The influences of these passive components are modeled by the biomechanical parameters described previously, namely, inertia, elasticity, and viscosity. Thus, when a mechanical system moves through a certain pattern of motion, these three **passive mechanical properties** influence the process in a particular manner, and each requires a special component of the applied force. Conceptually, if you think about a mass connected via a spring to a fixed point, the role of these various properties can be appreciated. When you first start to move the mass, the force required is primarily to overcome the inertia of the mass itself. Conversely, at the starting position, the stiffness of the spring is relatively insignificant. However, as the mass gets into motion and the spring gets stretched, the applied force is used more to overcome the stiffness of the spring, especially as it is stretched further and further. In this simple example, the passive resistance of the mass is proportional to how fast it is brought up to some speed (acceleration) and the passive resistance of the spring is related to the distance moved (displacement).

As noted earlier, components of elasticity and inertia are inherent energy storage devices, hence temporally redistribute the applied force in relation to the resultant motion. For example, in the respiratory system as it operates for both speech and other purposes, passive elasticity stored in the rib cage during inspiration generates respiratory volume reductions and produces air pressures for speech expiration. Indeed, only after the recoil forces were measured and incorporated into models of respiration were physiologists able to evaluate possible neural

control of respiration for speech (Mead, Bouhuys, and Proctor, 1968). It is probable that peripheral control of laryngeal and articulatory movements likewise depends on inherent passive properties. Unfortunately, they appear more complex than respiration, and our understanding of those properties has not progressed to the same degree. Study of the simpler respiratory system does, however, provide provocative clues. In any case, it is clear that one cannot understand movements and/or EMG patterns without an appreciation of these passive properties.

Simulation of Speech System Peripheral Biomechanics

There have been some reports of mathematically explicit models of the speech production periphery (Perkell, 1974; Abbs and Eilenberg, 1976). With such models one can presumably simulate the relations between motoneuron discharge and speech movements, including all biomechanical properties described here. In principle, we can learn whether our hypotheses regarding relationships between applied muscle force and movement are sound; that is, whether their measured values of system biomechanical variables and hypothesized interactions between these variables are reasonable approximations of the actual system. The biomechanical models generated admittedly have been simplistic and lack the isomorphism required for their optimal use as tools to explore system function. However, in the future, as these modeling efforts mature, one should be able (1) to provide a more meaningful representation of the several control signals that must be available to drive articulatory structures during speech production and (2) to assess some models of speech motor control.

While mechanical properties represent the most peripheral and accessible aspects of the speech system, it is on this peripheral keyboard that the nervous system maestro must play to generate the patterns we recognize as speech. If we are impressed with the peripheral complexity and elegance, they pale by comparison with the motor-sensory processes of the nervous system.

Motor-Sensory Programming, Execution, and Control

For a time the neural processes underlying speech production were conceptualized as a series of layers, with the upper layers seemingly reflecting the contribution of the nervous system. It was often implied and even at times explicitly stated that linguistically identified elements were pumped into the uppermost layer, and after some filtering these were transmitted in a recognizable fashion to the articulators. One sometimes still sees such explanations. However, from the standpoint of a modern neurobiologist, these are merely abstractions, with little support theoretically or empirically. Their inadequacy lies in the fact that the processes of speech motor control and execution are not simply filtering and transmitting linguistic entities. Rather, specific muscle contractions, movements, and forces involved in producing those elements are determined as part of a flexible and dynamic process. Because motor-sensory mechanisms appear to be the key elements in speech motor execution, programming, and control, those processes will be the focus of the remainder of this chapter.*

Speech scientists of the 1960s and 1970s debated whether in the most global sense sensorimotor processes contributed significantly to the moment-to-moment control of speech production. For over a decade that general issue has been settled. Starting in the early 1980s a series of experiments were conducted to show that (1) afferent projections from the jaw, lips, and tongue in particular, and most probably from laryngeal and respiratory muscles and sites, are continuously monitored by the nervous system as a basis for moment-to-moment adjustments and corrections in motor output; (2) the nature of this sensory-based regulation is complex, with sensory information from a given movement or site being used not only to make adjustments at that site but also to coordinate actions among movements and articulators; and (3) such sensory adjustments are involved not only in controlling the magnitude of movement or muscle contraction but also in the timing among the many actions necessary for speech (Abbs, Shaiman, Gracco, and Cole 1985; Shaiman,

*It has been popular in speech production to discuss the organization of phonetic elements as a motor programming process. This is at variance with how this term is used by the much larger group of neurobiologists who study motorsensory mechanisms. In the latter convention motor programming refers variously to the organization of multiple muscle contractions and movements underlying natural motor behavior. This chapter adopts the convention of the neurobiologists.

Abbs, and Gracco, 1985; Connor, 1989). Understanding these control mechanisms provides useful insight into both normal speech motor processes and disorders thereof.

Basic Sensorimotor Mechanisms

The change in perspective on how sensorimotor processes contribute to the control of speech movements was due to changes in basic research and to advances in available technology. For 40 years neurophysiologists concerned with how sensory input influenced motor output studied the microphysiology of various reflex arcs in the spinal motor system. This work provided very precise understanding of (1) the sensory information available on the length of a muscle, its tension, and the position of a joint and (2) the peripheral influence of this **afferent** activity on associated **efferent** fibers. To a large extent, however, these basic studies dealt with acute preparations in the spinal motor systems of anesthetized animals. That work did not provide the basis to document (to the satisfaction of most investigators dealing with voluntary motor control in waking organisms, especially humans) that afferent mechanisms were crucial elements in on-line motor control. The counterargument was that spindle, tendon, and joint receptor information was part of a long latency–slow monitoring system for control of involuntary postural or slow motor activities and/or to provide peripheral status information as a basis for centrally generated motor commands.

The principal studies that bridged the gap from anesthetized cats to waking, performing humans must be credited to the late Edward Evarts. Evarts, a psychiatrist with an interest in motor behavior, devised a technique that made it possible to record activity from individual neural **pyramidal cells** in the primary motor neocortex of monkeys while they performed certain kinds of movements. This technique immediately provided data on a question that heretofore was only the subject of speculation; that is, what kinds of brain activity were involved in movement planning, programming, and control? In those experiments Evarts developed a paradigm whereby he would interrupt ongoing movement, in effect creating a motor output error, and then observe motor cortex changes in response to the induced error. Consistently there was a relatively short latency response in the primary motor cortex, documenting the operation of central nervous system monitoring of sensory inputs and pyramidal cell correction of motor output errors. A flurry of experiments followed in waking animals and in human subjects, with the observation that unanticipated induced errors (perturbations) led to motor output corrections with latencies far shorter than conventional reaction times but longer than stretch reflexes. Moreover, there were corrections at several different latencies, possibly corresponding to multiple sensorimotor adjustments, via lower motoneurons, pyramidal cells of the primary motor cortex, and even pathways via the cerebellum and basal ganglia.

Since Evarts's initial observations, motor control studies of the arm, hand, eye, head, locomotion, and speech movements have increasingly indicated that these motor acts depend moment to moment on somatic sensory input. This work, ranging from studies in anesthetized animals to waking humans performing functional motor acts, thus changed the general view of sensorimotor contributions. Sensory information appears to project from peripheral sites to almost all motor centers in the central nervous system, with moment-to-moment modulations of motor output. It also was apparent that while general motor goals (e.g., speech acoustic outputs) were planned, the specific pattern of muscle contraction and individual joint movements to accomplish those goals were programmed flexibly in an on-line fashion. This framework offers a background upon which to consider motor-sensory processes in speech production.

Sensorimotor Contributions to Speech Motor Control

The role of sensory input in control of speech movements has been a scientific focus for at least 50 years. The first attempt to disrupt nonauditory afferent feedback in the speech system apparently was made by Guttman (1954), who bilaterally anesthetized touch and pain of the tongue, lower lip, and superficial tissues of the mandible, presumably via blockade of the inferior alveolar and lingual branches of the mandibular nerve. Subsequent studies by McCroskey (1958), McCroskey, Corley, and Jackson (1959), Weber (1961), Ringel and Steer (1963), Scott and Ringel (1971a, 1971b), and others involved similar anesthetization procedures, with some additions.

Unfortunately, because of methodological and conceptual difficulties, these studies did not provide much specific information concerning the sensorimotor control of speech. There is a serious difficulty with all experiments that use system disturbance as a manipulation. What we learn is how that system functions without the part that was removed, not necessarily what that part contributed; that is, how well speech could be produced without certain somatic sensory input. Because of an increased awareness of the plasticity and adaptation of the nervous system, it is believed that preservation of speech motor function in studies of experimental anesthetization was due to an ability to use different sensory inputs alternatively to accomplish the same motor goals. For example, while anesthetization techniques resulted in partial loss of sensation, seldom was the loss complete or without substantial residual to implement other processes to produce almost as good desired movements. Specifically, while anesthetization of the inferior alveolar branch of the trigeminal nerve (mandibular branch) yields loss of sensation in the lower face and lip, **spindles** in jaw-closing muscles, the tongue, and many other afferents remain intact, including cutaneous mechanoreceptors in the posterior third of the tongue, the hard palate, the upper face and lip, and baroreceptors in the pharynx. Claiming that sensation is not used in normal speech motor control from these experiments is analogous to claiming that vision is not important in upright posture and equilibrium, simply because the blind can stand and walk.

The techniques employed to assess speech motor changes with sensory deprivation also were somewhat inappropriate. Often, speech errors were counted and categorized to assess the influence of neural blockade. If one is attempting to analyze a neuromuscular control system that has muscle tension and/or structural movement as an output, judgments of remote end outcomes are inadequate for discerning subtle variations in the nature of that output. Likewise, the specific properties of the speech system's output that might be affected most directly by the anesthetization procedures (i.e., muscle tension, muscle length, joint position, movement) were not monitored. Measures such as the acoustic signal, phonetic transcription, and judged correctness of production are several complex steps removed from the motor output of the system and likely to be confounded by

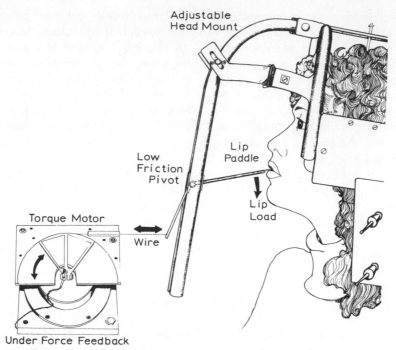

FIGURE 3-6   Subject with direct current brushless torque motor apparatus set up to apply unanticipated perturbations to the lower lip.

physical and perceptual distortion. Moreover, as we know of disordered speech, the compensatory capabilities of the speech system often lead to a speech output that is acoustically and perceptually acceptable, despite considerable compensatory reorganization in the individual motor activities that generated those productions.

Perturbation Analyses of Speech Motor-Sensory Processes

As reflected in the work of Evarts mentioned earlier, the litmus test of sensorimotor contributions to control of a particular motor act is to introduce an unanticipated error and examine the nature of the corrections, if any, to that disturbance. In speech this test was first conducted in an experiment published by Folkins and Abbs (1976). For this study a custom tooth splint permitted the application of loads to the jaw during speech. Resistive loads, albeit crude, were applied with a device that stopped upward jaw movement in the same manner that a bicycle brake stops a wheel: via activation of a solenoid. Movements of the upper lip, lower lip, and jaw were monitored. Subjects did not know when the jaw movement was to be interrupted. In all

cases of interruption, subjects produced adequate bilabial closure. Lip and jaw movements that accompanied interruptions demonstrated a clear pattern of on-line compensation. Specifically, when the jaw movement was reduced, both upper and lower lips compensated to avoid speech disruption.

Additional studies were subsequently undertaken with more sophisticated instruments (Abbs and Gracco, 1982, 1984; Gracco and Abbs, 1982, 1985, 1987, 1988, 1989). Some representative experiments in which the unanticipated perturbation technique has been used provide a number of useful insights. Figure 3-6 illustrates how a brushless DC torque motor was coupled to the lower lip to introduce unanticipated perturbations during speech. Loads from the torque motor were transmitted to the lower lip via a steel wire and a low friction lever. Similar coupling was used to apply loads to the upper lip or jaw. The torque motor was under force feedback control, permitting the motor to follow lower lip, upper lip, or jaw movements at low, constant tracking forces (3 to 5 g). According to subject reports and associated EMG and movement, these low tracking forces appear to offer indiscernible resistance to normal movements. For lower lip perturbations inferiorly

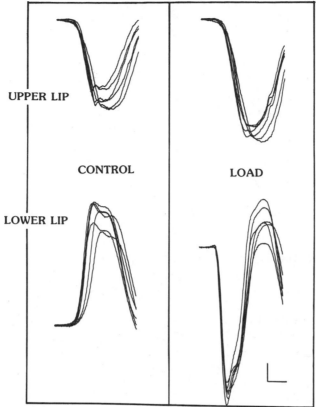

FIGURE 3-7 Lip movement adjustments in response to unanticipated perturbations of lower lip movements during speech.

directed loads ranging from 10 to 40 g were superimposed on the constant tracking forces. The load forces employed and the displacement perturbations they produced were within the physiological range of forces and displacements normally associated with lip movements in speech. Loads were applied in the 100-ms interval ranging from 50 ms prior to OOI contraction onset (the vertical lines in Figs. 3-7 and 3-8) to 50 ms after that onset. To eliminate confounding due to anticipation, loads were introduced randomly on only 10% to 15% of the movement trials.

The movement and EMG responses to these perturbations provided additional direct support for sensorimotor actions in speech movement control. As illustrated in Figure 3-7, velocity and displacement of both upper and lower lip movements were adjusted in response to the lower lip perturbation. That is, while the perturbation was applied to the lower lip, compensations were seen in both upper and lower lip muscles. Clear compensatory responses such as those shown in Figure 3-8

were observed even if the loads were introduced as late as 25 ms after the onset of the orbicularis oris inferior muscle burst. In the approximately 100 naive subjects studied with this paradigm in several different laboratories, quantitative analyses of kinematics and EMG revealed consistent, statistically significant changes to these loads (Folkins and Abbs, 1975; Abbs and Gracco, 1984; Gracco and Abbs, 1985, 1989).

In addition, these studies provided some important insights into sensorimotor actions for speech. First, despite some sizable movement perturbations (more than 15 mm in some studies), the intended speech motor objective was not disrupted in a discernible way (i.e., a listener could not distinguish acoustic speech patterns for loaded trials from those produced during normal, unloaded trials). Seemingly, the nervous system's objective was to occlude the vocal tract, with flexibility in lip and jaw movements that might be utilized in that process. Second, compensations such as the ones shown in Figures 3-7 and 3-8 were observed the

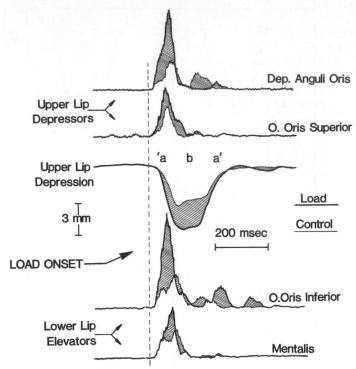

Dep. Anguli Oris

Upper Lip
Depressors

O. Oris Superior

Upper Lip
Depression

'a   b   a'

Load

Control

3 mm

200 msec

LOAD ONSET

O.Oris Inferior

Lower Lip
Elevators

Mentalis

FIGURE 3-8   Muscle activity (EMG) adjustments in response to unanticipated perturbations of lower lip movements during speech.

first time a load was introduced. These observations appear to indicate that the sensorimotor compensations reflect normal processes of speech movement control. Other results indicating that these sensorimotor processes are utilized in natural situations come from studies in which load magnitudes were limited to 10 to 15 g, producing perturbation displacements as small as 1 mm (Abbs and Gracco, 1984). Even with these small perturbations the EMG and movement responses were statistically significant and comparable to those illustrated in Figures 3-7 and 3-8. The suggestion that these sensorimotor processes are an integral component of speech movement control also is reflected in verbal reports of subjects in these experiments. When asked how many times their lip got stuck, subjects consistently underestimated the load occurrence by a factor of at least 5 to 1 (e.g., if 50 loads were introduced in a session, estimates never exceeded 10). Furthermore, when asked their reactions to the perturbations, a common response was that the loads were no problem; the subject ignored them. Finally, when subjects were instructed to stop all lip movements if they sensed a load, cessation of EMG and movement was never accomplished until compensation had occurred and lip closure was achieved.

Another interesting aspect of these speech sensorimotor processes was the fact that the response latencies in a particular muscle (either upper or lower lip) varied with the timing of the load onset and certain parameters of perturbation (Gracco and Abbs, 1985). For example, the mean latency of the compensatory increase in muscle activity varied from 72 ms with loads introduced 45 ms before OOS onset to 36 ms for loads introduced 15 ms after the onset of the muscle burst. For perturbations introduced at points even later, other forms of compensatory responses were observed, apparently depending upon the moment-to-moment dynamics of the motor execution process (Gracco and Abbs, 1985, 1989). Sensorimotor actions apparently were operating throughout the motor execution interval for these lip closures. That is, while the nature of these responses varied with perturbation timing and magnitude, functionally useful compensatory responses were always discernible, indicating that this complex behavior is never independent of on-line sensorimotor influence. The adaptive response latencies also indicate the operation of a flexible, task-dependent central nervous system control process. Indeed, in these various studies time-locked stereotypical muscle responses (as might be indicative of reflex mechanisms) were conspicuously absent. Of particular interest was the absence of short latency responses that might suggest peripheral reflex involvement (lower brain stem reflexes have a latency of 15 to 18 ms for facial muscles).

These and similar studies also demonstrate that the role of somatic sensory input in the control of speech movements is at least as important as in the control of similar movements of the hand, arms, head, and eyes. However, merely acknowledging that sensory mechanisms play an important role in these processes is not sufficient. Specifically, to begin to appreciate how deficits in sensory inputs and processes may contribute to speech disorders requires a refinement of our understanding and perhaps, as pointed out in the following comments, an awareness that such contributions are not likely to be simple.

Multiple Roles for Speech Motor-Sensory Mechanisms

In parallel with documentation that sensory mechanisms are likely to play a key role in the control of speech has also come increasing evidence of the complexity of that role. Since the early formulations of Grant Fairbanks (1954), we have operated under the shadow of the then popular notions of cybernetics and the classical feedback loop. However, in the past decade, the conceptualization of sensory input contributing to motor output via some sort of a closed-loop corrective or reactive feedback action in the minds of some has been a straw man with little likelihood of being correct in even the most limited manner. Indeed, even the first studies in which unanticipated mechanical disturbances were introduced upon speech movements indicated that the errors are seldom corrected as such but rather are canceled by short latency adjustments distributed throughout the speech motor system. For example, perturbations of lower lip movements during a speech gesture associated with labial closure yield functional compensatory actions in the upper lip and jaw in addition to adjustments in the lower lip itself; the corrections are not confined to lower lip adjustments, as would be predicted from a classical corrective feedback process. Many parallel experiments confirmed the ubiquity of a functionally distributed sensorimotor reorganization rather than a more focused response. For example, mechanical perturbations of the jaw during production of a labial or lingual consonant yield compensatory corrections in the lip and tongue muscles, respectively.

The role of such sensorimotor actions does not appear to be confined to adjustments of muscle contraction or movement. That is, subsequent experiments revealed that timing among speech actions (i.e., jaw, tongue, larynx, velum) as well as sequencing for the serial movements associated with speech likewise may rely upon sensory input (Shaiman, Abbs, and Gracco, 1985; Gracco and Abbs, 1988). In these simple cases it is apparent that sensory input from a given peripheral site is used to control movement at that site and to coordinate movements at other times and in other places within the vocal tract.

It might be tempting to suggest that, based upon experiments on the articulatory system, sensorimotor mechanisms are involved in controlling both the spatial and temporal coordination of speech movements. If researchers are to develop a substantive set of measures to detect functions and dysfunctions in the contribution of sensory input to the control of speech movements, the full scope of sensorimotor contributions must be evaluated. What is the range of such use in the control of speech production? The answer is not likely to be forthcoming in the near future without a more analytical approach to the specific biological and biomechanical actions of speech. Moreover, very little is gained and much can be lost by assuming that a few general principles will suffice to capture the nature of such use. At the least, different parts of the speech production system must be examined individually; there are a number of substantive biological bases to expect differences among parts of the speech production system. The control and generation of air pressures, transformation of that aerodynamic energy into sound, and finally, the manipulation of the size and shape of the vocal tract resonances are fundamentally different motor tasks. Therefore, contributions of sensory mechanisms or sensory dysfunction are almost certain to influence each in a substantially different manner, at least as these are manifested in the speech acoustic output. For example, the control of laryngeal movements and isometric muscle contractions of the vocalis and cricothyroid muscles associated with pitch control are unlikely to require the same sensory adjustments as movements of the tongue tip for labial stop consonant production. In this particular example, it has been argued that the former task is a continuous steady-state control effort, while the labial occlusion might be considered dynamic and binary. First, vocal pitch control may demand greater precision of muscle contraction than that required for labial occlusion. Second, the mechanical objective in pitch control presumably is the longitudinal tension in the vocal folds via isometric contraction (at least for sustained phonation with small pitch adjustments). By contrast, in actions of labial occlusion and opening, the labial muscles clearly are not contracting isometrically, and the mechanical variable being controlled is movement, with velocities and movement durations being key variables.

Another major difference between parts of the speech production system is in respect to the kinds of sensory information that is available. The muscle groups of the respiratory, laryngeal, lingual, labial, and masticatory systems are not endowed with the same kind of sensory monitoring apparatus (Abbs, Hunker, and Barlow, 1983; Abbs and Winstein, 1990). In this context it is likely that the muscle spindle afferent contributions from the jaw closing for example, intrinsic laryngeal, and lingual muscles) have influences that are quite different from the cutaneous **mechanoreceptor** afferent inputs that presumably provide proprioceptive information for the face and lips, motor systems devoid of muscle spindles. At the most superficial level, the central projections of these different kinds of afferents are unequivocally distinct, including connectivity to the brain stem motor nuclei, the somatic sensory cerebral neocortex, and the primary motor cortex. Undeniably, their influences on motor output thus must be correspondingly different as well.

With respect to different kinds of somatic sensory inputs, recent work suggests that cutaneous mechanoreceptors may play a key role, especially for control of orofacial and hand movements. Specifically, with the contractions of lip, jaw, tongue, pharyngeal, and velopharyngeal muscles, the tissues are compressed and stretched in their surface veneer, with the primary stimulus being mechanical shear within that connective tissue covering, where cutaneous mechanoreceptors are found. Based upon a study conducted on movement sensitivity of receptors in the dorsal skin of the human hand (Edin and Abbs, 1991), it is obvious that natural lip, tongue, and even jaw movements excite receptors from a widely distributed field. In that study using microneurographic recording of radial nerve cutaneous mechanoreceptor afferents, a number of mechanoreceptors with traditionally defined receptive fields as far away as the skin overlying the wrist were exquisitely sensitive to movements of a single finger. Remote mechanoreceptors of this kind could thus provide afferent signals not confounded by labial or lingual contact, or other stimulation not directly relevant to controlling the movements of interest.

Time-Varying Contributions of Motor-Sensory Processes

The differences in use of sensory input among parts of the speech production system are more than likely overshadowed by the fact that sensory information also is used in many different ways even in the control of a single movement. This can be discerned in studies in which mechanical errors or disturbances are introduced at various points prior to and following the generation of a movement. As illustrated by the findings of Gracco and Abbs (1985), sensory information is used differently at different phases of speech movement programming and execution. Specifically, it was shown that prior to movement initiation, sensory information seemingly is a means to determine the state of the motor system in programming the upcoming event. By contrast, at some point after the motor activity is initiated (viz., in activity of the pyramidal cells of the primary motor cortex), sensory input contributes in the on-line correction and shaping of the evolving motor output. While this kind of time-varying use of sensory information is illustrative, it is nevertheless extremely simplified with regard to the spectrum that is most probably operating.

Studies of sensory functions for control of reaching-grasping and pointing movements in human and nonhuman primates are quite illuminating. Because of the slower speed of these movements and the fact that they can be recorded easily, we have a more complete perspec-

TABLE 3-1 To grasp and lift an object, one must:

1. Assess object surface, size, shape, probable weight, center of mass, etc. (sensory processing of current conditions).
2. Recall properties of this or like objects (memory access of past sensory experience).
3. Evaluate prior grasping and lifting of like objects (learning and sensory generalization).
4. Select, sequence, and coordinate initial torso, shoulder, elbow, wrist, and finger actions (based upon sensory inputs).
5. Anticipate time when hand will contact the object (prediction via sensory input of evolving movement) and make necessary compensatory corrections.
6. Incorporate information from initial object contact and grasp regarding object characteristics so as to fine-tune adjustments for lifting (perception, integration, sensory-based adjustments).

tive on the contributions of sensory input. To amplify this point, Table 3-1 lists some of the brain functions that appear necessary for the simple movements for reaching toward, grasping, and lifting an object. All of these processes involve sensory inputs. While the illustration in the table is from a different motor system, it is not difficult to conceive of parallel planning, programming, coordinating, and execution underlying the generation of a speech motor event.

SUMMARY: MANY HYPOTHESES TO TEST

While it appears that sensorimotor contributions are critical in speech and similar motor behaviors, it is necessary to guard against conceptualizations of these important functions that are so oversimplified as to be counterproductive. The real progress in the next two decades will be by those who pursue some of the complexities revealed by the initial studies outlined previously. In that respect results from a combination of studies suggest that (1) sensorimotor processes are used in spatial coordination of multiple speech movements to control their sequential timing and to assist in planning and programming; (2) specific contributions of spindle, **tendon organ,** cutaneous mechanoreceptor inputs vary across speech motor subsystems as well as over the time course of a given speech gesture; and (3) different higher centers are likely to be involved as a natural consequence of variations in sensory input and at different instances in the time course of motor execution. While these are broad hypotheses, each requires elaboration with well-defined experiments aimed at underlying neural processes. At the same time, because it is virtually impossible to separate sensory and motor processes, it is likely to be fruitful to investigate whether many speech disorders of unknown or neurological origin are in fact impairments of sensorimotor function. Recent data suggest this, even in disorders that previously have defied understanding (DeNil and Abbs, 1991).

Finally, to avoid confusion, it is appropriate to restate a caution offered by Titze (1991) who noted that much of the research on speech production appears to reflect too much measurement and too little thought spent trying to determine what should be measured. Perhaps there should be a moratorium on gathering information for its own sake, just because an instrument has made it possible, or perhaps because careful testing of specific hypotheses carries high risk and requires hard thinking. It certainly is true that the literature on speech functions is burdened with a plethora of unfocused data sets trapped in theoretical purgatory, waiting for the salvation of even a weak hypothesis.

Review Questions

1. List the primary mechanical properties of speech motor systems.

2. Distinguish between passive and active mechanical properties.

3. Describe the stages and factors intervening between motoneuron firing and speech movement.

4. What are the contributions of sensory inputs to speech motor control?

5. List sources of sensory information for speech control.

References

Abbott, B.C., & Wilkie, D.R. (1953). The relation between velocity of shortening and the tension-length curve of skeletal muscle. *Journal of Physiology, 12,* 214-223.

Abbs, J. H., & Connor, N. P. (1989). Motor coordination for functional human behaviors: Perspectives from a speech motor data base. In Wallace, S. (Ed.), *Perspectives on the coordination of movement.* Amsterdam: Elsevier Science North-Holland (pp. 157-183).

Abbs, J. H., & Eilenberg, G. R. (1976). Peripheral mechanisms of speech motor control. In Lass, N. J. (Ed.), *Contemporary issues in experimental phonetics.* New York: Academic Press (pp. 139-168).

Abbs, J. H., & Gracco, V. L. (1982, November). *Motor control of multi-movement behaviors: Oro-facial muscle responses to load perturbations of the lips during speech.* Paper presented at the Society for Neuroscience Meeting, Minneapolis.

Abbs, J. H., & Gracco, V. L. (1984). Control of complex motor gestures: Orofacial muscle responses to load perturbations of the lip during speech. *Journal of Neurophysiology, 51*(4), 705-723.

Abbs, J. H., & Gracco, V. L. (1991, December). *Compensatory responses to low magnitude loads applied to the lower lip during speech.* Paper presented at the Acoustical Society of America meeting, Miami Beach.

Abbs, J. H., Gracco, V. L., & Cole, K. J. (1984). Control of multi-joint movement coordination: Sensorimotor mechanisms in speech motor programming. *Journal of Motor Behavior, 16,* 195-231.

Abbs, J. H., Hunker, C. J., & Barlow, S. M. (1983). Differential speech motor subsystem impairments with suprabulbar lesions: Neurophysiological framework and supporting data. In Berry, W. (Ed.), *Clinical dysarthria.* San Diego: College-Hill Press (pp. 21-56).

Abbs, J. H., Shaiman, S., Gracco, V. L., & Cole, K. J. (1985, October). *Task-dependent sensorimotor actions are inherent in speech motor programs.* Paper presented at the Society for Neuroscience Meeting, Dallas.

Abbs, J. H., & Welt, C. W. (1985). Structure and function of the lateral precentral cortex: Significance for speech motor control. In Daniloff, R. G. (Ed.), *Recent advances in speech science.* San Diego: College-Hill Press (pp. 155-191).

Abbs, J. H., & Winstein, C. J. (1990). Functional contributions of rapid and automatic sensory-based adjustments to motor output. In Jeannerod, M. (Ed.), *Attention and performance XIII. Motor representation and control.* Hillsdale, NJ: Erlbaum (pp. 627-652).

Alexander, R. M. (1981). Mechanics of skeletons and tendons. In Brooks, V. (Ed.), Handbook of physiology: Sec. 1. *The nervous system: vol. II. Motor control.* Bethesda, MD: The American Physiological Society (pp. 17-42).

DeNil L. S., & Abbs, J. H. (1991). Kinesthetic acuity of stutterers and non-stutterers for oral and non-oral movements. *Brain, 114,* 2145-2158.

Edin, B. B., & Abbs, J. H. (1991). Finger movement responses of cutaneous mechanoreceptors in the dorsal skin of the human hand. *Journal of Neurophysiology, 65,* 657-670.

Eilenberg, G., & Abbs, J. H. (1974, November). *Instantaneous center of rotation of the jaw during speech and non-speech tasks.* Paper presented at the Annual Convention of the American Speech and Hearing Association Convention, Las Vegas.

Fairbanks, G. (1954). Systematic research in experimental phonetics: A theory of the speech mechanism as a servosystem. *Journal of Speech and Hearing Research, 19,* 133-139.

Fenn, W. O., & Marsh, B. S. (1935). Muscular force at different speeds of shortening. *Journal of Physiology, 85,* 277-297.

Folkins, J. W., & Abbs, J. H. (1975). Lip and jaw motor control during speech: Responses to resistive loading of the jaw. *Journal of Speech and Hearing Research, 18,* 207-220.

Folkins, J. W., & Abbs, J. H. (1976). Additional observations on responses to resistive loading of the jaw. *Journal of Speech and Hearing Research, 19,*820-821.

Gracco, V. L., & Abbs, J. H. (1982, November). *Temporal response characteristics of the perioral system to load perturbations.* Paper presented at the Society for Neuroscience Meeting, Minneapolis.

Gracco, V. L., & Abbs, J. H. (1985). Dynamic control of the perioral system during speech: Kinematic analyses of autogenic and nonautogenic sensorimotor processes. *Journal of Neurophysiology, 54,* 418-432.

Gracco, V. L., & Abbs, J. H. (1987). Programming and execution processes of speech movement control: Potential neural correlates. In Keller, E., & Gopnik, M. (Eds.), *Motor and sensory processes of language.* Hilldale, NJ: Erlbaum (pp.163-201).

Gracco, V. L., & Abbs, J. H. (1988). Central patterning of speech movements. *Experimental Brain Research, 71,* 515-526.

Gracco, V. L., & Abbs, J. H. (1989). Sensorimotor characteristics of speech motor sequences. *Experimental Brain Research, 75,* 586-598.

Green, D. G. (1969). A note on modelling muscle in physiological regulators. *Medical and Biological Engineering, 7,* 41-47.

Guttman, N. (1954). Experimental studies of the speech control system. Unpublished doctoral dissertation, University of Illinois.

Hill, A. V. (1938). The heat of shortening and dynamic constant of muscle. *Proceedings of the Royal Society, B126,* 136-195.

Jewell, B.R., & Wilkie, D. R. (1958). An analysis of mechanical components in frog striated muscle. *Journal of Physiology, 143,* 515-540.

McCroskey, R. (1958). The relative contributions of auditory and tactile cues to certain aspects of speech. *Southern Speech Journal, 24,* 84-90.

McCroskey, R, Corley, N., & Jackson, G. (1959). Some effects of disrupted tactile cues upon the production of consonants. *Southern Speech Journal, 25,* 55-60.

Mead, J., Bouhuys, A., & Proctor, D. F. (1968). Mechanisms generating subglottal pressure. *Annals of the New York Academy of Science, 155,* 171-181.

Milhorn, H. T. (1966). *The application of control theory to physiological systems.* Philadelphia, Saunders.

Müller, E. M., Abbs, J. H., & Kennedy, J. G. III. (1981). Some system physiology considerations for vocal control. In Stevens, K. N., & Hirano, M. (Eds.), *Vocal fold physiology.* Tokyo: University of Tokyo Press (pp. 209-227).

Partridge, L. D., & Benton, L. A. (1981). Muscle, the motor. In Brooks, V. (Ed.), Handbook of physiology: Sec. 1. *The nervous system: vol. II. Motor control.* Bethesda, MD: The American Physiological Society (pp. 43-106).

Penrod, D. D., Davy, D. T., & Singh, D. P. (1972, December). *An optimization approach to tendon force analysis.* Paper presented at the 25th Annual Conference on Engineering in Medicine and Biology, Bal Harbour, California.

Perkell, J. S. (1974). Quasiphysiological tongue model. *Journal of the Acoustical Society of America, 55,* 578-579.

Ringel, R. L., & Steer, M. D. (1963). Some effects of tactile and auditory alterations on speech output. *Journal of Speech and Hearing Research, 6,* 369-378.

Scott, C. M., & Ringel, R. L. (1971a). Articulation without oral sensory control. *Journal of Speech and Hearing Research, 14,* 804-818.

Scott, C. M., & Ringel, R. L. (1971b). The effects of motor and sensory disruptions on speech: A description of articulation. *Journal of Speech and Hearing Research, 14,* 819-828.

Shaiman, S., Abbs, J. H., & Gracco, V. L. (1985, October). *Sensorimotor contributions to oral-laryngeal coordination for speech.* Paper presented at the Society for Neuroscience Meeting, Dallas.

Titze, I. (1991). Measurements for the assessment of voice disorders. In Cooper, J. (Ed.), *Assessment of speech and voice production: research and clinical applications.* Bethesda, MD: National Institutes of Health (pp. 42-49).

Weber, B. A. (1961). *Effect of high level masking and anesthetization of oral structures upon articulatory proficiency and voice characteristics of normal speakers.* Unpublished master's thesis, The Pennsylvania State University.

Welt, C., & Abbs, J. H. (1990). Musculotopic organization of the facial motor nucleus in *Macaca fascicularis:* A morphometric and retrograde tracing study with cholera toxin B-HRP. *Journal of Comparative Neurology, 291,* 621-636.

Wilkie, D. R. (1956). The mechanical properties of muscle. *British Medical Bulletin, 1200,* 177-182.

Suggested Readings

Basic Biomechanics of Motor Systems

Alexander, R. M. (1981). Mechanics of skeletons and tendons. In Brooks, V. (Ed.), *Handbook of physiology: Sec. 1. The nervous system: vol. II. Motor control.* Bethesda, MD: The American Physiological Society (pp. 17-42).

Müller, E. M., Abbs, J. H., & Kennedy, J. G. III. (1981). Some system physiology considerations for vocal control. In Stevens, K. N., & Hirano, M. (Eds.), *Vocal fold physiology,* Tokyo: University of Tokyo Press (pp. 209-227).

Partridge, L. D., & Benton, L. A. (1981). Muscle, the motor. In Brooks, V. (Ed.), *Handbook of physiology: Sec. 1. The nervous system: vol. II. Motor control.* Bethesda, MD: The American Physiological Society (pp. 43-106).

Sensorimotor Control

Abbs, J. H., & Cole, K. J. (1982). Consideration of bulbar and suprabulbar afferent influences upon speech motor coordination and programming. In Grillner, S., Lindblom, B., Lubker, J., & Persson, A. (Eds.), *Speech motor control: Vol. 36.* New York: Pergamon Press (pp. 159-186).

Abbs, J. H., & Welt, C. W. (1985). Structure and function of the lateral precentral cortex: Significance for speech motor control. In Daniloff, R. G. (Ed.), *Recent advances in speech science.* San Diego: College-Hill Press (pp. 155-191).

Abbs, J. H., & Winstein, C. J. (1990). Functional contributions of rapid and automatic sensory-based adjustments to motor output. In Jeannerod, M. (Ed.), *Attention and performance XIII. Motor Representation and Control.* Hillsdale, NJ: Erlbaum (pp. 627-652).

Gracco, V. L., & Abbs, J. H. (1987). Programming and execution processes of speech movement control: Potential neural correlates. In Keller, E., & Gopnik, M. (Eds.), *Motor and sensory processes of language.* Hillsdale, NJ: Erlbaum (pp. 163-201).

Chapter 4

Structure and Function of the Larynx

Robert F. Orlikoff, Joel C. Kahane

Chapter Outline

Key Terms

INTRODUCTION

Our earliest air-breathing ancestors, the African and Australian lungfishes, opened and closed the airway by sphincteric action (Negus, 1949; Hast, 1985). A sphincter is a muscular ring that encircles a bodily orifice. When a sphincter contracts, it acts like a purse string to close the lumen (the space inside a tube). Primitive respiratory sphincters evolved into the structure that we now colloquially call the "voice box" (Figure 4-1). However, the structure of the human larynx is far more elaborate and its function far more complex than its common nickname suggests, indeed, more than many medical texts imply.

THE LARYNX

Vegetative Laryngeal Function

Situated in the anterior neck between the upper and lower respiratory systems, the larynx is foremost a valve that regulates the flow of air to and from the lungs (Figure 4-2). Thus, while the human larynx has by no means remained a simple sphincter, it has preserved that function, upon which all others are overlaid. In humans, laryngeal valving, in addition to its respiratory function, may be protective, expectorative, supportive (fixative), or phonatory and may take the form of a complete, incomplete, or transitory constriction.

The trachea (windpipe) is a flexible tube that connects the larynx and upper airways with the lungs. It is composed of a series of C-shaped cartilaginous rings that are enclosed posteriorly by fibroelastic tissue and muscle. This arrangement ensures patency of the airway, which if unsupported would collapse under the negative pressures of inspiration. However, because the trachea is held open, there is free and easy access to the bronchi and lungs for any undesirable

substance. This is particularly serious because the lungs and stomach share a pathway, the pharynx. Thus, by its ability to close off the trachea from the pharynx, the larynx serves a vital protective function (Murakami and Kirchner, 1972). To perform this life-preserving task, the larynx is outfitted with some of the fastest muscles in the body, second only to those that control eye movement (Faaborg-Andersen, 1957, 1965; Mårtensson and Skoglund, 1964; Mårtensson, 1968).

Closure of the lower airway also allows for a volume of air to be trapped and, through biomechanical and muscular effort, pressurized. Thus, like an inflatable plastic air cushion, the lungs can be made stiffer and more resilient. This added support stabilizes the chest wall, allowing the muscles of the trunk and limbs to perform with greater efficiency, such as during heavy lifting, throwing, pushing, and pulling. Heavy work is not ordinarily performed without some laryngeal adjustment of one's breathing pattern; during particularly strenuous activity we tend first to inhale and then to suspend breathing to provide a greatly stiffened upper torso. (Grunting and sighing often result from an effort that exceeds our ability to maintain complete laryngeal closure.) Additionally, the buildup of intrathoracic pressure aids in the maintenance of intraabdominal pressure, which is important for such functions as childbirth, vomiting, sexual function, and forced urination and defecation.

Given that the tracheal ring cartilages allow for minimal movement, the larynx provides a quick and efficient way to regulate the resistance to the flow of air as it passes through the respiratory system. Laryngeal airway dilation during inspiration and slight narrowing during expiration may influence the pattern of breathing (Fink, Basek and Epanchin, 1956; Hast, 1967; Suzuki and Kirchner, 1969; Stanescu et al., 1972; Bartlett, Remmers and Gautier, 1973;

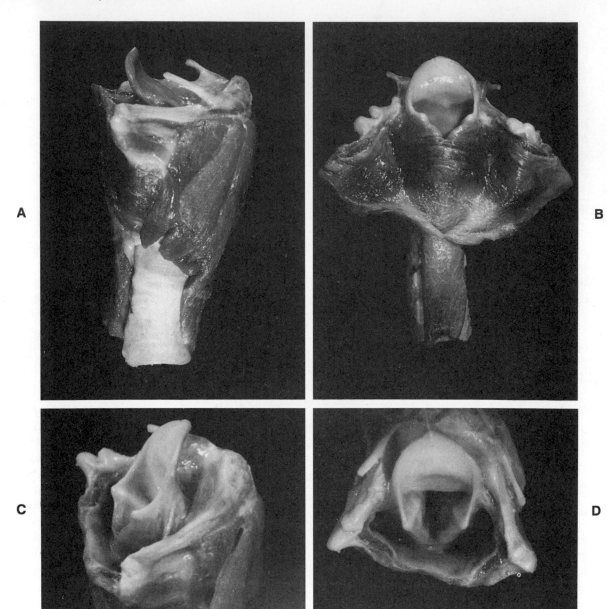

FIGURE 4-1 Dissections of the human larynx in lateral (*A*), posterior (*B*), oblique (*C*), and superior (*D*) views. (From Kahane, J. C., & Folkins, J.W. [1984]. *Atlas of speech and hearing anatomy*. Columbus, OH: Charles E. Merrill.)

Gautier, Remmers, and Bartlett, 1973; Baier et al., 1977; McCaffrey and Kern, 1980; Kosch et al., 1985; Mu and Yang, 1990) along with dynamic resistances provided by the rest of the upper respiratory tract (Davis, Bartlett, and Luschei, 1993). The nares, for instance, often exhibit a similar action during the breathing cycle.

The respiratory system is lined with pseudostratified *ciliated* columnar epithelium and mucus-producing glands. The sticky coating of mucus traps inhaled foreign particles, and the upward beating of the hairlike cilia propels the mucus away from the lungs. The expectorative function of the larynx is triggered whenever mucus or foreign material is present in the lower airway. This expulsive force is the result of an extremely rapid egressive airflow produced by a sudden release of high lung pressure. The ability both to generate high lung pressure and to release it quickly is achieved through a coordinated laryngeal gesture.

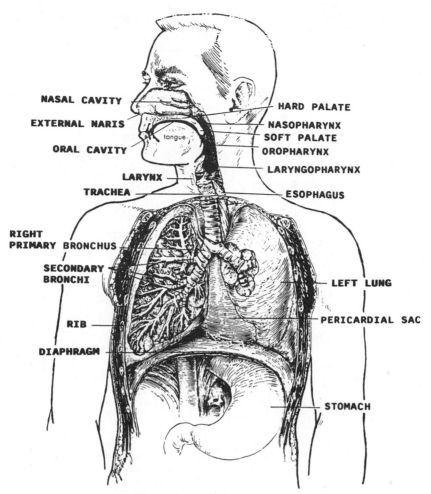

FIGURE 4-2 Relationship of the larynx to other structures of the head, neck and trunk. (Modified from Crouch, J. [1985]. *Functional human anatomy,* [4th ed.]. Philadelphia: Lea and Febiger.)

The Structure of the Human Larynx

The human larynx has evolved from a sphincter to a sophisticated shutter valve controlled by an intricate set of muscles and supported by a membranous and cartilaginous framework. The cartilagenous skeleton gives form and shape to the larynx and supports an otherwise collapsible tubular passageway, the laryngeal cavity. The laryngeal cartilages also serve as points of attachment for muscles and other connective tissues within the larynx. The cartilages are the phylogenetically oldest portions of the larynx (Negus, 1929; Wind, 1970), predating the intrinsic laryngeal muscles and the laryngeal cavity. The advent of each cartilage heralded significant evolutionary advances in the development of the upper and lower airways, influencing such functions as terrestrial breathing,

swallowing, sound production, locomotion, and prehension.

The laryngeal skeleton consists of five major cartilages: the *thyroid, cricoid,* one pair of *arytenoids,* and the *epiglottis.* The general shape of these cartilages and their relationship to one another within the larynx is illustrated in Figure 4-3. Except for the epiglottis and the vocal process of each arytenoid, the laryngeal cartilages are composed of *hyaline cartilage,* which is firm and resilient. The epiglottis and vocal processes are composed of a very flexible connective tissue, *elastic cartilage.* Changes in the size and constitution of the laryngeal cartilages occur throughout life. During infancy, they are pliable, and they become firmer throughout childhood and adolescence. Beginning in adulthood and continuing into old age, the cartilages become

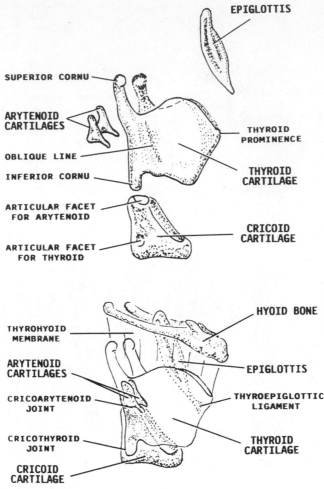

FIGURE 4-3 Laryngeal cartilages shown separately (top) and articulated (bottom) at the laryngeal joints and with the hyoid bone.

less resilient and harden as a consequence of progressive calcification and ossification. Although these changes occur in both sexes, they are greatest in the male, and they affect each cartilage to a different extent (Chamberlain and Young, 1935; Roncollo, 1949; Keen and Wainwright, 1958; Kahane, 1981, 1983a, 1983b).

Deep to the cartilaginous laryngeal skeleton are flexible fibroelastic connective tissues lined with epithelium. These tissues form the walls of the *laryngeal cavity*. The laryngeal cavity is traditionally divided into (1) a somewhat expanded upper *supraglottal* region defined by the *quadrangular membrane,* (2) a narrow middle *glottal* region bounded principally by the *vocal folds,* and (3) a lower *infraglottal* or *subglottal* region bordered by the *conus elasticus* (Figure 4-4). The area of primary laryngeal valving is the glottal region, where the shape and size of the *rima glottidis,* or **glottis** (the space between

the vocal folds), is modified during respiration, **vocalization,** and sphincteric valving (effort closure). The rima glottidis consists of an *intramembranous portion* bordered by the soft tissue of the vocal folds and encompassing the anterior three-fifths of the glottal airway and an *intracartilaginous portion,* the posterior two-fifths of the rima glottidis, between the vocal processes of the arytenoid cartilages. The posterior glottis is an area of dynamic change occasioned by the positioning and aerodynamic displacement of the vocal folds. The overall dimensions of the intramembraneous glottis remain relatively stable except in strenuous sphincteric valving.

Although the laryngeal cartilages do not directly contribute to the valving of the ventilatory airstream, the cartilaginous joints of the larynx directly influence the shape and size of the rima glottidis (and thus laryngeal airway

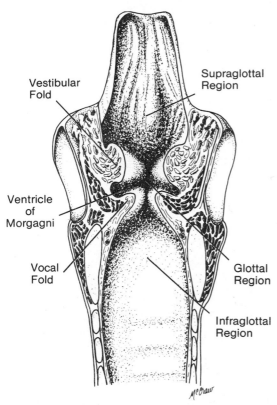

FIGURE 4-4   The laryngeal cavity.

Labels on figure:
Vestibular Fold
Supraglottal Region
Ventricle of Morgagni
Vocal Fold
Glottal Region
Infraglottal Region

resistance). In particular, the larynx has two pairs of movable (diarthrotic) joints that are morphologically specialized for different roles in laryngeal function.

The *cricoarytenoid joints* (CAJ) are formed by joining the articular facets of the cricoid and arytenoid carilages by a joint capsule and a short, broad cricoarytenoid ligament. The CAJ is highly symmetrical bilaterally (Maue, 1970). Detailed anatomical studies (von Leden and Moore, 1961; Sellers and Keen, 1978) have clarified the function of this joint. As shown in Figure 4-5, *A,* the principal movement of the CAJ is a rocking of the arytenoid cartilage around the longitudinal axis of the cricoid facet. This action abducts or adducts the vocal folds. *Abduction* is drawing the folds away from the midline, increasing the glottal area and decreasing glottal resistance. *Adduction* is drawing the vocal folds toward the midline, sealing the glottis. The detailed movements of the arytenoids are complex (Frable, 1961; Baken and Isshiki, 1977), consisting of simultaneous displacements of parts of the cartilage in horizontal, vertical, and depth planes. CAJ activity is essential to both respiratory and sound-producing functions

of the larynx. Specific age-related changes in the CAJ include involutional changes in the articular surfaces and in the synovial membranes that nourish and lubricate the joint (Kahane and Kahn, 1986; Kahn and Kahane, 1986; Kahane and Hammons, 1987).

The *cricothyroid joints* (CTJ) are formed by joining the articular facets on the thyroid and cricoid cartilages by three ligaments and a joint capsule (Mayet and Mundrich, 1958). The primary motion of the CTJ is rotation about a horizontal axis through the center of the joint, which approximates the thyroid and cricoid cartilages and alters the length, tension, and thickness of the vocal folds (Figure 4-5). The functional significance of both CAJ and CTJ will be discussed later.

The discrete and refined movements of the laryngeal cartilages are achieved primarily by a set of striated muscles that are among the smallest and fastest in the body. These *intrinsic laryngeal muscles* (Figure 4-6) (1) abduct and adduct the vocal folds, (2) change the position of the cartilages relative to each other, (3) transiently change the dimensions and physical properties of the vocal folds, and (4) modify laryngeal airway resistance. The intrinsic laryngeal muscles contain, in varying proportions, fibers that control fine movements for prolonged periods (type 1 fibers) and fibers that develop tension rapidly within a muscle (type 2 fibers) (Matzelt and Vosteen, 1963; Ganz, 1971; Tieg, Dahl, and Thorkelson, 1978; Malmgren and Gacek, 1981; Rosenfield et al., 1982; Cooper, Partridge, and Alipour-Haghighi, 1993). In particular, the striated muscles with origins and insertions on the laryngeal cartilages differ significantly from those in the limbs, the standard morphological reference for this tissue. Major differences include (1) the typically smaller mean diameter of the laryngeal muscles, (2) the less regular shape of laryngeal muscle fibers, (3) the generally uniform fiber diameter across laryngeal muscles, (4) the greater variability in the course of laryngeal muscle fibers within a facsimile owing to the tendency for intermingling of fibers in their longitudinal and transverse planes, and (5) the greater investment of laryngeal muscle fibers with nonmuscular connective tissue.

Most descriptions of intrinsic laryngeal muscle function are based on clinical observation, gross anatomy studies, electrostimulation of excised larynges, and biochemical analysis of

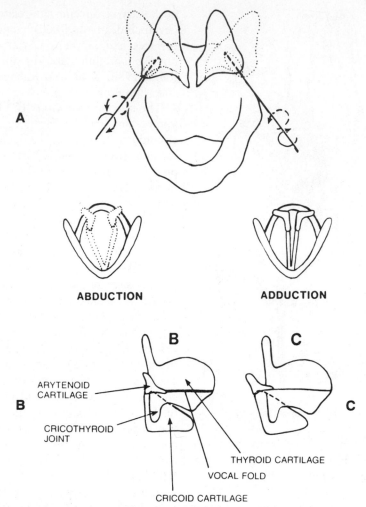

ABDUCTION   ADDUCTION

ARYTENOID
CARTILAGE

CRICOTHYROID
JOINT

THYROID CARTILAGE

VOCAL FOLD

CRICOID CARTILAGE

FIGURE 4-5   The laryngeal joints. The principal action of the cricoarytenoid joint (*A*) is a rocking motion that abducts and adducts the vocal folds. The orientation of the cricoid and thyroid cartilages at rest (*B*) changes with the rotary movement at the cricothyroid joint (*C*). Note the lengthening of the vocal folds and the approximation of the anterior portions of the cricoid and thyroid cartilages. (*A* from Kahane, J. C. [1986]. *Anatomy and physiology of the speech mechanism.* **Austin, TX: Pro-Ed. B and C from Kahane, J. C. [1988]. Anatomy of the organs of the peripheral speech mechanism. In Lass, N. J., Northern, J. L., McReynolds, L. V., & Yoder, D. C. [Eds.],** *Handbook of speech-language pathology and audiology.* **St. Louis: Mosby.)**

muscle tissue. From these diverse sources the intrinsic muscles are broadly classified into abductor (posterior cricoarytenoid), adductor (lateral cricoarytenoid and interarytenoids), and tensor (thyroarytenoid and cricothyroid) groups (Table 4-1).

Of all the intrinsic muscles of the larynx, the thyroarytenoid muscle (TA) has generated the most interest. It has been extensively studied during the past century, particularly in the past 40 years. It is well accepted that TA is the major constituent of the vocal folds and that some portions of TA are more involved in voice production than others. It is usually divided into *thyrovocalis* (or *vocalis*) fibers and *thyromuscularis* fibers, although no clear distinction exists between them. These names are derived from the fibers' different points of attachment to the arytenoid cartilage. The thyrovocalis fibers originate from the deep surface of the thyroid cartilage at midline, run parallel to a band of connective tissue, the *vocal ligament,* and insert at the vocal process of the arytenoid. The thyromuscularis fibers originate below those of the thyrovocalis and course superolaterally to insert at the base and muscular process of the

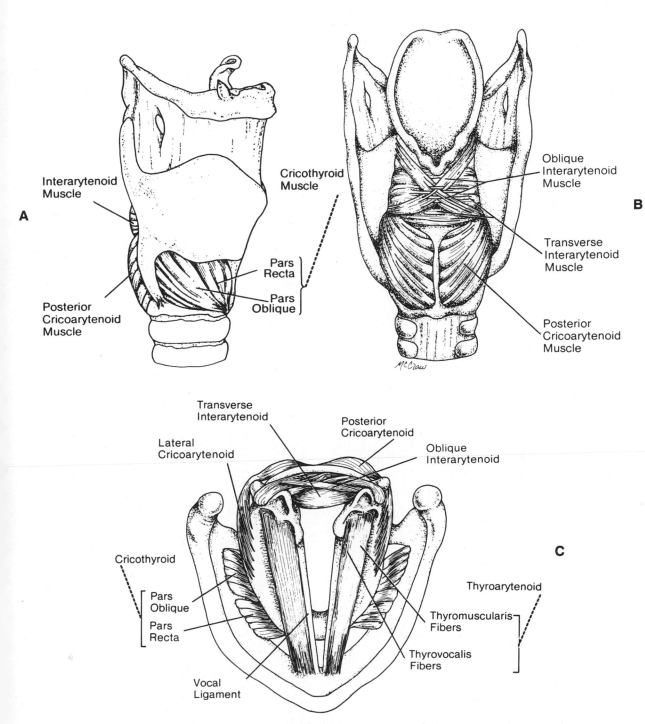

FIGURE 4-6   The intrinsic muscles of the larynx as shown in (A) lateral, (B) posterior, and (C) superior views. (From Kahane, J. C. [1988]. Anatomy of the organs of the peripheral speech mechanism. In Lass, N. J., Northern, J. L., McReynolds, L. V., & Yoder, D. C. [Eds.], *Handbook of speech-language pathology and audiology.* St. Louis: Mosby.)

TABLE 4-1   The morphology and general function of the intrinsic laryngeal muscles

Muscle	Origin	Insertion	Action	Innervation
Cricothyroid	Lateral surface of cricoid cartilage arch; fibers divide into upper portion (pars recta) and lower portion (pars oblique)	Pars recta fibers attach to anterior lateral half of inferior border of thyroid cartilage; pars oblique fibers attach to anterior margin of inferior cornu of thyroid cartilage	Rotational approximation of the cricoid and thyroid cartilages; lengthens and tenses vocal folds	External branch of the superior laryngeal nerve (CN X)
Lateral cricoarytenoid	Upper border of arch of cricoid cartilage	Anterior aspect of muscular process of arytenoid cartilage	Adducts vocal folds; closes rima glottidis	Recurrent laryngeal nerve (CN X)
Posterior cricoarytenoid	Cricoid lamina	Muscular process of arytenoid cartilage	Abducts vocal folds; opens rima glottidis	Recurrent laryngeal nerve (CN X)
Interarytenoid Transverse fibers	Horizontally coursing fibers extending between the dorsolateral ridges of each arytenoid cartilage	Dorsolateral ridge of opposite arytenoid cartilage	Approximates bases of arytenoid cartilages; assists vocal fold adduction	Recurrent laryngeal nerve (CN X)
Oblique fibers	Obliquely coursing fibers from base of one arytenoid cartilage	Inserts onto apex of opposite arytenoid cartilage	Same as transverse fibers	Recurrent laryngeal nerve (CNX)
Thyroarytenoid	Deep surface of thyroid cartilage at midline	Fovea oblonga of arytenoid cartilage; vocalis fibers attach close to vocal process; muscularis fibers attach more laterally	Tenses vocal folds (vocalis fibers); may assist vocal fold adduction (muscularis fibers)	Recurrent laryngeal nerve (CN X)

CN, cranial nerve.

arytenoid cartilage. Although the definitive functions of the vocalis and muscularis portions of TA have not been determined, van den Berg and Moll (1955) have suggested that thyrovocalis acts as a vocal fold tensor, and Wustrow (1952) has proposed that the thyromuscularis serves primarily as a vocal fold adductor. It has been suggested that the classic functional characterization of all of the intrinsic laryngeal muscles should be refined to explain their specific combined effects on the shaping of the rima glottidis and on the tissue layers of the vocal folds (Hirano, 1974; Koike, Hirano, and Morio, 1976).

The Neurology of the Larynx

The activities of the larynx are regulated or influenced by the nervous system. This control is derived from a network of neurological components that includes areas of the cerebral hemispheres, the brain stem, the cranial nerves, and end organs within the larynx. Our understanding of the complexities of the neural substrata underlying laryngeal control is incomplete, although significant advances have been made over the past quarter of a century (Wyke and Kirchner, 1976). Limitations inherent in the use of human subjects make the study of this area slow and difficult. Thus, much of the information available today is derived from experiments on dogs, cats, and higher primates, and so the validity of inferring human laryngeal (particularly vocal) function from infrahuman forms is still to be determined. The discussion that follows is drawn largely from human studies. When no information is available from human studies, animal studies will be cited and identified as such.

Central Nervous Control of the Larynx

Neural control of the larynx begins in the cerebral cortex bilaterally, principally from the *inferior precentral gyrus* and the *supplementary motor area* (Penfield and Roberts, 1959). Forming part of the *corticobulbar tract,* neurons (nerve fibers) from these areas pass through the internal capsule into the brain stem, where at the junction of the pons and medulla most fibers cross midline to enter the contralateral pool of laryngeal motor neurons (Figure 4-7). Some nerve fibers remain uncrossed, so that each cerebral cortex projects motor neurons to both sides of the brain stem. This ensures that

laryngeal function will be preserved in case of disease or trauma, unless a bilateral lesion affecting the cerebral cortex or corticobulbar tract has occurred. The corticobulbar fibers supplying the larynx and pharynx innervate the *nucleus ambiguus,* the main nucleus of the tenth cranial nerve (CN X), the *vagus nerve.* Other areas in the cerebrum also appear to contribute to laryngeal control. In humans the anterior *cingulate gyrus* may be important in the volitional control of voice intonation (Jürgens and von Cramon, 1982; Jürgens, 1983). In the monkey a wide variety of structures in the limbic system have been found to produce vocalizations when stimulated (Jürgens, 1976; Ploog, 1981; Larson, Yoshida, and Sessle, 1993).

The basal ganglia and thalamus undoubtedly contribute to laryngeal control, as evidenced by the effects of lesions in these structures (Aronson, 1990). The basal ganglia, an important motor control center, greatly influence the lower motor neurons that innervate the laryngeal musculature. The thalamus, a sensory control center, also contributes to the control and regulation of **phonation**. Broca's area receives connections from the dorsomedian and centromedian nuclei of the thalamus, and Botez and Barbeau (1971) noted that the ventrolateral nucleus connects with the precentral gyrus of the cortex through projection fibers. The ventrolateral nucleus is important to the initiation of speech movements as well as to the regulation of **pitch** and **loudness**. These motor and sensory centers probably influence laryngeal activity indirectly via inputs to motor neurons in the brainstem (Hassler, 1956; Rudomin, 1965; Dunker, 1968). Electrostimulation and ablation experiments in monkeys have identified three areas in the brainstem that appear to be particularly important for laryngeal and vocal function (Botez and Barbeau, 1971; Larson, Wilson, and Luschei, 1983; Larson, 1985; Jürgens and Richter, 1986; Larson and Kistler, 1986; Richter and Jürgens, 1986; Ortega et al., 1988; Larson et al., 1991). These areas include (1) the *nucleus tractus solitarius,* a primary center for sensory feedback from the larynx; (2) the *periaquaductal gray,* in the midbrain tectum below the inferior coliculus, a center for the control of vocalization*; and (3) the *nucleus parabrachealis,* a second-order processing center

---

*In humans, lesions in this area have been shown to cause mutism (Botez and Barbeau, 1971).

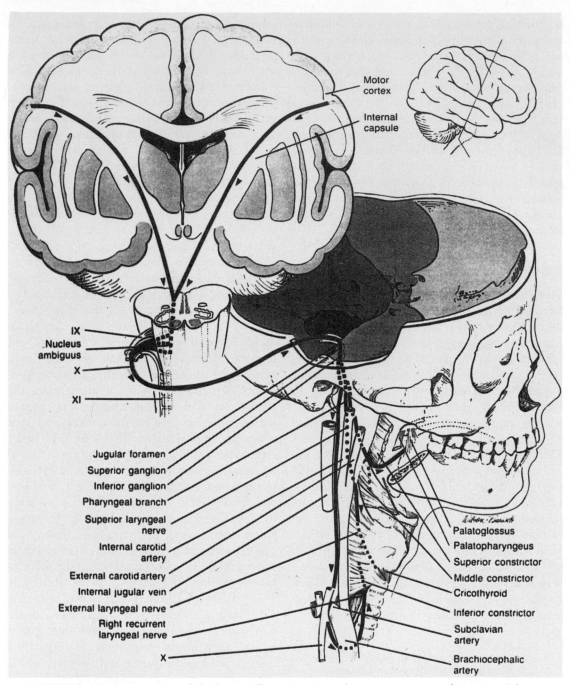

FIGURE 4-7 **Innervation of the larynx illustrating central nervous system and extracranial relationships.** (From Wilson-Pauls, L., Akesson, E. J., & Stewart, P. A. [1988]. *Cranial nerves: Anatomy and clinical comments.* St. Louis: Mosby.)

for somatosensory information from the larynx. In addition, inputs from the *lateral pontine* and *medullary reticular formation* may be important in the control of various vocal tract structures during vocalization (Thoms and Jürgens, 1987).

The cerebellum is involved not in the initiation of vocalization but in its governance

(Bender, 1928; Dunker, 1968). Inputs from the cerebellum to the laryngeal motor nuclei come from relay systems, apparently in the tectum of the midbrain, via the tubobulbar tract. These neurons pass through the anterior lobe of the cerebellum on their way to laryngeal motor neurons. These fibers may be reflexively influenced by afferent (sensory) inputs from the larynx (Lam and Ogura, 1952). While cerebellar inputs to the laryngeal motor nuclei are known to coordinate laryngeal muscle activity during voice production, the specific neurophysiological mechanisms and pathways are yet to be completely delineated.

Brainstem Nuclei and Lower Motor Neurons to the Larynx

Special visceral efferent (motor) nerve fibers from the vagus nerve control intrinsic laryngeal muscle activity. The nucleus ambiguus is a longitudinal column of cells in the ventrolateral part of the medulla. Histological studies have revealed that the cell bodies of efferent neurons that supply each of the intrinsic laryngeal muscles are topographically distributed within this nucleus (Gretz and Sirnes, 1949; Lawn, 1966). The axonal projections of these nerve fibers leave the medulla, and within the jugular foramen at the base of the skull, they join afferent fibers arising from the nodose and jugular ganglia. These neurons intermingle with those of the accessory cranial nerve (CN XI) and travel within the main body of the vagus nerve, which descends in the neck between the carotid artery and internal jugular vein. Together, the nerve and these vessels form the *carotid sheath*.

In the neck, CN X branches first go to the pharyngeal muscles. At the level of the thyrohyoid membrane, another branch, the *superior laryngeal nerve,* divides into smaller internal and external branches. The internal branch enters the larynx through the thyrohyoid membrane to supply all mucous membranes and glands in the supraglottal region down to the level of the vocal folds. The external branch of the superior laryngeal nerve continues to course caudally outside the larynx to innervate the cricothyroid muscle and the inferior pharyngeal constrictor muscle of the pharynx.

The main trunk of the vagus supplies viscera in the thoracic and abdominal cavities. However, as the nerve enters the root of the neck, the *inferior laryngeal nerve,* or *recurrent laryngeal nerve* (RLN), divides from the main trunk. The right RLN loops around the subclavian artery before ascending toward the larynx in the tracheoesophageal groove. The left RLN loops around the aorta just distal to the ligamentum arteriosum and travels up the tracheoesophageal groove to the larynx. Both RLNs enter the larynx posteriorly, in the vicinity of the cricothyroid joint, where each divides to supply all of the intrinsic musculature except the cricothyroid.

Both the SLN and RLN are composed of the axons of neurons whose cell bodies lie in the brainstem nuclei of CN X and XI. Branches of these nerves spread among the fascicles of the intrinsic laryngeal muscles and divide into microscopic endings terminated by motor end plates. Each terminal axonal ending and end plate innervates a muscle fiber. An efferent neuron, its end plates, and the muscle fibers they innervate form a *motor unit* (Figure 4-8). The motor unit is the smallest functional neuromuscular component of striated muscle, with each muscle containing several motor units. The strength of muscle contraction largely depends on how many motor units are activated, or *recruited,* in the muscular response. The size of the motor unit is also important. The fewer the muscle fibers supplied by a motor neuron, the greater the control over the muscle contraction. Thus, discrete or refined muscle actions are found in muscles with smaller motor units. Such muscles are said to have a small *innervation ratio*. The muscles of the larynx are known to have a particularly small innervation ratio (Faaborg-Andersen, 1957; Mårtensson and Skoglund, 1964; English and Blevins, 1969), especially compared with limb motor units.

The afferent fibers of the SLN and RLN supply sensory function to the larynx. Several types of small biological transducers, *mechanoreceptors,* have been identified in the larynx by morphological and/or electrophysiological methods. These sensory receptors are known to be located in the mucosa of the laryngeal cavity, within the movable joints, and in the intrinsic laryngeal muscles. An afferent neuron and its associated sensory receptors constitute a *sensory unit.*

Laryngeal Mechanoreceptors

Wyke (1967, 1969, 1973, 1974), a British neurologist working with cat larynges, advanced the idea that the larynx is supplied by many specialized receptors that influence laryngeal motor neurons by triggering coordinated reflexes. Though this position is intuitively attractive, since similar feedback and control mechanisms

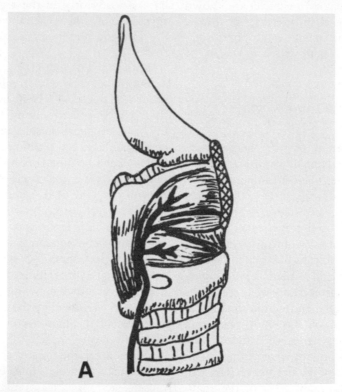

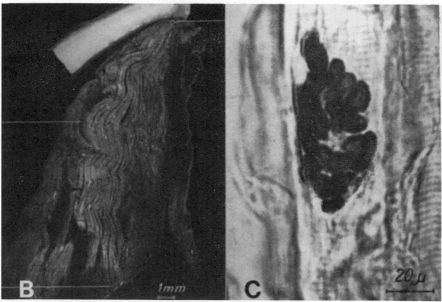

FIGURE 4-8   Details of the innervation of the intrinsic laryngeal muscles. *A,* The course and distribution of the recurrent laryngeal nerve and its branches to the thyroarytenoid and lateral cricoarytenoid muscles. *B,* A histochemically stained transverse section of the vocal fold showing the arrangement of end plates in the thyroarytenoid muscle, where they are arranged in a broad end plate zone in the middle of the vocal fold. *C,* A micrograph of a motor end plate in the vocalis muscle. A terminal axonal ending runs parallel to the muscle fiber and is contiguous to the end plate.   (B and C from Sonesson, B. [1960]. On the anatomy and vibratory pattern of the human vocal folds. *Acta Oto-laryngologica, 156* (Suppl.), 1-80.)

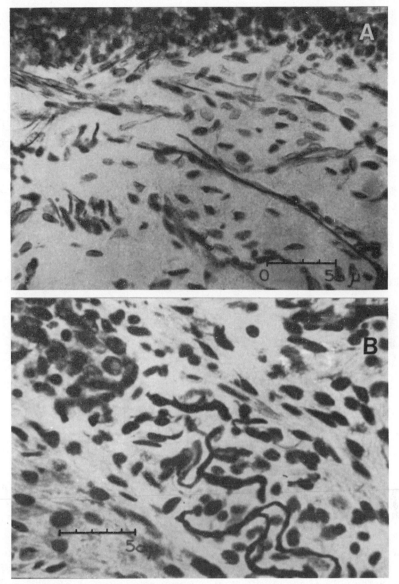

FIGURE 4-9   Mechanoreceptors in the human larynx. *A,* Subepithelial neurofibrils in the posterior third of the vocal fold. *B,* Fundiform corpuscular endings from epithelium overlying the corniculate cartilages. (A and B from König, W. F., & von Leden, H. [1961]. The peripheral nervous system of the human larynx: 1. The mucous membrane. *Archives of Otolaryngology, 73,* 1-14.)

exist elsewhere in the body, it has not been widely accepted in its native form for several reasons. Among these is the fact that not all of the mechanoreceptors in the human larynx have been identified. In addition to the fact that some of the physiological responses seen in the cat have not been verified in the human, the neurophysiological response times for some of these receptors appear too slow to serve the rapid mechanical and aerodynamic events associated with the human voice. Nonetheless, Wyke's model is valuable because it offers a framework within which to test and explain the various mechanisms of laryngeal control.

Corpuscular receptors have been found in the mucosa of the supraglottal and infraglottal regions (König and von Leden, 1961a). These receptors (Figure 4-9, *A* and *B*) respond to defor-

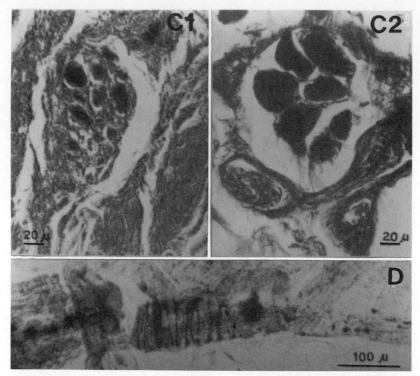

FIGURE 4-9, cont'd. *C1* and *C2,* Cross-sections of muscle spindles in the vocalis muscle. *D,* A spiral nerve ending around a vocalis muscle fiber. (C and D from Rossi, G., & Cortesina, G. [1965]. Morphological study of the laryngeal muscles in man. *Acta Otolaryngologica, 59,* 575-592.)

mation of the mucosa caused by tactile and aeromechanical stimuli. The mucosal receptors in the supraglottal region elicit an occlusive response (Sampson and Eyzaguirre, 1964). Stimulation of the infraglottal region increases tonicity in the adductor muscles while reciprocally decreasing abductor activity (Takenouchi et al., 1968). According to Kirchner and Suzuki (1968), these receptors are sensitive to the rate of airflow and influence muscle activity in the area of the glottis.

Specialized receptors, called *arthroreceptors,* have been identified in the joint capsules of the cricothyroid and cricoarytenoid joints (Jankovskaya, 1959; Gracheva, 1963). They were studied extensively in cat larynges by Kirchner and Wyke (1964). Sensitive to joint movement, these arthroreceptors are modified corpuscular receptors, similar to the pacinian pressure corpuscles found elsewhere in the body. Responses of these receptors may facilitate or inhibit laryngeal motor neurons (Kirchner and Suzuki, 1968). Joint receptors are thought to be particularly important for the precise positioning

of the vocal folds for respiration and voice production.

The intrinsic laryngeal muscles are supplied with a system of receptor nerve endings, the exact nature of which has yet to be delineated. Two forms of receptors, *muscle spindles* and *spiral nerve endings,* have been identified in the human larynx (Figure 4-9, *C* and *D*). Neuromuscular spindles are sensitive to a change in muscle length (i.e., stretch) and the velocity of that change. Small numbers of muscle spindles and their associated intrafusal fibers have been found in the intrinsic musculature, where they are arranged parallel to the extrafusal muscle fibers that make up the bulk of the muscle mass (Lucas-Keene, 1961; Voss, 1966; Grim, 1967; Baken, 1971; Baken and Noback, 1971; Okamura and Katto, 1988). However, no one author has reported finding spindle organs in each muscle. While Rossi and Cortesina (1965) maintain that muscle spindles can be found only in the vocalis muscle, Okamura and Katto (1988) reportedly observed these receptors in all laryngeal muscles except the lateral cricoarytenoid.

Other investigators maintain that there is not ample morphological evidence to support the existence of spindle organs in any of the intrinsic muscles, but instead that a number of spiral nerve endings coil around individual or paired muscle fibers and, as with spindle function, sense changes in muscle length (Rudolf, 1961; König and von Leden, 1961b; Gracheva, 1963; Nakamura, 1964; Abo-El-Enein and Wyke, 1966).

The case for a laryngeal feedback system is supported by the presence of several types of receptors and the observation that stimulation of these receptors gives rise to coordinated reflexive changes in the tonus of the intrinsic laryngeal muscles, at least in the cat (Kirchner and Wyke, 1965; Abo-El-Enein and Wyke, 1966). Determining how these reflexes may function during human voice production is one of the great challenges in voice science.

Phonatory Function

Sound is any audible pressure fluctuation. The larynx produces voice sound by converting a source of static potential energy (the volume of compressed air in the lower respiratory system) into the kinetic energy of a rapidly modulated egressive airflow, resulting in a series of airborne pressure waves.

While almost everyone feels comfortable with the term *voice,* it is difficult to propose a universally accepted definition. For some the voice is the signal produced by the larynx. For others the voice is the laryngeal signal altered by the vocal tract to shape a vowel or other voiced speech sound. [In this chapter *phonation* will refer to the production of a *laryngeal tone* or *buzz.* *] In the truest sense this tone is the vocal signal, but it does not sound like or even resemble a vowel sound. On the contrary, and for good reasons, the laryngeal tone sounds quite similar to the bilabial trill often called a "Bronx cheer" or "raspberry." This crude and undistinguished tone is rich in harmonic energy and is the primary sound source for speech. The nature of the vocal signal heavily influences our perception of pitch and loudness, and thus the *prosody* of speech, as well as certain qualities such as hoarseness and breathiness. Further-

more, *voicing,* the presence or absence of the laryngeal tone during consonant articulation, has great phonemic importance. The remainder of this chapter will focus on these highly specialized and uniquely human functions of the laryngeal valve.

PHONATION: HOW IS IT ACHIEVED?

Despite new experimental methods and the increased precision of measurement that has followed major technological advances over the past half century, some fundamental questions concerning phonation remain largely unanswered. The act of producing voice is not a simple one; its complexity is responsible for the wide range of phonatory behaviors that characterize the human voice. Thus, present theories of voice production have arisen from the efforts of many types of voice scientists, including those with training in anatomy, physiology, neurology, vocal music, linguistic phonetics, physics, engineering, medicine, and speech pathology.

Preliminaries To A Myoelastic-Aerodynamic Theory

The myoelastic-aerodynamic theory of phonation maintains that the vocal folds vibrate as the result of a dynamic competition involving opposing and complementary muscular, biomechanical, and aerodynamic forces that act at the rima glottidis. This characterization forms the foundation of all modern descriptions of phonatory function.

Myoelastic Factors

The first myoelastic theory was advanced by the French physician Antoine Ferrein (1746), who also coined the term *vocal cords.* Although Ferrein was a professor of anatomy, he failed to recognize that what he called the vocal cords were *folds* of tissue. Ferrein viewed voice production as a process in which the airstream plucks or bows the vocal ligament, which vibrates much like a harpsichord or violin string. In this scheme, phonation results as the vibration of the "cords" is transmitted to the surrounding air. While his theory is now known to be in error, Ferrein made important statements regarding the mass, length, and tension of the vocal folds. Just as a uniform tube model is a useful but highly simplified model of vocal tract function

---

*The larynx may also produce an aperiodic, turbulent sound source, as in whispered speech. Both whisper and the glottal fricative [h] result from a relatively high airflow through a relatively static and incomplete glottal occlusion.

during vowel production, the string model is a useful but rudimentary model of vocal fold vibration. String factors of particular interest are tension and stiffness as they relate to elasticity and mass as it relates to inertia.

Stiffness is a structure's resistance to displacement, and *elasticity* is its tendency to return to its rest position following displacement (elastic recoil). A rubber band, for instance, is elastic not because it can be stretched but because it snaps back to its original condition. *Compliance* is the inverse of stiffness; that is, it is the ease with which a body can be deformed. Glass marbles, for example, are less compliant than rubber balls. When two glass marbles strike, they keep their shape and almost immediately bounce off each other. However, when two rubber balls strike, they deform one another and maintain a longer period of contact before rebounding. If two balls of modeling clay collide, they deform themselves with minimal recovery. Although elastic media may be solid, liquid, or gaseous, elasticity is usually modeled as a simple spring. After all, the resilience of an air mattress or water bed is equivalent to that provided by a box spring mattress.

We can also view elasticity in terms of the *tension* generated within a structure; the more taut a body is, the faster it will recover from displacement. Both the resistance to movement and the speed of recovery are directly proportional to the tension of an elastic medium. The degree of stretch and the magnitude of tension generated will depend on the *stress-strain* relationship. The tensile coefficient of elasticity, *Young's modulus,* is the ratio of stress to strain, where stress is a force divided by the cross-sectional area perpendicular to the direction of force, and strain is the elongation of the body in the direction of the force divided by its resting length. Tension and elongation are not linearly related; tension grows faster than length. As a body (such as a spring) is stretched by equal increments, the passive tension will tend to increase exponentially.

Mass is the amount of matter in a body. It is not, strictly speaking, equivalent to its weight, which is a function of gravitational force. More effort is required to move a large mass than a small one. In addition, it is more difficult to stop the larger mass. *Inertia* is the tendency for objects at rest to stay at rest and for objects that are moving to continue moving. The inertia of an object is directly proportional to its mass.

When a string is stretched, it not only tenses but becomes thinner, so that its mass and inertia decrease *at each point* along the string but not for the string as a whole.

The mass and elasticity of a medium determine its vibratory characteristics. Figure 4-10 shows the behavior of a mass coupled to a spring. For any such system there is a point of equilibrium with the mass at rest and the spring unperturbed. At point A the transient force is great enough to displace the mass and stretch the spring. The elasticity of the spring will work to restore the mass to its rest position (point B), but inertia will keep the mass moving and compress the spring (point C). Having again been deformed, the spring will move the mass toward its rest position (point D), but inertia will again move the mass past the point of equilibrium (point A). In this "ideal" model no frictional forces dissipate energy, and this action will continue indefinitely with the same amplitude of displacement in each cycle. This is *simple harmonic motion.* The rate of oscillation is directly proportional to the elasticity (speed of restoration) and inversely proportional to the mass (degree of inertia). The amplitude of oscillation is inversely proportional to the mass and elasticity. In a real system friction will dampen the oscillation, so that the amplitude of displacement will grow less and less until the mass-spring system reaches its point of equilibrium, the system's *operating point,* and stops.

Aerodynamic Factors

The German physiologist Johannes Müller (1839) suggested that it was not the vibration of the vocal folds per se but the modulation of the expiratory airstream by vocal fold vibration that produces voice. Although incorrect in likening the larynx to a reed instrument, Müller nonetheless laid the foundation for modern aerodynamic theory of voice production. The exact mechanism by which vocal fold vibration chops the subglottal airstream was argued through the middle of this century, when Janwillem van den Berg formulated a cohesive myoelastic-aerodynamic theory of phonation in 1958. Like Ferrein and Müller before him, van den Berg used data derived from experiments with excised cadaveric larynges (Figure 4-11) to support his theory (van den Berg and Tan, 1959).

For air to flow it must be pushed along; that is, there must be an energy source. *Pressure,*

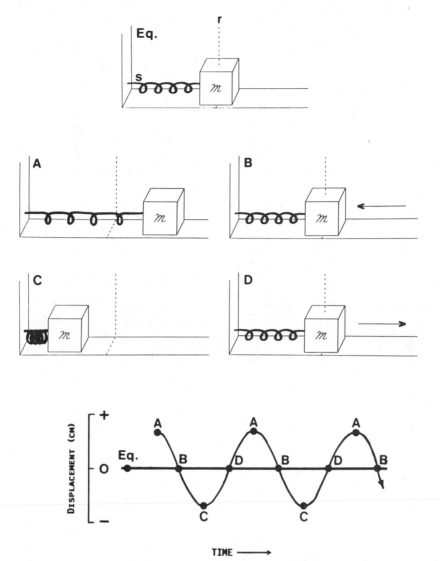

FIGURE 4-10   The vibration of an ideal mass-spring system (*Eq.,* equilibrium; *r,* rest position, *m,* mass). (See text for more information).

defined as a force per unit area, is the static energy source from which the flowing kinetic energy is drawn. The force exerted by pressure acts perpendicularly to the surface to which it is applied. Air pressure can be thought of as an aerodynamic system's battery. Air will flow if there is a conduit connecting an area of high pressure to one of low pressure. Phonation requires the pressure below the vocal folds to be higher than that above so that an egressive airflow ensues. All of the acoustic energy in the vocal signal is derived from this **transglottal pressure,** which is the relative difference between the subglottal (lung) and supraglottal (pharyngeal) pressures. Thus, the transglottal pressure drop is often called the *driving pressure*

of phonation. Since the supraglottal pressure approximates that of the atmosphere during vowel production, the subglottal pressure is the *effective driving pressure.*

The volume of air flowing through a constricted tube per unit of time is determined by the magnitude of the supply pressure relative to the resistance offered by the obstruction to the flow. If 125 ml of air enters the tube per second, it follows that the same volume of air per second must exit the tube. At the constriction, the volume of air that can pass through at a given speed is reduced. To maintain the flow rate through the narrowed portion, the velocity must increase in proportion to the degree of constriction. This explains why the water from a garden

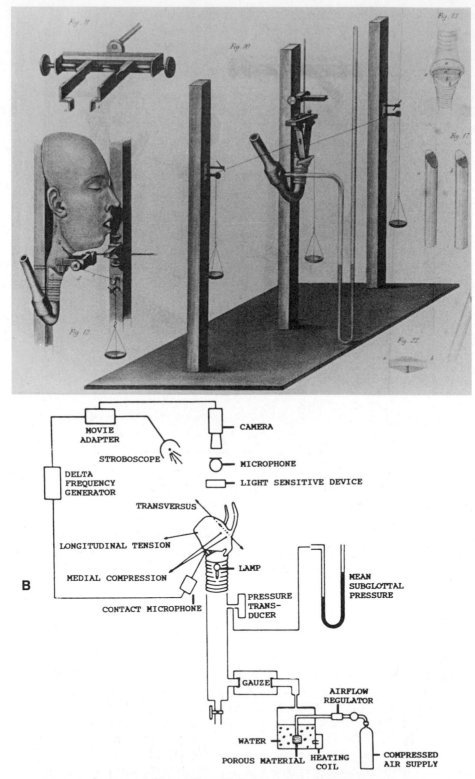

FIGURE 4-11 Apparatus used by Müller (1839) (*A*) and van den Berg and Tan (*B*) to investigate the mechanisms of human voice production using insufflated excised larynges. (A from Müller, J. [1839]. *Üeber die Compensation der physischen Kräfte am menschlichen Stimmorgan.* Berlin: A. Hirschwald. B from van den Berg, Jw., & Tan T. S. [1959]. Results of experiments with human larynxes. *Practica Oto-Rhino- Laryngologica, 21,* 425-450.)

hose travels farther and faster when you put your finger over the opening and occlude part of the aperture (Walker, 1987).

The total energy in an ideal system is equal to the sum of the potential energy of pressure (P) and the kinetic energy (KE) of motion. KE is related to the density of the flowing medium (ρ) and to the velocity with which it flows (v):

$$KE = \tfrac{1}{2}\rho\, v^2.$$

It follows that the total energy (E) available to a system may be represented as

$$E = P + \tfrac{1}{2}\rho\, v^2.$$

Assuming that the density of air is constant (about 0.0012 g/cm^3), if the velocity of the flowing medium increases, KE increases. A basic law of physics is that the total energy of a system is conserved (neither created nor destroyed). Thus, with an increase in KE, P must decrease proportionately, since the sum of potential and kinetic energy must remain constant. Therefore, if air is flowing through a tube that narrows at some point, its velocity will increase as a function of the degree of constriction. The energy needed to increase air velocity cannot be simply created; it is drained from the potential energy available at that point in the tube. For this reason, the pressure at the constriction will be lower than that on either the upstream or downstream side of the narrows. The fall in pressure will be inversely proportional to the velocity of flow at that point. The phenomenon by which airflow generates negative pressure at a tube constriction is called the **Bernoulli effect**, after the eighteenth century Swiss mathematician who first described it. Tonndorf (1925) was the first to apply the Bernoulli principle to the glottal airstream.

Classical Myoelastic-Aerodynamic Theory

At its core the myoelastic-aerodynamic theory maintains that the aerostatic lung pressure works to open the glottis as the myoelastic recoil force and aerodynamic Bernoulli force work to seal the glottis, resulting in vocal fold vibration.

According to the traditional account, at the onset of phonation, the adducted vocal folds are pushed apart by the buildup of subglottal pressure. This pressure must overcome both vo-

cal fold stiffness and inertia. A minimum of about 3 to 5 cm H$_2$O of pressure appears to be necessary to begin phonation (van den Berg, 1956; Isshiki, 1964; Kunze, 1964), but vibration can be sustained on pressures as low as 1 or 2 cm H$_2$O (van den Berg and Tan, 1959; Draper, Ladefoged, and Witteridge, 1960; Lieberman, Knudson, and Mead, 1969; Sawashima et al., 1988). With the separation of the vocal folds and the formation of a glottis, transglottal airflow will ensue. The glottis is a tube constriction for which the Bernoulli principle is applicable (Stevens and Klatt, 1974). As soon as the vocal folds allow an airflow, the increased air velocity through the glottis and the resulting intraglottal pressure drop suck the folds back together (van den Berg, Zantema, and Doornenbal, 1957). The elastic recoil of the tissue is strongest, and the Bernoulli force weakest, at the vocal fold's widest excursion from the midline. However, as the folds approach one another, the air velocity increases and the Bernoulli suction grows stronger. Once the glottis closes and airflow ceases, the Bernoulli effect disappears, leaving the vocal folds again at the mercy of the subglottal pressure drive, and the cycle begins anew.

Toward a Myomucoviscoelastic-Aerodynamic Theory

Unfortunately, the traditional account of the myoelastic-aerodynamic theory does not adequately describe self-sustained oscillation of the vocal folds (Broad, 1979; Titze, 1980). This does not mean that the myoelastic-aerodynamic theory is wrong; it simply means that the necessary details have not been adequately delineated. For instance, opposite forces compete in many bodily systems, from the graded contraction of agonist and antagonist muscle groups to the regulation of the heart and breathing rates by the autonomic nervous system. In normal function these and other systems do not result in instability and oscillation but rather in a summation of influences, hence a dynamic compromise (Figure 4-12). The details necessary to describe self-oscillation (that is, factors that prevent a static compromise from being reached) came largely in the 1970s with a greater understanding of vocal fold ultrastructure and with an appreciation of the complex relationship between vocal fold mechanics and glottal aerodynamics.

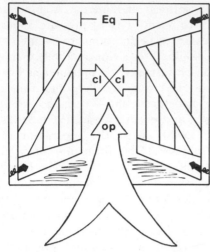

FIGURE 4-12 The degree to which saloon doors are held open depends on the sum of the opening and closing forces. Here, air pressure from a steady wind forces the doors open as the Bernoulli force and elastic recoil of the spring hinge work to close them, producing a static compromise (*Eq*, equilibrium; *op*, opening force; *cl*, closing force).

Cover-Body Characterization of Vocal Fold Ultrastructure

The vocal folds are not merely shelves of homogeneous tissue that move toward and away from each other as units. Despite earlier notions that the vocal folds were relatively uniform structures largely composed of a ligament and muscle, Hirano (1974) showed that each vocal fold consists of several layers, each layer distinct in histological structure and vibromechanical characteristics. In general, the outer nonmuscular mucosal cover is more compliant than the inner muscular body and is responsible for most of the vibratory movement (Hirano, 1977). The malleability of the epithelium and underlying connective tissues that support it accounts for much of the complex vibration of phonation (Figure 4-13). The wavelike motion of the vocal folds results from the interactive properties of the tissue layers within the mucosa (McGowan, 1990). Although the mucosa is only a small portion of the total mass of the vocal folds, ultrahigh-speed motion pictures taken during phonation clearly indicate the critical role of the most superficial fold layers. The relationships between the gross anatomical and histological characteristics of the vocal folds and the functional morphology of the fold layers are summarized in Table 4-2.

Figure 4-14 illustrates the organization and general composition of the vocal fold layers,

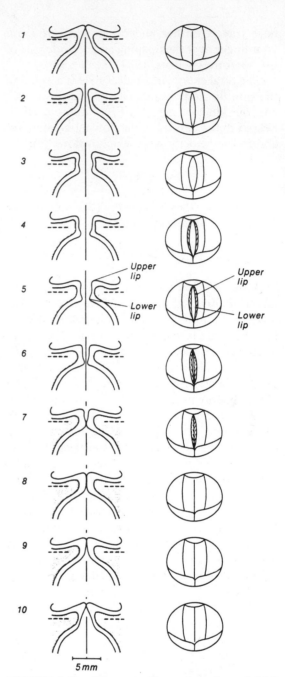

FIGURE 4-13 Schematic illustration of vocal fold vibration. At left the folds are shown in frontal section. At right they are viewed from above. A similar characterization was proposed by Schönhärl (1960). (From Hirano, M. [1981]. *Clinical examination of voice.* New York: Springer-Verlag.)

includng the epithelium, connective tissue (lamina propria), and muscle (vocalis muscle fibers).

EPITHELIUM Except for a small area on the medial and superior edge, the vocal fold is covered by pseudostratified ciliated columnar

TABLE 4-2 Gross anatomy and histology of the vocal folds

Gross Anatomy	Histologic Structure	Functional Division	Biomechanical Property[a]	Vibration
Mucosa				
Epithelium	Stratified squamous type[b]	Cover	Behaves like "a thin and stiff capsule"	Greatest
Connective Tissue	Superficial lamina propria	Cover	Consistency of "a mass of soft gelatin"	Greatest
	Intermediate lamina propria	Transition	Consistency of "a bundle of soft rubber bands"	Intermediate
	Deep lamina propria	Transition	Consistency of "a bundle of cotton thread"	Intermediate
Muscle	Vocalis fibers of the thyroarytenoid muscle	Body	Consistency of "a bundle of rather stiff rubber bands"	Least

[a]Description used by Hirano (1981a).
[b]Contacting portion of the vocal folds.

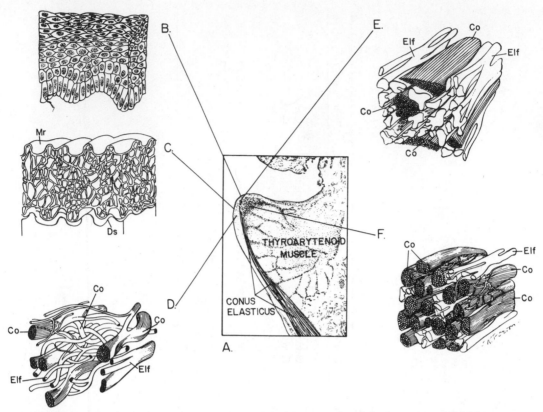

FIGURE 4-14 Composite figure illustrates the ultrastructure of the human vocal folds, particularly of the lamina propria. *A,* Schematic coronal section showing the macroscopic relationship between the nonmuscular and muscular portions of the vocal fold. *B,* Layers of vocal fold epithelium. *C,* Ultrastructure of the epithelial cell showing upper and lower layers interconnected by minute cellular projections called tonofilaments. *D,* Superficial layer of the lamina propria. *E,* Intermediate layer of the lamina propria. *F,* Deep layer of the lamina propria. (*Mr,* microridges on the surface of the squamous epithelial cell. *Ds,* desmozome. *Co,* collagenous fibers. *Elf,* elastic fibers.) (Adapted from Hirano, M. [1975]. Phonosurgery. Basic and clinical investigations. *Otologia Fukuoka, 21,* 239-440.)

epithelium like that found lining the rest of the respiratory system. At the midportion of the fold, which makes contact with the opposite fold during vocal vibration, the epithelium is stratified and squamous. The area covered with squamous epithelium is approximately 4 mm (Hirano, 1975). This epithelium covering is especially well adapted to protecting wet surfaces from the kind of friction and pounding associated with voice production. The epithelium is composed of eight layers with a combined thickness of only about 0.05 mm (Hirano, 1975, 1977). The upper and lower surfaces of each epithelial cell are connected by minute cellular projections called *tonofilaments.*

LAMINA PROPRIA The lamina propria is a common connective tissue underlying many simple epithelia. Its primary function is to bind epithelia to underlying muscle, providing support for blood vessels and nerve fibers. However, the lamina propria in the human vocal fold has a far more elaborate structure than that in most other parts of the body. The vocal fold lamina propria consists of three layers, histologically distinguishable by the distribution, weave, and density of elastic and collagenous connective tissue fibers. Progressing from the epithelium to the muscle, the lamina propria is divided into a *superficial, intermediate,* and *deep* layer. Their combined thickness is about 1.2 mm (Hirano, 1975, 1977).

The superficial lamina propria (SLP) is separated from the overlying epithelium by a basement membrane. Composed of scant amounts of loosely woven elastic and collagenous fibers, the SLP is about 0.3 mm thick. The small amount of dense connective tissue and the generally loose weave within the layer give it greater mobility than the deeper layers of the lamina propria.

The intermediate layer of the lamina propria (ILP) is readily distinguishable from the SLP in its stiffness and density. The ILP is composed mainly of greatly interwoven elastic fibers, although small amounts of dense collagenous fibers are also present. The collagenous fibers of the ILP largely form the conus elasticus, the principal fibroelastic membrane of the infraglottis.

The deep layer of the lamina propria (DLP) lies between the ILP and the vocalis fibers of the thyroarytenoid muscle. Fibers of the deeper portion of the ILP intermix with fibers of the DLP to form the *vocal ligament*. The vocal ligament, about 0.8 mm thick, is composed principally of tightly woven, dense collagenous fibers that course anteroposteriorly parallel to the adjacent muscle. Collagenous fibers from the DLP intermix with the perimysium (connective tissue) of the underlying muscle, forming a linkage between the nonmuscular and muscular portions of the vocal fold. The DLP is the least mobile of the layers of connective tissue in the vocal fold.

MUSCULAR BODY   The TA alone forms the muscular portion of the vocal fold. It courses anteroposteriorly from the deep surface of the thyroid cartilage to the arytenoid cartilage. The most medial TA fibers, the vocalis muscle, are systematically active during voice production, whereas other portions of the muscle, particularly the thyromuscularis fibers, do not appear to be nearly so important in voice production.

Observation of the vocal folds with ultrahigh-speed motion pictures and stroboscopy suggests that functionally the different layers of the vocal folds operate not as separate entities but as an integrated unit composed of a *cover, transition, and body* (Hirano, 1977).

The cover of the vocal folds, consisting of the epithelium and the SLP, is the portion of the folds most pliant and most accessible to aerodynamic forces. While the epithelium has a high Young's modulus, it is a very small proportion of the cover. When lax, the encapsulating epithelium serves to maintain vocal fold contour. However, when the vocal fold is pulled taut, the epithelium contributes greatly to the stiffness of the cover (Kakita, Hirano, and Ohmaru, 1981).

The transition of the vocal folds, composed of the ILP and DLP, is less mobile than the cover but appears to influence the longitudinal stability of the vocal folds during vibration. The muscular body is the least movable portion of the vocal folds. Because it exerts a substantial influence on biomechanical properties distributed along the longitudinal axis of the fold, it has a significant effect on the vibration of the transition and cover.

The Mucosal Wave

In the most common modes of phonation the vocal folds first lose medial contact at the inferior margins and peel away from bottom to top (Figure 4-13). As the superior portions of the folds lose contact, the bottom "lips" once again begin to move toward closure. The sealing of the glottis likewise progresses from bottom to top. This delay between the upper and lower medial surfaces of the folds during glottal opening and closing is called the *vertical phase difference* (Schönhärl, 1960; Vennard, 1967; Hollien, Coleman, and Moore, 1968; Hirano, 1975; Matsushita, 1975; Hirano, Yoshida, and Tanaka, 1991). The result of this phase difference is a wavelike motion of the vocal fold cover, the **mucosal wave**. The rippling effect of the mucosal wave can usually be seen on the superior surfaces of the folds as well (Hirano et al., 1981).

Viscosity, a property of matter that inhibits flow, is associated with the degree of resistance to a shearing stress (a force applied at an angle). For instance, imagine blowing on a block of gelatin from above and behind. The upper layers of the gelatin will be pushed away from you in the direction of the flow, which will tend to drag the lower layers along. *Viscoelasticity* is both the resistance of a body to such a shearing force and its tendency to rebound from an angular deformation (as will the gelatin in this case). The functional importance of the viscoelastic properties of the vocal fold mucosal cover has been highlighted by Hiroto (1966) and subsequently employed by Ishizaka and Matsudaira (1972) and Ishizaka and Flanagan (1972) in their two-mass models of vocal fold mechanics.

Mechanical Coupling of Vocal Fold Tissue

The two-mass model takes into account not only a vertical phase difference but also a nonuniform

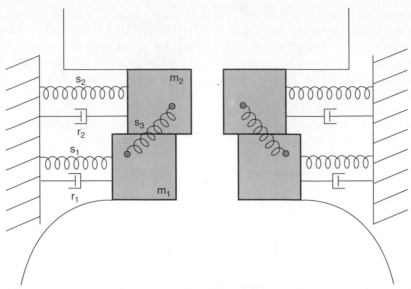

FIGURE 4-15   A two-mass model of vocal fold mechanics, as proposed by Ishizaka and Matsudaira (1972) (See text for more information).

glottal width; that is, the convergence of the inferior glottis represented by the conus elasticus. Not surprisingly, the model (Figure 4-15) employs two masses, one representing the lower margin (m_1) and the other the upper margin (m_2) of the mucosa. Each mass is associated with its own elastic spring (s_1 and s_2) and its own viscous resistance (r_1 and r_2), represented by a dashpot. (A dashpot works something like a shock absorber and is found on many storm doors and automatic doors to prevent them from closing too rapidly.) While the two masses can move independently, a third spring (s_3) couples the masses. Figure 4-15, shows the model at its operating point. Soon after the lower mass is displaced outward, the mechanical coupling will displace the upper mass in the same direction. The lower spring will compress earlier than the upper spring, and the elastic rebound of the two masses will be delayed. The strength of the mechanical coupling of the mucosa has been demonstrated by Fukuda et al. (1987) when they induced external neck vibrations on nonphonating subjects. By attaching a mechanical vibrator to the thyroid prominence, they drove the tissue longitudinally but nonetheless elicited strong vertical vibrations of the vocal fold surface similar to those seen during phonation.

The two-mass model is also called the two degrees of freedom model, since it allows for only horizontal, inward-outward movement of the tissue masses. The vibrations of the vocal

folds are far more complex than suggested by this simple model. Data derived from excised larynges (Baer, 1975, 1981a; Matsushita, 1975; Saito et al., 1981; Fukuda et al., 1983) indicate that the vocal folds undergo a fair amount of vertical displacement during phonation, so they tend to vibrate in a somewhat elliptical manner. The noncolliding portions of the folds (covered by ciliated columnar epithelium) move mostly horizontally, whereas the tissue trajectory of the medial mucosal edge is primarily circular (Figure 4-16). The muscular body of the vocal folds, on the other hand, shows an almost completely vertical displacement. In composite form, Figure 4-17 shows the dynamic nature of the vocal fold contour during a single vibratory cycle (Saito et al., 1981; Fukuda et al., 1983).

Other important shortcomings of the two-mass model are that it fails to represent the mechanical properties of the muscular body of the vocal folds and that it does not consider differences in mass and viscoelasticity along the length of the folds (Titze, 1976, 1981). There also may be horizontal phase differences, in that the vocal folds do not open or close simultaneously along their length (Rothenberg, 1981; Childers and Krishnamurthy, 1985; Hirano et al., 1985; Childers et al., 1986). Evidence from Hirano, Yoshida, and Tanaka (1991) indicates that the posterior portions of the vocal folds make contact much higher in the glottis than the anterior portions. Such considerations have prompted refinements to

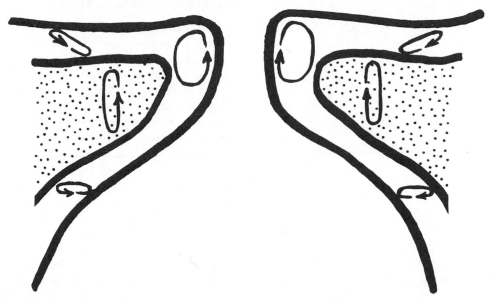

FIGURE 4-16   Typical tissue trajectories within the vocal folds during phonation. (Adapted from Baer, T. [1975]. *Investigation of phonation using excised larynxes.* Unpublished doctoral dissertation, Massachusetts Institute of Technology, Cambridge, MA; Baer, T. [1981]. Observation of vocal fold vibration: Measurement of excised larynges. In Stevens, K. N., & Hirano, M. [Eds.], *Vocal fold physiology.* Tokyo: University of Tokyo Press [pp. 119-133]; Saito, S., Fukuda, H., Isogai, Y., & Ono, H. [1981]. X-ray stroboscopy. In Stevens, K. N., & Hirano, M. [Eds.], *Vocal fold physiology.* Tokyo: University of Tokyo Press [pp. 95-106].)

this type of model. Titze (1973, 1974), for instance, has developed a 16-mass model, later supplanting that with a 64-component characterization (Titze and Talkin, 1979, 1981) (Figure 4-18).

Aerodynamic Coupling

The vibration of the vocal folds during phonation creates a constantly changing glottal geometry (Hiroto, 1966; Hollien, Coleman, and Moore, 1968; Hirano, 1977; Baer, 1981a; Saito et al., 1981) which allows for interplay of aerodynamic forces (Flanagan, 1959; Stevens, 1977; Titze, 1980, 1985; Scherer and Titze, 1983). The pressure differential between the trachea and the pharynx is critical because this pressure drives the transglottal airflow, and the transglottal airflow drives the fold tissues so that self-oscillation can occur (Ananthapadmanabha and Gauffin, 1985; Titze, 1986).

Ishizaka and Matsudaira (1972) introduced their two-mass representation of the vocal folds primarily to model the response of the tissue to the glottal airstream. When the folds are separated, the total glottal space is a function of the relative displacement of the upper and lower margins of the vocal folds. When the folds are

approximated, the subglottal pressure works to push the lower edges apart. As the folds lose contact, the intraglottal pressure on the convergent fold surface is relatively high. Indeed, data derived from miniaturized pressure transducers placed directly below the folds indicate that the subglottal pressure varies over the glottal cycle and is highest just before a glottis emerges (Perkins and Koike, 1969; Koike and Hirano, 1973; Koike, 1981; Koike et al., 1983). On the fold's return trip to midline, the upper edges are farther apart than the lower edges. The mean intraglottal pressure applied to this divergent glottis is relatively low, as the Bernoulli force works differentially to suck the inferior portions of the vocal folds together. According to Gauffin et al. (1983), aerodynamic forces work primarily on the lower margins of the glottis, allowing the upper edges of the vocal folds to be driven mainly by their mechanical coupling to the lower edges.

The mass inertia of air, however, provides for an aerodynamic mechanism that contributes to the closing of the upper portions of the folds. Upon the loss of vocal fold contact, the driving pressure overcomes the inertia of the air mass within the vocal tract and sets it in motion. As the lower glottis closes, the forward momentum

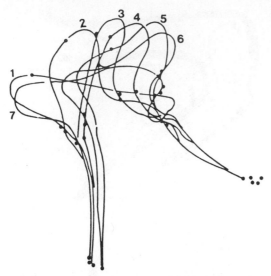

FIGURE 4-17 Successive vocal fold contours in a single vibratory cycle. Small lead pellets were implanted under the epithelium of an excised larynx. The trajectories of the pellets were tracked with x-ray stroboscopy, in this case during a 200-Hz phonation maintained at middle-range intensity. Baer (1975, 1981) was the first to employ a pellet-tracking technique. (From Fukuda, H., Saito, S., Kitahara, S., Isogai, Y., Makino, K., Tsuzuki, T., Kogawa, N., & Ono, H. [1983]. Vocal fold vibration in excised larynges viewed with an x-ray stroboscope and an ultra-high-speed camera. In Bless, D. M., & Abbs, J. H. [Eds.], *Vocal fold physiology: Contemporary research and clinical issues.* San Diego, CA: College-Hill Press [pp. 238-252].)

of the supraglottal air keeps it moving toward the upper airway. In this way, inertia leads to a pressure rise in the subglottal space and a pressure drop in that region above the constriction upon closure. The rarefied air within the upper glottis is thus thought to aid the approximation of the upper vocal fold margins (Titze, 1986, 1988a).

Because the aerodynamic coupling to the upper and lower fold masses works opposite to that of the mechanical viscoelastic coupling, the glottal airstream is said to provide a negative coupling stiffness. It is primarily due to this temporospatial coupling of oppositional forces that the vocal folds fail to reach static equilibrium during phonation. Viscous losses are counteracted by the fact that the aerodynamic forces acting on the vocal folds are in phase with the tissue velocity, so aerodynamic forces add energy to the vibration of the tissue during each oscillatory cycle (Stevens and Klatt, 1974; Stevens, 1977; Titze, 1985, 1986).

Current and Future Directions

Research continues to delineate glottal dynamics during phonation and its influence on the distribution of intraglottal pressures and the mechanical stresses on the tissues. Further elaboration of laryngeal structure, cover-body coupling, and improvement in measurement technology will aid research. In particular, the interplay of muscular and nonmuscular forces in phonatory function should be outlined in greater detail. Lauth (1835) advanced a hypothesis that the displacement of fibroelastic tissues in the larynx by muscular effort could provoke passive movements through elastic recoil forces. This concept has been advanced by Fink (1975), who described mechanisms of folding within the laryngeal cavity during a variety of functions, including voice production. He posited that reconstitution of laryngeal dimensions is possible by "elastic springs" that shorten, enlarge, widen, and narrow various laryngeal structures and dimensions. In this way, tissues displaced by muscular activity, aerodynamic forces, or passive stretch may be restored to resting or preadjustment states by nonmuscular forces. Such a mechanism would be biomechanically efficient and energy conserving. However, more study must be undertaken to define the possible contribution of these elastic forces to laryngeal and phonatory function.

Two avenues of investigation likely to be pursued with great vigor over the next several years are application of fluid mechanics and its recent offspring, deterministic chaos, to the study of phonatory processes. Work in these areas may well lead to enhanced mathematical models, to an improved ability to synthesize natural-sounding speech, and ultimately to a greater understanding of normal and abnormal phonatory function.

Theoretical Fluid Mechanics

Fluid mechanics describes the static and dynamic behavior of liquids and gases. Until fairly recently, theories of phonation have assumed a laryngeal airflow that closely conforms to an ideal, unidirectional flow. Ishizaka and Matsudaira (1972) first formally questioned this notion in their flow-separation theory.

Flow remains largely laminar as it traverses the uniform trachea and inferior glottis. A laminar flow travels in distinct tubular layers, with each layer sliding under or over the adjacent layer and remaining separate from it

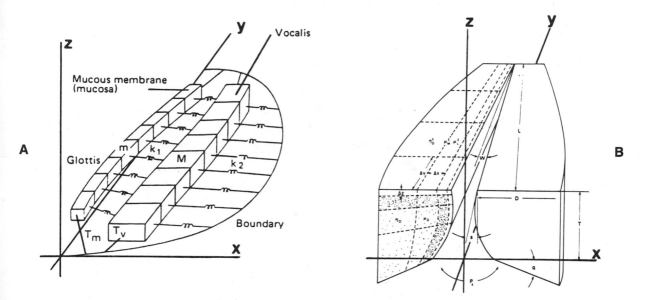

FIGURE 4-18 Two computational models of the vocal folds. *A,* a 16-mass model. *B,* a 64-element model. (A from Titze, I. R. [1973]. The human vocal cords: A mathematical model: 1. *Phonetica, 28,* 129-170. B from Titze, I. R., & Talkin, D. [1979]. A theoretical study of the effect of various laryngeal configurations on the acoustics of phonation. *Journal of the Acoustical Society of America, 66,* 60-86.)

(Warren, 1982, 1988). The outermost layer is said to be attached to the inner walls of the channel, which is called the *boundary*. In real flows, the friction of the boundary tends to retard the outer layers, disrupting the flow. For all intents and purposes, such behavior appears to be negligible until the flow passes over the medial surface of the vocal folds and enters the supraglottal space. At this point, the abrupt change in boundary geometry is thought to separate the outer layer from the boundary, producing turbulence and vortices, or eddies, in the flow (Figure 4-19). The effects are that the location and motion of any individual air particle cannot be precisely determined and flow lines become difficult to track. Fluid mechanical models employ a multidimensional view of the vocal tract and concern themselves not with the air *volume* velocity but with the specific air *particle* velocity in a vector field (Gauffin and Liljencrants, 1988; McGowan, 1988; Liljencrants, 1991). In addition, since fluid mechanical systems do not lend themselves well to computer simulation (Ishizaka and Matsudaira, 1972), physical analog models are often used to build, test, and refine theory (Teager and Teager, 1983; Gauffin and Liljencrants, 1988; Kakita, 1988).

Since the Bernoulli principle presupposes that

there are no energy losses due to turbulent or rotational flow, the effect does not hold for flows downstream of the glottis, at least not until the flow reattaches itself to the boundary (Ishizaka and Matsudaira, 1972; Broad, 1979; Kaiser, 1985). However, there is an exchange of energy as flows alternate between being irrotational and rotational. As a vortex tends to store kinetic energy, this alternation results in pressure fluctuations. Such aerodynamic phenomena have led to a search for ancillary sound sources (McGowan, 1988; Davies, McGowan, and Shadle, 1993), and has even resulted in aeroacoustic theories that call into question the very foundations of the traditional characterization of speech production as a function of a glottal sound source and a passive vocal tract filter (Kaiser, 1985; Teager and Teager, 1985a, 1985b).

Another recent theory of note is the collapsible tube model of the larynx advanced by Conrad (1980, 1983, 1987). He suggested that supraglottal resistances, such as those represented by the vestibular folds or supralaryngeal articulators, may generate a negative differential resistance within the glottis. This phenomenon has been modeled by physicists and engineers using collapsible rubber tubes with a fixed resistance somewhere beyond the tube outlet.

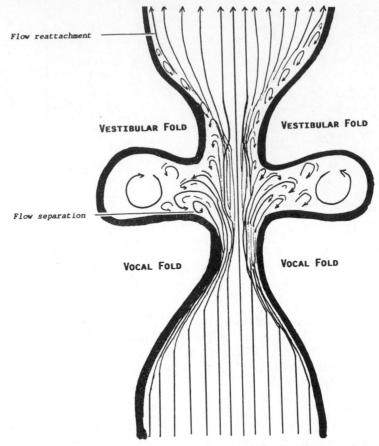

FIGURE 4-19 Frontal schematic drawing of the larynx showing the separation of the flow boundary layer at the glottal outlet and the resulting airflow turbulences and vortices. Boundary reattachment is presumed to occur somewhere within the supraglottal laryngeal cavity.

When air under constant pressure is blown through the tube, downstream resistance generates back pressure. Under specific circumstances this back pressure will lead to an increase in flow through the tube constriction associated with a decrease in the pressure drop across the tube. Such a condition has been shown to lead to instability and oscillation in the tube walls (Griffiths, 1975). Conrad and McQueen (1987) suggested that the upper margins of the vocal folds, while separating, may act as a downstream resistance and thus help drive vocal fold oscillation. However, such phenomena would only hold for phonation produced with relatively lax vocal folds and with a minimal coupling stiffness between the upper and lower mucosal margins.

Indeed, little is known about how changing glottal geometry may influence fluid mechanical phenomena (Ananthapadmanabha and Gauffin, 1985; Gauffin and Liljencrants, 1988; Titze, 1988a; Berke et al., 1989). At present the

applicability, potency, and utility of such aerodynamic models remain to be demonstrated.

Chaos Theory

The development of *deterministic chaos* (also known as *nonlinear dynamics*) in the 1970s revolutionized both physics and mathematics (Prigogine and Stengers, 1984; Gleick, 1987; Grebogi, Ott, and Yorke, 1987; Lauterborn and Parlitz, 1988; Pagels, 1988; Ruelle, 1989) and has begun to make major inroads in our understanding of physiological control processes as well (Mackey and Glass, 1977; Kelso and Tuller, 1984; Olsen and Degn, 1985; Kleiger et al., 1987; Mayer-Kress and Layne, 1987; Glass and Mackey, 1988; Rapp et al., 1989). For instance, chaos theory describes how a relatively stable system, such as that regulating heart or ventilatory function, makes the transition to complete irregularity and instability, as with cardiac fibrillation and Cheyne-Stokes respiration (Glass,

Guevara, and Shrier, 1987; Goldberger and West, 1987a; Kleiger et al., 1987; Mackey and Milton, 1987; Goldberger and Rigney, 1990; Coumel and Maison-Blanche, 1991; Kryger and Millar, 1991). Traditional scientific thought dictates that such behaviors are tied to the many degrees of freedom associated with each system. If the system is typically regular in its function but becomes unpredictable, one normally looks for uncontrolled intervening variables. That is, such behavior does not fit within the theory of normal function. Chaos theory, on the other hand, posits that because of inherent nonlinearities such systems can produce unpredictable irregular behavior even if all of the necessary control variables have been accounted for and there are no random or unpredictable inputs (Devaney, 1987, 1990; Moon, 1987; Chernikov, Sagdeev, and Zaslavsky, 1988; Olsen and Schaffer, 1990).

There is little doubt that chaos theory will become an exciting and integral part of our description of phonatory behavior. For instance, for the first time there is a method to describe the nature of the whorl, swirl, and tumble of the airstream turbulence before, beyond, or within the glottis. Nonlinearities in vocal fold tissue dynamics allow vibration to be portrayed in a similar manner (Awrejcewicz, 1990; Titze, 1990a). Chaos theory may lead toward the development of a unified model of voice production that explains both normal phonatory function and the failure of function (Baken, 1990; Mende, Herzel, and Wermke, 1990; Herzel et al., 1991; Lucero, 1993; Titze, Baken, and Herzel, 1993; Berry et al., 1994). Such characterizations would represent an evolution from a correlative approach (which relates variables) to an explanatory approach (which ascribes causation). Since nonlinearity and irregularity are undoubtedly part of the phonatory system, it is not surprising that aphonia can spring from normal phonation. There is some evidence, however, that a system's ability to regulate and control itself depends on its nonlinearities (Mackey and Glass, 1977; Prigogine and Stengers, 1984; Goldberger and West, 1987a; Pool, 1989; Baken, 1990; Mandell and Shlesinger, 1990). Linear feedback systems, when perturbed, tend to remain out of kilter, whereas nonlinear systems tend to adapt fairly quickly to quite a range of stimuli. At present, the nonlinear dynamical view of phonatory function appears to hold great but guarded promise.

THE SOURCE OF THE VOICE

Much information regarding glottal and vocal fold behavior has come from ultrahigh-speed films of the superior surface of the vocal folds during phonation. Analysis of these films frame by frame has allowed researchers to chart changes in vocal fold excursion and glottal area over the course of a vibratory cycle (Moore and von Leden, 1958; Timcke, von Leden, and Moore, 1958, 1959; Tanabe et al., 1975; Hirano et al., 1981). The recent development and accessibility of new instruments and techniques has led to a greater understanding of vocal physiology. The diverse outputs of these modern instrumental systems describe or measure glottal or vocal fold behavior and fall under the general term of *glottographic waveforms* (Titze and Talkin, 1981). A thorough review of voice instrumentation and measurement is available in Baken (1987). We will briefly describe the various types of glottographic waveforms being studied and their salient characteristics.

Glottographic Waveforms

First employed by Sonesson (1959, 1960), photoglottography measures the amount of light passing through the glottis during phonation. The resulting waveform, the *photoglottogram* (PGG), varies proportionately with changes in glottal area and is thus a continuous and automated representation of what would otherwise have to be painstakingly plotted from high-speed film data (Harden, 1975; Baer, Löfqvist, and McGarr, 1983). The PGG waveform is rather symmetrical and triangular, indicating that glottal area tends to increase and decrease fairly uniformly. However, the PGG relays no information once the light path is obstructed by the lower margins of the vocal folds; information related to the closure of the upper glottis is not transmitted.

A complementary waveform represents the vibratory pattern of the vocal folds (Kelman, 1981). Electroglottograpy is the detection of impedance changes in a small electric current as it flows across the neck at the level of the vocal folds (Fabre, 1957; Chevrie-Muller, 1967; Fourcin, 1974, 1981; Baken, 1987). Since the electrical impedance is inversely proportional to the extent of tissue contact in the horizontal and vertical planes, the *electroglottogram* (EGG) plots changes in vocal fold medial contact area (Gilbert, Potter, and Hoodin, 1984; Scherer,

Druker, and Titze, 1988; Baken, 1992). Unlike the PGG, the EGG is typically asymmetrical. Once contact between the lower margins of the vocal folds is made, maximal fold contact is achieved relatively quickly. The loss of contact is a slower process. Since the EGG is sensitive to contact changes in the vertical plane, it provides information during the portion of the oscillatory cycle when the PGG is silent. Insight regarding possible horizontal phase differences might be obtained by the nature and degree of overlap between a concurrent PGG and EGG (Baer et al., 1983). The simultaneous measurement of the PGG and EGG thus improves the utility of either in isolation, providing a great deal of information about both glottal and vibratory dynamics (Baer, Titze, and Yoshioka, 1983).

A glottographic waveform of particular significance is associated with the flow of air through the glottis during phonation. It is usually approximated by inverse-filtering the oral airflow to subtract the effect of the supraglottal resonances (Miller, 1959; Rothenberg, 1973, 1981). The resulting signal is called the **glottal volume velocity**, or glottal flow waveform or, more recently, the *flow glottogram* (Fritzell et al., 1986; Sundberg, 1987; Gauffin and Sundberg, 1989), abbreviated FLOGG (Sundberg, 1990).

Because the laryngeal tone is tied to the modulation of the expiratory flow, the FLOGG can be considered the waveform of the glottal sound source. One might expect the FLOGG and PGG to be quite similar to each other. After all, if the driving pressure is constant, as the glottal area increases, the resistance to the flow of air should decrease. Nevertheless, the two glottograms are by no means identical. When the glottis first opens, the inertia of the subglottal air mass retards the transglottal flow. As the glottis closes, the generated momentum of the air mass retards the fold's ability to stop the glottal flow (Rothenberg, 1973, 1983). The delay in air acceleration and deceleration results in a FLOGG phase lag with respect to the PGG (glottal area) and a skewing of the waveform (Figure 4-20). Other possible influences on the glottal flow include pressure fluctuations associated with the resonant properties of the subglottal and supraglottal airway and with horizontal phase differences in vocal fold movement (Flanagan, 1968; Rothenberg, 1981, 1983).

Figure 4-21 shows the lip-radiated acoustic (sound pressure) signal with several simultaneous glottographic waveforms as might be obtained during vowel production. Notice that each glottogram repeats itself each cycle and that

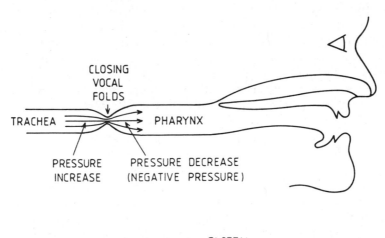

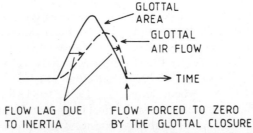

FIGURE 4-20 The effects of inertia on glottal airflow. (From Rothenberg [1983]. An interactive model for the voice source. In Bless, D.M., & Abbs, J. H. [Eds.], *Vocal fold physiology: contemporary research and clinical issues.* San Diego, CA: College Hill Press [pp. 155-165].)

the major acoustic pressure disturbance corresponds to a *closure* of the vocal folds. Thus, phonation is not like a series of quick coughs but rather it is the sudden stoppage of flow and subsequent drop in supraglottal pressure that results in the acoustic excitation of the vocal tract. As such, the rate of the FLOGG airflow "plunge" is critical to the nature and quality of the sound produced by the larynx (Rosenberg, 1971; Fant, 1979; Gauffin and Sundberg, 1989; Price, 1989).

Glottal and Vocal Efficiency

The efficiency of any mechanical system is simply the ratio of input power to output power. As far as the laryngeal generator is concerned, this is the amount of physical or bodily effort required to produce a given amount of acoustic energy at the glottal outlet. Since physiological power cannot be measured in a practical manner, we typically substitute pulmonic or subglottal power (van den Berg, 1956; Isshiki, 1964). *Subglottal power* is the product of the static subglottal air

pressure and the kinetic tracheal airflow. Because it is difficult to measure acoustic energy at the level of the glottis (Koyama, Harvey, and Ogura, 1972), researchers have substituted the lip-radiated acoustic energy (that is, the vowel **intensity** measured at a fixed distance from the mouth) for the measure of power output. Therefore, such measurements relate to vocal rather than glottal efficiency. Both van den Berg (1956) and Cavagna and Margaria (1968) found that vocal efficiency increases with the amount of subglottal power spent. Unfortunately, the vocal tract is known to absorb a variable amount of acoustic energy, and the degree of mouth opening surely affects the intensity detected at the microphone (Fairbanks, 1950; House, 1959; Ladefoged and McKinney, 1963; Isshiki, 1964; Baken and Orlikoff, 1992). Accordingly, Isshiki (1964) has recommended that a mouthpiece be used to stabilize the configuration of the vocal tract during phonation.

While the utility of vocal efficiency measures in the description of normal phonatory function has yet to be demonstrated, their application to

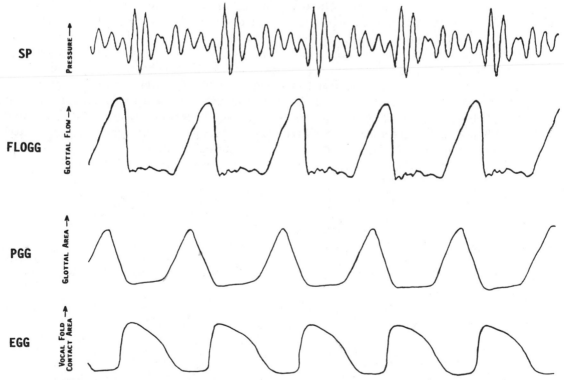

FIGURE 4-21 A representation of typical acoustic (*SP*), flow glottographic (*FLOGG*), photoglottographic (*PGG*), and electroglottographic (*EGG*) waveforms obtained simultaneously during a prolonged phonation. There is a short delay as the acoustic signal travels from the larynx to the microphone.

dysphonic populations is self-evident. Since subglottal pressure cannot be easily measured in a clinical setting, Isshiki (1981, 1985) has proposed a pseudoefficiency measure, the vocal efficiency index, or AC/DC ratio, based on airflow alone. In short, the measure compares the *effective* (that is, the root mean square) glottal flow with the mean expiratory flow rate, reflecting the ability of the glottis to convert an unmodulated, or DC, pulmonary airflow into a modulated, or AC, supraglottal airstream.

If the vocal folds do not make complete contact over their entire length, the unmodulated airflow emerging from the glottis may increase, producing an abnormally low AC/DC ratio. Unmodulated airflow does not contribute to the glottal signal and thus is wasted air and energy. Excessive DC flow may result in unwanted turbulence noise (Yanagihara, 1967, 1970), a decrease in relative acoustic energy (Fant, 1979; Holmberg, Hillman, and Perkell, 1988; Gauffin and Sundberg, 1989), and a breathy voice (Fritzell et al., 1986; Södersten and Lindestad, 1990). Even subjects with an apparently normal voice may have incomplete vocal fold contact, especially at the posterior glottis (Schönhärl, 1960; Koike and Hirano, 1973; Cavagna and Camporesi, 1974; Biever and Bless, 1989; Holmberg, Hillman, and Perkell, 1989; Södersten and Lindestad, 1990; Linville, 1992). On the other hand, normal to high AC/DC ratios can be obtained from an inefficient, so-called hyperfunctional voice (Isshiki, 1981; Hillman et al., 1989). These factors, coupled with the high intrasubject variability typically observed in efficiency measures, have severely limited their ability to discriminate pathology when used alone (Wilson and Starr, 1985; Schutte, 1986; Hillman et al., 1989) but in conjunction with other measures may more accurately describe both normal and abnormal phonatory function (Schutte and van den Berg, 1976; Hiki, 1983; Tanaka and Gould, 1985; Schutte, 1986; Hillman et al., 1989). Feasible

efficiency measures and various indices of glottal efficiency (such as phonation quotient, phonation time, and mean airflow measures) continue to be developed, tested, and modified using a wide variety of subjects (Isshiki, Okamura, and Morimoto, 1967; Hirano, Koike, and von Leden, 1968; Hirano, 1981a; Baken, 1987).

Vocal Stability

In addition to the turbulence noise and reduced intensity that may be associated with inefficient phonation, the degree of cycle-to-cycle variability of the vocal fold vibratory rate (fundamental frequency) and acoustic amplitude (sound pressure) have been shown to be closely allied with perceived voice quality (Heiberger and Horii, 1982).

Fundamental Frequency Perturbation (Vocal Jitter)

Scripture (1904, 1906) noted that the normal voice is associated with a variable and irregular vocal **period,** the time it takes to complete a single glottal cycle; the reciprocal of the frequency of phonation. Simon (1927) later extended Scripture's observation to sustained phonations in which the speaker maintained as steady a pitch as possible in an attempt to produce a maximally constant vocal period (Figure 4-22). However, it is only in the past 30 years that there has been much research on this cycle-to-cycle period variability (known as **fundamental frequency perturbation** or **vocal jitter**) in the normal voice.

While early attempts at synthesizing speech indicated that some degree of jitter is needed for listeners to perceive a natural-sounding voice (Schroeder and David, 1960; Rozsypal and Millar, 1979), others have related the excessive short-term frequency variability common in vocal pathology to the perception of a harsh, hoarse, or rough voice (Lieberman, 1963;

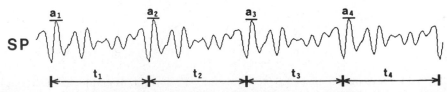

FIGURE 4-22 Sequential vocal periods (*t*) and amplitudes (*a*) marked on an acoustic sound pressure (*SP*) waveform of a prolonged vowel. Although the vocal period and intensity appear uniform, perceptually significant differences (typically on the order of a fraction of a millisecond or a fraction of a decibel) exist for any two contiguous cycles.

Wendahl, 1963; 1966; Bowler, 1964; Moore and Thompson, 1965; Takahashi and Koike, 1975; Hillenbrand, 1988). It is not surprising, if normal voices are never perfectly stable, that such imperfection is generally amplified in disorder. As a rule of thumb, a mean cycle-to-cycle period difference under 100 microseconds or variation less than 1% of the mean frequency is characteristic of a controlled, sustained phonation produced by the normal voice.

Several physiological mechanisms have been proposed to account for jitter in normal voices. For instance, there is a certain degree of asymmetry in the structure and biomechanical properties of a given individual's vocal folds, just as no one has perfect structural or functional symmetry of the two halves of the face. The unpredictable effects of laryngeal mucus and airflow on glottal and laryngeal behavior have also been implicated (Broad, 1979; Fukuda et al., 1988). Based on electromyographic (EMG) data, Baer (1980, 1981b) has advanced the hypothesis that the inherent random muscle activity associated with the noisy integration of laryngeal motor units contributes to an imperfect stability of vocal fold tension. This notion has been supported and extended by subsequent EMG studies (Larson and Kempster, 1985; Larson, Kempster, and Kistler, 1987). Normal cardiovascular function also appears to affect short-term frequency variability (Orlikoff and Baken, 1989a). Heartbeat or vascular pulse may cause periodic fluctuations in subglottal pressure or influence the biomechanical properties of the vocal folds through a blood volume-related increase in vocal fold mass or a blood pressure-related increase in muscular and/or mucosal stiffness (Orlikoff, 1989; Orlikoff and Baken, 1989b). An improved understanding of such mechanisms may ultimately help explain the intricacies of voice control and changes in voice quality associated not only with pathology but with normal physiological aging as well (Wilcox and Horii, 1980; Benjamin, 1981; Ramig and Ringel, 1983; Linville and Fisher, 1985; Orlikoff, 1990a).

Amplitude Perturbation (Vocal Shimmer)

While measures of jitter are primarily thought to characterize the stability of vocal fold vibration, measures of cycle-to-cycle amplitude perturbation (vocal shimmer) are generally believed to reflect the regularity of glottal airway dynamics (Koike, Takahashi, and Calcaterra, 1977). Like fundamental frequency perturbation, excessive vocal shimmer seems to be tied to the perception of a noisy voice, but the roughness or hoarseness may be qualitatively different from that attributed to immoderate levels of jitter (Hillenbrand, 1988).

Mean amplitude variation less than 7% or a mean cycle-to-cycle amplitude difference under 0.7 **decibels (dB)** may be expected in normal young adult voices. Like jitter, mean shimmer tends to be higher in vocal pathology and in normal phonations sustained at low fundamental frequencies and intensities (Jacob, 1968; Hollien, Michel, and Doherty, 1973; Horii, 1979, 1980; Pabon and Plomp, 1988; Orlikoff and Baken, 1990; Orlikoff and Kahane, 1991). Although many of the mechanisms contributing to jitter variability are thought to be related to the shimmer of normal and pathologic voices (Horii, 1980; Heiberger and Horii, 1982; Orlikoff, 1990b; Orlikoff and Kahane, 1991), our understanding of short-term amplitude perturbation remains incomplete.

Current And Future Directions

Work continues toward the detailed physiological, acoustic, and perceptual characterization of jitter and shimmer in normal young, geriatric, and pathologic voices. These efforts have been impeded by a lack of standardization of procedure and measure (e.g., Pinto and Titze, 1990; Laver, Hiller, and Beck, 1992). Progress in this area will improve our ability to compare data between studies and perhaps lead to more valid and reliable conclusions.

Developments in nonlinear dynamics and in the geometric mathematical structures that support it offer considerable potential for altering our approach to and deepening our comprehension of vocal phenomena. For example, the prevalent methods of assessing vocal perturbation necessarily confound the contributions of regular variations (such as result from small-amplitude tremor) and truly erratic random irregularity. In a series of compelling demonstrations, Baken (1990) has shown that relatively simple analyses using the methods of fractal geometry (Mandelbrot, 1967, 1982; Goldberger and West, 1987b; Moon, 1987; Barnsley, 1988; Jürgens, Peitgen, and Saupe, 1990) can quantify irregularity while essentially ignoring regular variability. The analytical techniques of nonlinear dynamics theory thus may provide more powerful descriptive systems and so lead to the sources of phonatory irregularity and to an improved understanding of voice control and regulation.

The detection and processing of glottographic waveforms and their physiological interpretation also are widely studied (Köster and Smith, 1970; Kitzing, 1977, 1986, 1990; Gauffin et al., 1983; Baken, 1987, 1992; Kempster et al., 1987; Titze, 1989a, 1990b; Slavit, Lipton, and McCaffrey, 1990; Löfqvist and McGowan, 1991; Ursino et al., 1991). Such research is designed to identify artifact and outline salient glottographic features that may best relay information about glottal and laryngeal configuration and vocal fold status (Rothenberg, 1972; Ono et al., 1976; Kitzing and Löfqvist, 1979; Titze and Talkin, 1981; Fourcin, 1982; Kitzing, 1982, 1990; Dejonckere and Lebacq, 1985; Childers et al., 1986; Scherer and Titze, 1987; Painter, 1988; Rothenberg and Mahshie, 1988; Schutte and Seidner, 1988; Abberton, Howard, and Fourcin, 1989; Price, 1989; Colton and Conture, 1990; Howard, Lindsey, and Allen, 1990; Motta et al., 1990; Robb and Simmons, 1990; Orlikoff, 1991). In particular, glottographic waveforms allow a greater understanding of frequency and intensity control and regulation, the physiological nature of various modes of phonation, and factors contributing to the efficiency of voice production.

PHONATION: HOW IS IT MODIFIED?

The dynamic nature of speech is largely born of our ability to modify various vocal parameters quickly and precisely. To do this, several adjustments of the ventilatory, laryngeal, and/or extralaryngeal systems are employed simultaneously in a highly coordinated manner. Such adjustments influence voice characteristics by regulating the manner in which phonation is initiated as well as the intensity, frequency, and mode of phonation. While a good deal of information is known about these processes, our knowledge of the physiology, acoustics, and perceptual significance of phonatory adjustment is far from complete. The following discussion summarizes salient information on these issues.

Prephonatory Laryngeal Adjustment And Vocal Attack

Much understanding of the muscular events associated with voice production can be traced to Faaborg-Andersen's (1957, 1965) classic

EMG investigation of the intrinsic laryngeal muscles (Figure 4-23). One of his particularly interesting observations was that the dimensions of the glottal aperture and the tension, length, and mass of the vocal folds (and thus their vibratory characteristics) are preset as much as half a second before phonation, well in advance of acoustic feedback. The adductory presetting of the vocal folds is accomplished primarily via lateral cricoarytenoid (LCA) activity, which helps close the membranous glottis, assisted by the transverse and oblique interarytenoid muscles (IA), which act largely to narrow the cartilagenous glottis (Hirano, Kiyokawa, and Kurita, 1988). These subtle but critical events, along with the simultaneous generation of appropriate aerodynamic forces, comprise the *prephonatory adjustment phase*.

Immediately following the prephonatory phase is the *phonatory attack phase* at the initiation of the laryngeal tone. Faaborg-Andersen (1957, 1965) found that the vocal folds begin their adduction to midline about 50 to 100 ms before the onset of expiration. The speed and extent of vocal fold adduction chiefly determine the nature of the attack phase (Luchsinger and Arnold, 1965; Koike, 1967; Koike, Hirano, and von Leden, 1967). Vocal fold vibration is typically observed before the folds meet at midline. Although it has not been explicitly studied, the role of the Bernoulli force may be more important to the initiation than to the maintenance of vocal fold vibration.

Moore (1938) identified three basic types of *vocal attack*. In *simultaneous* (or *normal*) vocal attack, an expiratory airstream is established about the same time the vocal folds make contact at midline. Simultaneous vocal attack is associated with a gradual and well-regulated buildup of subglottal pressure and a fairly stable onset of vocal fold vibration. With a *hard glottal attack* (also known as *coup de glotte*) the vocal folds are firmly compressed against each other at midline before phonation. There may be increased supraglottal laryngeal constriction as well (Moore, 1938). Because of the increased medial compression of the vocal folds, a higher subglottal pressure is necesary to initiate phonation. The sudden release of this elevated pressure results in the perception of a transient rise and fall in pitch and loudness as phonation begins. At the other extreme of the continuum, a *breathy* (or *aspirate*) *attack* is associated with the initiation of expiration before the completed adduction of

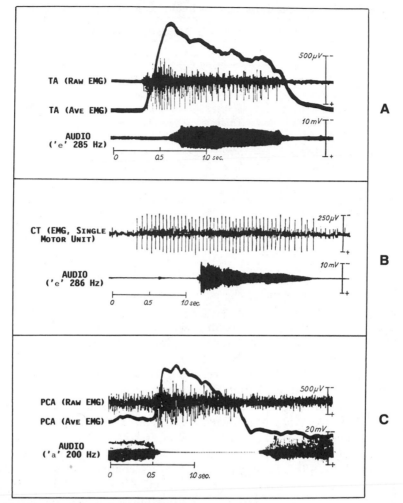

FIGURE 4-23   Electromyographic (*EMG*) and acoustic (*AUDIO*) signals. *A*, Raw and averaged thyroarytenoid (*TA*) muscle EMG activity. *B*, Cricothyroid (*CT*) muscle activity within a single motor unit. *C*, Raw and averaged posterior cricoarytenoid (*PCA*) muscle EMG activity associated with the termination and initiation of phonation. (Adapted from Faaborg-Andersen [1965]. Electromyography of laryngeal muscles in humans. Technics and results. In *Current problems in phoniatrics and logopedics*, Vol. 3. Basel: Karger.)

the vocal folds. A turbulent airstream may be audible before a periodic vocal signal is produced. A given individual is likely to use a wide variety of vocal attacks when speaking. The type of voice onset used is most likely influenced by a number of factors, including the phonetic context and the nature of the utterance.

Conventional descriptions of intrinsic laryngeal muscle function are inadequate to explain their specific effects on the vocal folds during the initiation and maintenance of voice production. Such information is very difficult to obtain in vivo, though much knowledge has been gleaned from the study of excised larynges (Hirano, 1974; Koike, Hirano, and Morio, 1976). Although relatively crude, data derived from

cadaveric specimens underscore the subtle effects of the intrinsic muscles on the geometry and physical properties of the vocal folds and the complexity of their interaction. A differential involvement of one or more of the intrinsic muscles thus provides a precise sculpturing action on the rima glottidis (Table 4-3). This coordinated activity seems to be strongly influenced by cricothyroid (CT) action, though the effects of the CT muscle on glottal shaping appears to be greater in women than in men (Hirano et al., 1988). The reasons for this have not been determined, but this sex difference may have important physiological and clinical implications.

The degree of glottal constriction maintained for the duration of the phonation may dramati-

TABLE 4-3 Characteristic functions of the laryngeal muscles in vocal fold adjustment

Vocal Fold	Muscles and Their Actions				
Change	CT	VOC	LCA	IA	PCA
Position	Paramed	*Adduct*	*Adduct*	*Adduct*	*Abduct*
Level	Lower	Lower	*Lower*	0	*Elevate*
Length	*Elongate*	*Shorten*	Elongate	(Shorten)	*Elongate*
Thickness	*Thin*	*Thicken*	Thin	(Thicken)	Thin
Edge	*Sharpen*	*Round*	Sharpen	0	Round
Muscle (body)	*Stiffen*	*Stiffen*	Stiffen	(Slacken)	Stiffen
Mucosa (cover and transition)	*Stiffen*	*Slacken*	Stiffen	(Slacken)	Stiffen

0, no effect; Parentheses, slight effect; italics, marked effect.
CT, cricothyroid muscle; VOC, vocalis muscle; LCA, lateral cricoarytenoid muscle; IA, interarytenoid muscle; PCA, posterior cricoarytenoid muscle. (From Hirano, M., & Kakita, Y. (1985). Cover-body theory of vocal fold vibration. In Daniloff, R.G. [Ed.], *Speech Science: Recent Advances*. San Diego, CA: College-Hill Press.)

cally affect the acoustic and perceptual characteristics of the voice and the vibratory behavior of the vocal folds. *Adducted hyperfunction* seems to be associated with an increased vibrational amplitude and a higher velocity of vocal fold collision (Hillman et al., 1989). Relative vocal fold contact duration, as determined from the observation of EGG signals (Figure 4-24), increases with progression from loosely adducted breathy to tightly adducted pressed phonation (Painter, 1988; Rothenberg and Mahshie, 1988; Scherer, Druker, and Titze, 1988; Scherer et al., 1988).

Fundamental Frequency Control

The rate of vocal fold vibration, the **fundamental frequency (F_o)**, is the primary physical correlate of perceived pitch. (Perceived pitch is secondarily influenced by vocal intensity and vowel, that is, spectral, characteristics.) Frequency is measured in **hertz (Hz)**, or cycles per second (cps). The F_o of the voice is altered by influencing the rate of fold separation, approximation, or both.

Subglottal Adjustment

Since Müller in the 1830s, the control of F_o has been linked to the regulation of subglottal pressure. Augmenting the subglottal pressure not only speeds glottal opening but also increases the amplitude of fold displacement (Titze and Durham, 1987; Titze, 1989b). It is not surprising, then, that the **open quotient (OQ)**, the percentage of the vocal cycle occupied by an open glottis, tends to increase with rising frequency

(Moore and von Leden, 1958; Timcke, von Leden, and Moore, 1958; Kitzing and Sonesson, 1974).

Increased vibrational amplitude is also associated with greater stretch of the vocal folds as they bow away from each other. This produces a larger transitory increase in lengthwise tension and thus in elastic recoil (Titze, 1987b; Titze and Durham, 1987). The typical voice produces about a 3- to 5-Hz change in F_o for each cm H_2O of subglottal pressure change (van den Berg, 1957; Lieberman, Knudson, and Mead, 1969; Hixon, Klatt, and Mead, 1971; Baer, 1979; Rothenberg and Mahshie, 1986; Baken and Orlikoff, 1987a). However, F_o variations on the order of 75 to 100 Hz are common during spoken utterances, so sole reliance on transglottal pressure adjustments would require an exorbitant amount of breath to be spent on frequency control. Furthermore, chest-wall adjustments are relatively slow (Baken et al., 1979; Baken and Orlikoff, 1987a), and measures of subglottal pressure during speech have revealed a surprising degree of long-term constancy (Draper, Ladefoged, and Witteridge, 1960; Mead, Bouhuys, and Proctor, 1968; Netsell, 1973; Gelfer, Harris, and Baer, 1987). Nevertheless, some investigators have emphasized the importance of subglottal pressure control at particularly low F_os when fold tension is reduced (Atkinson, 1978; Holmberg, Hillman, and Perkall, 1989; Titze, 1989b).

Laryngeal Adjustment

Adjustment of the mechanical properties of the vocal folds alters the rate of vibration quite

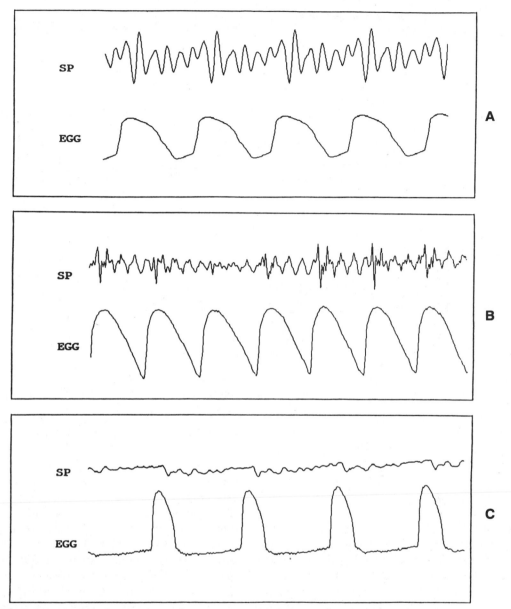

FIGURE 4-24 Simultaneous sound pressure (*SP*) and electroglottographic (*EGG*) signals during (*A*) normal, (*B*) constricted, and (*C*) breathy phonations.

dramatically (van den Berg and Tan, 1959). Increases in vocal F_o have long been tied to an increase in vocal fold length (Moore, 1937; Sonninen, 1954; Hollien, 1960a, 1960b; Hollien and Moore, 1960; Nishizawa, Sawashima, and Yonemoto, 1988), which both raises mean longitudinal tension (Colton, 1988) and thins the folds, decreasing the effective vibratory mass (Hollien, 1962). (The fact that men tend to have more massive vocal folds than women explains the lower F_o characteristic of the male voice.)

The longitudinal tension of the vocal folds is changed primarily by the visorlike action of the CTJ. Figure 4-25 presents a simplified two-dimensional mechanical model of the larynx. A contraction of the two portions of the cricothyroid muscle (CT) will rotate the thyroid cartilage downward and forward. The distance between the thryoid prominence and the arytenoid cartilages is increased as the cricoid and thyroid cartilages approximate, lengthening the vocal folds (Arnold, 1961). Thus, the isotonic (muscle shortening) contraction of the CT generates passive tension in both the muscular and nonmuscular tissues of the vocal fold (Titze and Durham, 1987; Colton, 1988). Active vocal fold tension can be generated by a contraction of the TA *against* the CT. Because the muscular por-

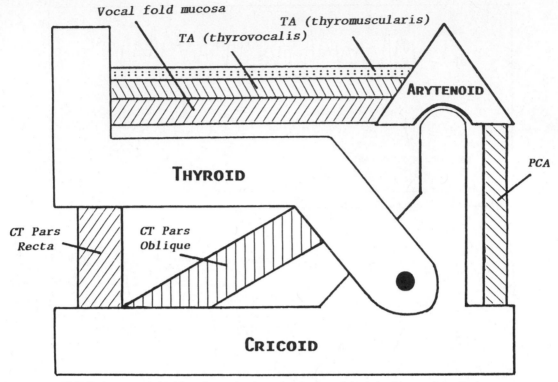

FIGURE 4-25   A highly schematized mechanical model of the larynx (lateral view).

tions of the folds are being stretched, the TA contraction may be primarily isometric (non-shortening) but will increase fold tension. It is a characteristic of muscle physiology that the force of contraction and the isometric tension will be greater if the muscle is initially stretched beyond its resting length (Hast, 1966).

It appears that this fine antagonistic interplay between the CT and the TA is largely responsible for our quick and versatile regulation of longitudinal tension (Faaborg-Andersen, Yanagihara, and von Leden, 1967; Hirano, Vennard, and Ohala, 1970; Titze, Jiang, and Drucker, 1987; Tanaka and Tanabe, 1989; Titze, Luschei, and Hirano, 1989). Furthermore, extreme vocal fold tension will tend to tax the CAJ by pulling the arytenoids away from their respective cricoid facets. Thus, at high phonatory frequencies, the posterior cricoarytenoid muscle (PCA) tends to brace the arytenoid cartilages against the anterior pull of the folds and thus maintain or even increase longitudinal tension (Gay et al., 1972; Baer, Gay, and Niimi, 1976; Harris, 1981). Interarytenoid and lateral cricoarytenoid muscle activity increase at high F_os, perhaps to counteract the abductory influence of PCA (Hirano, Vennard, and Ohala, 1970; Hirano, 1988a). Nonetheless, a posterior glottal gap or chink is often associated with high-frequency phonations.

As a consequence of their manipulation of insufflated excised larynges, van den Berg and Tan (1959) proposed that the degree to which the vocal processes are medially compressed influences the vibratory frequency. Broad (1973) has likened this ancillary F_o-regulating mechanism to pressing a guitar string against a fret. In the larynx such action does not substantially alter the longitudinal tension of the vocal folds, but it does reduce the amount of effective vibratory mass by largely stopping the vibration in the folds near the vocal processes (Honda, 1985).

Vocal Fold Adjustment

There is yet no consensus as to the exact role of the TA in F_o control. While the TA is generally regarded as a vocal fold tensor and thus a frequency-elevating muscle, some investigators have argued its role in F_o depression (Hardcastle, 1976; Harvey and Howell, 1980; Fujimura, 1981). In EMG studies, Larson et al. (1985, 1987) stimulated the TA at various locations and found that although F_o usually increased, in several trials it fell substantially. In light of Hirano's (1974) cover-body functional characterization of the vocal fold, it has been postulated that while an isotonic contraction of TA may stiffen the vocal fold, it will also shorten and thicken the muscular body and slacken the mucosal cover. It is not known whether the thyromuscularis and thyrovocalis portions of the TA serve different functions in this regard; that is, one portion may be largely responsible for active body tension and the other, for the manipulation of passive mucosal stiffness. Titze, Jiang, and Drucker (1987) and Titze, Luschei, and Hirano (1989) emphasized that if the mucosal cover is relatively lax, as when producing a low F_o, TA activity will most likely raise the vibratory frequency by stiffening the muscular body. When the cover is quite tense, as with high-frequency phonations, TA may primarily depress F_o.

Extralaryngeal Adjustment

The *extrinsic laryngeal muscles* are divided into *suprahyoid* and *infrahyoid* groups. The suprahyoid muscles, consisting of the anterior and posterior digastrics, mylohyoid, geniohyoid, and stylohyoid muscles, lie between the mandible or skull and the hyoid. The hyoid is a nonarticulated bone in the anterior neck, from which the thyroid cartilage is suspended and to which much of the tongue is anchored. The suprahyoids may depress or retract the mandible when the hyoid is stabilized or may elevate the hyoid and therefore the larynx, as it does during swallowing, when the position of the mandible is fixed. The infrahyoid muscle group, the *strap muscles* of the neck, consist of the sternothyroid, thyrohyoid, sternohyoid, and omohyoid muscles. The strap muscles allow both laryngeal depression and fixation of the hyoid bone against suprahyoid influence. Muscles such as the cricopharyngeus and thyropharyngeus may also displace the larynx posteriorly.

Since the rotation of the thyroid cartilage is critical to the control of longitudinal vocal fold tension, various extrinsic forces, particularly the action of the sternothyroid and thyrohyoid muscles, have been implicated as an ancillary F_o control mechanism (Figure 4-26). The larynx is typically elevated within the neck for very high F_o and depressed for very low F_o, and extrinsic muscle activity often corresponds with extreme frequency change (Faaborg-Andersen and Sonninen, 1960; Shipp, 1975; Baer, Gay, and Niimi, 1976). The external frame function theory,

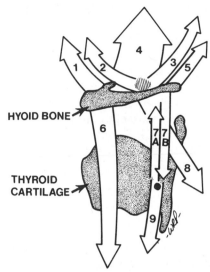

FIGURE 4-26 The force vectors of the suprahyoid and infrahyoid (extrinsic laryngeal) muscles. *1,* Geniohyoid. *2,* Anterior digastric. *3,* Posterior digastric. *4,* Mylohyoid. *5,* Stylohyoid. *6,* Sternohyoid. *7,* thyrohyoid as an elevator (*A*) and depressor (*B*) of the thyroid cartilage. *8,* Omohyoid. *9,* Sternohyoid. (From Kahane, J. C. [1988]. Anatomy of the organs of the peripheral speech mechanism. In Lass, N. J., Northern, J. L., McReynolds, L. V., & Yoder, D. C. [Eds.], *Handbook of speech-language pathology and audiology.* St. Louis: Mosby.)

originally proposed by Aatto Sonninen (1956, 1968) and subsequently investigated by Zenker and Zenker (1960), Faaborg-Andersen and Vennard (1964), Sonesson (1968), Shipp (1975), Shipp and Izdebski (1975), Ewan (1979, 1980), Shin et al. (1981), Erickson, Baer, and Harris (1983), Honda (1983), Sundberg and Askenfelt (1983), Vilkman and Karma (1989), and Zawadzki and Gilbert (1989), attributes F_o changes to a manipulation of the cricoid-thyroid complex through laryngeal height changes and isometric contractions of the infrahyoid or suprahyoid muscles. The influence of tongue position and movement on the hyoid bone may help explain the observation that high vowels tend to be associated with a higher mean frequency than low vowels produced within a similar context (Black, 1949; House and Fairbanks, 1953; Lehiste and Peterson, 1961; Sapir, 1989). Some investigators have recently attributed this "intrinsic vowel pitch" to a highly complex and variable interaction between the intrinsic and extrinsic musculature rather than ascribing a purely extralaryngeal cause (Honda, 1985; Vilkman et al., 1989; Vilkman and Karma, 1989).

It appears that extrinsic laryngeal activity supplies a small or negligible F_o-regulating influence within the range of frequencies usually employed in speech. Since the extrinsic laryngeal musculature has so many points of attachment, the relative position of the head, mandible, and shoulder appear to introduce a great deal of variability into external frame function and its influence on voice frequency. Nonetheless, extralaryngeal control seems to help regulate exceptionally high and low frequencies.

Intensity Control

The amplitude of radiated acoustic energy, in conjunction with the vocal F_o and vocal tract resonance associated with a given vowel production, strongly influences our perception of loudness. Measured in decibels, the intensity of the voice may be altered via independent or concurrent adjustments of the breath, glottal airway resistance, and configuration of the vocal tract.

Subglottal Adjustment

Vocal intensity is proportional to the square of the sound pressure, so voice intensity may be changed by adjusting the aerodynamic power used in phonation. Indeed, mean subglottal pressure affects vocal intensity quite directly (Ladefoged and McKinney, 1963; Isshiki, 1964; Kunze, 1964; Cavagna and Margaria, 1968). There also appears to be a general but variable tendency for mean airflow to increase as vocal intensity rises (Isshiki, 1964, 1965; Bouhuys, Proctor, and Mead, 1966; Yanagihara and Koike, 1967; Cavagna and Margaria, 1968; Koyama, Kawasaki, and Ogura, 1969; McGlone, 1970; Schneider and Baken, 1984; Colton, 1985). Airflow depends not only on the aerodynamic force of expiration but also on the resistance in the glottis. Much of the variability in the relationship between airflow and intensity seems to be tied to changes in glottal resistance associated with F_o regulation (Arnold, 1961; Hirano et al., 1969; Hirano, 1981b; Colton, 1985; Lindestad, Fritzell, and Persson, 1990). Thus, the driving pressure of phonation and glottal adjustments share allegiance between frequency and intensity control. This accounts for the fact that phonatory frequency tends to covary with intensity during prolonged phonations and spoken utterances.

Laryngeal Adjustment

Vocal intensity may be regulated by laryngeal adjustments designed to vary the amount of aerodynamic power converted to acoustic power. This is largely a function of the medial compression of the vocal folds during phonation. This power conversion seems to depend on the degree to which the vocal processes are adducted relative to the amplitude of vocal fold vibration (Titze, 1988b). Indeed, increases in vocal intensity tend to be associated with a reduction in OQ (Timcke, von Leden, and Moore, 1958; Cavagna and Camporesi, 1974) and an increased vocal fold contact duration (Orlikoff, 1991). Glottographic records indicate that the energy in the vocal signal strongly depends on the maximal rate of glottal airflow decrease during the vocal cycle (Fant, 1979; Gauffin and Sundberg, 1989). Rothenberg (1981), Colton (1985), and Kakita (1988) indicate that the negative slope of the FLOGG is steepest at the latter stages of glottal closure, as the vocal folds approximate at their lower margins and rapidly increase in medial contact. Thus both the negative slope of the FLOGG and the positive slope of the EGG strongly tend to increase as vocal intensity rises (Colton, 1985; Holmberg, Hillman, and Perkell, 1988; Gauffin and Sundberg, 1989; Orlikoff, 1991).

Supralaryngeal Adjustment

Lip-radiated acoustic energy differs from that radiated from the larynx. Traditionally the vocal tract has been considered a filter of the vocal signal, absorbing varying amounts of energy. Subglottal and laryngeal factors aside, vocal intensity will vary as a function of vowel characteristics. In particular, intensity will increase as more of the higher-energy harmonics, especially the F_o, correspond to the vocal tract resonant (formant) frequencies. Furthermore, certain vowels are associated with greater or lesser degrees of vocal tract constriction, and these adjustments also affect the radiated energy. Thus the generation of vocal intensity has many degrees of freedom. House (1959) cited these considerations as reasons the concept of optimal pitch (that vocal F_o produced with "optimal" laryngeal efficiency as determined largely by loudness changes) is an invalid measure of laryngeal function.

Voice Range Profiles

At a comfortable F_o the typical voice can produce phonations ranging from about 55 dB to a maximum of approximately 110 dB SPL (Colton, 1973; Coleman, Mabis, and Hinson, 1977). However, the actual dynamic intensity range of the voice will vary greatly according to the frequency of phonation. Because the mechanisms of frequency and intensity control are inextricably related, the assessment of the *maximum phonational frequency range* (MPFR) and *dynamic intensity range* are often combined in a *voice range profile,* also known as a phonetogram or F_o-SPL plot. Such a profile (Figure 4-27) is produced by having the subject phonate at fixed intervals within the MPFR and sustain the vowel as loudly and as softly as possible (Damsté, 1970; Coleman, Mabis, and Hinson, 1977; Schutte, 1980; Komiyama, Watanabe, and Ryu, 1984;

Seidner, Krueger, and Wernecke, 1985; Gramming et al., 1988; Pabon and Plomp, 1988; Gramming, 1991). The voice range is the best indication of the physiological limits of phonatory function; that is, the profile indicates the degree to which the subglottal, glottal, and supraglottal systems can be adjusted and coordinated so as to produce the widest range of frequencies and intensities. Because of the influence of vocal tract configuration on radiated acoustic energy, several vowels (usually /a/, /i/, and /u/) are profiled (Gramming and Sundberg, 1988; Titze, 1992).

Voice Registers

Voice registers are various modes of phonation. There has been a great deal of debate concerning the exact number of distinct mechanical modes of vibration produced by the normal larynx. This has been complicated by the fact that there is no one universally accepted definition of a voice register. For the past 20 years, Hollien's (1972, 1974) characterization of registers has

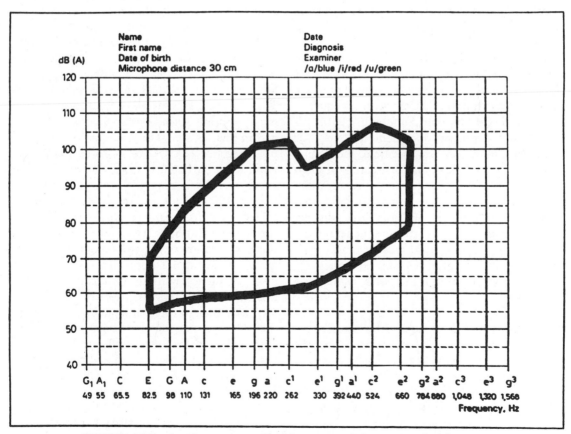

FIGURE 4-27   A voice range profile (phonetogram) for a normal male voice.

generally been followed by researchers and clinicians primarily because it is founded on experimentally derived, quantifiable data and does not rely solely on the perception of either the listener or the speaker. According to Hollien, a voice register is a range of consecutive vocal F_os that can be produced with a perceptually distinct voice quality. Furthermore, the series of frequencies associated with a register should have little if any overlap with any other register. Of particular importance is the fact that the registers must differ from one another on the basis of laryngeal events and must be operationally defined according to unequivocal perceptual, acoustic, and physiological evidence that differentiates them on the basis of vocal fold status, vibratory pattern, driving pressure, and mean phonatory airflow.

A great deal of the contradiction and complication associated with the voice register controversy can be avoided by describing only the speaking voice and omitting the singing voice. Many of the registers identified by singers may differ because of a supralaryngeal (resonance) adjustment rather than a vibromechanical modification (Hollien, 1974; Hollien, Gould, and Johnson, 1976; Estill et al., 1985; Hollien and Schoenhard, 1985; Welch, Sargeant, and Mac-Curtain, 1988). Furthermore, many singers are trained to reduce or eliminate distinct register transitions and to produce a variety of voice qualities, or timbres, at a given frequency (Hertegård, Gauffin, and Sundberg, 1990). Although not explicitly documented, "true" or "primary" voice registers specific to the singing voice may indeed exist, and the search for them is a particularly active area of investigation. Nevertheless, along the restricted guidelines proposed by Hollien (1974), three distinct speaking voice registers are now generally acknowledged. As the typical speaker ranges from his or her physiologically lowest to highest F_o, the voice passes through the *pulse, modal,* and *loft registers.*

PULSE REGISTER Encompassing the lowest range of frequencies that can be produced by the human voice, the **pulse register** is characterized by a coarse and bubbly quality. It has been called glottal fry or vocal fry in the United States and creaky voice in most other English-speaking countries. Compared with the higher-frequency registers, pulse phonation is associated with

shorter (Hollien, Damsté, and Murry, 1969) and thicker (Allen and Hollien, 1973) vocal folds and a significantly reduced airflow rate (McGlone, 1967; McGlone and Shipp, 1971; Murry, 1971; Allen and Hollien, 1973). It is not clear whether the subglottal pressure is reduced as well (Hollien et al., 1966; McGlone and Shipp, 1971; Murry, 1971; Murry and Brown, 1971a; Zemlin, 1988; Holmberg, Hillman, and Perkell, 1989). The two sexes can produce approximately the same range of pulse frequencies (Hollien and Michel, 1968), the upper F_o limit appearing to reside somewhere about 80 ± 10 Hz (McGlone, 1967; Hollien and Michel, 1968; Murry, 1971; Allen and Hollien, 1973).

Certainly, of all the speaking voice registers, pulse phonation is the least understood. Pulse register is produced with a fair amount of medial compression but minimal vocal fold tension (McGlone and Shipp, 1971), and it takes a relatively long time for the subglottal pressure to separate the thick and lax folds. It is thought that once a glottis appears, the reduction in driving pressure produces a short-lived open period. The folds open only a short distance and not along their entire length. Because the vocal folds are approximated for so long, the acoustic energy generated at closure is completely or almost completely damped by the time of the next excitation (Coleman, 1963; Wendahl, Moore, and Hollien, 1963; Hollien and Wendahl, 1968; Titze, 1988c). This gives rise to the discrete pulsing or popping sound of phonations maintained within this register. The spectrum of the typical pulse-register FLOGG tends to be rich in harmonics but particularly low in energy. Thus the vocal intensity is generally reduced (Murry and Brown, 1971b; Hollien, 1974). Because the vocal folds are maximally relaxed, subglottal pressure adjustment appears to take precedence in the F_o regulation of pulse phonations. Thus, it is quite difficult if not impossible to increase the pulse frequency without a concomitant rise in intensity and vice versa (Murry and Brown, 1971b). Much of the rough quality attributed to the pulse register may be a consequence of the extremely high frequency and amplitude perturbation associated with sustained pulse productions (Cavallo, Baken, and Shaiman, 1984; Horii, 1985).

Several early investigations of pulse register identified a peculiar vibratory pattern whereby the folds approximate twice per cycle (Moore

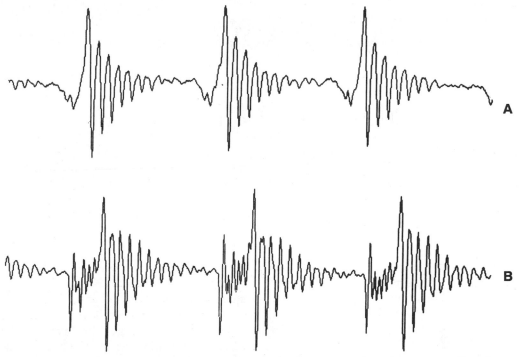

FIGURE 4-28 Characteristic acoustic waveforms of pulse register phonation. *A,* Nondicrotic pulsatile pattern. *B,* Typical dicrotic pattern; short, low-amplitude waves are immediately followed by larger waves of longer duration.

and von Leden, 1958; Timcke, von Leden, and Moore, 1959; Wendahl, Moore, and Hollien, 1963). Called **dicrotic pulse phonation,** the rapid double opening of the folds is followed by a long closure with almost complete acoustic damping before each excitation (Figure 4-28). The initial excitation is almost always of lesser amplitude than the one that follows. While dicrotic phonation is only poorly understood, possible mechanisms have been suggested by Moore and von Leden (1958) and by Cavallo, Baken, and Shaiman (1984). Many individuals seem able to produce both dicrotic and nondicrotic (single-pulse) waveforms at low F_o (Cavallo, Baken, and Shaiman, 1984).* This leads to some confusion, as some investigators accept only nondicrotic phonation as "true" pulse register productions (e.g., Hollien, Girard, and

Coleman, 1977), while others reject anything but dicrotic vibratory patterns as characteristic of the register (e.g., Sorensen and Horii, 1984).

Fourcin (1974, 1981) reports that the perceptual character of the double pulse is markedly different from that of the single pulse and therefore uses the term *creaky voice* for dicrotic phonation and *vocal fry* for nondicrotic phonation. Both creaky voice and vocal fry may then be considered varieties of pulse register phonation. However, certain dysphonias produce a perceptually frylike or creaky-type phonation but are nonetheless produced abnormally and independent of register. True pulse phonation is physiologically normal (Hollien et al., 1966; Hollien and Michel, 1968; Hollien and Wendahl, 1968) and is acoustically and perceptually distinct from the "harshness" of vocal pathology (Michel, 1968; Michel and Hollien, 1968). In fact, pulse register is often employed in speech (Figure 4-29), especially at lower vocal intensities such as at the end of breath groups, and is even used in some West African and American Indian languages as a phonetic feature (Catford, 1968, 1983; Ladefoged, 1983). For these reasons it is probably best to avoid the terms fry and creaky voice when referring to

---

*A few studies have documented the relatively rare multiple pulses in pulse register (Hollien, Girard, and Coleman, 1977; Whitehead, Metz, and Whitehead, 1984). Our experience is that occasionally the normal pulse-register voice produces as many as four discrete pulses per cycle. In addition, the voice sometimes shifts repeatedly and unpredictably between single, double, and even multiple pulses within a given sustained pulse phonation.

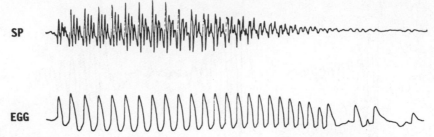

FIGURE 4-29 Sound pressure (*SP*) and electroglottographic (*EGG*) signal associated with the word "oh," produced by a male speaker using a rising and falling intonation. Note the transition from a modal register to a dicrotic pulse register. (From Abberton, E., & Fourcin, A. J. [1975]. Visual feedback and the acquisition of intonation. In Lenneberg, E. H., & Lenneberg, E. [Eds.], *Foundations of language development: A multidisciplinary approach,* Vol. 2. New York: Academic Press [pp. 157-165].)

normal vibratory modes and to identify such phenomena as either dicrotic or nondicrotic pulse register phonation.

Modal Register

The most common type of phonation occurs in what Hollien (1972) calls the **modal register.** *Modal* refers to the statistical mode, that which occurs most often. Occasionally *chest register* is used synonymously, but this can lead to confusion, since some authors identify chest and head voice as separate entities within the modal range (Faaborg-Andersen et al., 1967; Hirano, Vennard, and Ohala, 1970; Hollien, 1974; Hirano, 1981b; Schutte and Seidner, 1988; Hirano, Hibi, and Sanada, 1989).

The shift from pulse register to modal register involves what Titze (1988c) calls a *periodicity transition.* This transition is associated with a shift from a mode of phonation producing complete acoustic decay between pulses to one in which the acoustic energy fails to die out before the next excitation event. The perception is of a more continuous tone. Most of this chapter addresses this manner of phonation. As distinguished from the other registers, modal phonations are characterized by moderate levels of vocal fold length (Hollien, 1960a, 1960b; Hollien and Moore, 1960; Hollien, Brown, and Hollien, 1971), thickness (Hollien and Curtis, 1960; Hollien, 1962; Hollien and Colton, 1969), subglottal pressure (van den Berg, 1956; Murry and Brown, 1971a), and transglottal airflow (Shipp and McGlone, 1971). However, phonations within the modal register also represent the greatest variation in these parameters,

as well as in CT, LCA, and TA activity (Hirano, Vennard, and Ohala, 1970). The expansive range and interplay of myoviscoelastic and aerodynamic forces employed in the modal voice register allow for the fastest and most versatile regulation of vocal F_o and intensity during spoken utterances.

For men the typical range of modal-register F_o runs from those that may abut or slightly overlap the upper pulse register to frequencies on the order of 450 Hz (Hollien and Michel, 1968; Murry, 1971). Women can produce modal-register frequencies ranging from around 130 Hz to about 525 Hz (Hollien and Michel, 1968; Colton and Hollien, 1972). There is no frequency overlap between the pulse and modal registers in women's voices; instead there seems to be a range of intermediate F_os within about 90 to 130 Hz that physiologically cannot be produced by most women.

Loft Register

The **loft register,** or falsetto, is the uppermost range of voice frequencies. Phonations in this register are produced with thin and generally elongated vocal folds (Hollien and Moore, 1960). No systematic length or thickness changes are associated with loft frequency change (Hollien and Colton, 1969; Hollien, Brown, and Hollien, 1971). Both subglottal pressure and mean airflow rate tend to be higher in loft register (Large, Iwata, and von Leden, 1970; McGlone, 1970; Shipp and McGlone, 1971; Shipp et al., 1972). An increase in airflow is associated with elevations in loft-register intensity (Isshiki, 1964, 1965; Kunze, 1964; Yanagihara and Koike, 1967; McGlone, 1970). Based on the work of Hirano, Ohala, and Vennard (1969) and others, Hollien (1972, 1974) has commented that while vocal fold vibratory characteristics have prime importance in pulse register and vibratory and aerodynamic characteristics share importance in modal register, "aerodynamic relationships" largely govern phonations in the loft register.

The shift from modal to loft register is difficult to identify accurately (McGlone and Brown, 1969), and there is a fair amount of frequency overlap between the two in the typical voice. Data indicate that the loft register ranges roughly from 300 to 700 Hz for men and from about 450 to 1100 Hz for women (Hollien and Michel, 1968; Hollien, Dew, and Philips, 1971; Colton and Hollien, 1972). The frequency at which a register shift occurs appears to be highly sensitive to the concomitant vocal intensity (Damsté, 1970), and a notch in the maximum intensity contour in the voice range profile is thought to indicate the shift between the modal and loft registers (Giger, 1985).

While thyroarytenoid activity is often reported to be reduced, mucosal tension appears to be near maximal levels in loft register (Sawashima, Gay, and Harris, 1969; Hirano, Vennard, and Ohala, 1970; Gay et al., 1972; Hirano, 1974, 1988b). However, the vocal processes are less firmly adducted than in the lower registers, resulting in a very high open quotient (Rubin and Hirt, 1960) or even in a complete failure of glottal closure (OQ = 1). This may be associated with the reedy and breathy quality of loft-register phonations. Cinematographic and stroboscopic observations of the vocal folds have revealed diminished or absent vertical and horizontal phase differences during the vibratory cycle. Instead the folds exhibit a uniform, primarily horizontal movement for which a single-mass model seems most appropriate.

The crossover from modal to loft register appears to be signaled by a *timbre transition* (Titze, 1988c). The loft-register FLOGG is much more symmetrical than in either of the other registers. Because of the more gradual fall of glottal airflow, the higher harmonic energy is reduced, resulting in a less rich laryngeal tone (van den Berg, 1968a, 1968b; Colton, 1972). Loft phonations also tend to have lower vocal intensity and a more restricted intensity range than those produced in modal register. Furthermore, because the harmonics are few and necessarily widely spaced (because of the high F_o), it is more difficult for the listener to differentiate loft-register vowels (Figure 4-30).

Current and Future Directions

The ability of investigators to reproduce all three major modes of phonation in excised larynges by altering aerodynamic parameters and simulating various muscle forces (van den Berg, 1960; Slavit, Lipton, and McCaffrey, 1990) highlights the laryngeal nature of the voice register distinction. Such data led Isshiki (1969) to speculate that the differences among the registers is tied to the amount of vocal fold tissue employed in the vibration. It seems clear that any vibratory mode engages the entire mucosal cover. In pulse register, minimal muscular tension results in a strong coupling of the cover-body complex, so that both participate substantially in the vibration. In modal register vibration penetrates only a short distance into the muscular body. The depth of penetration varies according to the generated active and passive muscle tension (Titze, Jiang, and Drucker, 1987). For loft-register phonations, extreme mucosal tension and reduced TA activity result in a near decoupling of the cover and body with severely limited participation of the muscular layer in the vibratory movement. A highly tenuous but working hypothesis is that the adjustment of vocal fold body tension alters the degree of penetration of the vibration into the muscle and thus influences the mode of phonation. Hirano (1981b) has suggested that the TA is primarily involved in register regulation, whereas CT is largely responsible for frequency variation within a register, especially in pulse and modal phonations (Hirano et al., 1969; Shipp and McGlone, 1971). The complete characterization of voice registers will continue to be an intriguing, frustrating, and controversial area of investigation that may ultimately provide a great deal of insight regarding how phonation is maintained and how vocal frequency, intensity, and efficiency are controlled.

PHONATORY BEHAVIOR IN SPEECH

Consonants differ from vowels primarily by the amount of vocal tract constriction employed in their production. Consonants have lesser inten-

sity than vowels, largely because they are produced with a more fully occluded vocal tract.
Speech can be considered to be an overlay of
consonants on the vocal signal. The dispersion
of consonants results in an amplitude modulation of the acoustic energy that, for the most
part, gives rise to our perception of syllables. We
may also vary the acoustic characteristics of the
raw vocal signal to alter the meaning and emotional content of the utterance. Suprasegmental
features are prosodic elements that determine
the linguistic stress, lexical prominence, and in-
tonations of a language. Chapter 6 more completely addresses the complex issue of suprasegmentals, but we will briefly outline the gross
aspects of phonatory dynamics during running
speech.

Intonation Contours and Syllable Stress

The mean *speaking fundamental frequency*
(SF_o), or the average vocal frequency used

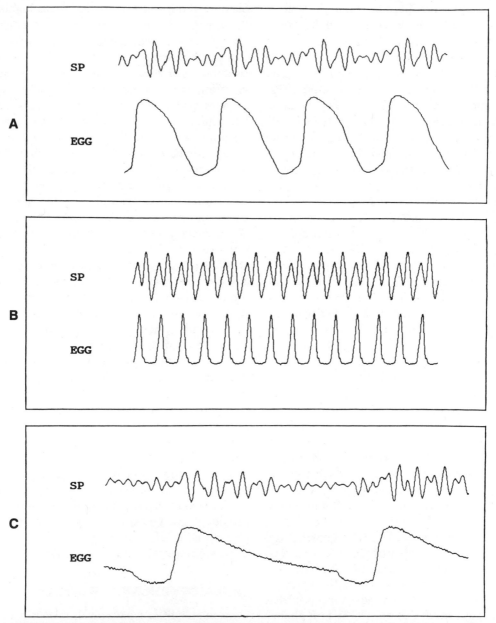

FIGURE 4-30   Simultaneous sound pressure (*SP*) and electroglottographic (*EGG*) signals
typical of the (*A*) modal, (*B*) loft, and (*C*) pulse registers.

during a spoken utterance, is on the order of 110 and 225 Hz for men and women, respectively. During senescence, the average man's SF_o rises to about 140 Hz, and the woman's SF_o tends to drop slightly (Mysak, 1959; McGlone and Hollien, 1963; Hollien and Shipp, 1972; Stoicheff, 1981). The extent of variability of spoken F_o during speech depends on the emotional and linguistic content of the utterance and is somewhat language specific (Cooper and Sorenson, 1981). F_o variability during speech is measured as the standard deviation of the frequencies about the mean SF_o and is called the **pitch sigma** (Figure 4-31). As expressed in the relative frequency scale of **semitones** (ST), the pitch sigmas used by men and women tend to be quite similar, averaging about 3 ST.

Frequency variability in speech is primarily linguistically driven. The generated F_o pattern is called the *intonation contour* (Figure 4-32). However, a fairly consistent feature of this contour is a gradual fall of F_o across breath groups and over the course of the utterance, regardless of the speaker's native language (Cohen, Collier, and 't Hart, 1982; Kutik,

Cooper, and Boyce, 1983; Anderson and Cooper, 1986).* The *fundamental frequency declination,* or the tendency toward a decreasing F_o, is thought to be largely a consequence of a progressively decreasing subglottal pressure (Collier, 1975, 1987), but the declination slope also appears to be substantially influenced by various linguistic and biomechanical factors in a highly complicated manner (Lehiste and Peterson, 1961; Atkinson, 1978; O'Shaughnessy, 1979; Fujisaki, 1983; Gelfer et al., 1985; Anderson and Cooper, 1986; Titze and Durham, 1987).

In conjunction with vocal intensity and durational cues, short-lived frequency rises within an intonation contour signal syllable stress and lexical emphasis (Fry, 1955, 1968; Lehiste and Peterson, 1959; Lieberman, 1960; Lieberman and Michaels, 1962; Ladefoged and McKinney, 1963; Terken, 1991). Local syllable stress is primarily a result of CT activity that may on occasion be accompanied by a slight transient augmentation of subglottal pressure (Netsell,

---

*Hauser and Fowler (1992) provide evidence of F_o declination in the vocalizations of monkeys!

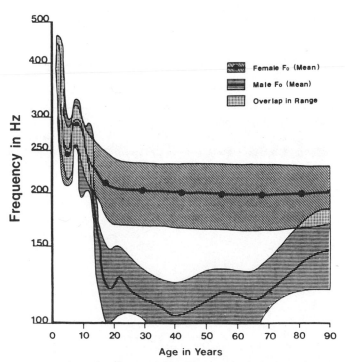

FIGURE 4-31 **Mean speaking fundamental frequency and pitch sigma by age and sex.** (From Hollien, H., and Massey, K. [1986]. A male-female coalescence model of vocal change. In V. L. Lawrence [Ed.], *Transcripts of the Fourteenth Symposium: Care of the Professional Voice.* New York: Voice Foundation [pp. 57-60].)

1970, 1973; Brown and McGlone, 1974; Aaltonen, Vilkman, and Raimo, 1988).

The Larynx as an Articulator

Consonants are distinguishable not only by the degree, locus, and time course of the vocal tract constrictions that produce them but by whether such articulatory gestures are accompanied by vocal fold vibration. Voicing is laryngeal sound attending consonant production. Consonants such as /b/, /z/, and /dʒ/ are said to be voiced, and their voiceless cognates, /p/, /s/, and /tʃ/, respectively, are produced with exactly the same manner and place of articulation but without laryngeal vibration. A substantial amount of back pressure is necessary to produce turbulent (fricative) and transient (plosive) articulatory sound sources. The vocal folds themselves may be the principal site of articulation, using an intricate set of gestures that carefully regulate glottal resistance (Sawashima et al., 1970; Stevens, 1971; Hirose, Sawashima, and Yoshioka, 1983).

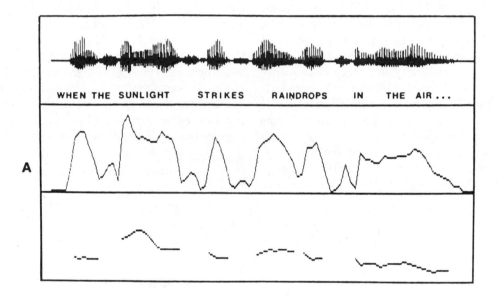

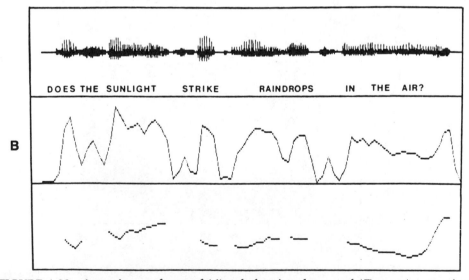

FIGURE 4-32 Acoustic waveforms of (*A*) a declarative phrase and (*B*) a yes/no question spoken by a man. Shown below each are the relative intensity and fundamental frequency of the acoustic signal.

Primary glottal turbulence distinguishes the glottal fricative /h/, and a forceful stoppage and release of subglottal pressure is used to produce the glottal plosive /ʔ/, as used in "uh oh" ([ʔʌʔoʊ]) and as an allophone of /t/ in some dialects of English. For voiceless supralaryngeal consonants, strong PCA activity widely abducts the vocal folds (Hiroto et al., 1967; Hirose and Gay, 1972; Hirose, 1976; Sawashima and Hirose, 1983). Antagonistic CT activity tenses the fold mucosa (Löfqvist et al., 1989) so that a sufficient amount of pressure can be generated quickly and efficiently at the point of constriction without interference from fold oscillation. During the production of such sounds the intraoral pressure more or less approximates the lung pressure (Smitheran and Hixon, 1981; Löfqvist, Carlborg, and Kitzing, 1982; but see also Rothenberg [1982] and Kitajima and Fujita [1990]). It is not clear how the timing of such gestures varies with the class of speech sound, the lexical context, and the nature of the syllabic stress (Löfqvist and Yoshioka, 1984; Munhall and Ostry, 1985; Löfqvist and McGarr, 1987; Löfqvist and McGowan, 1991; Stevens, 1991).

During the production of voiced consonants, intraoral pressure is substantially lower than the lung pressure because of the pressure drop across the adducted vocal folds (Arkebauer, Hixon, and Hardy, 1967). Vocal fold vibration associated with high-pressure consonants is profoundly affected by dynamically changing vocal tract aerodynamics. Figure 4-33 is a simultaneous record of percent F_o change and intraoral pressure as a man attempted to produce a prolonged phonation at a constant pitch while overlaying repeated but discrete productions of /z/. As the intraoral pressure rises for the fricative articulation, F_o drops proportionally. Since subglottal pressure remains relatively constant during speech, the intraoral pressure rise represents a fall in the transglottal pressure that drives phonation. Baken and Orlikoff (1987b, 1988) found that the ratio of vocal frequency change with transglottal pressure change during spoken and sung utterances is equivalent to that of responses to passive manipulations of driving pressure. Chollet and Kahane (1979) also investigated the effects of such constrictions on the vibration of the vocal folds, and Bickley and Stevens (1986, 1987) provide some evidence that intraglottal pressures and radiated acoustic energy are affected as well.

In the case of plosive supralaryngeal consonants the complete vocal tract constriction results in a precipitous fall of transglottal pres-

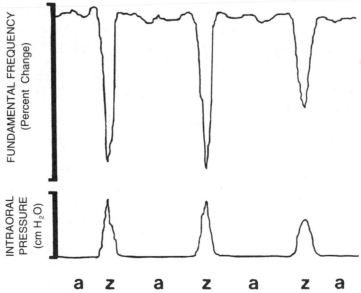

FIGURE 4-33   Percent fundamental frequency change and intraoral pressure during repeated articulations of /z/ on a sustained vowel production. The speaker is attempting to sustain a stable pitch.   (From Baken, R. J., & Orlikoff, R. F. [1987]. The effect of articulation on fundamental frequency in speakers and singers. *Journal of Voice, 1,* 68-76.)

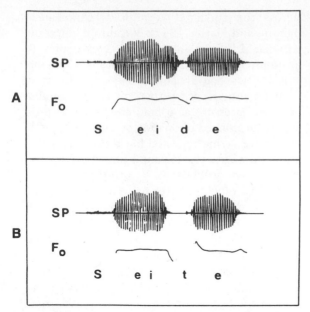

FIGURE 4-34   A stylized sound pressure (*SP*) waveform and associated F_o contour during production of the German words (*A*) Seide and (*B*) Seite spoken in monotone. (From Kohler, K. J. [1982]. F_o in the production of lenis and fortis plosives. *Phonetica, 39,* 199-218.)

sure that may preclude continued phonation. For this class of consonant, voicing is determined primarily by the voice onset time (VOT), the interval between the quick release of the vocal tract occlusion and the onset (or resumption) of glottal vibration (Lisker and Abramson, 1964). Although language and context specific, plosives produced with uninterrupted voicing or a short VOT (generally less than 20 ms) are perceived as voiced, whereas those produced with relatively long VOTs (typically greater than 25 ms) are perceived as voiceless. The voicing of plosives thus requires an extremely quick and precise coordination of laryngeal and supralaryngeal activity. Figure 4-34 shows the typical pattern of F_o change before and after phonation is squelched by the dramatic shift in transglottal pressure. The tendencies toward F_o depression and elevation after voiceless and voiced plosives, respectively, were identified by House and Fairbanks (1953) and described in some detail by Lehiste and Peterson (1961). Such F_o characteristics subsequently have been shown to be used as a subordinate perceptual cue to the voicing of plosives (Haggard, Ambler, and Callow, 1970; Lisker and Abramson, 1971; Haggard,

Summerfield, and Roberts, 1981; Abramson and Lisker, 1985; Kohler, 1985).

Current and Future Directions

The larynx is both an articulatory and a phonatory organ. Much of the difficulty in describing laryngeal behavior during running speech is the dauntingly difficult problem of separating inherent physical responses from those that have a learned linguistic base. This is particularly true for spontaneous utterances. Furthermore, mechanisms that contribute to the production, control, and regulation of sustained phonation may be quite different from those employed during speech. Nonetheless, an increased understanding of basic phonatory processes and the development of more refined measurement techniques and mathematical models will shed light on this fascinating but poorly understood area of laryngeal function.

SUMMARY

This chapter provides a working understanding of the human larynx with particular attention to its role in voice production. In general, it relates how the interplay of laryngeal tissue with the expiratory airstream affects vocal function and how that function contributes to the acoustic end product. However, because of the great flexibility and diversity of phonatory function, such charaterizations are neither simple nor straightforward and are considerably incomplete. Therefore, our intent is to provide a basic understanding of the germinal concepts of vocal function and to show how these principles shape and govern contemporary thought in voice science. Additionally, we have surveyed the contribution of various glottographic measures to the understanding of the phonatory process.

While we have not directly addressed how pathology may corrupt the phonatory system, a firm comprehension of the principles in this chapter is essential to the delineation of vocal dysfunction. This also applies to the exceptional or highly trained speaking or singing voice. Thus, as voice scientists acquire more information concerning the intricacies of normal vocal function, our understanding of poor and extraordinary voice use will improve, as will the techniques of voice therapy and training.

Review Questions

1. What are the vegetative (nonspeech) functions of the human larynx?

2. Identify the major cartilages, muscles, and membranes of the larynx. Describe their location, orientation and morphology.

3. As a group, the intrinsic laryngeal muscles perform what functions that are critical to voice production?

4. Describe the neural structures that appear to be important to the central and peripheral control of vocalization.

5. What types of mechanoreceptors have been identified in the human larynx? What possible functions may they serve?

6. How has the cover-body characterization of vocal fold structure modified our understanding of vocal fold physiology?

7. What significance has the mucosal wave for the maintenance of vocal fold vibration?

8. Describe the three basic types of vocal attack.

9. What subglottal, laryngeal, and extralaryngeal adjustments may contribute to the control and regulation of fundamental frequency?

10. What sort of evidence is necessary to differentiate among the speaking voice registers?

References

Aaltonen, O., Vilkman, E., & Raimo, I. (1988). Laryngeal adjustments or subglottal pressure? Studies on sentence stress production with excised human larynges. *Journal of Phonetics, 16*, 349-353.

Abberton, E. R. M., Howard, D. M., & Fourcin, A. J. (1989). Laryngographic assessment of normal voice: A tutorial. *Clinical Linguistics and Phonetics, 3*, 281-296.

Abo-El-Enein, M. A., & Wyke, B. D. (1966). Laryngeal myotatic reflexes. *Nature, 209*, 682-686.

Abramson, A. S., & Lisker, L. (1985). Relative power of cues: F_o shift versus voice timing. In Fromkin, V. A. (Ed.), *Phonetic linguistics: Essays in honor of Peter Ladefoged.* New York: Academic Press (pp. 25-33).

Allen, E. L., & Hollien, H. (1973). Vocal fold thickness in pulse (vocal fry) register. *Folia Phoniatrica, 25*, 241-250.

Ananthapadmanabha, T., & Gauffin, J. (1985). Some results on the acoustic and aerodynamic factors in phonation. In Titze, I. R., & Scherer, R. C. (Eds.), *Vocal fold physiology: Biomechanics, acoustics and phonatory control.* Denver, CO: The Denver Center for the Performing Arts (pp. 402-413).

Anderson, S. W., & Cooper, W. E. (1986). Fundamental frequency patterns during spontaneous picture description. *Journal of the Acoustical Society of America, 79*, 1172-1174.

Arkebauer, H., Hixon, T., & Hardy, J. (1967). Peak intraoral air pressures during speech. *Journal of Speech and Hearing Research, 10*, 196-208.

Arnold, G. E. (1961). Physiology and pathology of the cricothyroid muscle. *Laryngoscope, 71*, 687-753.

Aronson, A. E. (1990). *Clinical voice disorders,* 3rd ed. New York: Thieme.

Atkinson, J. E. (1978). Correlation analysis of the physiological factors controlling fundamental voice frequency. *Journal of the Acoustical Society of America, 63*, 211-222.

Awrejcewicz, J. (1990). Bifurcation portrait of the human vocal cord oscillations. *Journal of Sound and Vibration, 136*, 151-156.

Baer, T. (1975). *Investigation of phonation using excised larynxes.* Unpublished doctoral dissertation, Massachusetts Institute of Technology, Cambridge.

Baer, T. (1979). Reflex activation of laryngeal muscles by sudden induced subglottal pressure changes. *Journal of the Acoustical Society of America, 65*, 1271-1275.

Baer, T. (1980). Vocal jitter: A neuromuscular explanation. In Lawrence, V. L., & Weinberg, B. (Eds.), *Transcripts of the eighth symposium: care of the professional voice.* New York: The Voice Foundation (pp. 19-24).

Baer, T. (1981a). Observation of vocal fold vibration: Measurement of excised larynges. In Stevens, K. N., & Hirano, M. (Eds.), *Vocal fold physiology.* Tokyo: University of Tokyo Press (pp. 119-133).

Baer, T. (1981b). Investigation of the phonatory mechanism. *ASHA Reports, 11*, 38-47.

Baer, T., Gay, T., & Niimi, S. (1976). Control of fundamental frequency, intensity, and register of phonation. *Haskins Laboratories Status Report on Speech Research* (New Haven, CT), SR-45/46 (pp. 175-185).

Baer, T., Löfqvist, A., & McGarr, N. S. (1983). Laryngeal vibrations: A comparison between high-speed filming and glottographic techniques. *Journal of the Acoustical Society of America, 73,* 1304-1308.

Baer, T., Titze, I. R., & Yoshioka, H. (1983). Multiple simultaneous measures of vocal fold activity. In Bless, D. M., & Abbs, J. H. (Eds.), *Vocal fold physiology: Contemporary research and clinical issues.* San Diego, CA: College-Hill Press (pp. 229-237).

Baier, H., Wanner, A., Zarzecki, S., & Sackner, M. A. (1977). Relationships among glottis opening, respiratory flow, and upper airway resistance in humans. *Journal of Applied Physiology, 43,* 603-611.

Baken, R. J. (1971). Neuromuscular spindles in the intrinsic laryngeal muscles in man. *Folia Phoniatrica, 23,* 204-210.

Baken, R. J. (1987). *Clinical measurement of speech and voice.* Boston: Little, Brown.

Baken, R. J. (1990). Irregularity of vocal period and amplitude: a first approach to the fractal analysis of voice. *Journal of Voice, 4,* 185-197.

Baken, R. J. (1992). Electroglottography. *Journal of Voice, 6,* 98-110.

Baken, R. J., Cavallo, S. A., and Weissman, K. L. (1979). Chest wall movements prior to phonation. *Journal of Speech and Hearing Research, 22,* 862-872.

Baken, R. J., and Isshiki, N. (1977). Arytenoid displacement by simulated muscle contraction. *Folia Phoniatrica, 29,* 206-216.

Baken, R. J., & Noback, C. (1971). Neuromuscular spindles in the intrinsic muscles of the human. *Journal of Speech and Hearing Research, 14,* 513-518.

Baken, R. J., & Orlikoff, R. F. (1987a). Phonatory response to a step-function change in supraglottal pressure. In Baer, T., Sasaki, C. T., & Harris, K. S. (Eds.), *Laryngeal function in phonation and respiration.* Boston: College-Hill Press (pp. 273-290).

Baken, R. J., & Orlikoff, R. F. (1987b). The effect of articulation on fundamental frequency in speakers and singers. *Journal of Voice, 1,* 68-76.

Baken, R. J., & Orlikoff, R. F. (1988). Changes in vocal fundamental frequency at the segmental level: Control during voiced fricatives. *Journal of Speech and Hearing Research, 31,* 207-211.

Baken, R. J., & Orlikoff, R. F. (1992). Acoustic assessment of vocal function. In Blitzer, A., Sasaki, C. T., Fahn, S., Brin, M., & Harris, K. S. (Eds.), *Neurological disorders of the larynx.* New York: Thieme-Stratton (pp. 124-134).

Barnsley, M. (1988). *Fractals everywhere.* Boston: Academic Press.

Bartlett, D. A., Jr., Remmers, J. E., & Gautier, H. (1973). Laryngeal regulation of respiratory airflow. *Respiratory Physiology, 18,* 194-204.

Bender, L. (1928). The cerebellar control of the vocal organs. *Archives of Neurology and Psychiatry, 19,* 796-833.

Benjamin, B. J. (1981). Frequency variability in the aged voice. *Journal of Gerontology, 36,* 722-726.

Berke, G. S., Moore, D. M., Monkewitz, P. A., Hanson, D. G., & Gerratt, B. R. (1989). A preliminary study of particle velocity during phonation in an in vivo canine model. *Journal of Voice, 3,* 306-313.

Berry, D. A., Herzel, H., Titze, I. R., and Kirscher, K. (1994). Interpretation of biomechanical simulations of normal and chaotic vocal fold oscillations with empirical eigenfunctions. *Journal of the Acoustical Society of America, 95,* 3595-3604.

Bickley, C. A., and Stevens, K. N. (1986). Effects of a vocal-tract constriction on the glottal source: Experimental and modelling studies. *Journal of Phonetics, 14,* 373-382.

Bickley, C. A., & Stevens, K. N. (1987). Effects of a vocal-tract constriction on the glottal source: Data from voiced consonants. In Baer, T., Sasaki, C., & Harris, K. S. (Eds), *Laryngeal function in phonation and respiration.* Boston: College-Hill Press (pp. 239-253).

Biever, D. M., and Bless, D. M. (1989). Vibratory characteristics of the vocal folds in young adult and geriatric women. *Journal of Voice, 3,* 120-131.

Black, J. W. (1949). Natural frequency, duration, and intensity of vowels in reading. *Journal of Speech and Hearing Disorders, 14,* 216-221.

Botez, M. I., & Barbeau, A. (1971). Role of subcortical structures, and particularly of the thalamus, in the mechanism of speech and language. *International Journal of Neurology, 8,* 300-320.

Bouhuys, A., Proctor, D., & Mead, J. (1966). Kinetic aspects of singing. *Journal of Applied Physiology, 21,* 483-496.

Bowler, N. W. (1964). Fundamental frequency analysis of harsh voice quality. *Speech Monographs, 31,* 129-134.

Broad, D. J. (1973). Phonation. In Minifie, F. D., Hixon, T. J., & Williams, F. (Eds.), *Normal aspects of speech, hearing, and language.* Englewood Cliffs, NJ: Prentice-Hall (pp. 127-167).

Broad, D. J. (1979). The new theories of vocal fold vibration. In Lass, N. J. (Ed.), *Speech and language: Advances in basic research and practice,* Vol. 2. New York: Academic Press (pp. 203-256).

Brown, W. S., Jr., & McGlone, R. E. (1974). Aerodynamic and acoustic study of stress in sentence productions. *Journal of the Acoustical Society of America, 56,* 971-974.

Catford, J. C. (1968). The articulatory possibilities of man. In Malmberg, B. (Ed.), *Manual of phonetics.* Amsterdam: North-Holland (pp. 309-333).

Catford, J. C. (1983). Pharyngeal and laryngeal sounds in Caucasian languages. In Bless, D. M., &

Abbs, J. H. (Eds.), *Vocal fold physiology: Contemporary research and clinical issues.* San Diego, CA: College-Hill Press (pp. 343-350).

Cavagna, G. A., & Camporesi, E. (1974). Glottal aerodynamics and phonation. In Wyke, B. (Ed.), *Ventilatory and phonatory control systems.* New York: Oxford University Press (pp. 76-92).

Cavagna, G. A., & Margaria, R. (1968). Airflow rates and efficiency changes during phonation. *Annals of the New York Academy of Sciences, 155,* 152-163.

Cavallo, S. A., Baken, R. J., & Shaiman, S. (1984). Frequency perturbation characteristics of pulse register phonation. *Journal of Communication Disorders, 17,* 231-243.

Chamberlain, W. E., & Young, B. R. (1935). Ossification (so-called calcification) of normal laryngeal cartilages mistaken for foreign bodies. *American Journal of Roentgenology, 33,* 441-450.

Chernikov, A. A., Sagdeev, R. Z., & Zaslavsky, G. M. (1988). Chaos: How regular can it be? *Physics Today, 41*(11), 27-35.

Chevrie-Muller, C. (1967). Contribution à l'étude des traces glottographiques chez l'adulte normal. *Revue de Laryngologie, 88,* 227-243.

Childers, D. G., Hicks, D. M., Moore, G. P., & Alsaka, Y. A. (1986). A model for vocal fold vibratory motion, contact area, and the electroglottogram. *Journal of the Acoustical Society of America, 80,* 1309-1320.

Childers, D. G., & Krishnamurthy, A. K. (1985). A critical review of electroglottography. *CRC Critical Review of Biomedical Engineering, 12,* 131-161.

Chollet, G. F., & Kahane, J. C. (1979). Laryngeal patterns of consonant productions in sentences observed with an impedance glottograph. In Hollien, H., & Hollien, P. (Eds.), *Current issues in the phonetic sciences.* Amsterdam: John Benjamins B. V. (pp. 119-128).

Cohen, A., Collier, R., & 't Hart, J. (1982). Declination: Construct or intrinsic feature of speech pitch? *Phonetica, 39,* 254-273.

Coleman, R. F. (1963). Decay characteristics of vocal fry. *Folia Phoniatrica, 15,* 256-263.

Coleman, R. Mabis, J., & Hinson, J. (1977). Fundamental frequency - sound pressure level profiles of adult male and female voices. *Journal of Speech and Hearing Research, 20,* 197-204.

Collier, R. (1975). Physiological correlates of intonation patterns. *Journal of the Acoustical Society of America, 58,* 249-255.

Collier, R. (1987). F₀ declination: The control of its setting, resetting, and slope. In Baer, T., Sasaki, C. T., & Harris, K. S. (Eds.), *Laryngeal function in phonation and respiration.* Boston: College-Hill Press (pp. 403-421).

Colton, R. H. (1972). Spectral characteristics of the modal and falsetto registers. *Folia Phoniatrica, 24,* 337-344.

Colton, R. H. (1973). Vocal intensity in the modal and falsetto registers. *Folia Phoniatrica, 25,* 62-70.

Colton, R. H. (1985). Glottal waveform variations associated with different vocal intensity levels. In Lawrence, V. L. (Ed.), *Transcripts of the thirteenth symposium on the care of the professional voice.* New York: Voice Foundation (pp. 39-47).

Colton, R. H. (1988). Physiological mechanisms of vocal frequency control: the role of tension. *Journal of Voice, 2,* 208-220.

Colton, R. H., & Conture, E. G. (1990). Problems and pitfalls of electroglottography. *Journal of Voice, 4,* 10-24.

Colton, R. H., & Hollien, H. (1972). Phonational range in the modal and falsetto registers. *Journal of Speech and Hearing Research, 15,* 708-713.

Conrad, W. A. (1980). A new model of the vocal cords based on a collapsible tube analogy. *Medical Research Engineering, 13,* 7-10.

Conrad, W. A. (1983). Collapsible tube model of the larynx. In Titze, I. R., & Scherer, R. C. (Eds.), *Vocal fold physiology: Biomechanics, acoustics and phonatory control.* Denver, CO: The Denver Center for the Performing Arts (pp. 328-348).

Conrad, W. A. (1987). Simplified one-mass model with supraglottal resistance: A testable hypothesis. In Baer, T., Sasaki, C. T., & Harris, K. S. (Eds.), *Laryngeal function in phonation and respiration.* Boston: College-Hill Press (pp. 320-338).

Conrad, W. A., & McQueen, D. M. (1987). The two-mass and one-mass models and supraglottal resistance. Paper presented at the 16th Symposium on the Care of the Professional Voice, June 1-5, New York.

Cooper, D. S., Partridge, L. D., & Alipour-Haghighi, F. (1993). Muscle energetics, vocal efficiency, and laryngeal biomechanics. In Titze, I. R. (Ed.), *Vocal fold physiology: Frontiers in basic science.* San Diego, CA: Singular Publishing Group (pp. 37-92).

Cooper, W. E., & Sorenson, J. M. (1981). *Fundamental frequency in sentence production.* New York: Springer-Verlag.

Coumel, P., & Maison-Blanche, P. (1991). Complex dynamics of cardiac arrhythmias. *Chaos, 1,* 335-342.

Damsté, H. (1970). The phonetogram. *Practica Oto-Rhino-Laryngologica, 32,* 185-187.

Davies, P. O. A. L., McGowan, R. S., & Shadle, C. H. (1993). Practical flow duct acoustics applied to the vocal tract. In Titze, I. R. (Ed.), *Vocal fold physiology: Frontiers in basic science.* San Diego, CA: Singular Publishing Group (pp. 93-142).

Davis, P. J., Bartlett, D. A., Jr., & Luschei, E. S. (1993). Coordination of the respiratory and laryngeal systems in breathing and vocalization. In Titze, I. R. (Ed.), *Vocal fold physiology: Frontiers in basic science.* San Diego, CA: Singular Publishing Group (pp. 189-226).

Dejonckere, P. H., & Lebacq, J. (1985). Electroglottography and vocal nodules: An attempt to quantify the shape of the signal. *Folia Phoniatrica, 37,* 195-200.

Devaney, R. L. (1987). Chaotic bursts in nonlinear dynamical systems. *Science, 235,* 342-345.

Devaney, R. L. (1990). Chaotic explosions in simple dynamical systems. In Krasner, S. (Ed.), *The ubiquity of chaos.* Washington, DC: American Association for the Advancement of Science (pp. 1-9).

Draper, M. H., Ladefoged, P., & Witteridge, D. (1960). Expiratory pressure and airflow during speech. *British Medical Journal, 1,* 1837-1843.

Dunker, E. (1968). The central control of laryngeal function. *Annals of the New York Academy of Sciences, 155,* 112-121.

English, D. T., & Blevins, C. E. (1969). Motor units of laryngeal muscles. *Archives of Otolaryngology, 89,* 778-784.

Erickson, D., Baer, T., & Harris, K. S. (1983). The role of the strap muscles in pitch lowering. In Bless, D. M., & Abbs, J. H. (Eds.), *Vocal fold physiology: Contemporary research and clinical issues.* San Diego, CA: College-Hill Press (pp. 279-285).

Estill, J., Baer, T., Honda, K., & Harris, K. S. (1985). Supralaryngeal activity in a study of six voice qualities. In Askenfelt, A., Felicetti, S., Jansson, E., & Sundberg, J. (Eds.), *Proceedings of the Stockholm music acoustics conference.* Stockholm: Royal Swedish Academy of Music (pp. 152-174).

Ewan, W. G. (1979). Can intrinsic vowel F_o be explained by source/tract coupling? *Journal of the Acoustical Society of America, 66,* 358-362.

Ewan, W. G. (1980). Aspects of speech and orthognathic surgery. In Lass, N. J. (Ed.), *Speech and language: Advances in basic research and practice,* Vol. 4. New York: Academic Press (pp. 239-289).

Faaborg-Andersen, K. (1957). Electromyographic investigation of intrinsic laryngeal muscles in humans. *Acta Physiologica Scandinavica, 41,* (Suppl. 140), 1-150.

Faaborg-Andersen, K. (1965). Electromyography of laryngeal muscles in humans. Technics and results. In *Current problems in phoniatrics and logopedics,* Vol. 3. Basel: Karger.

Faaborg-Andersen, K., & Sonninen, A. (1960). The function of the extrinsic laryngeal muscles at different pitch. *Acta-Otolaryngologica, 51,* 89-93.

Faaborg-Andersen, K., & Vennard, W. (1964). Electromyography of the extrinsic laryngeal muscles during phonation of different vowels. *Annals of Otology, Rhinology and Laryngology, 73,* 248-254.

Faaborg-Andersen, K., Yanagihara, N., and von Leden, H. (1967). Vocal pitch and intensity regulation. A comparative study of electrical activity in the cricothyroid muscle and the airflow rate. *Archives of Otolaryngology, 85,* 448-454.

Fabre, P. (1957). Un procédé électrique percutané d'inscription de l'accolement glottique au cours de la phonation: Glottographie de haut fréquence. Premiers résultats. *Bulletin de l'Académie Nationale de Médecine, 141,* 66-69.

Fairbanks, G. (1950). A physiological correlative of vowel intensity. *Speech Monographs, 17,* 390-395.

Fant, G. (1979). Glottal source and excitation analysis. *Speech Transmission Laboratory Quarterly Progress and Status Report* (Royal Institute of Technology, Stockholm, Sweden), *1,* 85-107.

Ferrein, A. (1746). De la formation de la voix de l'homme. *Mémoires de mathématique et de physique tirés des registres de l'Académie Royale des Sciences de l'année MDCCXLI.* Amsterdam: Pierre Mortier (pp. 545-579).

Fink, B. R. (1975). *The human larynx: A functional study.* New York: Raven Press.

Fink, B. R., Basek, M., & Epanchin, V. (1956). The mechanism of opening of the human larynx. *Laryngoscope, 66,* 410-425.

Flanagan, J. L. (1959). Estimates of intraglottal pressure during phonation. *Journal of Speech and Hearing Research, 2,* 168-172.

Flanagan, J. L. (1968). Source-system interaction in the vocal tract. *Annals of the New York Academy of Sciences, 155,* 9-17.

Fourcin, A. J. (1974). Laryngographic examination of vocal fold vibration. In Wyke, B. (Ed.), *Ventilatory and phonatory control systems.* New York: Oxford University Press (pp. 315-333).

Fourcin, A. J. (1981). Laryngographic assessment of phonatory function. *ASHA Reports, 11,* 116-127.

Fourcin, A. J. (1982). Electrolaryngographic assessment of vocal fold function. *Journal of Phonetics, 14,* 435-442.

Frable, M. A. (1961). Computation of motion at the cricoarytenoid joint. *Archives of Otolaryngology, 73,* 551-556.

Fritzell, B., Hammarberg, B., Gauffin, J., Karlsson, I., & Sundberg, J. (1986). Breathiness and insufficient vocal fold closure. *Journal of Phonetics, 14,* 549-553.

Fry, D. B. (1955). Duration and intensity as physical correlates of linguistic stress. *Journal of the Acoustical Society of America, 27,* 765-768.

Fry, D. B. (1968). Prosodic phenomena. In Malmberg, B. (Ed.), *Manual of phonetics.* Amsterdam: North-Holland (pp. 365-410).

Fujimura, O. (1981). Body-cover theory of the vocal fold and its phonetic implications. In Stevens, K. N., & Hirano, M. (Eds.), *Vocal fold physiology.* Tokyo: University of Tokyo Press (pp. 271-288).

Fujisaki, H. (1983). Dynamic characteristics of voice fundamental frequency in speech and singing. In MacNeilage P. F. (Ed.), *The production of speech.* New York: Springer-Verlag (pp. 39-55).

Fukuda, H., Kawaida, M., Tatehara, T., Ling, E., Kita,

K., Ohki, K., Kawasaki, Y., & Saito, S. (1988). A new concept of lubricating mechanisms of the larynx. In Fujimura, O. (Ed.), *Vocal physiology: Voice production, mechanisms and functions.* New York: Raven Press (pp. 83-91).

Fukuda, H., Muta, H., Kanou, S., Takayama, E., Fujioka, T., Kawaida, T., Tatehara, T., & Saito, S. (1987). Response of vocal folds to externally induced vibrations: Basic study and its clinical application. In Baer, T., Sasaki, C. T., & Harris, K. S. (Eds.), *Laryngeal function in phonation and respiration.* Boston: College-Hill Press (pp. 366-377).

Fukuda, H., Saito, S., Kitahara, S., Isogai, Y., Makino, K., Tsuzuki, T., Kogawa, N., & Ono, H. (1983). Vocal fold vibration in excised larynges viewed with an x-ray stroboscope and an ultra-high-speed camera. In Bless, D. M., & Abbs, J. H. (Eds.), *Vocal fold physiology: Contemporary research and clinical issues.* San Diego, CA: College-Hill Press (pp. 238-252).

Ganz, H. (1971). The metabolism of laryngeal muscles. *Archives of Otolaryngology, 94,* 97-107.

Gauffin, J., Binh, N., Ananthapadmanabha, T. V., & Fant, G. (1983). Glottal geometry and volume velocity waveform. In Bless, D. M., & Abbs, J. H. (Eds.), *Vocal fold physiology: Contemporary research and clinical issues.* San Diego, CA: College-Hill Press (pp. 194-201).

Gauffin, J., & Liljencrants, J. (1988). The role of convective acceleration in glottal aerodynamics. In Fujimura, O. (Ed.), *Vocal physiology: Voice production, mechanisms and functions.* New York: Raven Press (pp. 219-226).

Gauffin, J., & Sundberg, J. (1989). Spectral correlates of glottal voice source waveform characteristics. *Journal of Speech and Hearing Research, 32,* 556-565.

Gautier, H., Remmers, J. E., & Bartlett, D. A., Jr. (1973). Control of the duration of expiration. *Respiratory Physiology, 18,* 205-221.

Gay, T., Hirose, H., Strome, M., & Sawashima, M. (1972). Electromyography of the intrinsic laryngeal muscles during phonation. *Annals of Otology, Rhinology and Laryngology, 81,* 401-409.

Gelfer, C. E., Harris, K. S., & Baer, T. (1987). Controlled variables in sentence intonation. In Baer, T., Sasaki, C., & Harris, K. S. (Eds.), *Laryngeal function in phonation and respiration.* Boston: College-Hill Press (pp. 422-435).

Gelfer, C. E., Harris, K. S., Collier, R., & Baer, T. (1985). Is declination actively controlled? In Titze, I. R., & Scherer, R. C. (Eds.), *Vocal fold physiology: Biomechanics, acoustics and phonatory control.* Denver, CO: Denver Center for the Performing Arts (pp. 113-126).

Giger, H. L. (1985). The value of phonetogram studies in clinical work. In Lawrence, V. L. (Ed.), *Transcripts of the thirteenth symposium on the care of the professional voice. Part II: Vocal therapeutics-Medical.* New York: The Voice Foundation (pp. 367-369).

Gilbert, H. R., Potter, C. R., & Hoodin, R. (1984). Laryngograph as a measure of vocal fold contact area. *Journal of Speech and Hearing Research, 27,* 173-178.

Glass, L., Guevara, M. R., & Shrier, A. (1987). Universal bifurcations and the classification of cardiac arrhythmias. *Annals of the New York Academy of Sciences, 504,* 168-178.

Glass, L., & Mackey, M. C. (1988). *From clocks to chaos: The rhythms of life.* Princeton, NJ: Princeton University Press.

Gleick, J. (1987). *Chaos: Making a new science.* New York: Viking Press.

Goldberger, A. L., & Rigney, D. R. (1990). Sudden death is not chaos. In Krasner, S. (Ed.), *The ubiquity of chaos.* Washington, DC: American Association for the Advancement of Science (pp. 23-34).

Goldberger, A. L. & West, B. J. (1987a). Applications of nonlinear dynamics to clinical cardiology. *Annals of the New York Academy of Sciences, 504,* 195-213.

Goldberger, A. L., & West, B. J. (1987b). Fractals in physiology and medicine. *Yale Journal of Biology and Medicine, 60,* 421-435.

Gracheva, M. S. (1963). Sensory innervation of locomotor apparatus of the larynx. *Arkhiv Anatomii, Gistologii l'Enbriologii, 44,* 77-83.

Gramming, P. (1991). Vocal loudness and frequency capabilities of the voice. *Journal of Voice, 5,* 144-157.

Gramming, P., & Sundberg, J. (1988). Spectrum factors relevant to phonetogram measurement. *Journal of the Acoustical Society of America, 83,* 2352-2360.

Gramming, P., Sundberg, J., Ternström, S., Leanderson, R., & Perkins, W. H. (1988). Relationship between changes in voice pitch and loudness. *Journal of Voice, 2,* 118-126.

Grebogi, C., Ott, E., & Yorke, J. A. (1987). Chaos, strange attractors, and fractal basin boundaries in nonlinear dynamics. *Science, 238,* 632-638.

Gretz, B., & Sirnes, T. (1949). The localization within the dorsal motor vagal nucleus: An experimental investigation. *Journal of Cooperative Neurology, 90,* 95-110.

Grim, M. (1967). Muscle spindles in the posterior cricoarytenoid muscles of the human larynx. *Folia Morphologica, 15,* 124-131.

Griffiths, D. J. (1975). Negative-resistance effects in flow through collapsible tubes: 1. Relaxation oscillations. *Medical and Biological Engineering, 13,* 785-790.

Haggard, M., Ambler, S., & Callow, M. (1970). Pitch as a voicing cue. *Journal of the Acoustical Society of America, 47,* 613-617.

Haggard, M., Summerfield, Q., & Roberts, M. (1981). Psychoacoustical and cultural determinants of phoneme boundaries: Evidence from trading F_o cues in the voiced-voiceless distinction. *Journal of Phonetics, 9,* 49-62.

Hardcastle, W. J. (1976). *Physiology of speech production.* New York: Academic Press (p. 80).

Harden, R. J. (1975). Comparison of glottal area changes as measured from ultrahigh-speed photographs and photoelectric glottographs. *Journal of Speech and Hearing Research, 18,* 728-738.

Harris, K. S. (1981). Electromyography as a technique for laryngeal investigation. *ASHA Reports, 11,* 70-87.

Harvey, N., & Howell, P. (1980). Isotonic vocalis contraction as a means of producing rapid decreases in F_o. *Journal of Speech and Hearing Research, 23,* 576-592.

Hassler, R. (1956). Die extraphyramidalen Rindensysteme und die zentrale Regelung der Motoril. *Deutsche Zeitschrift für Nervenheilkunde, 175,* 233-258.

Hast, M. H. (1966). Physiological mechanisms of phonation: Tension of the vocal fold muscle. *Acta Oto-laryngologica, 62,* 309-318.

Hast, M. H. (1967). The respiratory muscle of the larynx. *Annals of Otology, Rhinology, and Laryngology, 76,* 489-497.

Hast, M. H. (1985). Comparative anatomy of the larynx: Evolution and function. In Titze, I. R., & Scherer, R. C. (Eds.), *Vocal fold physiology: Biomechanics, acoustics and phonatory control.* Denver, CO: Denver Center for the Performing Arts (pp. 3-14).

Hauser, M. D., & Fowler, C. A. (1992). Fundamental frequency declination is not unique to human speech: Evidence from nonhuman primates. *Journal of the Acoustical Society of America, 91,* 363-369.

Heiberger, V. L., and Horii, Y. (1982). Jitter and shimmer in sustained phonation. In Lass, N. J. (Ed.), *Speech and language: advances in basic research and practice,* vol. 7. New York: Academic Press (pp. 299-332).

Hertegård, S., Gauffin, J., & Sundberg, J. (1990). Open and covered singing as studied by means of fiberoptics, inverse filtering, and spectal analysis. *Journal of Voice, 4,* 220-230.

Herzel, H., Steinecke, I., Mende, W., & Wermke, K. (1991). Chaos and bifurcations during voiced speech. In Mosekilde, E. (Ed.), *Complexity, chaos, and biological evolution.* New York: Plenum.

Hiki, S. (1983). Relationship between efficiency of phonation and the tonal quality of speech. In Bless, D. M., & Abbs, J. H. (Eds.), *Vocal fold physiology: Contemporary research and clinical issues.* San Diego, CA: College-Hill Press (pp. 333-343).

Hillenbrand, J. (1988). Perception of aperiodicities in synthetically generated voices. *Journal of the Acoustical Society of America, 83,* 2361-2371.

Hillman, R. E., Holmberg, E. B., Perkell, J. S., Walsh, M., & Vaughan, C. (1989). Objective assessment of vocal hyperfunction: An experimental framework and initial results. *Journal of Speech and Hearing Research, 32,* 373-392.

Hirano, M. (1974). Morphological structure of the vocal cord as a vibrator and its variations. *Folia Phoniatrica, 26,* 89-94.

Hirano, M. (1975). Phonosurgery: Basic and clinical investigations. *Otologia Fukuoka, 21,* 239-440.

Hirano, M. (1977). Structure and vibratory behavior of the vocal folds. In Sawashima, M., & Cooper, F. S. (Eds.), *Dynamic aspects of speech production.* Tokyo: University of Tokyo Press (pp. 13-30).

Hirano, M. (1981a). *Clinical examination of voice.* New York: Springer-Verlag.

Hirano, M. (1981b). The function of the intrinsic laryngeal muscles in singing. In Stevens, K. N., & Hirano, M. (Eds.), *Vocal fold physiology.* Tokyo: University of Tokyo Press (pp. 155-170).

Hirano, M. (1988a). Vocal mechanisms in singing: Laryngological and phoniatric aspects. *Journal of Voice, 2,* 51-69.

Hirano, M. (1988b). Behavior of laryngeal muscles of the late William Vennard. *Journal of Voice, 2,* 291-300.

Hirano, M., Hibi, S., & Sanada, T. (1989). Falsetto, head/chest, and speech mode: An acoustic study with three tenors. *Journal of Voice, 3,* 99-103.

Hirano, M., Kakita, Y., Kawasaki, H., Gould, W. J., & Lambiase, A. (1981). Data from high-speed motion picture studies. In Stevens, K. N., & Hirano, M. (Eds.), *Vocal fold physiology.* Tokyo: University of Tokyo Press (pp. 85-93).

Hirano, M., Kiyokawa, K., & Kurita, S. (1988). Laryngeal muscles and glottic shaping. In Fujimura, O. (Ed.), *Vocal physiology: Voice production, mechanisms and functions.* New York: Raven Press (pp. 49-65).

Hirano, M., Koike, Y., & von Leden, H. (1968). Maximum phonation time and air usage during phonation. *Folia Phoniatrica, 20,* 185-201.

Hirano, M., Matsuo, K., Kakita, Y., Kawasaki, H., & Kurita, S. (1985). Vibratory behavior versus the structure of the vocal fold. In Titze, I. R., & Scherer, R. C. (Eds.), *Vocal fold physiology: Biomechanics, acoustics and phonatory control.* Denver, CO: Denver Center for the Performing Arts (pp. 26-40).

Hirano, M., Ohala, J., and Vennard, W. (1969). The function of laryngeal muscles in regulating fundamental frequency and intensity of phonation. *Journal of Speech and Hearing Research, 12,* 616-627.

Hirano, M., Vennard, W., & Ohala, J. (1970).

Regulation of register, pitch and intensity of voice. *Folia Phoniatrica, 22,* 1-20.

Hirano, M., Yoshida, T., & Tanaka, S. (1991). Vibratory behavior of human vocal folds viewed from below. In Gauffin, J., & Hammarberg, B. (Eds.), *Vocal fold physiology: Acoustic, perceptual, and physiological aspects of voice mechanisms.* San Diego, CA: Singular Publishing Group (pp. 1-6).

Hirose, H. (1976). Posterior cricoarytenoid as a speech muscle. *Annals of Otology, Rhinology and Laryngology, 85,* 334-342.

Hirose, H. (1977). Laryngeal adjustments in consonant production. *Phonetica, 34,* 289-294.

Hirose, H., & Gay, T. (1972). The activity of the intrinsic laryngeal muscles in voicing control: An electromyographic study. *Phonetica, 25,* 140-164.

Hirose, H., Sawashima, M., & Yoshioka, H. (1983). Laryngeal adjustment for initiation of utterances: A simultaneous EMG and fiberscopic study. In Bless, D. M., & Abbs, J. H. (Eds.), *Vocal fold physiology: Contemporary research and clinical issues.* San Diego, CA: College-Hill Press (pp. 253-263).

Hiroto, I. (1966). Pathophysiology of the larynx from the viewpoint of the vocal mechanism. *Practica Otologica Kyoto, 59,* 229-292.

Hiroto, I., Hirano, M., Toyozumi, Y., & Shin, T. (1967). Electromyographic investigation of the intrinsic laryngeal muscles related to speech sounds. *Annals of Otology, Rhinology and Laryngology, 76,* 861-872.

Hixon, T. J., Klatt, D. H., & Mead, J. (1971). Influence of forced transglottal pressure changes on vocal fundamental frequency. *Journal of the Acoustical Society of America, 49,* 105 (Abstract).

Hollien, H. (1960a). Some laryngeal correlates of vocal pitch. *Journal of Speech and Hearing Research, 3,* 52-58.

Hollien, H. (1960b). Vocal pitch variation related to changes in vocal fold length. *Journal of Speech and Hearing Research, 3,* 150-156.

Hollien, H. (1962). Vocal fold thickness and fundamental frequency of phonation. *Journal of Speech and Hearing Research, 5,* 237-243.

Hollien, H. (1972). Three major vocal registers: A proposal. In Rigault, A., & Charbonneau, R. (Eds.), *Proceedings of the Seventh International Congress of Phonetic Sciences.* The Hague: Mouton (pp. 320-331).

Hollien, H. (1974). On vocal registers. *Journal of Phonetics, 2,* 125-143.

Hollien, H., Brown, W. S., Jr., & Hollien, K. (1971). Vocal fold length associated with modal, falsetto and varying vocal intensity phonations. *Folia Phoniatrica, 23,* 66-78.

Hollien, H., Coleman, R., & Moore, P. (1968). Stroboscopic laminagraphy of the larynx during phonation. *Acta Otolaryngologica, 65,* 209-215.

Hollien, H., & Colton, R. H. (1969). Four laminagraphic studies of vocal fold thickness. *Folia Phoniatrica, 21,* 179-198.

Hollien, H., & Curtis, J. F. (1960). A laminagraphic study of vocal pitch. *Journal of Speech and Hearing Research, 3,* 362-371.

Hollien, H., Damsté, H., & Murry, T. (1969). Vocal fold length during vocal fry phonation. *Folia Phoniatrica, 21,* 257-265.

Hollien, H., Dew, D., & Philips, P. (1971). Phonational frequency ranges of adults. *Journal of Speech and Hearing Research, 14,* 755-760.

Hollien, H., Girard, G. T., & Coleman, R. F. (1977). Vocal fold vibratory patterns of pulse register phonation. *Folia Phoniatrica, 29,* 200-205.

Hollien, H., Gould, W. J., & Johnson, B. (1976). A two-level concept of vocal registers. In Loebell, E. (Ed.), *Proceedings of the Sixteenth International Congress of Logopedics and Phoniatrics.* Basel: Karger (pp. 188-194).

Hollien, H., & Michel, J. F. (1968). Vocal fry as a phonational register. *Journal of Speech and Hearing Research, 11,* 600-604.

Hollien, H., & Michel, J., & Doherty, E. T. (1973). A method for analyzing vocal jitter in sustained phonation. *Journal of Phonetics, 1,* 85-91.

Hollien, H., & Moore, P. (1960). Measurements of the vocal folds during changes in pitch. *Journal of Speech and Hearing Research, 3,* 157-163.

Hollien, H., Moore, P., Wendahl, R. W., & Michel, J. F. (1966). On the nature of vocal fry. *Journal of Speech and Hearing Research, 9,* 245-247.

Hollien, H., & Schoenhard, C. (1985). The riddle of the "middle" register. In Titze, I. R., & Scherer, R. C. (Eds.), *Vocal fold physiology: Biomechanics, acoustics and phonatory control.* Denver, CO: Denver Center for the Performing Arts (pp. 256-269).

Hollien, H., & Shipp, T. (1972). Speaking fundamental frequency and chronologic age in males. *Journal of Speech and Hearing Research, 15,* 155-159.

Hollien, H., & Wendahl, R. W. (1968). Perceptual study of vocal fry. *Journal of the Acoustical Society of America, 43,* 506-509.

Holmberg, E. B., Hillman, R. E., & Perkell, J. S. (1988). Glottal airflow and transglottal air pressure measurement for male and female speakers in soft, normal, and loud voice. *Journal of the Acoustical Society of America, 84,* 511-529.

Holmberg, E. B., Hillman, R. E., & Perkell, J. S. (1989). Glottal airflow and transglottal air pressure measurements for male and female speakers in low, normal, and high pitch. *Journal of Voice, 3,* 294-305.

Honda, K. (1983). Relationship between pitch control and vowel articulation. In Bless, D. M., & Abbs, J. H. (Eds.), *Vocal fold physiology: Contem-*

porary research and clinical issues. San Diego, CA: College-Hill Press (pp. 286-297).

Honda, K. (1985). Variability analysis of laryngeal muscle activities. In Titze, I. R., & Scherer, R. C. (Eds.), *Vocal fold physiology: Biomechanics, acoustics and phonatory control.* Denver, CO: Denver Center for the Performing Arts (pp. 128-137).

Horii, Y. (1979). Fundamental frequency perturbation observed in sustained phonation. *Journal of Speech and Hearing Research, 22,* 5-19.

Horii, Y. (1980). Vocal shimmer in sustained phonation. *Journal of Speech and Hearing Research, 23,* 202-209.

Horii, Y. (1985). Jitter and shimmer differences in sustained vocal fry phonation. *Folia Phoniatrica,* 37, 81-86.

House, A. S. (1959). A note on optimal vocal frequency. *Journal of Speech and Hearing Research, 2,* 55-60.

House, A. S., & Fairbanks, G. (1953). The influence of consonant environment upon the secondary characteristics of vowels. *Journal of the Acoustical Society of America, 25,* 105-113.

Howard, D. M., Lindsey, G. A., & Allen, B. (1990). Toward the quantification of vocal efficiency. *Journal of Voice, 4,* 205-212.

Ishizaka, K., & Flanagan, J. L. (1972). Synthesis of voiced sounds from a two-mass model of the vocal cords. *Bell System Technical Journal, 51,* 1233-1268.

Ishizaka, K., & Matsudaira, M. (1972). Fluid mechanical considerations of vocal cord vibration. *SCRL Monograph* (Santa Barbara, CA: Speech Communications Research Laboratory), *8,* 1-72.

Isshiki, N. (1964). Regulatory mechanism of vocal intensity variation. *Journal of speech and Hearing Research, 7,* 17-29.

Isshiki, N. (1965). Vocal intensity and air flow rate. *Folia Phoniatrica, 17,* 92-104.

Isshiki, N. (1969). Remarks on mechanism for vocal intensity variation. *Journal of Speech and Hearing Research, 12,* 665-672.

Isshiki, N. (1981). Vocal efficiency index. In Stevens, K. N., & Hirano, M. (Eds.), *Vocal fold physiology.* Tokyo: University of Tokyo Press (pp. 193-207).

Isshiki, N. (1985). Clinical significance of a vocal efficiency index. In Titze, I. R., & Scherer, R. C. (Eds.), *Vocal fold physiology: Biomechanics, acoustics and phonatory control.* Denver, CO: Denver Center for the Performing Arts (pp. 230-238).

Isshiki, N., Okamura, H., & Morimoto, M. (1967). Maximum phonation time and air flow rate during phonation: Simple clinical tests for vocal function. *Annals of Otology, Rhinology and Laryngology, 76,* 998-1007.

Jacob, L. A. (1968). *A normative study of laryngeal jitter.* Unpublished master's thesis, University of Kansas, Lawrence.

Jankovskaya, N. F. (1959). The receptor innervation of the perichondrium of the laryngeal cartilages. *Arkhiv Anatomii, Gistologii l'Enbriologii, 37,* 70-75.

Jürgens, H., Peitgen, H.-O., & Saupe, D. (1990). The language of fractals. *Scientific American, 263*(2), 60-67.

Jürgens, U. (1976). Projections from the cortical larynx area in the squirrel monkey. *Experimental Brain Research, 25,* 401-411.

Jürgens, U. (1983). Afferent fibers to the cingular vocalization region in the squirrel monkey. *Experimental Neurology, 80,* 395-409.

Jürgens, U., & Richter, K. (1986). Glutamate-induced vocalization in the squirrel monkey. *Brain Research, 373,* 349-358.

Jürgens, U., & von Cramon, D. (1982). On the role of the anterior cingulate cortex in phonation: A case report. *Brain and Language, 15,* 234-238.

Kahane, J. C. (1981). Age related histological changes in the human male and female laryngeal cartilages: Biological and functional implications. In Lawrence, V., & Weinberg, B. (Eds.), *Transcripts of the ninth symposium: care of the professional voice: I. Physical factors, vocal function and control.* New York: Voice Foundation (pp. 11-20).

Kahane, J. C. (1983a). Postnatal development and aging of the human larynx. *Seminars in Speech and Language, 4,* 189-203.

Kahane, J. C. (1983b). Survey of age related changes in the connective tissues of the adult human larynx. In Bless, D. M., & Abbs, J. H. (Eds.), *Vocal fold physiology: Contemporary research and clinical issues.* San Diego, CA: College-Hill Press (pp. 44-49).

Kahane, J. C., & Hammons, J.-A. (1987). Developmental changes in the articular cartilage of the human cricoarytenoid joint. In Baer, T., Sasaki, C., & Harris, K. S. (Eds.), *Laryngeal function in phonation and respiration.* Boston: College-Hill Press (pp. 14-28).

Kahane, J. C., & Kahn, A. (1986). India ink pinprick experiments on surface organization of cricoarytenoid joints. *Journal of Speech and Hearing Research, 29,* 544-548.

Kahn, A., & Kahane, J. C. (1986). India ink pinprick assessment of age related changes in the cricoarytenoid joint articular surfaces. *Journal of Speech and Hearing Research, 29,* 536-543.

Kakita, Y. (1988). Simultaneous observation of the vibratory pattern, sound pressure, and airflow signals using a physical model of the vocal folds. In Fujimura, O. (Ed.), *Vocal physiology: Voice production, mechanisms and functions.* New York: Raven Press (pp. 207-218).

Kakita, Y., Hirano, M., & Ohmaru, K. (1981). Physical properties of the vocal fold tissue: Measurement on excised larynges. In Stevens, K. N., & Hirano, M. (Eds.), *Vocal fold physiology.* Tokyo: University of Tokyo Press (pp. 377-396).

Keen, J. A., & Wainwright, J. (1958). Ossification of

the thyroid, cricoid and arytenoid cartilages. *South African Journal of Laboratory and Clinical Medicine, 4,* 83-108.

Kelman, A. W. (1981). Vibratory pattern of the vocal folds. *Folia Phoniatrica, 33,* 73-99.

Kelso, J. A. S., & Tuller, B. (1984). Converging evidence in support of common dynamical principles for speech and movement coordination. *American Journal of Physiology, 246,* R928-R935.

Kempster, G., Preston, J., Mack, R., & Larson, C. (1987). A preliminary investigation relating laryngeal muscle activity to changes in EGG waveforms. In Baer, T., Sasaki, C., & Harris, K. S. (Eds.), *Laryngeal function in phonation and respiration.* Boston: College-Hill Press (pp. 339-348).

Kirchner, J. A., & Suzuki, M. (1968). Laryngeal reflexes and voice production. *Annals of the New York Academy of Sciences, 155,* 98-109.

Kirchner, J. A., & Wyke, B. D. (1964). The innervation of laryngeal joints in the cat. *Journal of Anatomy, 98,* 684 (Abstract).

Kirchner, J. A., & Wyke, B. D. (1965). Articular reflex mechanisms in the larynx. *Annals of Otology, Rhinology and Laryngology, 74,* 749-768.

Kitajima, K., & Fujita, F. (1990). Estimation of subglottal pressure with intraoral pressure. *Acta Oto-laryngologica, 109,* 473-478.

Kitzing, P. (1977). Methode zur kombinierten photo- und elekroglottographischen Registrierung von Stimmlippen-schwingungen. *Folia Phoniatrica, 29,* 249-260.

Kitzing, P. (1982). Photo- and electroglottographical recording of the laryngeal vibratory pattern during different registers. *Folia Phoniatrica, 34,* 234-241.

Kitzing, P. (1986). Glottography, the electrophysical investigation of phonatory biomechanics. *Acta Otorhinolaryngologica Belgica, 40,* 863-878.

Kitzing, P. (1990). Clinical applications of electroglottography. *Journal of Voice, 4,* 238-249.

Kitzing, P., & Löfqvist, A. (1979). Evaluation of voice therapy by means of photoglottography. *Folia Phoniatrica, 31,* 103-109.

Kitzing, P., and Sonesson, B. (1974). A photoglottographical study of the female vocal folds during phonation. *Folia Phoniatrica, 31,* 138-149.

Kleiger, R. E., Miller, J. P., Bigger, J. T., Jr., & Moss, A. J. (1987). Decreased heart rate variability and its association with increased mortality after acute myocardial infarction. *American Journal of Cardiology, 59,* 256-262.

Kohler, K. J. (1982). F_o in the production of lenis and fortis plosives. *Phonetica, 39,* 199-218.

Kohler, K. J. (1985). F_o in the perception of lenis and fortis plosives. *Journal of the Acoustical Society of America, 78,* 21-32.

Koike, Y. (1967). Experimental studies on vocal attack. *Practica Otologica Kyoto, 60,* 663-688.

Koike, Y. (1981). Sub- and supraglottal pressure variation during phonation. In Stevens, K. N., &

Hirano, M. (Eds.), *Vocal fold physiology.* Tokyo: University of Tokyo Press (pp. 181-191).

Koike, Y., & Hirano, M. (1973). Glottal area time function and subglottal pressure variation. *Journal of the Acoustical Society of America, 54,* 1618-1627.

Koike, Y., Hirano, M., & Morio, M. (1976). Function of the laryngeal muscles on the position and shape of the vocal cord. In Loebell, E. (Ed.), *Proceedings of the Sixteenth International Congress of Logopedics and Phoniatrics.* Basel: Karger (pp. 257-263).

Koike, Y., Hirano, M., & von Leden, H. (1967). Vocal initiation: Acoustic and aerodynamic investigations of normal subjects. *Folia Phoniatrica, 19,* 173-182.

Koike, Y., Imaizumi, S., Kitano, Y., Kawasaki, H., & Hirano, M. (1983). Glottal area time function and supraglottal pressure variation. In Bless, D. M., & Abbs, J. H. (Eds.), *Vocal fold physiology: Contemporary research and clinical issues.* San Diego, CA: College-Hill Press (pp. 300-306).

Koike, Y., Takahashi, H., & Calcaterra, T. C. (1977). Acoustic measures for detecting laryngeal pathology. *Acta Otolaryngologica, 84,* 105-117.

Komiyama, S., Watanabe, H., & Ryu, S. (1984). Phonographic relationship between pitch and intensity of the human voice. *Folia Phoniatrica, 36,* 1-7.

König, W. F., & von Leden, H. (1961a). The peripheral nervous system of the human larynx: 1. The mucous membrane. *Archives of Otolaryngology, 73,* 1-14.

König, W. F., & von Leden, H. (1961b). The peripheral nervous system of the human larynx: 2. The thyroarytenoid (vocalis) muscle. *Archives of Otolaryngology, 74,* 153-163.

Kosch, P. C., Hutchison, A. A., Wozniak, J. A., & Stark, A. R. (1985). Expiratory airflow control mechanisms in term infants. *Federation Proceedings, 44,* 1002 (Abstract).

Köster, J.-P., & Smith, S. (1970). Zur Interpretation elektrischer und photoelektrischer Glottogramme. *Folia Phoniatrica, 22,* 92-99.

Koyama, T., Harvey, J. E., & Ogura, J. H. (1972). Mechanics of voice production: 3. Efficiency of voice production. *Laryngoscope, 82,* 210-217.

Koyama, T., Kawasaki, M., & Ogura, J. (1969). Mechanics of voice production: 1. Regulation of vocal intensity. *Laryngoscope, 79,* 337-354.

Kryger, M. H., & Millar, T. (1991). Cheyne-Stokes respiration: Stability of interacting systems in heart failure. *Chaos, 1,* 265-269.

Kunze, L. E. (1964). Evaluation of methods of estimating subglottal air pressure. *Journal of Speech and Hearing Research, 7,* 151-164.

Kutik, E. J., Cooper, W. E., & Boyce, S. (1983). Declination of fundamental frequency in speakers' production of parenthetical and main clauses. *Journal of the Acoustical Society of America, 73,* 1723-1730.

Ladefoged, P. (1983). The linguistic use of different phonation types. In Bless, D. M., & Abbs, J. H. (Eds.), *Vocal fold physiology: Contemporary research and clinical issues.* San Diego, CA: College-Hill Press (pp. 351-360).

Ladefoged, P., & McKinney, N. P. (1963). Loudness, sound pressure, and subglottal pressure in speech. *Journal of the Acoustical Society of America, 35,* 454-460.

Lam, R. L., & Ogura, J. H. (1952). An afferent representation of the larynx in the cerebellum. *Laryngoscope, 62,* 486-495.

Large, J., Iwata, S., & von Leden, H. (1970). The primary female register transition in singing: An aerodynamic study. *Folia Phoniatrica, 22,* 385-396.

Larson, C. R. (1985). The midbrain periaquaductal gray: A brainstem structure involved in vocalization. *Journal of Speech and Hearing Research, 28,* 241-249.

Larson, C. R., DeRosier, E., & West, R. (1991). Comparison of physiological properties of PAG and medullary neurons involved in vocalization. In Gauffin, J., & Hammarberg, B. (Eds.), *Vocal fold physiology: Acoustic, perceptual, and physiological aspects of voice mechanisms.* San Diego, CA: Singular Publishing Group (pp. 167-173).

Larson, C. R., & Kempster, G. B. (1985). Voice fundamental frequency changes following discharge of laryngeal motor units. In Titze, I. R., & Scherer, R. C. (Eds.), *Vocal fold physiology: Biomechanics, acoustics, and phonatory control.* Denver, CO: Denver Center for the Performing Arts (pp. 91-104).

Larson, C. R., Kempster, G. B., & Kistler, M. K. (1987). Changes in voice fundamental frequency following discharge of single motor units in cricothyroid and thyroarytenoid muscles. *Journal of Speech and Hearing Research, 30,* 552-558.

Larson, C. R., & Kistler, M. K. (1986). The relationship of the periaquaductal gray neurons in vocalization and laryngeal EMG in the behaving monkey. *Experimental Brain Research, 63,* 595-606.

Larson, C. R., Wilson, K. E., and Luschei, E. S. (1983). Preliminary observations on cortical and brainstem mechanisms of laryngeal control. In Bless, D. M., and Abbs, J. H. (Eds.), *Vocal fold physiology: contemporary research and clinical issues.* San Diego, CA: College-Hill Press (pp. 82-95).

Larson, C. R., Yoshida, Y., & Sessle, B. J. (1993). Higher level motor and sensory organization. In Titze, I. R. (Ed.), *Vocal fold physiology: Frontiers in basic science.* San Diego, CA: Singular Publishing Group (pp. 227-275).

Lauterborn, W., & Parlitz, U. (1988). Methods of chaos physics and their application to acoustics. *Journal of the Acoustical Society of America, 84,* 1975-1993.

Lauth, E. A. (1835). Remarques sur las structure du larynx et de la trachée-artère. *Mémoires de L'Académie Royale de Médecine, 4,* 95-116.

Laver, J., Hiller, S., & Beck, J. M. (1992). Acoustic waveform perturbations and voice disorders. *Journal of Voice, 6,* 115-126.

Lawn, A. M. (1966). The localization, in the nucleus ambiguus of the rabbit, of the cells of origin of motor fibers in the glossopharyngeal nerve and various branches of the vagus nerve by means of retrograde degeneration. *Journal of Comparative Neurology, 127,* 293-305.

Lehiste, I., & Peterson, G. E. (1959). Vowel amplitude and phonemic stress in American English. *Journal of the Acoustical Society of America, 31,* 428-435.

Lehiste, I., & Peterson, G. E. (1961). Some basic considerations in the analysis of intonation. *Journal of the Acoustical Society of America, 33,* 419-425.

Lieberman, P. (1960). Some acoustic correlates of word stress in American English. *Journal of the Acoustical Society of America, 32,* 451-454.

Lieberman, P. (1963). Some acoustic measures of the fundamental periodicity of normal and pathologic larynges. *Journal of the Acoustical Society of America, 35,* 344-353.

Lieberman, P., Knudson, R., & Mead, J. (1969). Determination of the rate of change of fundamental frequency with respect to subglottal air pressure during sustained phonation. *Journal of the Acoustical Society of America, 45,* 1537-1543.

Lieberman, P., & Michaels, S. B. (1962). Some aspects of fundamental frequency envelope amplitude as related to the emotional content of speech. *Journal of the Acoustical Society of America, 34,* 922-927.

Liljencrants, J. (1991). Numerical simulations of glottal flow. In Gauffin, J., & Hammarberg, B. (Eds.), *Vocal fold physiology: Acoustic, perceptual, and physiological aspects of voice mechanisms.* San Diego, CA: Singular Publishing Group (pp. 99-104).

Lindestad, P.-Å., Fritzell, B., & Persson, A. (1990). Evaluation of laryngeal muscle function by quantitative analysis of the EMG interference pattern. *Acta Oto-Laryngologica, 109,* 467-472.

Linville, S. E. (1992). Glottal gap configurations in two age groups of women. *Journal of Speech and Hearing Research, 35,* 1209-1215.

Linville, S. E., & Fisher, H. B. (1985). Acoustic characteristics of women's voices with advancing age. *Journal of Gerontology, 40,* 324-330.

Lisker, L., & Abramson, H. (1964). A cross-language study of voicing in initial stops: Acoustical measurements. *Word, 20,* 384-442.

Lisker, L., & Abramson, A. S. (1971). Distinctive features and laryngeal control. *Language, 47,* 767-785.

Löfqvist, A., Baer, T., McGarr, N. S., & Story, R. S. (1989). The cricothyroid muscle in voicing control. *Journal of the Acoustical Society of America, 85,* 1314-1321.

Löfqvist, A., Carlborg, B., & Kitzing, P. (1982). Initial validation of an indirect measure of subglottal pressure during vowels. *Journal of the Acoustical Society of America, 72*, 63-65.

Löfqvist, A., & McGarr, N. S. (1987). Laryngeal dynamics in voiceless consonant production. In Baer, T., Sasaki, C., & Harris, K. S. (Eds.), *Laryngeal function in phonation and respiration.* Boston: College-Hill Press (pp. 391-402).

Löfqvist, A., & McGowan, R. S. (1991). Voice source variations in running speech. In Gauffin, J., & Hammarberg, B. (Eds), *Vocal fold physiology: Acoustic, perceptual, and physiological aspects of voice mechanisms.* San Diego, CA: Singular Publishing Group (pp. 113-120).

Löfqvist, A., & Yoshioka, H. (1984). Intrasegmental timing: Laryngeal-oral coordination in voiceless consonant production. *Speech Communication, 3*, 279-289.

Lucas-Keene, M. F. (1961). Muscle spindles in the human laryngeal muscles. *Journal of Anatomy, 95*, 25-29.

Lucero, J. C. (1993). Dynamics of the two-mass model of the vocal folds: Equilibria, bifurcations, and oscillation region. *Journal of the Acoustical Society of America, 94*, 3104-3111.

Luchsinger, R., & Arnold, G. (1965). *Voice-speech-language.* Belmont, CA: Wadsworth.

Mackey, M. C., & Glass, L. (1977). Oscillation and chaos in physiological control systems. *Science, 197*, 287-289.

Mackey, M. C., & Milton, J. G. (1987). Dynamical diseases. *Annals of the New York Academy of Sciences, 504*, 16-32.

Malmgren, L. T., & Gacek, R. R. (1981). Histochemical characteristics of muscle fiber types in the posterior cricoarytenoid muscle. *Annals of Otology, Rhinology and Laryngology, 90*, 423-429.

Mandelbrot, B. (1967). How long is the coast of Britain? Statistical self-similarity and fractional dimension. *Science, 156*, 636-638.

Mandelbrot, B. (1982). *The fractal geometry of nature.* San Francisco: W. H. Freeman.

Mandell, A. J., & Shlesinger, M. F. (1990). Lost choices: Parallelism and topological entropy decrements in neurobiological aging. In Krasner, S. (Ed.), *The ubiquity of chaos.* Washington, DC: American Association for the Advancement of Science (pp. 36-47).

Mårtensson, A. (1968). The functional organization of the intrinsic laryngeal muscles. *Annals of the New York Academy of Sciences, 155*, 91-97.

Mårtensson, A., & Skoglund, C. R. (1964). Contraction properties of intrinsic laryngeal muscles. *Acta Physiologica Scandinavica, 60*, 318-336.

Matsushita, H. (1975). The vibratory mode of the vocal folds in the excised larynx. *Folia Phoniatrica, 27*, 7-18.

Matzelt, D., & Vosteen, K. H. (1963). Electroenop-

tische und enzymatische Untersuchungen an menchlicher Kehlkopfmuskulatur. *Archiv für Ohren-, Nasen- und Kehlkopfheilkunde, 181*, 447-457.

Maue, W. (1970). *Cartilages, ligaments, and articulations of the adult human larynx.* Unpublished doctoral dissertation, University of Pittsburgh.

Mayer-Kress, G., & Layne, S. P. (1987). Dimensionality of the human electroencephalogram. *Annals of the New York Academy of Sciences, 504*, 62-87.

Mayet, V. A., & Mundrich, K. (1958). Beitrag sur Anatomie und zur Funktion des M. Cricothyreoideus und der Cricothyreoidgelenke. *Acta Anatomica, 33*, 273-288.

McCaffrey, T. V., & Kern, E. B. (1980). Laryngeal regulation of airway resistance: 1. Chemoreceptor reflexes. *Annals of Otology, Rhinology, and Laryngology, 89*, 209-214.

McGlone, R. E. (1967). Air flow during vocal fry. *Journal of Speech and Hearing Research, 10*, 299-304.

McGlone, R. E. (1970). Air flow in the upper register. *Folia Phoniatrica, 22*, 231-238.

McGlone, R. E., & Brown, W. S., Jr. (1969). Identification of the shift between vocal registers. *Journal of the Acoustical Society of America, 46*, 1033-1036.

McGlone, R., & Hollien, H. (1963). Vocal pitch characteristics of aged women. *Journal of Speech and Hearing Research, 6*, 165-170.

McGlone, R. E., & Shipp, T. (1971). Some physiologic correlates of vocal fry phonation. *Journal of Speech and Hearing Research, 14*, 769-775.

McGowan, R. S. (1988). An aeroacoustic approach to phonation. *Journal of the Acoustical Society of America, 83*, 696-704.

McGowan, R. S. (1990). An analogy between the mucosal waves of the vocal folds and wind waves on water. *Haskins Laboratories Status Report on Speech Research* (New Haven, CT), SR-101/102 (pp. 243-249).

Mead, J., Bouhuys, A., & Proctor, D. F. (1968). Mechanisms generating subglottic pressure. *Annals of the New York Academy of Sciences, 155*, 177-181.

Mende, W., Herzel, H., & Wermke, K. (1990). Bifurcations and chaos in newborn infant cries. *Physics Letters A, 145*, 418-424.

Michel, J. F. (1968). Fundamental frequency investigation of vocal fry and harshness. *Journal of Speech and Hearing Research, 11*, 590-594.

Michel, J. F., & Hollien, H. (1968). Perceptual differentiation in vocal fry and harshness. *Journal of Speech and Hearing Research, 11*, 439-443.

Miller, R. L. (1959). Nature of the vocal cord wave. *Journal of the Acoustical Society of America, 31*, 667-677.

Moon, F. C. (1987). *Chaotic vibrations: An introduction for applied scientists and engineers.* New York: John Wiley.

Moore, P. (1937). Vocal fold movement during vocalization. *Speech Monographs, 4,* 44-55.

Moore, P. (1938). Motion picture studies of the vocal folds and vocal attack. *Journal of Speech and Hearing Disorders, 3,* 235-238.

Moore, P., & Thompson, C. L. (1965). Comments on physiology of hoarseness. *Archives of Otolaryngology, 81,* 97-102.

Moore, P., & von Leden, H. (1958). Dynamic variations of the vibratory pattern in the normal larynx. *Folia Phoniatrica, 10,* 205-238.

Motta, G., Cesari, U., Iengo, M., & Motta, G., Jr. (1990). Clinical application of electroglottography. *Folia Phoniatrica, 42,* 111-117.

Mu, L., & Yang, S. (1990). The respiratory function of the cricothyroid muscle: An electromyographic investigation in dogs. *Journal of Voice, 4,* 250-255.

Müller, J. (1839). *Ueber die Compensation der physischen Kräfte am menschlichen Stimmorgan.* Berlin: A. Hirschwald.

Munhall, K., & Ostry, D. (1985). Ultrasonic measurement of laryngeal kinematics. In Titze, I. R., & Scherer, R. C. (Eds.), *Vocal fold physiology: Biomechanics, acoustics and phonatory control.* Denver, CO: Denver Center for the Performing Arts (pp. 145-161).

Murakami, Y., & Kirchner, J. A. (1972). Mechanical and physiological properties of reflex laryngeal closure. *Annals of Otology, Rhinology, and Laryngology, 81,* 59-71.

Murry, T. (1971). Subglottal pressure airflow measures during vocal fry phonation. *Journal of Speech and Hearing Research, 14,* 544-551.

Murry, T., & Brown, W. S., Jr. (1971a). Regulation of vocal intensity in vocal fry phonation. *Journal of the Acoustical Society of America, 49,* 1905-1907.

Murry, T., & Brown, W. S., Jr. (1971b). Subglottal air pressure during two types of vocal activity: Vocal fry and modal phonation. *Folia Phoniatrica, 23,* 440-449.

Mysak, E. D. (1959). Pitch and duration characteristics of older males. *Journal of Speech and Hearing Research, 2,* 46-54.

Nakamura, F. (1964). Movement of the larynx induced by electrical stimulation of the laryngeal nerves. In Brewer, D. W. (Ed.), *Research potentials in voice physiology.* New York: State University of New York Press (pp. 129-135).

Negus, V. E. (1929). *The mechanism of the larynx.* St. Louis: Mosby.

Negus, V. E. (1949). *The comparative anatomy and physiology of the larynx.* London: W. Heinemann Medical Books.

Netsell, R. (1970). Underlying physiological mechanisms of syllable stress. *Journal of the Acoustical Society of America, 47,* 103 (Abstract).

Netsell, R. (1973). Speech physiology. In Minifie, F. D., Hixon, T. J., & Williams, F. (Eds.), *Normal aspects of speech, hearing, and language.* Englewood Cliffs, NJ: Prentice-Hall (pp. 211-234).

Nishizawa, N., Sawashima, M., & Yonemoto, K. (1988). Vocal fold length in vocal pitch change. In Fujimura, O. (Ed.), *Vocal physiology: Voice production, mechanisms and functions.* New York: Raven Press (pp. 75-82).

Okamura, H., & Katto, Y. (1988). Fine structure of muscle spindle in interarytenoid muscle of the human larynx. In Fujimura, O. (Ed.), *Vocal physiology: Voice production, mechanisms and functions.* New York: Raven Press (pp. 135-143).

Olsen, L. F., & Degn, H. (1985). Chaos in biological systems. *Quarterly Review of Biophysics, 18,* 165-225.

Olsen, L. F., & Schaffer, W. M. (1990). Chaos versus noisy periodicity: Alternative hypotheses for childhood epidemics. *Science, 249,* 499-504.

Ono, H., Saito, S., Fukuda, H., & Tamura, H. (1976). Observation of the vocal cord vibration by glottal waves using on-line-computer system and clinical application. In Loebell, E. (Ed.), *Proceedings of the Sixteenth International Congress of Logopedics and Phoniatrics.* Basel: Karger (pp. 357-365).

Orlikoff, R. F. (1989). Vocal jitter at different fundamental frequencies: A cardiovascular-neuromuscular explanation. *Journal of Voice, 3,* 104-112.

Orlikoff, R. F. (1990a). The relationship of age and cardiovascular health to certain acoustic characteristics of male voices. *Journal of Speech and Hearing Research, 33,* 450-457.

Orlikoff, R. F. (1990b). Vowel amplitude variation associated with the heart cycle. *Journal of the Acoustical Society of America, 88,* 2091-2098.

Orlikoff, R. F. (1991). Assessment of the dynamics of vocal-fold contact from the electroglottogram: Data from normal male subjects. *Journal of Speech and Hearing Research, 34,* 1066-1072.

Orlikoff, R. F., & Baken, R. J. (1989a). The effect of the heartbeat on vocal fundamental frequency perturbation. *Journal of Speech and Hearing Research, 32,* 576-582.

Orlikoff, R. F., & Baken, R. J. (1989b). Fundamental frequency modulation of the human voice by the heartbeat: Preliminary results and possible mechanisms. *Journal of the Acoustical Society of America, 85,* 888-893.

Orlikoff, R. F., & Baken, R. J. (1990). Consideration of the relationship between the fundamental frequency of phonation and vocal jitter. *Folia Phoniatrica, 42,* 31-40.

Orlikoff, R. F., & Kahane, J. C. (1991). Influence of mean sound pressure level on jitter and shimmer measures. *Journal of Voice, 5,* 113-119.

Ortega, J. D., DeRosier, E., Park, S., & Larson, C. R. (1988). Brainstem mechanisms of laryngeal control as revealed by microstimulation studies. In

Fujimura, O. (Ed.), *Vocal physiology: Voice production, mechanisms and functions.* New York: Raven Press (pp. 19-28).

O'Shaughnessy, D. (1979). Linguistic features in fundamental frequency patterns. *Journal of Phonetics, 7,* 119-145.

Pabon, J. P. H., and Plomp, R. (1988). Automatic phonetogram recording supplemented with acoustical voice-quality parameters. *Journal of Speech and Hearing Research, 31,* 710-722.

Pagels, H. R. (1988). *The dreams of reason: The computer and the rise of the sciences of complexity.* New York: Bantam.

Painter, C. (1988). Electroglottogram waveform types. *Archives of Oto-Rhino-Laryngology, 245,* 116-121.

Penfield, W., & Roberts, L. (1959). *Speech and brain mechanisms.* Princeton, NJ: Princeton University Press.

Perkins, W. H., & Koike, Y. (1969). Patterns of subglottal pressure variations during phonation. *Folia Phoniatrica, 21,* 1-8.

Pinto, N. B., & Titze, I. R. (1990). Unification of perturbation measures in speech signals. *Journal of the Acoustical Society of America, 87,* 1278-1289.

Ploog, D. (1981). Neurobiology of primate audio-vocal behavior. *Brain Research, 228,* 35-61.

Pool, R. (1989). Is it healthy to be chaotic? *Science, 243,* 604-607.

Price, P. J. (1989). Male and female voice source characteristics: Inverse filtering results. *Speech Communication, 8,* 261-277.

Prigogine, I., & Stengers, I. (1984). *Order out of chaos: Man's new dialogue with nature.* New York: Bantam.

Ramig, L. A., & Ringel, R. L. (1983). Effects of physiological aging on selected acoustic characteristics of voice. *Journal of Speech and Hearing Research, 26,* 22-30.

Rapp, P. E., Bashore, T. R., Martinerie, J. M., Albano, A. M., Zimmerman, I. D., & Mees, A. I. (1989). Dynamics of electrical activity. *Brain Topography, 2,* 99-118.

Richter, K., & Jürgens, U. (1986). A comparative study on the excitability of vocalization by electrical stimulation, glutamate, aspartate and quisqualate in the squirrel monkey. *Neuroscience Letters, 66,* 239-244.

Robb, M. P., & Simmons, J. O. (1990). Gender comparisons of children's vocal fold contact behavior. *Journal of the Acoustical Society of America, 88,* 1318-1322.

Roncollo, P. (1949). Researches about ossification and conformation of the thyroid cartilage in man. *Acta Oto-laryngologica, 103,* 169-171.

Rosenberg, A. E. (1971). Effect of glottal pulse shape on the quality of natural vowels. *Journal of the Acoustical Society of America, 49,* 583-590.

Rosenfield, D. B., Miller, R. H., Sessions, R. B., & Patten, B. M. (1982). Morphologic and histochemical characteristics of laryngeal muscle. *Archives of Otolaryngology, 108,* 662-666.

Rossi, G., & Cortesina, G. (1965). Morphological study of the laryngeal muscles in man. *Acta Oto-laryngologica,* 575-592.

Rothenberg, M. (1972). The glottal volume velocity waveform during loose and tight voiced glottal adjustments. In Rigault, A., & Charbonneau, R. (Eds.), *Proceedings of the Seventh International Congress of Phonetic Sciences.* The Hague: Mouton (pp. 380-388).

Rothenberg, M. (1973). A new inverse-filtering technique for deriving the glottal airflow waveform during voicing. *Journal of the Acoustical Society of America, 53,* 1632-1645.

Rothenberg, M. (1981). Some relations between glottal air flow and vocal fold contact area. *ASHA Reports, 11,* 88-96.

Rothenberg, M. (1982). Interpolating subglottal pressure from oral pressure. *Journal of Speech and Hearing Disorders, 47,* 219-223.

Rothenberg, M. (1983). An interactive model for the voice source. In Bless, D. M., & Abbs, J. H. (Eds.), *Vocal fold physiology: contemporary research and clinical issues.* San Diego, CA: College-Hill Press (pp. 155-165).

Rothenberg, M., & Mahshie, J. (1986). Induced transglottal pressure variations during voicing. *Journal of Phonetics, 14,* 365-371.

Rothenberg, M., & Mahshie, J. J. (1988). Monitoring vocal fold abduction through vocal fold contact area. *Journal of Speech and Hearing Research, 31,* 338-351.

Rozsypal, A. J., & Millar, B. F. (1979). Perception of jitter and shimmer in synthetic vowels. *Journal of Phonetics, 7,* 343-355.

Rubin, H., & Hirt, C. C. (1960). The falsetto, a high speed cinematographic study. *Laryngoscope, 70,* 1305-1324.

Rudolf, G. (1961). Spiral nerve endings (proprioceptors) in the human vocal muscle. *Nature, 190,* 726-727.

Rudomin, P. (1965). The influence of the motor cortex upon the vagal motorneurons of the cat. *Acta Physiologica Latino-America, 15,* 171-179.

Ruelle, D. (1989). *Chaotic evolution and strange attractors.* New York: Cambridge University Press.

Saito, S., Fukuda, H., Isogai, Y., & Ono, H. (1981). X-ray stroboscopy. In Stevens, K. N., & Hirano, M. (Eds.), *Vocal fold physiology.* Tokyo: University of Tokyo Press (pp. 95-106).

Sampson, S., & Eyzaguirre, C. (1964). Some functional characteristics of mechanoreceptors in the larynx of the cat. *Journal of Neurophysiology, 27,* 464-480.

Sapir, S. (1989). The intrinsic pitch of vowels:

Theoretical, physiological, and clinical considerations. *Journal of Voice, 3,* 44-51.

Sawashima, M., Abramson, A. S., Cooper, F. S., & Lisker, L. (1970). Observing laryngeal adjustments during running speech by use of a fiberoptics system. *Phonetica, 22,* 193-201.

Sawashima, M., Gay, T., & Harris, K. S. (1969). Laryngeal muscle activity during vocal pitch and intensity changes. *Haskins Laboratories Status Report on Speech Research* (New Haven, CT), SR-19/20 (pp. 211-220).

Sawashima, M., & Hirose, H. (1983). Laryngeal gestures in speech production. In MacNeilage, P. F. (Ed.), *The production of speech.* New York: Springer-Verlag (pp. 11-38).

Sawashima, M., Niimi, S., Horiguchi, S., & Yamaguchi, H. (1988). Expiratory lung pressure, airflow rate, and vocal intensity: Data on normal subjects. In Fujimura, O. (Ed.), *Vocal physiology: Voice production, mechanisms and functions.* New York: Raven Press (pp. 415-422).

Scherer, R. C., Druker, D. G., & Titze, I. R. (1988). Electroglottography and direct measurement of vocal fold contact area. In Fujimura, O. (Ed.), *Vocal physiology: Voice production, mechanisms and functions.* New York: Raven Press (pp. 279-291).

Scherer, R. C., & Titze, I. R. (1983). Pressure-flow relationships in a model of the laryngeal airway with a diverging glottis. In Bless, D. M., and Abbs, J. H. (Eds.), *Vocal fold physiology: contemporary research and clinical issues.* San Diego, CA: College-Hill Press (pp. 179-193).

Scherer, R. C., & Titze, I. R. (1987). The abduction quotient related to vocal quality. *Journal of Voice, 1,* 246-251.

Schneider, P., & Baken, R. J. (1984). Influence of lung volume on the airflow-intensity relationship. *Journal of Speech and Hearing Research, 27,* 430-435.

Schönhärl, E. (1960). *Die Stroboskopie in der praktischen Laryngologie.* Stuttgart: Thieme Verlag.

Schroeder, M. R., & David, E. E., Jr. (1960). A vocoder for transmitting 10 kc/s speech over a 3.5 kc/s channel. *Acustica, 10,* 35-43.

Schutte, H. K. (1980). Untersuchungen von Stimmqualitaten durch Phonetographie. *HNO Praxis, 5,* 132-139.

Schutte, H. K. (1986). Aerodynamics of phonation. *Acta Oto-Rhino-Laryngologica Belgica, 40,* 344-357.

Schutte, H. K., & Seidner, W. W. (1988). Registerabhängige Differenzierung von Elektroglottogrammen. *Sprache-Stimme-Gehör, 12,* 59-62.

Schutte, H. K., & van den Berg, Jw. (1976). Determination of the subglottic pressure and the efficiency of sound production in patients with disturbed voice production. In Loebell, E. (Ed.), *Proceedings of the Sixteenth International Congress of Logopedics and Phoniatrics.* Basel: Karger (pp. 415-420).

Scripture, E. W. (1904). *Elements of experimental phonetics.* New York: Scribner.

Scripture, E. W. (1906). *Researches in experimental phonetics.* Washington, DC: Carnegie Institute.

Seidner, W., Krueger, H., & Wernecke, K.-D. (1985). Numerische Auswertung spektraler Stimmfelder. *Sprache-Stimme-Gehör, 9,* 10-13.

Sellers, I. E., & Keen, E. N. (1978). The anatomy and movements of the cricoarytenoid joint. *Laryngoscope, 88,* 667-674.

Shin, T., Hirano, M., Maeyama, T., Nozoe, I., & Ohkubo, H. (1981). The function of the extrinsic laryngeal muscles. In Stevens, K. N., & Hirano, M. (Eds.), *Vocal fold physiology.* Tokyo: University of Tokyo Press (pp. 171-180).

Shipp, T. (1975). Vertical laryngeal position during continuous and discrete vocal frequency change. *Journal of Speech and Hearing Research, 18,* 707-718.

Shipp, T., & Izdebski, K. (1975). Vocal frequency and vertical laryngeal positioning by singers and nonsingers. *Journal of the Acoustical Society of America, 58,* 1104-1106.

Shipp, T., & McGlone, R. E. (1971). Laryngeal dynamics associated with vocal frequency change. *Journal of Speech and Hearing Research, 14,* 761-768.

Shipp, T., McGlone, R., & Morrissey, P. (1972). Some physiologic correlates of voice frequency change. In Rigault, A., & Charbonneau, R. (Eds.), *Proceedings of the 7th International Congress of Phonetic Sciences.* The Hague: Mouton (pp. 407-411).

Simon, C. (1927). The variability of consecutive wavelengths in vocal and instrumental sounds. *Psychological Monographs, 36,* 41-83.

Slavit, D. H., Lipton, R. J., & McCaffrey, T. V. (1990). Glottographic analysis of phonation in the excised canine larynx. *Annals of Otology, Rhinology and Laryngology, 99,* 396-402.

Smitheran, J. R., & Hixon, T. J. (1981). A clinical method for estimating laryngeal airway resistance during vowel production. *Journal of Speech and Hearing Disorders, 46,* 138-146.

Södersten, M., & Lindestad, P.-Å. (1990). Glottal closure and perceived breathiness during phonation in normally speaking subjects. *Journal of Speech and Hearing Research, 33,* 601-611.

Sonesson, B. (1959). A method for studying the vibratory movements of the vocal folds. *Journal of Laryngology and Otology, 73,* 732-737.

Sonesson, B. (1960). On the anatomy and vibratory pattern of the human vocal folds. *Acta Otolaryngologica 156* (Suppl.), 1-80.

Sonesson, B. (1968). The functional anatomy of the speech organs. In Malmberg, B. (Ed.), *Manual of phonetics.* Amsterdam: North-Holland (pp. 45-75).

Sonninen, A. (1954). Is the length of the vocal cords

the same at all different levels of singing? *Acta Oto-laryngologica, 118* (Suppl.), 219-231.

Sonninen, A. (1956). The role of the external laryngeal muscles in length-adjustment of the vocal cords in singing. *Acta Oto-laryngologica, 130* (suppl.).

Sonninen, A. (1968). The external frame function in the control of pitch in the human voice. *New York Academy of Sciences, 155,* 68-90.

Sorensen, D., & Horii, Y. (1984). Frequency characteristics of male and female speakers in the pulse register. *Journal of Communication Disorders, 17,* 65-73.

Stanescu, D. C., Pattijn, J., Clement, J., & van de Woestijne, K. P. (1972). Glottis opening and airway resistance. *Journal of Applied Physiology, 32,* 460-466.

Stevens, K. N. (1971). Airflow and turbulence noise for fricative and stop consonants: static considerations. *Journal of the Acoustical Society of America, 50,* 1180-1192.

Stevens, K. N. (1977). Physics of laryngeal behavior and larynx modes. *Phonetica, 34,* 264-279.

Stevens, K. N. (1991). Vocal-fold vibration for obstruent consonants. In Gauffin, J., & Hammarberg, B. (Eds.), *Vocal fold physiology: Acoustic, perceptual, and physiological aspects of voice mechanisms.* San Diego, CA: Singular Publishing Group (pp. 29-36).

Stevens, K. N., & Klatt, D. H. (1974). Current models of sound sources for speech. In Wyke, B. (Ed.), *Ventilatory and phonatory control systems.* New York: Oxford University Press (pp. 279-298).

Stoicheff, M. L. (1981). Speaking fundamental frequency characteristics and phonational frequency ranges of non-smoking female adults. *Journal of Speech and Hearing Research, 24,* 437-441.

Sundberg, J. (1987). *The science of the singing voice.* DeKalb: Northern Illinois University Press.

Sundberg, J. (1990, June). Loudness regulation in male singers. Paper presented at the Nineteenth Annual Symposium of the Voice Foundation: Care of the Professional Voice, Philadelphia.

Sundberg, J., & Askenfelt, A. (1983). Larynx height and voice source: A relationship? In Bless, D. M., & Abbs, J. H. (Eds.), *Vocal fold physiology: Contemporary research and clinical issues.* San Diego, CA: College-Hill Press (pp. 307-316).

Suzuki, M., & Kirchner, J. A. (1969). The posterior cricoarytenoid as an inspiratory muscle. *Annals of Otology, Rhinology, and Laryngology, 78,* 849-864.

Takahashi, H., & Koike, Y. (1975). Some perceptual dimensions and acoustical correlates of pathologic voices. *Acta Oto-laryngologica, 338* (Suppl.), 1-24.

Takenouchi, S., Koyama, T., Kawasaki, M., & Ogura, J. (1968). Movements of the vocal cords. *Acta Oto-laryngologica, 65,* 33-50.

Tanabe, M., Kitajima, K., Gould, W. J., & Lambiase, A. (1975). Analysis of high-speed motion pictures of the vocal folds. *Folia Phoniatrica, 27,* 77-87.

Tanaka, S., & Gould, W. J. (1985). Vocal efficiency and aerodynamic aspects in voice disorders. *Annals of Otology, Rhinology and Laryngology, 94,* 29-33.

Tanaka, S., & Tanabe, M. (1989). Experimental study on regulation of vocal pitch. *Journal of Voice, 3,* 93-98.

Teager, H. M., & Teager, S. M. (1983). The effects of separated airflow on vocalization. In Bless, D. M., & Abbs, J. H. (Eds.), *Vocal fold physiology: Contemporary research and clinical issues.* San Diego, CA: College-Hill Press (pp. 124-143).

Teager, H. M., & Teager, S. M. (1985a). Active fluid dynamic voice production models, or, There is a unicorn in the garden. In Titze, I. R., & Scherer, R. C. (Eds.), *Vocal fold physiology: Biomechanics, acoustics and phonatory control.* Denver, CO: Denver Center for the Performing Arts (pp. 387-401).

Teager, H. M., & Teager, S. M. (1985b). A phenomenological model for vowel production in the vocal tract. In Daniloff, R. G. (Ed.), *Speech science: recent advances.* San Diego, CA: College-Hill Press (pp. 73-101).

Terken, J. (1991). Fundamental frequency and perceived prominence of accented syllables. *Journal of the Acoustical Society of America, 89,* 1768-1776.

Thoms, G., & Jürgens, U. (1987). Common input of the cranial motor nuclei involved in phonation of the squirrel monkey. *Experimental Neurology, 95,* 85-99.

Tieg, E., Dahl, H. A., & Thorkelsen, H. (1978). Actomyosin ATPase activity in human laryngeal muscles. *Acta Oto-laryngologica, 85,* 272-281.

Timcke, R., von Leden, H., & Moore, P. (1958). Laryngeal vibrations: Measurements of the glottic wave: I. The normal vibratory cycle. *Archives of Otolaryngology, 68,* 1-19.

Timcke, R., von Leden, H., & Moore, P. (1959). Laryngeal vibrations: Measurements of the glottic wave: II. Physiologic variations. *Archives of Otolaryngology, 69,* 438-444.

Titze, I. R. (1973). The human vocal cords: A mathematical model: I. *Phonetica, 28,* 129-170.

Titze, I. R. (1974). The human vocal cords: a mathematical model: II. *Phonetica, 29,* 1-21.

Titze, I. R. (1976). On the mechanics of vocal-fold vibration. *Journal of the Acoustical Society of America, 60,* 1366-1380.

Titze, I. R. (1980). Comments on the myoelastic-aerodynamic theory of phonation. *Journal of Speech and Hearing Research, 23,* 495-510.

Titze, I. R. (1981). Biomechanics and distributed-mass models of vocal fold vibration. In Stevens, K. N., & Hirano, M. (Eds.), *Vocal fold physiology.* Tokyo: University of Tokyo Press (pp. 245-270).

Titze, I. R. (1985). Mechanisms of sustained oscillation of the vocal folds. In Titze, I. R., & Scherer, R. C. (Eds.), *Vocal fold physiology: Biomechanics, acoustics and phonatory control*. Denver, CO: Denver Center for the Performing Arts (pp. 349-357).

Titze, I. R. (1986). Mean intraglottal pressure in vocal fold oscillation. *Journal of Phonetics, 14*, 359-364.

Titze, I. R. (1988a). The physics of small-amplitude oscillation of the vocal folds. *Journal of the Acoustical Society of America, 83*, 1536-1552.

Titze, I. R. (1988b). Regulation of vocal power and efficiency by subglottal pressure and glottal width. In Fujimura, O. (Ed.), *Vocal physiology: Voice production, mechanisms and functions*. New York: Raven Press (pp. 227-238).

Titze, I. R. (1988c). A framework for the study of vocal registers. *Journal of Voice, 2*, 183-194.

Titze, I. R. (1989a). A four parameter model of the glottis and vocal fold contact area. *Speech Communication, 8*, 191-201.

Titze, I. R. (1989b). On the relation between subglottal pressure and fundamental frequency in phonation. *Journal of the Acoustical Society of America, 85*, 901-906.

Titze, I. R. (1990a, June). Nonlinearities in airflow and tissue mechanics leading to chaotic vocal fold vibration. Paper presented at the Nineteenth Annual Symposium of the Voice Foundation: Care of the Professional Voice, Philadelphia.

Titze, I. R. (1990b). Interpretation of the electroglottographic signal. *Journal of Voice, 4*, 1-9.

Titze, I. R. (1992). Acoustic interpretation of the voice range profile. *Journal of Speech and Hearing Research, 35*, 21-34.

Titze, I. R., Baken, R. J., & Herzel, H. (1993). Evidence of chaos in vocal fold vibration. In Titze, I. R. (Ed.), *Vocal fold physiology: Frontiers in basic science*. San Diego, CA: Singular Publishing Group (pp. 143-188).

Titze, I. R., & Durham, P. L. (1987). Passive mechanisms influencing fundamental frequency control. In Baer, T., Sasaki, C., & Harris, K. S. (Eds.), *Laryngeal function in phonation and respiration*. Boston: College-Hill Press (pp. 304-319).

Titze, I. R., Jiang, J., & Drucker, D. G. (1987). Preliminaries to the body-cover theory of pitch control. *Journal of Voice, 1*, 314-319.

Titze, I. R., Luschei, E. S., & Hirano, M. (1989). Role of the thyroarytenoid muscle in regulation of fundamental frequency. *Journal of Voice, 3*, 213-224.

Titze, I. R., & Talkin, D. (1979). A theoretical study of the effect of various laryngeal configurations on the acoustics of phonation. *Journal of the Acoustical Society of America, 66*, 60-86.

Titze, I. R., & Talkin, D. (1981). Simulation and interpretation of glottographic waveforms. *ASHA Reports, 11*, 48-54.

Tonndorf, W. (1925). Die Mechanik bei der Stimmlippenschwingungen und beim Schnarchen.

Zeitschrift für Hals-Nasen-Ohrenheilkunde, 12, 241-245.

Ursino, F., Pardini, L., Panattoni, G., Matteucci, F., & Grosjacques, M. (1991). A study of EGG and simultaneous subglottal pressure signals. *Folia Phoniatrica, 43*, 220-225.

van den Berg, Jw. (1956). Direct and indirect determination of the mean subglottic pressure. *Folia Phoniatrica, 8*, 1-24.

van den Berg, Jw. (1957). Subglottal pressure and vibrations of the vocal folds. *Folia Phoniatrica, 9*, 65-71.

van den Berg, Jw. (1958). Myoelastic-aerodynamic theory of voice production. *Journal of Speech and Hearing Research, 1*, 227-244.

van den Berg, Jw. (1960). Vocal ligaments versus registers. *Current Problems in Phoniatrics and Logopedics, 1*, 19-34.

van den Berg, Jw. (1968a). Mechanism of the larynx and the laryngeal vibrations. In Malmberg, B. (Ed.), *Manual of phonetics*. Amsterdam: North-Holland (pp. 278-308).

van den Berg, Jw. (1968b). Register problems. *Annals of the New York Academy of Sciences, 155*, 129-134.

van den Berg, Jw., & Moll, J. (1956). Zur Anatomie des menschlichen Musculus vocalis. *Zeitschrift für Anatomie und Entwicklungsgeschichte, 118*, 465-470.

van den Berg, Jw., & Tan, T. S. (1959). Results of experiments with human larynxes. *Practica Oto-Rhino-Laryngologica, 21*, 425-450.

van den Berg, Jw., Zantema, J. T., & Doornenbal, P. (1957). On the air resistance and the Bernoulli effect of the human larynx. *Journal of the Acoustical Society of America, 29*, 626-631.

Vennard, W. (1967). *Singing: The mechanism and the technic*, 4th ed., New York: Carl Fischer.

Vilkman, E., Aaltonen, O., Raimo, I., Arajärvi, P., & Oksanen, H. (1989). Articulatory hyoid-laryngeal changes vs. cricothyroid muscle activity in the control of intrinsic F_o of vowels. *Journal of Phonetics, 17*, 193-203.

Vilkman, E., & Karma, P. (1989). Vertical hyoid bone displacement and fundamental frequency of phonation. *Acta Oto-laryngologica, 108*, 142-151.

von Leden, H., & Moore, P. (1961). The mechanics of the crico-arytenoid joint. *Archives of Otolaryngology, 73*, 541-550.

Voss, H. (1966). Untersuchungen uber Vorkommen Zahl und individuelle Variation der Mukelspindeln in den Muskeln des menschlichen Kehlkopfes. *Anatomischer Anzeiger, 118*, 305-309.

Walker, J. (1987). Why a fluid flows faster when the tube is pinched. *Scientific American, 257*, 104-107.

Warren, D. W. (1982). Aerodynamics of speech. In Lass, N. J., McReynolds, L. V., Northern, J. L., & Yoder, D. E. (Eds.), *Speech, language and hearing*. Vol I. Normal processes. Philadelphia: Saunders (pp. 219-245).

Warren, D. W. (1988). Aerodynamics of speech. In Lass, N. J., McReynolds, L. V., Northern, J. L., & Yoder, D. E. (Eds.), *Handbook of speech-language pathology and audiology*. St. Louis: Mosby (pp. 191-214).

Welch, G. F., Sargeant, D. C., & MacCurtain, F. (1988). Some physical characteristics of the male falsetto voice. *Journal of Voice, 2*, 151-163.

Wendahl, R. (1963). Laryngeal analog synthesis of harsh voice quality. *Folia Phoniatrica, 15*, 241-250.

Wendahl, R. (1966). Some parameters of auditory roughness. *Folia Phoniatrica, 18*, 26-32.

Wendahl, R. W., Moore, P., & Hollien, H. (1963). Comments on vocal fry. *Folia Phoniatrica, 15*, 251-255.

Whitehead, R. L., Metz, D. E., & Whitehead, B. H. (1984). Vibratory patterns of the vocal folds during pulse register phonation. *Journal of the Acoustical Society of America, 75*, 1293-1297.

Wilcox, K. A., & Horii, Y. (1980). Age and changes in vocal jitter. *Journal of Gerontology, 35*, 194-198.

Wilson, F. B., & Starr, C. D. (1985). Use of the phonation analyzer as a clinical tool. *Journal of Speech and Hearing Disorders, 50*, 351-356.

Wind, J. (1970). *On the phylogeny and ontogeny of the human larynx*. Groningen: Wolter-Noordhoff.

Wustrow, F. (1952). Bau and Funktion des Menschlichen Musculus vocalis. *Zeitschrift für Anatomie und Entwicklungsgeschichte, 116*, 506-522.

Wyke, B. D. (1967). Recent advances in the neurology of phonation: Phonatory reflex mechanisms in the larynx. *British Journal of Disorders of Communication, 2*, 2-14.

Wyke, B. D. (1969). Deus ex machina vocis: Analysis of the laryngeal reflex mechanisms of speech. *British Journal of Disorders of Communication, 4*, 3-35.

Wyke, B. D. (1973). Myotatic reflexogenic systems in the intrinsic muscles of the larynx. *Folia Morphologica, 21*, 113-119.

Wyke, B. D. (1974). Laryngeal myotatic reflexes and phonation. *Folia Phoniatrica, 26*, 249-264.

Wyke, B. D., & Kirchner, J. A. (1976). Neurology of the larynx. In Hinchcliffe, R., & Harrison, D. (Eds.), *Scientific foundations of otolaryngology*. London: Heinemann (pp. 546-574).

Yanagihara, N. (1967). Hoarseness: Investigation of the physiological mechanisms. *Annals of Otology, Rhinology and Laryngology, 76*, 472-489.

Yanagihara, N. (1970). Aerodynamic examination of the laryngeal function. *Studia Phonologica, 5*, 45-51.

Yanagihara, N., & Koike, Y. (1967). The regulation of sustained phonation. *Folia Phoniatrica, 19*, 1-18.

Zawadzki, P. A., and Gilbert, H. R. (1989). Vowel fundamental frequency and articulator position. *Journal of Phonetics, 17*, 159-166.

Zemlin, W. R. (1988). *Speech and hearing science: Anatomy and physiology*, 3rd ed. Englewood Cliffs, NJ: Prentice-Hall (pp. 166-167).

Zenker, W., & Zenker, A. (1960). Über die Regelung der Stimmlippenspannung durch von aussen eingreifende Mechanismen. *Folia Phoniatrica, 12*, 1-36.

Suggested Readings

Laryngeal Structure

Bach, A. C., Lederer, R. L., & Dinolt, R. (1941). Senile changes in the laryngeal musculature. *Archives of Otolaryngology, 34*, 47-56.

Hast, M. H. (1970). The developmental anatomy of the larynx. *Otolaryngology Clinics of North America, 3*, 413-438.

Hirano, M. (1974). Morphological structure of the vocal cord as a vibrator and its variations. *Folia Phoniatrica, 26*, 89-94.

Hirano, M., Kakita, Y., Ohmaru, K., & Kurita, S. (1982). Structure and mechanical properties of the vocal fold. In Lass, N. J. (Ed.), *Speech and language: Advances in basic research and practice*, Vol. 7. New York: Academic Press (pp. 271-297).

Kahane, J. C. (1978). A morphological study of the human prepubertal and pubertal larynx. *American Journal of Anatomy, 151*, 11-20.

Kahane, J. C. (1982). Growth of the human prepubertal and pubertal larynx. *Journal of Speech and Hearing Research, 25*, 446-455.

Kahane, J. C. (1983). Postnatal development and aging of the human larynx. *Seminars in Speech and Language, 4*, 189-203.

Kahane, J. C. (1987). Connective tissue changes in the larynx and their effects on voice. *Journal of Voice, 1*, 27-30.

König, W. F., and von Leden, H. (1961). The peripheral nervous system of the human larynx: 1. The mucous membrane. *Archives of Otolaryngology, 73*, 1-14.

König, W. F., & von Leden, H. (1961). The peripheral nervous system of the human larynx: 2. The thyroarytenoid (vocalis) muscle. *Archives of Otolaryngology, 74*, 153-163.

Negus, V. E. (1949). *The comparative anatomy and physiology of the larynx*. London: W. Heinemann Medical Books.

Rossi, G., & Cortesina, G. (1965). Morphological study of the laryngeal muscles in man: Insertions and courses of the muscle fibres, motor end-plates and proprioceptors. *Acta Otolaryngologica, 59*, 575-592.

Sellars, I. E., & Keen, E. N. (1978). The anatomy and movements of the cricoarytenoid joint. *Laryngoscope, 88,* 667-674.

Tucker, J. A., & O'Rahilly, R. (1972). Observations on the embryology of the human larynx. *Annals of Otology, Rhinology and Laryngology, 81,* 520-523.

Wind, J. (1970). *On the phylogeny and the ontogeny of the human larynx.* Groningen: Wolter-Noordhoff Publishing.

Laryngeal Function

Atkinson, J. E. (1978). Correlation analysis of the physiological factors controlling fundamental voice frequency. *Journal of the Acoustical Society of America, 63,* 211-222.

Baer, T., Sasaki, C. T., & Harris, K. S. (Eds.). (1987). *Laryngeal function in phonation and respiration.* Boston: Little, Brown.

Baken, R. J. (1991). An overview of laryngeal function for voice production. In Sataloff, R. T. (Ed.), *Professional voice: The science and art of clinical care.* New York: Raven Press (pp. 19-47).

Berke, G. S., & Gerratt, B. R. (1993). Laryngeal biomechanics: An overview of mucosal wave mechanics. *Journal of Voice, 7,* 123-128.

Bless, D. M., & Abbs, J. H. (Eds.). (1983). *Vocal fold physiology: Contemporary research and clinical issues.* San Diego, CA: College-Hill Press.

Broad, D. J. (1979). The new theories of vocal fold vibration. In Lass, N. J. (Ed.), *Speech and language: advances in basic research and practice,* Vol. 2. New York: Academic Press (pp. 203-256).

Collier, R. (1975). Physiological correlates of intonation patterns. *Journal of the Acoustical Society of America, 58,* 249-255.

Colton, R. H. (1988). Physiological mechanisms of vocal frequency control: The role of tension. *Journal of Voice, 2,* 208-220.

Davis, S. B. (1979). Acoustic characteristics of normal and pathological voices. In Lass, N. J. (Ed.), *Speech and language: Advances in basic research and practice,* Vol. 1. New York: Academic Press (pp. 271-335).

Faaborg-Andersen, K. (1957). Electromyographic investigation of intrinsic laryngeal muscles in humans. *Acta Physiologica Scandinavica, 41* (Suppl. 140), 1-150.

Faaborg-Andersen, K. (1965). Electromyography of laryngeal muscles in humans: Technics and results. In *Current problems in phonetics and logopedics,* Vol. 3. Basel: Karger.

Faaborg-Andersen, K., Yanagihara, N., and von Leden, H. (1967). Vocal pitch and intensity regulation: At comparative study of electrical activity in the cricothyroid muscle and the airflow rate. *Archives of Otolaryngology, 85,* 448-454.

Fink, B. R. (1975). *The human larynx: A functional study.* New York: Raven Press.

Fujimura, O. (Ed.). (1988). *Vocal physiology: Voice production, mechanisms and functions.* New York: Raven Press.

Fujimura, O., & Hirano, M. (Eds.). (1995). *Vocal fold physiology: Voice quality control.* San Diego, CA: Singular Publishing Group.

Gauffin, J., & Hammarberg, B. (Eds.). (1991). *Vocal fold physiology: Acoustic, perceptual, and physiological aspects of voice mechanisms.* San Diego, CA: Singular Publishing Group.

Gay, T., Hirose, H., Strome, M., & Sawashima, M. (1972). Electromyography of the intrinsic laryngeal muscles during phonation. *Annals of Otology, Rhinology and Laryngology, 81,* 401-409.

Hast, M. H. (1966). Phyiological mechanism of phonation: Tension of the vocal fold muscle. *Acta Oto-laryngologica, 62,* 309-318.

Hast, M. H. (1967). Mechanical properties of the vocal fold muscle. *Practica Oto-Rhino-Laryngologica, 29,* 53-56.

Heiberger, V. L., & Horii, Y. (1982). Jitter and shimmer in sustained phonation. In Lass, N. J. (Ed.), *Speech and language: Advances in basic research and practice,* Vol. 7. New York: Academic Press (pp. 299-332).

Hirano, M., & Kakita, Y. (1985). Cover-body theory of vocal fold vibration. In Daniloff, R. G. (Ed.), *Speech science: Recent advances.* San Diego, CA: College-Hill Press (pp. 1-46).

Hirano, M., Ohala, J., & Vennard, W. (1969). The function of laryngeal muscles in regulating fundamental frequency and intensity of phonation. *Journal of Speech and Hearing Research, 12,* 616-627.

Hirano, M., Vennard, W., & Ohala, J. (1970). Regulation of register, pitch and intensity of voice. *Folia Phoniatrica, 22,* 1-20.

Hirose, H., & Gay, T. (1972). The activity of the intrinsic laryngeal muscles in voicing control: An electromyographic study. *Phonetica, 25,* 140-164.

Hollien, H. (1974). On vocal registers. *Journal of Phonetics, 2,* 125-143.

Isshiki, N. (1964). Regulatory mechanism of voice intensity variation. *Journal of Speech and Hearing Research, 7,* 17-29.

Isshiki, N. (1965). Vocal intensity and air flow rate. *Folia Phoniatrica, 17,* 92-104.

Isshiki, N. (1969). Remarks on mechanism for vocal intensity variation. *Journal of Speech and Hearing Research, 12,* 665-672.

Klatt, D. H., & Klatt, L. C. (1990). Analysis, synthesis, and perception of voice quality variations among female and male talkers. *Journal of the Acoustical Society of America, 87,* 820-857.

Larson, C. R. (1988). Brain mechanisms involved in the control of vocalization. *Journal of Voice, 2,* 301-311.

Moore, G. P. (1971). The physiology of phonation. In *Organic voice disorders.* Englewood Cliffs, NJ: Prentice-Hall (pp. 53-83).

Shipp, T. (1975). Vertical laryngeal position during continuous and discrete vocal frequency change. *Journal of Speech and Hearing Research, 18,* 707-718.

Shipp, T., & McGlone, R. E. (1971). Laryngeal dynamics associated with vocal frequency change. *Journal of Speech and Hearing Research, 14,* 761-768.

Stevens, K. N. (1977). Physics of laryngeal behavior and larynx modes. *Phonetica, 34,* 264-279.

Stevens, K. N., & Hirano, M. (Eds.). (1981). *Vocal fold physiology.* Tokyo: University of Tokyo Press.

Timcke, R., von Leden, H., & Moore, P. (1958). Laryngeal vibrations: Measurements of the glottic wave: 1. The normal vibratory cycle. *Archives of Otolaryngology, 68,* 1-19.

Timcke, R., von Leden, H., & Moore, P. (1959). Laryngeal vibrations: measurements of the glottic wave: 2. Physiologic variations. *Archives of Otolaryngology, 69,* 438-444.

Titze, I. R. (1980). Comments on the myoelastic-aerodynamic theory of phonation. *Journal of Speech and Hearing Research, 23,* 495-510.

Titze, I. R. (1986). Mean intraglottal pressure in vocal fold oscillation. *Journal of Phonetics, 14,* 359-364.

Titze, I. R. (1989). On the relation between subglottal pressure and fundamental frequency in phonation. *Journal of the Acoustical Society of America, 85,* 901-906.

Titze, I. R. (Ed.). (1993). *Vocal fold physiology: Frontiers in basic science.* San Diego, CA: Singular Publishing Group.

Titze, I. R., & Scherer, R. C. (Eds.). (1985). *Vocal fold physiology: Biomechanics, acoustics and phonatory control.* Denver, CO: Denver Center for the Performing Arts.

van den Berg, Jw. (1958). Myoelastic-aerodynamic theory of voice production. *Journal of Speech and Hearing Research, 1,* 227-244.

Wyke, B. D., & Kirchner, J. A. (1976). Neurology of the larynx. In Hinchcliffe, R., & Harrison, D. (Eds.), *Scientific foundations of otolaryngology.* London: Heinemann (pp. 546-574).

General Readings

Baken, R. J. (1987). *Clinical measurement of speech and voice.* Boston: Little, Brown.

Baken, R. J., & Daniloff, R. G. (Eds.). (1991). *Readings in clinical spectrography of speech.* San Diego, CA: Singular Publishing Group and Kay Elemetrics Corporation.

Bouhuys, A. (Ed.). (1968). *Sound production in man. Annals of the New York Academy of Sciences.*

Broad, D. J. (1973). Phonation. In Minifie, F. D., Hixon, T. J., & Williams, F. (Eds.), *Normal aspects of speech, hearing, and language.* Englewood Cliffs, NJ: Prentice-Hall (pp. 127-167).

Hess, W. (1983). The human voice source. In *Pitch determination of speech signals: Algorithms and devices.* New York: Springer (pp. 38-62).

Hirano, M. (1981). *Clinical examination of voice.* New York: Springer-Verlag.

Ludlow, C. L., & Hart, M. O. (Eds.) (1981). *Proceedings of the conference on the assessment of vocal pathology,* ASHA Reports No. 11. Rockville, MD: American Speech-Language-Hearing Association.

Negus, V. E. (1929). *The mechanism of the larynx.* St. Louis: Mosby.

Orlikoff, R. F., & Baken, R. J. (1993). *Clinical speech and voice measurement: Laboratory exercises.* San Diego, CA: Singular Publishing Group.

Sundberg, J. (1987). *The science of the singing voice.* DeKalb: Northern Illinois University Press.

Titze, I. R. (1993). Current topics in voice production mechanisms. *Acta Otolaryngologica, 113,* 421-427.

Titze, I. R. (1994). *Principles of voice production.* Englewood Cliffs, NJ: Prentice Hall.

Zemlin, W. R. (1988). Phonation. In *Speech and hearing science: Anatomy and physiology,* 3rd ed. Englewood Cliffs, NJ: Prentice-Hall (pp. 99-192).

Part II

THE SPEECH SIGNAL

Chapter 5

The Acoustic Characteristics of American English

Ray D. Kent, James Dembowski, Norman J. Lass

Key Terms

affricate 196
amplitude 187
antiformant 194
antinode 190
articulatory undershooting 215
bandwidth 188-189
Bark scale 200
burst 204
coupling 193
damping 203
diphthong 200
fast Fourier transform (FFT) 207
filter 187
formant 188
formant transition 197

THE ACOUSTIC STUDY OF SPEECH SOUNDS

The acoustic speech wave is the primary medium through which a talker's message is communicated to a listener. Thus, analysis of the acoustic signal provides insight into both the production processes of speech and the processes by which the listener perceives speech. And so it is that through study of the mediating acoustic signal we infer physiological phenomena that generate the signal on the one hand and perceptual phenomena whereby the signal is interpreted as linguistically meaningful on the other. Additionally, understanding the fundamental acoustic characteristics of speech is vital for an informed and critical use of tools for acoustic analyses of speech. Through broadly accessible microcomputer technology, such tools have proliferated in recent years and are no longer limited to research laboratories. Increasingly, clinics, schools, private practice settings, and rehabilitation centers incorporate acoustic analyses into their assessment and therapy programs. Acoustic analyses of speech are ever more widely applied in the fields of phonetics, speech synthesis, automatic speech recognition, speaker identification, communication aids, instructional programs, speech pathology, and machine translation, among others. Moreover, some forms of acoustic analysis are making their way into home computers for general educational or entertainment purposes.

The application of acoustic analysis to speech requires an appreciation of the interrelationships among (1) the theory underlying the acoustic analysis of speech (the acoustic theory of speech production), (2) instruments used to analyze speech acoustics, and (3) the measures resulting from those analyses (Kent, 1993). Ideally, understanding and interpreting acoustic measures of speech means understanding the advantages and limitations of the technology by which these measures are derived. It also means understanding the theory that has driven the derivation of those measures. Because of space limitations, this chapter will focus on two general issues, acoustic theory and acoustic measures. For a discussion of instruments and analysis procedures, see Kent and Read (1992), Read, Buder, and Kent (1992), and relevant chapters in this volume (Chapters 7, 11, and 13).

ACOUSTIC THEORY OF SPEECH PRODUCTION

Gunnar Fant's *Acoustic Theory of Speech Production* (1960) laid the foundations for current interpretations of speech acoustic analyses. The essential tenet of the theory is that characteristics of the speech production system (the vocal tract) may be inferred from analyses of the acoustic output of that system. That is, we may infer certain systematic articulatory-acoustic relationships. The validity of these inferences depends

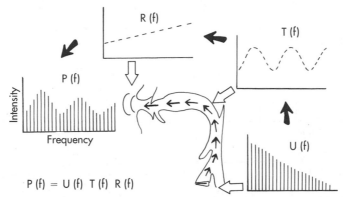

FIGURE 5-1 Source-filter theory for vowels. U(F) is the source spectrum, T(F) is the vocal tract transfer function, R(f) is the radiation characteristic, and P(F) is the radiated sound spectrum. (Redrawn from Kent, R. D., & Read, C. (1992). *The acoustic analysis of speech.* San Diego: Singular; with permission.)

on certain basic assumptions about the system, specifically that it is (1) linear and (2) time invariant. The assumption of linearity posits a linear relationship between the input to the system and the output from the system: if values describing the output of the system are graphed against values describing the input, the result is a straight line. Another way of defining linearity is that the sum of the output responses of a system to a series of individual inputs is equal to the response to the sum of the inputs. The assumption of time invariance means that the system will produce a consistent response to a consistent input across different points in time. Advances or delays in the input are reflected by commensurate advances or delays in the output. In fact, these simplifying assumptions do not reflect vocal tract characteristics with ideal accuracy. The vocal tract is known to be nonlinear and dynamic (time variant) in many respects. Despite this, many characteristics of the vocal tract are usefully approximated by modeling it as a linear, time-invariant system, as empirical studies have shown.

The acoustic theory of speech production posits that the vocal tract sound production system may be decomposed into two primary components: a source, which provides the input to the system, and a **filter,** which modulates the input. Thus, the acoustic theory is alternatively known as the **source-filter theory.** The filter is a frequency-dependent transmission system, meaning that different **frequency** components of the source are passed through the filter with varying degrees of **amplitude** reduction. The task of speech analysis is largely one of identifying sound sources and describing a corresponding filter function (also called the *transfer function*). Speech production involves three primary sound sources: (1) a quasiperiodic laryngeal voicing source, typified in the phonation of vowels, (2) a transient aperiodic noise source, exemplified by the release burst of **stop** consonants, and (3) a continuous aperiodic turbulent (noise) source used in the production of fricatives. Alone or in combination, these sources provide the vocal tract input for the sounds that make up the phonetic system of English and many other languages as well. Source-filter theory may be applied to any of the phonetic segments of English, but it is most often presented, and perhaps most easily understood, as a way of conceptualizing vowel production. It may be generalized to **obstruents, nasals,** glides, and liquids.

Source-Filter Theory for Vowels

Figure 5-1 illustrates source-filter theory for vowels. The figure shows the way the spectra (that is, the frequency domain representations) of source and filter interact to produce speech sounds radiated from the mouth. The following discussion assumes familiarity with the basic physics of sound as well as with the conventional representations of sound in the time domain (the **waveform**) and frequency domain (the **spectrum**).

The interaction of spectra to produce sound is expressed by this equation:

$$P(f) = U(f)\ T(f)\ R(f)$$

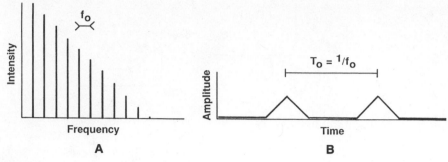

FIGURE 5-2 *A,* **Idealized glottal volume velocity waveform and** *B,* **its equivalent spectrum, or Fourier transform.** (From Kent, R. D., & Read, C. (1992). *The acoustic analysis of speech.* San Diego: Singular; reprinted with permission.)

The variable (f) indicates that all parameters are expressed as a function of frequency rather than time. The term P represents the radiated sound pressure spectrum at the mouth; U is the glottal volume velocity spectrum. T is the transfer function of the vocal tract filter, and R indicates another part of the overall filter function that results from radiating the sound beyond the vocal tract. The equation states that the spectrum of the radiated sound pressure equals the product of the glottal source spectrum, the vocal tract transfer function, and the **radiation characteristic**. The multiplication of terms in the frequency domain is the equivalent of convolution in the time domain. This discussion focuses on frequency domain (spectral) analysis, but each term in the equation could be expressed equally well as a time function. For example, P(f) in the frequency domain could be expressed as p(t) in the time domain.

The vowel source is typically generated by the periodic vibration of the vocal folds. Because a periodic sound pressure wave is generated by alternately stopping and releasing the flow of air through the glottis, the glottal source is conventionally represented as a volume velocity wave, where volume velocity is equal to the particle velocity of air times the varying area of the glottis during vibration. Figure 5-2 shows an idealized volume velocity waveform and its equivalent spectrum, or **Fourier transform.** The idealized waveform time history has a series of triangular pulses representing alternately increasing and decreasing volume velocity of air as the folds open and close, spaced at a fundamental period, T_0, which is equal to the reciprocal of the **fundamental frequency,** f_0. This triangular waveform may be considered a complex periodic sound with **harmonics** at integer multiples

of the fundamental frequency, as illustrated by the spectrum. The difference in frequency between any two adjacent harmonics equals the fundamental frequency. The source spectrum has a characteristic roll-off of 12 dB per octave. That is, the amplitude of the harmonics decreases 12 dB for every doubling of the fundamental frequency.

This is an illustrative ideal. In fact, the waveform may vary in shape, becoming more or less rounded, or more or less symmetric, with consequent effects on the spectrum, particularly on the roll-off (Fant, 1986). For example, the volume velocity waveform for a breathy voice may be less sharply defined and less distinctly triangular, resulting in a steeper roll-off, so that higher harmonics have a reduced amplitude. The glottal wave for a **strident** voice may take a sharply defined but asymmetric form, resulting in a more gradual roll-off, so that higher harmonics have a relatively greater amplitude. These varying source characteristics provide different sorts of raw material to be acted upon by the vocal tract filter, with corresponding consequences for the quality of the final output. Additionally, the source in natural speech production is never perfectly periodic (that is, there are continuous small variations in the periodicity of vibration) and so is often called a *quasi-periodic signal.*

The vocal tract filter selectively passes energy in the harmonics of the source. The size and shape of the vocal tract determine which harmonic frequencies will be passed with reduced amplitude and which will be passed with maximum amplitude (as described later). Frequencies resonated by the vocal tract are its characteristic resonances, or **formants.** The vocal tract transfer function is defined by the frequency and **band-**

width of these formants, where frequency means the center frequencies of the resonances (the frequencies of greatest amplitude) and band-width is the range of frequencies having amplitude no less than 3 dB of a given center frequency's amplitude. In theory, resonators such as the vocal tract have an infinite number of resonances, but in practical speech research only the lowest three or four formants are conventionally regarded as important for acoustic analysis of phonetic segments or for perceptual identification of speech sounds. Remember, formants do not supply energy; they only modify the energy supplied by the source. This means that the filter spectrum (i.e., the transfer function) indicates resonances *potentially* associated with peaks in the final output spectrum. However, if the source does not supply energy at the frequencies corresponding to the formants (the filter resonances), the peaks in the transfer function will not be reflected in the output spectrum.

This distinction between the energy of the source and the potential for energy modification by the vocal tract filter has led to the conventional characterization of source and filter as independent. This supposed independence is illustrated by the fact that glottal sources drastically different in frequency (e.g., the different vibratory frequencies of men, women, and children) or in quality (e.g., breathy or strident voices) may result in perceptually equivalent sound outputs. Therefore, we may perceive consistent vowels (characterized by consistent relationships among formant frequencies) produced by different speakers with different voice qualities. Given a particular set of formant relationships, we hear the "same" vowel, whether produced by a man, woman, or child, whether the voice is normal, breathy, or harsh, and so on. This independence of source and filter is even more vividly illustrated by the use of an artificial larynx to produce speech. However, recent research has shown that in natural speech production the source and filter are not truly independent. As the glottis opens with each cycle of vibration, the glottal source is coupled to the resonating cavities both above and below. This interdependence of source and filter may affect the intelligibility of speakers with voice or articulation disorders and the perceived vocal quality of singers. However, for this discussion of normal speech acoustics, the source and filter may be considered relatively independent.

The final term in the equation representing the source-filter theory is the radiation characteristic. This additional filtering effect occurs when the sound is radiated beyond the mouth into the atmosphere. The spectrum of the radiation characteristic shows that the coupling of the mouth to the atmosphere behaves like a high-pass filter: high frequencies are resonated more than low frequencies. In our ideal case the sound output increases at 6 dB per octave. If this is combined with the 12 dB per octave roll-off of the laryngeal source spectrum, the final output spectrum of this theoretical source-filter system has a high frequency roll-off of 6 dB per octave.

For the purposes of our idealized model of vowel production, the terms U(f) and R(f) may be considered constant across vowels. Thus, the salient changes in the output spectrum, P(f), for different vowels result from variations in the transfer function, T(f). Consequently, a description of different vowels amounts to a description of varying vocal tract resonances, or formant patterns.

Resonating Tube Model for Vowels

Normally, when we phonate a vowel, we spatially approximate the vocal folds to initiate and sustain vibration. Therefore, the vocal tract is nearly closed at the glottis. However, farther up in the vocal tract we articulate vowels with a relatively open mouth (compared with all other phonetic classes, obstruents in particular). The vocal tract forms a tube open at one end (the mouth) and closed at the other (the glottis) (Fig. 5-3, top). If we phonate a mid-central vowel (e.g., schwa), the vocal tract tube has a relatively uniform cross-sectional area over its length. The resonating characteristics of this uniform tube are well known. The curve of the tube as exemplified by a curving human vocal tract is relatively unimportant and may be ignored for practical purposes (Sondhi, 1986). The resonances of the tube are a function of its length and may be calculated according to the *odd-quarter wavelength* relationship:

$$F_n = (2n - 1)\ c/4l,$$

where F_n is a particular formant frequency, $(2n - 1)$ generates the series of odd integers, c is the velocity of sound (approximately 35,000 cm/sec), and l is the length of the vocal tract tube.

This formula generates a series of tube resonances, which occur at odd integer multiples of the first resonance. In theory, the tube has an infinite number of resonances, but for practical purposes only the first three will be considered here. Applying the formula to an average man's vocal tract 17.5 cm long results in an F_1 equal to 500 Hz. Higher resonances would thus occur at 1500 Hz and 2500 Hz. Applying the formula to a child's vocal tract of 8.75 cm produces $F_1 = 1000$ Hz, $F_2 = 3000$ Hz, and $F_3 = 5000$ Hz. Note that not only are the child's resonances higher than the man's but the spacing between resonances is wider. Thus, the longer the vocal tract, the lower the characteristic resonances and the narrower the spacing between resonances. Conversely, the shorter the vocal tract, the higher the resonances and the wider the spacing between them. And so it is that formant frequencies vary with age and gender, because these factors influence vocal tract length. Moreover, not only does vocal tract length vary across individuals, it may also vary within individuals. For example, speakers may lengthen the vocal tract by protruding the lips or by lowering the larynx. These adjustments lower all formant frequencies and reduce the differences among them. This illustrates that in natural speech vocal tract length is not a fixed property; however, for the purposes of analysis, it may be considered to have a characteristic length for a given articulation.

The tube resonances derived from this formula arise from the characteristic *standing wave distribution* of the tube. The propagation of sound through a medium (e.g., the air in the vocal tract acoustic tube) is the longitudinal propagation of the alternating volume velocity maxima and minima (points of maximum and minimum particle vibration respectively) generated by the opening and closing of the glottis. Alternatively, it may be thought of as the propagation of alternating pressure minima and maxima, where pressure minima are volume velocity maxima and vice versa. Thus, a point of maximum volume velocity, where air particle vibration is of greatest amplitude, is a point of minimum pressure and vice versa. The nature of the tube is such that at the resonance frequencies it facilitates particle vibration at some points and inhibits it at others. Points where vibration is facilitated so that particles vibrate with maximum amplitude (i.e., regions of volume velocity maxima) are called **nodes**. Regions of volume

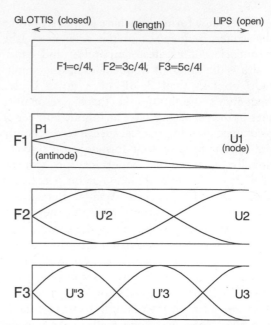

FIGURE 5-3   **A simplified model of the vocal tract as a tube, open at one end (the mouth) and closed at the other (the glottis), with the distribution of nodes and antinodes.**

velocity minima are called **antinodes**. Each resonance of the vocal tract has a characteristic distribution of nodes and antinodes.

The distribution of nodes and antinodes for the tube model of the vocal tract is illustrated in Figure 5-3. For a tube open at one end and closed at the other, movement must be minimal where the tube is closed, since the air molecules are constrained in their movement by the closure. At the open end, particle vibration is not constrained. Thus, there is a node at the open end (the lips) and an antinode at the closed end (the glottis). This represents the characteristic standing wave distribution for the first resonance, which has a wavelength four times the length of the tube. All higher resonances also have nodes at the open end and antinodes at the closed end but have additional nodes and antinodes in between. The presence of theoretically derived standing wave distributions in the vocal tract was empirically demonstrated by von Békésy (1960), who located nodes and antinodes by moving a miniature microphone through the vocal tract of a phonating subject.

Perturbation Theory

The relevance of a tube's standing wave distribution to vowel production is that constriction

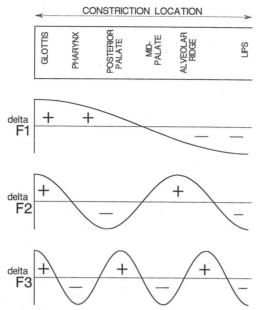

FIGURE 5-4 Effects of tube perturbation on the first three formant frequencies. A positive sign means that a constriction near that area raises the formant frequency; a negative sign means that a constriction near that area lowers the formant frequency.

of the tube near a node or antinode for a particular formant (resonance) alters the frequency of that formant. In other words, perturbing (constricting) the tube resonator will systematically alter the frequency of the resonances. The general relationship is that (1) a constriction near a node (volume velocity maximum) lowers the formant frequency, and (2) a constriction near an antinode (volume velocity minimum) raises the formant frequency. Since the first formant has a node at the lips and an antinode at the glottis, a narrowing at the lips lowers F_1, and a narrowing at the pharynx just above the glottis raises F_1. Actually, since all formants have a node at the lips, all formants are lowered by a labial constriction. Figure 5-4 illustrates the effects of tube **perturbation** on the first three formants. A positive sign means that a constriction near that area raises the frequency of that formant; a negative sign means that a constriction near that area lowers the frequency of the formant. It is possible to derive from these relationships a set of rules predicting changes in formant frequencies according to place of constriction in the vocal tract. In turn, these changes of formant frequency relations describe the acoustic characteristics of individual vowels. Formant frequency rules may be summarized as

follows (see Figure 5-4 to visualize these places of constriction in the vocal tract tube and their effects).

F_1 Frequency

The frequency of F_1 is lowered by a constriction near the front half of the vocal tract (i.e., the oral cavity). This happens, for example, when the lips are closed to form /u/ or when the tongue is raised near the alveolar ridge to form /i/. Its frequency is raised by a constriction in the posterior-inferior vocal tract (i.e., the pharynx). This occurs for the vowel /ɑ/.

F_2 Frequency

Frequency of F_2 is lowered by a constriction at the lips or at the rear of the oral cavity just above the pharynx. This occurs for /u/, which is produced by many speakers with constrictions at both these sites simultaneously. Frequency of F_2 is raised by a constriction in the anterior oral cavity behind the lips and teeth. This occurs for the vowel /i/. In theory, F_2 may also be raised by a constriction immediately above the glottis, but since most of these constrictions are conventionally made with the tongue and lips, that place is not a common perturbation site for manipulation of F_2 in English.

F_3 Frequency

Frequency of F_3 is lowered by a constriction at the lips, in the mid-oral cavity, or in the upper pharynx. This occurs for production of /r/ or for r-colored vowels such as /ɝ/. Frequency of F_3 is raised by a constriction near the anterior oral cavity such as we produce for the semivowel /j/ or near the area of the posterior oral cavity–upper pharynx such as we make for /ɑ/.

Remember, all formants are lowered by (1) lengthening the vocal tract tube and (2) forming a constriction at the lips. Both of these events occur in English production of high back vowels, which are conventionally rounded in English, and therefore have the lowest formant frequencies of all vowels.

Some early literature on vowel acoustics associates F_1 frequency with vowel height (i.e., the relative degree of tongue-palate constriction in the oral cavity) and F_2 frequency with anterior-posterior place of constriction in the oral cavity. The general rule for F_1 is that its

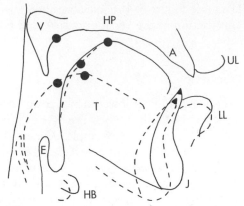

FIGURE 5-5   A mid-sagittal section of the vocal tract showing the articulatory configurations for the two vowels /i/ (solid line) and /ɑ/ (broken line). The filled circles represent the positions of three radiopaque pellets, two pellets attached to the tongue and one to the undersurface of the velum. The tip of the lower central incisor has been blackened to serve as an index of jaw position. Note a palatal constriction for /i/ and a pharyngeal constriction for /ɑ/. UL, upper lip; LL, lower lip; J, jaw; A, alveolar ridge; HP, hard palate; V, velum; T, tongue; E, epiglottis; HB, hyoid bone.

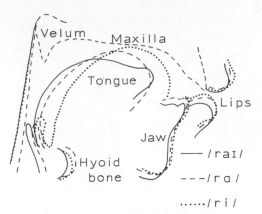

FIGURE 5-6   X-ray tracings showing different tongue configurations that produce a perceptually consistent /r/.

frequency is inversely proportional to tongue height. Thus, low vowels such as /ɑ/ have high F_1, and high vowels such as /i/ have low F_1 (see Fig. 5-5 for the vocal tract shapes of these vowels). It is not the case that there is no constriction for a vowel like /ɑ/, as a frontal view into someone's vocal tract might superficially suggest. Rather, because the tongue behaves as a flexible but incompressible mass, lowering the tongue in the oral cavity forces it to bulge out into the pharynx and form the constriction there. Retracting the tongue, as for /u/, also forms a constriction sufficiently posterior to lower F_1. Raising the tongue to approximate the alveolar ridge for /i/ widens the pharynx and moves the constriction anteriorly into the vicinity of the node for the first resonance. Thus, what we conventionally call low vowels are open in the vicinity of the anterior vocal tract but form a more posterior (pharyngeal) constriction, while those we call high vowels are formed with a more anterior constriction. The general rule for F_2 is that its frequency decreases as place of constriction moves from anterior to posterior in the oral cavity. This is easily understood with reference to the perturbation diagram in Figure 5-4 and the standing-wave distribution in Figure 5-3. Moving a constriction along the palate from front to back means moving from the site of an antinode for F_2 to the site of a node for F_2.

These rules illustrate that some characteristic formant positions for vowels or vowel-like segments may be produced in more than one way. Most notably, three different perturbation sites generate the characteristic low F_3 for /r/. These are the lips, the midpalatal region, and the pharynx. The functional consequence of being able to lower F_3 by any one of three different constrictions is variability in the production of /r/ across individuals, languages, and phonetic contexts. Production of the phoneme labeled /r/ may sound distinctively different when uttered by a French, a Spanish, and a North American speaker. In addition, variability in /r/ production may also contribute to confusion between /r/ and other phonemes with a similarly low F_3, such as /w/. Young children often fail to produce the adult distinction between /r/ and /w/, which is one of the last adult phonetic distinctions to emerge in speech development (Sander, 1972). Furthermore, some speakers never make the distinction ideally clear: one famous North American newscaster is notable for producing /r/ phonemes with a /w/ color to them. It is easy to see how the acoustic similarity in these phonemes, coupled with multiple movement options for generating their distinctive acoustic features, make /r/ and /w/ difficult to distinguish, especially for an immature speaker. Figure 5-6 shows cinefluorographic tracings that exemplify some of the tongue configurations possible for generating a perceptually consistent /r/ phoneme.

Source-Filter Theory for Obstruents

The concept that output from the vocal tract is the combined result of a sound source and a

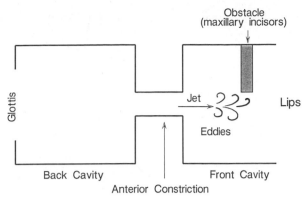

FIGURE 5-7   Schematized acoustic tube model of the vocal tract for a fricative such as /s/. The articulatory constriction divides the tube into back and front cavities. The incisors function as an obstacle.

resonating filter is applicable to **obstruents** (fricatives, stops) and sonorant consonants (**nasals**) as well as to vowels. However, there are complications. For stops and fricatives, a sound source is usually created by a severe constriction within the vocal tract, rather than just at one end of the vocal tract. This divides the resonating space into two cavities, which may be either **coupled** (i.e., the cavities interact to determine the resonances) or **uncoupled** (do not interact). Also, the resonating cavities may or may not interact with the source-producing constriction itself, depending on the relative shapes of the various cavities and constriction. The sound source within the vocal tract may be the sole source (as for voiceless obstruents) or it may combine with the glottal source (as for some voiced fricatives and stops) in which case there are two sources simultaneously providing energy to the divided vocal tract filter. Additionally, the sound source associated with a vocal tract constriction is an aperiodic source (a noise source) rather than the quasi-periodic source produced by the vibrating vocal folds. As such, the source spectrum is considerably different than it is for vowels.

Source-Filter Characteristics of Fricatives

Figure 5-7 presents a schematized acoustic tube model of the vocal tract as it might be for a **fricative** such as /s/. Note the back cavity, the anterior constriction, and the front cavity. The fricative source is generated by forcing air through the anterior constriction. Air exiting the constriction forms a jet, which mixes with the surrounding air of the anterior cavity. Under

certain conditions the flow of air into the front cavity ceases to be **laminar** (smoothly layered) and becomes turbulent, with complex rotations of air flow. That is, the mixing air forms eddies, which are high-frequency fluctuations of velocity and pressure. When the high-frequency flow velocity exceeds a critical point, noise results. That critical point is quantitatively defined by the **Reynolds number** (Re):

$$Re = vh/v,$$

where v is the flow velocity, v is the kinematic coefficient of viscosity (about 0.15 cm^2/s for air), and h is the characteristic dimension of the constriction (approximately the constriction diameter). Flow velocity is affected by volume velocity and area of the constriction ($v = U/A$); volume velocity in turn is affected by driving pressure. Thus, all these parameters interact in the generation of **turbulence,** which results when the Reynolds number exceeds a critical value of about 1800.

Fricative noise, that is, a continuous aperiodic source, is conventionally defined as possessing all frequencies at approximately equal amplitude. In theory, then, the spectrum is a straight line at some arbitrary amplitude level (as in Figure 5-8, *A*). In nature, however, fricative source spectra may vary in shape, depending on how the fricative is formed. Shadle (1990) showed through modeling studies that there are at least two classes of fricative sources which have distinctive spectra. She termed these *obstacle sources* and *wall sources*. An obstacle source results when the turbulent flow from a constriction encounters a rigid body normal to the flow. This occurs in English, for example,

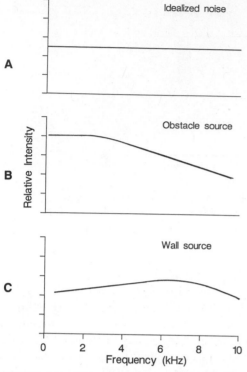

FIGURE 5-8 Examples of spectra for fricative sounds, including an idealized noise with *A*, a flat spectrum, *B*, an obstacle source with energy primarily in the low frequencies, and *C*, wall source with energy primarily in the higher frequencies.

when flow through an alveolar constriction for /s/ encounters the upper teeth. Similarly, the lower teeth are hypothesized to provide the obstacle for the palatal fricative /ʃ/. The spectrum for an obstacle source is illustrated in Fig. 5-8, *B*. The shape of the spectrum has a gradually falling profile at higher frequencies. Also, the overall source amplitude is relatively high and is notably affected by changes in flow rate. A wall source results when turbulence is generated along a structure parallel to the airflow. This occurs for uvular and pharyngeal fricatives, which are not phonemic in English and so will not be addressed in detail here. The spectral shape for a wall source differs from that of an obstacle source in that it possesses a broad peak in the vicinity of 4 to 9 kHz (Figure 5-8, *C*). Moreover, it is generally lower in amplitude than an obstacle source spectrum and less affected by changes in flow rate. The functional importance of an obstacle in the generation of some fricative sources is illustrated by the perceivable acoustic changes in children's /s/ production when they lose their front baby teeth. The fricative /s/ is articulatorily defined as

having a linguaalveolar, not linguadental, constriction, yet an appropriately articulated /s/ sounds abnormal when the front teeth are missing. This probably accounts for the assumption of some phonetically naive listeners that /s/ is formed at the teeth. The sound is generated in part at the dental obstacle, even though the actual point of articulation is posterior to the teeth.

Heinz and Stevens (1961) addressed fricative resonance in detail. Like vowels, fricatives have a mathematically defined transfer function (or vocal tract filter):

$$T(f) = [P(f)\ Z(f)]\ R(f),$$

where $T(f)$ is the transfer function defined in the frequency domain, $P(f)$ represents the formants, or *poles,* $Z(f)$ represents **antiformants,** or zeros, and $R(f)$ is the radiation characteristic.

The major difference between the fricative transfer function and the vowel transfer function is the presence of zeros. Zeros may be considered the opposite of resonances: they are frequencies of sound energy loss rather than sound energy transmission. In other words, they are points of maximum sound energy impedance. They are frequencies at which the sound is not transmitted through the vocal tract but is trapped, or short-circuited, in the back cavity. They arise in two circumstances: (1) when the vocal tract is bifurcated, or split into two passages such as an oral passage and a nasal passage, as occurs for nasal production, and (2) when the vocal tract is radically constricted. The latter case occurs when a fricative is produced. The poles for a given fricative are determined by the length of the entire vocal tract from glottis to lips. Thus, they are approximately the same as vowel formants for a vowel with a similar place of articulation. The zeros, however, are determined by the size of the back cavity and the size of the constriction itself. Since these cavities are smaller than the vocal tract as a whole, the zeros are more widely spaced than the poles. When a pole and a zero occur close to each other in frequency, their effects cancel each other. Also, because zeros are more widely spaced than poles, poles and zeros tend to occur close to each other at low frequencies but diverge at higher frequencies. Thus, their effects cancel at low frequencies but not at higher frequencies, where they are more widely separated. As a general rule the poles and zeros tend to cancel at frequencies below the frequency for which the constriction length is a quarter wavelength. Thus, for a fricative constriction approximately 2 cm long, effects of poles and zeros cancel at or below frequencies with a wavelength of 4 × 2 cm (or 8 cm), that is, frequencies below 4375 Hz. Frequencies in the source spectrum below 4375 Hz are relatively unaffected by the overall vocal tract resonances and the zeros of the back cavity. Another way to view this is that the back cavity is decoupled from the source and the front cavity, leaving the front cavity alone as the primary resonator. This decoupling occurs when the constriction area is small compared with the area of the cavities before and behind it, as occurs for most normal fricative productions.

The front cavity behaves like a half-open tube, with resonances determined by the odd-quarter wavelength relationship. Thus, small front cavities have high and more widely spaced resonances. In cases like /f v/ these are too high to shape the noise energy notably, and so the output spectrum tends to be relatively flat and diffuse. However, as place of articulation moves back in the vocal tract, the front cavity size increases and the lowest resonance frequency decreases. For a man's production of /s/, with a front cavity length of approximately 2 cm, the lowest resonance is about 4000 Hz. If place of constriction moves another centimeter back (e.g., for /ʃ/, the lowest resonance descends to about 3000 Hz (see Figure 5-20 for contrastive spectra from /s/ and /ʃ/).

When the cavities are coupled, vocal tract resonances vary from those of the uncoupled condition. Coupled, the output spectrum is more affected by the resonances of the back cavity and of the constriction itself. These cavities behave like acoustic tubes closed (or open) at both ends. For this type of tube, the resonances are given by

$$F_n = (n) (c/2l); \text{ for example, } 1c/2l, c/l, 3c/2l.$$

Thus, a back cavity with a length of 10 cm contributes resonances of about 1750 Hz, 3500 Hz, and so on. The chief functional effect of coupling the vocal tract cavities during fricative production (for example, by increasing the area of the constriction) is to separate resonances that converge in the uncoupled case. Stevens (1989) has shown that in the normally uncoupled case, at particular points of articulation the resonances of the front and back cavities converge

and thereby reinforce each other. They provide particularly salient resonance peaks. When the cavities become coupled, perhaps because the fricative constriction is insufficiently small, the resonances of the cavities diverge and do not reinforce each other. Thus, there may be an acoustic-perceptual advantage to producing fricatives with small constrictions, which uncouple the cavities and allow perceptually important resonances to be reinforced. Failure to do so, as in the case of an articulatorily disordered speaker, may result in the production of divergent resonance patterns that do not provide normal acoustic cues.

Source-Filter Characteristics of Stops and Affricates

Stop consonants are acoustically complex because of the fast articulatory and acoustic transitions inherent in their production. Classic descriptions of stops (Halle, Hughes, and Radley, 1957; Fant, 1973; Klatt, 1975) describe five articulatory-acoustic states that may be included in stop production: (1) a period of articulatory closure generally resulting in acoustic silence, or **stop gap,** except in the case of some voiced stops whose voicing energy is maintained during the closure; (2) an articulatory release from closure producing an acoustic aperiodic transient sound conventionally called the *release burst*; (3) a brief period of varying upper vocal tract constriction following release resulting in a post-release fricative-like aperiodic sound; (4) a period of turbulent airflow through the glottis (aspiration) just prior to onset of vocal fold vibration; and (5) a period of articulatory transition to another vocal tract configuration resulting in shifting formant frequencies. These stages are temporally overlapping rather than discrete, and not all stages are necessarily evident in any individual stop token. The evident acoustic-articulatory states vary with phonetic context and voicing characteristics. For instance, the period of vocal tract closure is not necessarily silent in voiced stops; the release burst and aspiration may not be evident in syllable-final stops; and in English, voiceless stops following /s/ have a release burst but no aspiration, in conformance with the phonological rules of the language.

In the case of voiceless stops there may be multiple acoustic sources: a transient aperiodic noise produced by the release, a continuous aperiodic noise produced by air flowing through the small articulatory constriction immediately following release, and an additional continuous aperiodic noise produced by air flowing through the glottis just prior to voicing. With voiced stops there is also the quasi-periodic source generated by vocal fold vibration. Of course, during the period of vocal tract closure, there is generally no source (i.e., no vocal tract excitation), especially with voiceless stops, because the airflow that produces sound is briefly stopped altogether. With voiced stops, air may continue to flow through the glottis, maintaining low-amplitude quasi-periodic vocal fold vibration (see Westbury, 1983, for a detailed description), though airflow will be stopped further along in the vocal tract and may be briefly stopped through the glottis as well if the subglottal and supraglottal pressures equalize during the period of closure. In the ideal (theoretical) case, the source spectrum for the transient stop release contains an infinitely broad range of frequencies at approximately equal amplitudes for an infinitely brief period of time (Halle, Hughes, and Radley, 1957). In nature, of course, the frequency and time parameters of the spectrum are neither infinitely broad nor infinitely short. The source spectra for frication and aspiration are grossly the same as for fricatives.

These multiple sources suggest some of the acoustic complexity of stops, particularly considering that the noise-generating aerodynamic conditions change continuously and quickly and that the noise sources may overlap each other in time. For example, the vocal tract constriction that generates post-release frication widens at 10 to 80 cm^2 per second and furthermore changes rate nonlinearly (Fant, 1960; Fujimura, 1961; Scully, 1990). The postrelease frication noise generated at an upper vocal tract constriction may temporally overlap the aspiration generated at the glottis, and aspiration in turn may temporally overlap the onset of periodic vocal fold vibration. Additionally, the quick articulations associated with stops require that the vocal tract resonating system be continuously changing, along with the changing sound sources.

Grossly, the shape and locus of energy of the stop release output spectrum (described in detail later) are affected by the size of the resonating cavity anterior to the place of articulation. Output spectra of post-release frication are roughly similar to the spectra of homorganic fricatives, with the provision that the spectra of

post-release stop frication change much more rapidly than the spectra of fricatives and that the spectrum of prevocalic aspiration is at least as likely to be affected by the vocal tract shape for the following vowel as by the place of stop release. Complete closure of the upper vocal tract means that the frequency of F_1 decreases to zero in the ideal case but to a value near zero in natural speech; this decrease in F_1 is easily seen in spectrograms of voiced stops. The closure of the vocal tract also introduces zeros into the transfer function and affects the acoustic coupling of the vocal tract resonating chambers in ways similar to those of fricatives. This likely contributes to the reduction of overall intensity of consonants relative to vowels and to consonants' less well defined formant structure.

The combination of sources and resonating filters for **affricates** may be inferred from these descriptions of stops and fricatives, bearing in mind that the primary distinction of affricates from the other two consonant classes is in the temporal progress of articulatory-acoustic events, as detailed later. For example, the rise time of affricate frication is faster than for fricatives but slower than for stops.

Source-Filter Theory for Nasals

The sound source for nasals, as for vowels, is quasi-periodic vocal fold vibration. The vocal tract filter, however, is affected by opening the velopharyngeal port. Thus, sound passes through the oral and nasal tracts for nasal vowels or through the nasal tract alone for nasal consonants. These two vocal tract configurations are illustrated in Figure 5-9. In both cases the long acoustic tube formed by the combined pharyngeal and nasal cavities is coupled to the shorter tube formed by the oral cavity (a *side-branch resonator*), which is open at both ends for nasal vowels and open only at one end for nasal consonants. Thus, in both cases the vocal tract is bifurcated, which generates zeros in the transfer function.

In the case of nasal vowels, the transfer function results from a complex interaction of oral formants (resonances), **nasal formants**, and antiformants introduced by the vocal tract bifurcation. The nasal cavities affect the acoustic output not only through the length of the tube but through the shape and tissue quality of the passages. Specifically, the soft and convoluted mucous membranes of the nasal cavity absorb

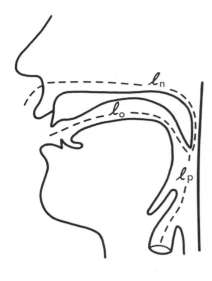

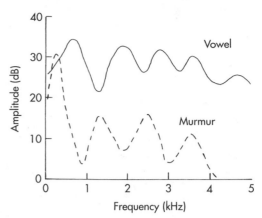

FIGURE 5-10 Contrasting vowel and nasal spectra, showing a dominant low frequency formant for the nasal (nasal murmur) and a reduction in higher formant energy relative to a vowel.

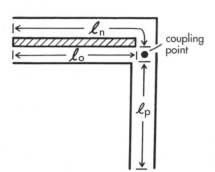

FIGURE 5-9 Vocal tract configurations for nasal vowels (sound passes through the oral and nasal tracts) and nasal consonants (sound passes through the nasal tract alone). Key: l_n is the length of the nasal cavity, l_o is the length of the oral cavity, and l_p is the length of the pharyngeal cavity. Note the coupling point at the velopharynx (lower figure).

sound. The general result of these interactions is a reduction in the overall energy of the vowel and a widening of the formant bandwidths.

In the case of nasal consonants, closure of the oral tract contributes distinctive antiformants as the oral cavity short-circuits sound energy from the larynx, preventing its radiation through the nasal passages. As with the zeros formed by the back-cavity resonators for fricatives, the zeros of the vocal tract during nasal consonant production are determined by the length of the cavity. Thus, characteristic antiformants (frequencies of energy minima in the output spectrum) are lowest and most narrowly spaced for /m/, which has the longest oral tract side branch resonator (with the first antiformant around 1000 Hz) and higher and more widely spaced for /n/ (the first

antiformant around 2000 Hz). The highest, widest antiformants are produced by the short oral side branch for /ŋ/ (the first antiformant at about 3000 Hz). In addition to introducing antiformants, the coupling of the nasal passages to the vocal tract increases the overall length of the tract, lowering formant frequencies generally and creating a distinctive low F_1 in the vicinity of 250 to 300 Hz (for normal adult male speakers). This distinctive low resonance is called the *nasal murmur* or nasal formant. Unlike antiformants, it varies little with change in place of articulation, since the combined length of the nasal-pharyngeal tube is stable across changes in oral articulation. Thus, relative to vowels, the output spectra of nasal consonants have a distinctive low-frequency formant peak with higher formants of markedly lower amplitude (Fig. 5-10).

Source-Filter Theory for Glides and Liquids

Source and filter characteristics for the **glides** /w/ and /j/ are essentially those of vowels /u/ and /i/, respectively. The major articulatory-acoustic distinctions between the glides and vowels are greater rate of change in articulator position for glides, and thus greater rate of change in **formant transitions**, and somewhat more extreme formant values for glides than for vowels, resulting from glides' smaller articulatory constrictions. The liquid /r/ has been discussed in the context of source-filter theory for vowels. The liquid /l/ is generally considered to have a lateral articu-

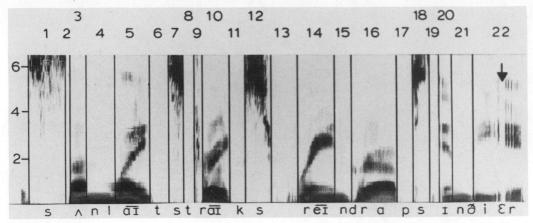

FIGURE 5-11 Spectrogram marked with vertical lines that represent our attempts to identify successive units. The utterance is derived from the first sentence of the Rainbow Passage and includes the words "sunlight strikes raindrops in the air." The speaker is a young woman. The phonetic transcription at the bottom of the spectrogram indicates the approximate location of phonetic units. The numbered segments are acoustic-phonetic intervals: *1,* frication; *2,* silence; *3,* short vowel; *4,* low-frequency resonance energy; *5,* diphthongal formant pattern; *6,* stop gap; *7,* frication; *8,* stop gap; *9,* noise burst plus aspiration; *10,* diphthongal formant pattern; *11,* stop gap; *12,* frication; *13,* silent pause; *14,* formant pattern for liquid and diphthong; *15,* nasal murmur; *16,* formant pattern for stop + liquid + vowel; *17,* stop gap; *18,* frication; *19,* silence; *20,* short vowel; *21,* nasal murmur; *22,* vocalic sequence with glottalization marked by arrow.

lation in that the tongue tip makes a midline closure near the alveolar ridge but airflow continues lateral to the occlusion. Thus, /l/ articulation bifurcates the vocal tract (as nasal articulations do) and introduces zeros into the transfer function. The acoustic consequence is a spectrum similar to that of nasals: most of the energy is in the low frequencies, with damped higher formants (i.e., the formants have low intensity and wide bandwidths) and frequencies of energy minima resulting from antiformants. As expected with an alveolar constriction, F_2 and F_3 for /l/ are relatively high, especially in contrast with the notably low F_3 for /r/.

ACOUSTIC CHARACTERISTICS OF THE SOUNDS OF AMERICAN ENGLISH

The perceptual impression of speech is that it consists of a series of individual sounds strung together to form words. A linguist might call these individual sounds *phonemes* or *phonetic segments.* However compelling this perceptual impression may be, the individual units of speech are not always readily identified at the physiologic or acoustic level of speech production. At the physical levels of articulation and acoustics, speech is not readily segmented into units such as phonemes. One of the major

long-standing challenges to the laboratory study of speech is precisely this problem of **segmentation,** or the identification of boundaries for the successive units in the speech stream. Articulatory studies, such as x-ray motion pictures, disclose that the movements of the various articulators, especially the tongue, jaw, lips, and velum, are not transparently organized into units such as phonemes. Rather, the movements overlap one another, frustrating attempts to establish boundaries between sound units. Likewise, acoustic studies reveal a variety of spectral-temporal patterns, but these do not necessarily align themselves into intervals that can be readily identified as phonemes. The problem of acoustic segmentation is described by some writers as the difficulty of drawing lines perpendicular to the time axis of a spectrogram to mark segment boundaries. Figure 5-11 is a spectrogram of the utterance "The sunlight strikes raindrops in the air." A phonetic transcription is provided at the bottom of the spectrogram. The lines corresponding to acoustic discontinuities do not always indicate a phonetic boundary, and phonetic segmentation of this phrase may be a challenge.

The difficulties associated with segmentation raise the question of whether phonemes have any physical or psychological reality besides

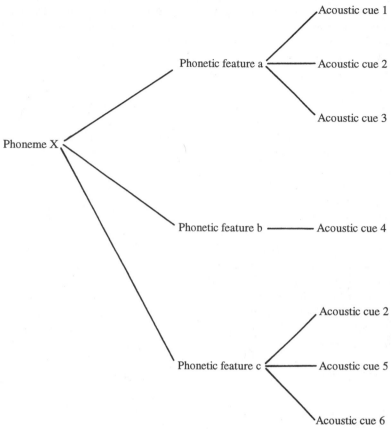

FIGURE 5-12 Hierarchical relationship among phoneme, phonetic feature, and acoustic cues. A phoneme is associated with a set of phonetic features, and a phonetic feature in turn is associated with one or more acoustic cues.

their usefulness in linguistic analysis. This complicated issue is outside the scope of this chapter. Some experts have come to doubt that the phoneme has psychological reality. However, no generally accepted alternative has been described. Given the lack of a good alternative and given the usefulness of phonemic analysis for a variety of purposes in linguistics, especially phonology and morphology, this chapter will assume the existence of the phoneme for discussion purposes. One advantage of the phoneme is that it provides an effective organizational scheme.

One of the complications in discussing acoustic phonetics is that what is considered to be the same phoneme can take quite different acoustic characteristics in different phonetic contexts. For this reason it is necessary to discuss acoustic characteristics of speech sounds with respect to phonetic context. This makes for somewhat lengthy descriptions, but it is necessary for the sake of accuracy. Neglect of this variance results in an incomplete or misleading account. Usually

a single phoneme will be associated with two or more acoustic events, so that acoustic description often entails a kind of inventory. Moreover, the acoustic events associated with a given phoneme may change with phonetic context.

It is helpful to keep in mind the following relation: A phoneme is associated with a set of phonetic features, and a phonetic feature in turn is associated with one or more acoustic cues. This relation is illustrated in Figure 5-12.

The following discussion of the acoustic characteristics is organized hierarchically as follows:

1. Phoneme class. Each class is a family of phonemes that share an important property or properties. The front vowels and the stop consonants are classes of phonemes.
2. The phonemes within the class. For example, /b d g p t k/ are the consonants in the class of stops. The individual sounds are distinguished within the class by place of articulation and voicing.
3. The phonetic features pertinent to the class.

These features describe the class and distinguish one phoneme from another. Unfortunately, no one set of phonetic features is universally accepted by phoneticians and linguists. This chapter will use the traditional vowel quadrilateral (front versus back, high versus low) for vowels and the traditional place-manner descriptions for consonants.

4. The acoustic cues for major allophones. These cues are the primary acoustic events or properties that signal the phonetic distinctions. These are frequently context sensitive. For example, cues will be given for stops that follow /s/ in a syllable-initial combination. To a degree each phoneme can be associated with a general set of acoustic cues, but the actual cues often vary with the phonetic context, especially syllable position. Therefore, the acoustic cues will be discussed with respect to the context in which a sound occurs.

The hierarchical discussion of phoneme class, phoneme, phonetic features, and acoustic cues is designed to show how linguistic and physical descriptions are related. The following information is essentially an acoustic taxonomy for the segments of American English. The discussion is organized by phoneme and phonetic features; the underlying concept is to describe the salient acoustic properties within the phonemic and phonetic organization. The acoustic description does not by any means exhaust the literature; it is intended to identify the major acoustic cues. To streamline the text, references have been compiled by speech sound type in the Suggested Readings section at the end of this chapter. Only selected references are included in the body of the paper.

Vowels

The vowels will be discussed in three categories: front, back, and central. For each category the major acoustic description will be in terms of formant pattern, specifically the frequencies of the first three formants, F_1, F_2, and F_3. These three formants typically are sufficient for the identification of a vowel sound in American English. Formant pattern is the classical acoustic description of vowels, but other descriptions have been proposed (Carlson, Fant, and Granstrom, 1975; Bladon, 1983; Strange, 1987). For present purposes, formant pattern will be taken as the essential acoustic feature of vowels. Formant pattern continues to be the most commonly used acoustic measure of vowel production and is the key factor in many speech synthesis systems. Indeed, a large class of these systems is called *formant synthesizers* in recognition of the role formants play in the synthesis procedure. **Diphthongs** (vowel-to-vowel glide-like sounds in words such as "bye" and "boy") can be understood as special cases of vowel production and will not be considered in detail here.

Front Vowels

Phonemes: /i I e ɛ æ/.

Key words: /i/—beat, /I/—bit, /e/—bate, /ɛ/—bet, /æ/—bat.

Phonetic features: front tongue position; various degrees of **tongue height**.

Acoustic cues: Large separation between F_1 and F_2 and a relatively close positioning of F_2 with F_3. The front vowels vary among themselves in formant pattern; particular attention will be given to F_1 frequency, which reflects tongue height. The frequency of F_1 varies inversely with tongue height; the lower the tongue in the oral cavity, the higher the F_1 frequency.

FORMANT PATTERN   The front vowels are illustrated in Figure 5-13. Although they differ in formant pattern, one shared characteristic is a large separation between F_1 and F_2. Thus, a simple articulatory-acoustic relation emerges: fronting of the tongue is associated with a relatively large F_2 to F_1 difference. Another formant characteristic of front vowels is a relative closeness of F_2 and F_3. This feature was noted by Syrdal and Gopal (1986), who suggested that front vowels have F_3 to F_2 differences of less than 3 Bark (the **Bark scale** is a nonlinear transform of frequency based on psychoacoustic studies).

The front vowels vary in their F_1 frequency, and here another articulatory-acoustic relation obtains: tongue height is associated with F_1 frequency; the higher the tongue position, the lower the F_1 value. The frequency value of F_1 for a given speaker is a gauge of relative tongue height for the vowel. Note in Figure 5-13 that the F_1 frequency roughly increases in the order /i I e ɛ æ/. Syrdal and Gopal (1986) showed that vowel height is correlated with the F_1 to fundamental frequency (f_o) difference, with high vowels having a small difference (less than 3 Bark) and low vowels having a large difference

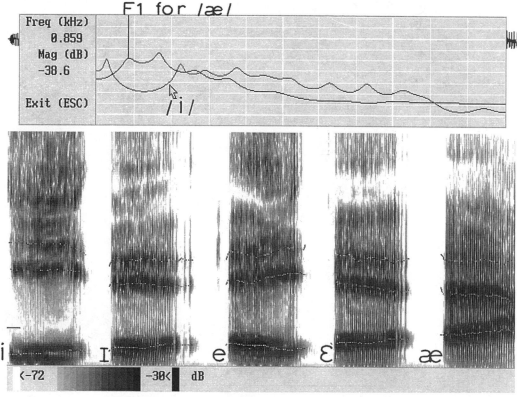

FIGURE 5-13 The front vowels. The spectrogram at the bottom shows the formant patterns for the vowels /i/, /I/, /e/, /ɛ/, /æ/. The linear predictive coding spectra at the top pertain to /i/ and /æ/. The arrow points to the spectrum for /i/, while the vertical marker indicates F_1 for /æ/. In general, note the relatively wide separation between F_1 and F_2.

(more than 3 Bark). On the average, high vowels have a higher f_o than low vowels, and this feature contributes to the small F_1 to f_o difference for the high vowels. (However, f_o can vary with many aspects of speech, especially intonation, and the f_o of any particular vowel can reflect more than tongue height.)

DURATION   The front vowels also differ in their inherent durations, or the relative durations of the vowel across various phonetic contexts. The vowels /i e æ/ (the long, or tense, vowels) have a long inherent duration, whereas the vowels /I ɛ/ (the short, or lax, vowels) have a short inherent duration.

Back Vowels

Phonemes: /u ʊ o ɔ ɑ/.

Key words: /u/—hoot, /ʊ/—hood, /o/—hoe, /ɔ/—hawed, /ɑ/—hot.

Phonetic features: Back tongue position; various degrees of tongue height.

Acoustic cues: Small separation between F_2 and F_1, large separation between F_2 and F_3. They vary among themselves primarily in the frequency of F_1, which varies with vowel height.

FORMANT PATTERN   The back vowels have a narrow separation between F_1 and F_2 (Fig. 5-14). Therefore, a small F_2 to F_1 difference is an acoustic correlate of backing in vowels. In addition, the F_3 to F_2 difference is large for back vowels. The back vowels vary among themselves with respect to the F_1 frequency, which varies inversely with tongue height. The lower the tongue position, the higher the F_1 frequency. This same relation holds for the front vowels. As Syrdal and Gopal (1986) observed, the F_1 to f_o difference also varies with tongue height, with high vowels having a small difference (less than 3 Bark) and low vowels having a large difference.

DURATION   The vowels /u o ɔ ɑ/ have an inherently long duration, whereas the vowel /ʊ/ has an inherently short duration. The former are sometimes called long, or tense, and the latter is termed short, or lax.

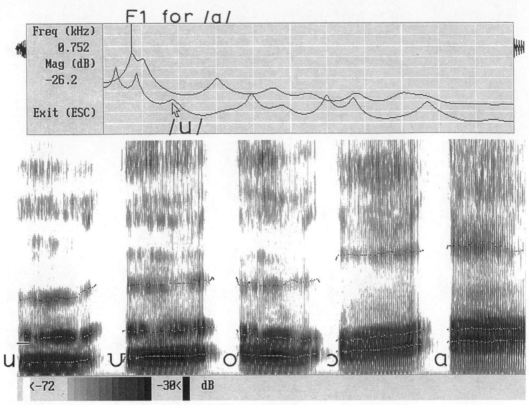

FIGURE 5-14 The back vowels. The spectrogram at the bottom shows the formant patterns for the vowels /u/, /ʊ/, /o/, /ɔ/, and /ɑ/. The linear predictive coding spectra at the top pertain to /u/ and /ɑ/. The arrow points to the /u/ spectrum, while the vertical marker indicates F₁ for /ɑ/. In general, note the relatively small separation between F₁ and F₂ (compare with Fig. 5-13).

Central Vowels

Phonemes: /ʌ ə ɝ ɚ/.

Key words: /ʌ/ — hut, /ə/ — first vowel in about, /ɝ/ — heard, /ɚ/ — second vowel in mother.

Phonetic features: Central tongue position.

Acoustic cues: The primary cue for centrality is a uniform formant pattern; that is, a pattern in which the formant frequencies tend to be nearly equally spaced, with the exception of a low F_3 for the rhotic (/r/-colored) /ɚ/ and /ɝ/.

FORMANT PATTERN   The major correlate of central tongue position is a rather uniform spacing of formants (Fig. 5-15). The left side of the spectrogram shows the vowel /ʌ/, and the right side shows that vowel with /r/-color added, and a consequent lowering of F_3. As described earlier, the formant frequencies of a vocal tract that has nearly constant cross-sectional diameter along its length is given by the odd-quarter wavelength relationship. Recall that for a vocal tract length of 17.5 cm, the formant frequencies will be about F_1, 500 Hz; F_2, 1500 Hz; and F_3,

2500 Hz. The average separation between adjacent formants is 1000 Hz. The formant frequencies in the example spectrogram of natural speech match these theoretically derived tube resonances very closely; the arrow on the spectral display of Figure 5-15 points to F_3 of /ʌ/, about 2500 Hz. The rhotic vowels /ɚ/ and /ɝ/ differ somewhat from this pattern in having a very low F_3 frequency, which is a consistent correlate of /r/-coloring in English. The vertical marker on the spectral display of Figure 5-15 indicates the F_3 of /ɝ/, at 2074 Hz.

DURATION   The vowels /ə ɚ/ tend to be inherently short, with schwa /ə/ and schwar /ɚ/ having the shortest average durations of all English vowels. Vowel /ʌ/ tends to be longer and is described by some phoneticians as tense.

Vowel Summary

Table 5-1 summarizes some of the major acoustic differences between classes of vowels. In

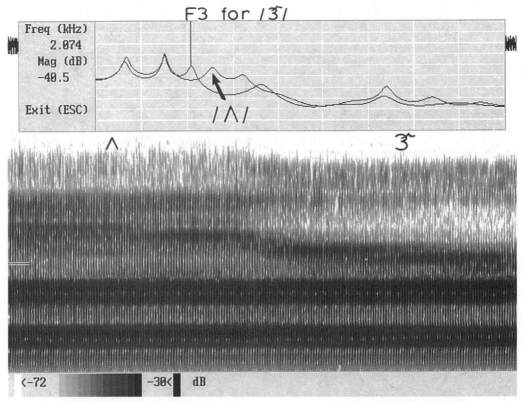

FIGURE 5-15 The central vowels. The spectrogram at the bottom shows the formant patterns for the vowels /ʌ/ and /ɝ/. The linear predictive coding spectra at the top pertains to /ʌ/ and /ɝ/. The arrow points to the /ʌ/ spectrum, while the vertical marker indicates F₃ for /ɝ/. Note in the spectrogram the decrease in F₃ as the central vowel becomes /r/-colored.

addition to the differences in formant pattern related to tongue position discussed so far, vowels have acoustic characteristics that vary with lip **rounding** and nasality. As discussed earlier, lip rounding lowers the frequencies of all formants. Nasalization introduces a low-frequency nasal formant as well as higher frequency nasal resonances and antiresonances. In addition, nasalization reduces the overall energy because of **damping** by the nasal cavities and increases the formant bandwidths. Table 5-2 contains the average formant frequencies of selected vowels produced by adult males and females.

Consonants

Stop Consonants

Phonemes: Voiced /b d g/ and voiceless /p t k/.

  Key words: /b/—bee, /d/—day, /g/—go, /p/—pay, /t/—toe, /k/—key.

  Phonetic features: Manner—stop or plosive; Place—bilabial, alveolar, or velar.

Acoustic cues: Silence, burst, transition, and various cues associated with the voicing feature. Important context conditions for phonetic description of the stops are syllable-initial position, syllable-final position, and voiceless stops after /s/. Figure 5-16 shows the sound pressure wave (A) and spectrogram (B) for syllable-initial stops in the context of consonant-vowel (CV) nonsense syllables, in the order /pʌ tʌ kʌ bʌ dʌ gʌ/.

Silence, or low-energy interval, corresponds to the period of oral constriction. This is also called a stop gap. Virtual silence may occur for voiceless stops, but voiced stops may have voicing energy during part or all of the interval of oral constriction. Therefore, voiced stops may have a low-energy interval rather than genuine silence. The voicing energy, especially the first harmonic, can be detected at low frequencies. This energy, sometimes called the *voice bar,* is evident in the spectrogram of Figure 5-16, preceding the voiced stops. Quasi-periodic, low-intensity voicing is also visible in the waveform above the spectrogram, especially preceding /b/. Note that the silence, or low-energy interval,

TABLE 5-1 Selected acoustic differences for certain vowel contrasts

Measure	Low-high Difference
Mean f_0	Low < High
Intensity	Low > High
Duration	Low > High
F_1 frequency	Low > High
$F_1 - f_0$ difference	Low > High

Measure	Front-back Difference
$F_2 - F_1$ difference	Back < Front
$F_3 - F_2$ difference	Back > Front

Measure	Tense-lax Difference
Duration	Tense > Lax

Measure	Rounded-unrounded Difference
$F_1 + F_2 + F_3$	Rounded < Unrounded

Measure	Nasal-nonnasal Difference
Formant bandwidth	Nasal > Nonnasal
Intensity	Nasal < Nonnasal
F_1 frequency	Nasal > Nonnasal
$F_2 + F_3$ frequency	Nasal < Nonnasal

may be continuous with a preceding or following silence for pauses of any kind, e.g., juncture, breathing, conversational rest, and so on. Therefore, the silent or low-energy interval may not be readily measured for utterance-initial stops or for unreleased utterance-final stops.

Burst corresponds to the articulatory release of the oral constriction and to the aerodynamic release of the impounded air pressure. The burst is a brief acoustic transient, typically 10 to 30 msec, with longer durations for voiceless stops. Bursts are reliable features of syllable-initial stops and are fairly common for medial stops. However, they are a variable feature of stops in final position.

The spectrum of the burst may signal place of articulation. The nature of this spectral information has been the subject of several studies, some of which are summarized below for each place of articulation. Classically, the burst spectrum was described in terms of prominent peaks or bands of spectral energy; for example, the typical burst for /t/ has energy prominence around 4 kHz. Stevens and Blumstein (1978)

and Blumstein and Stevens (1979) explored the use of templates to describe burst spectra. Each template is a kind of abstract depiction of the spectral envelope. More recently, Forrest, Weismer, Milenkovic, and Dougall (1988) applied statistical techniques to burst spectra. In this kind of analysis, any of the first four spectral moments can be calculated. The spectral moments can be interpreted approximately as follows: first moment, mean of spectrum; second moment, standard deviation or spread of energy around the mean; third moment, skewness of energy around the mean; and fourth moment, kurtosis, or peakedness of energy (kurtosis reflects other distributional properties as well). Both the template and spectral moment descriptions according to Stevens and Blumstein (1978), Blumstein and Stevens (1979), and Forrest, Weismer, Milenkovic, and Dougall (1988) are summarized next for each place of stop articulation. Figure 5-17 shows schematic illustrations of bilabial, alveolar, and velar burst spectra, to which template and spectral moment descriptions may be related.

Bilabial: Template—diffuse, flat or falling spectrum. Spectral moment: relatively low spectral mean, high skewness, and low kurtosis.

Alveolar: Template—diffuse, rising spectrum. Spectral moment: relatively high spectral mean, low skewness, and low kurtosis.

Velar: Template—compact (mid-frequency emphasis) spectrum. Spectral moment: relatively low spectral mean, high skewness, and high kurtosis, probably reflecting compact spectrum.

Aspiration is a diffuse noise generated at the larynx and possibly the lower pharynx. Its spectrum resembles that for the fricative /h/. Aspiration noise is generated during the interval in which the vocal folds move from an abducted state for the voiceless stop to an adducted state for a following voiced sound. As air passes through the adducting vocal folds, turbulence noise is generated. Voiceless stops in initial position typically are aspirated; however, voiced stops in English are not aspirated in any position. The degree of aspiration for voiceless stops varies with position and may be lacking altogether for stops in final position. In addition, aspiration is lost in voiceless stops that follow the fricative /s/, as in consonant sequences such as /sp/, /st/, and /sk/.

Transition corresponds to the articulatory movement from oral constriction for the stop to

TABLE 5-2   Formant frequencies in kHz for the first three formants (F1, F2, and F3) of selected vowels produced by adult males and females.

Vowel	Males			Females		
	F1	F2	F3	F1	F2	F3
/i/	.27	2.3	3.0	.30	2.8	3.3
/ɪ/	.40	2.0	2.6	.43	2.5	3.1
/ɛ/	.53	1.8	2.5	.60	2.4	3.0
/æ/	.66	1.7	2.4	.86	2.0	2.8
/a/	.73	1.1	2.4	.85	1.2	2.8
/ʊ/	.44	1.0	2.2	.47	1.2	2.7
/u/	.30	.85	2.2	.37	.95	2.6
/ʌ/	.64	1.2	2.4	.76	1.4	2.8
/ɝ/	.49	1.4	1.7	.50	1.6	2.0

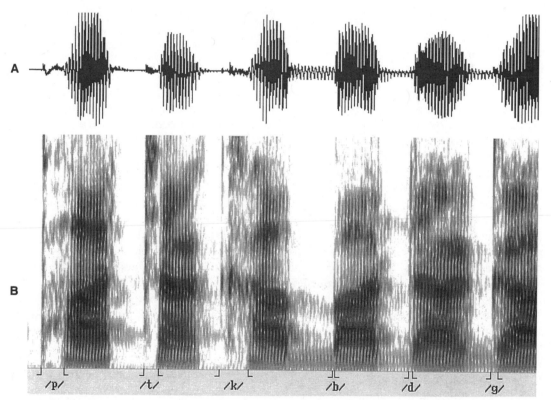

FIGURE 5-16   *A,* Sound pressure waveform and *B,* spectrogram illustrating oral stops, showing noise bursts and formant patterns for the syllables /pʌ tʌ kʌ bʌ dʌ gʌ/.

a more open vocal tract for a following sound, especially a vowel. Transition generally refers to formant transitions, or bends in the formant pattern. Formant transitions tend to be easier to identify for voiced stops because the voicing energy for these sounds is continuous with that for a following vowel. Most of the formant transition patterns described here are visible in the spectrogram of Figure 5-16, particularly for the voiced stops. A particular formant (F_1, F_2, or F_3) may have rising, falling, or relatively flat frequency shifts during the stop-to-vowel transition. In general, the direction of frequency shift is determined by both the place of articulation for the stop and the following vowel. The general rules are as follows for stop + vowel

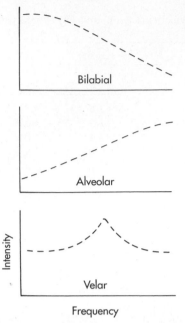

FIGURE 5-17 Schematized spectral envelopes for the bursts of bilabial, alveolar, and velar stops.

transitions (vowel + stop transitions are simply the reverse, although the dynamics may be somewhat different).

Bilabial: F_1 increases from a near-zero value to the F_1 frequency for the vowel. (Note: the F_1 frequency for vowels is always higher than the F_1 frequency for an occlusive segment.) F_2 increases from a low frequency of about 800 Hz to the F_2 for the vowel; except for some productions of the vowel /u/, vowel F_2 frequencies are always higher than the F_2 locus for bilabial consonants. F_3 increases from a low-frequency value of about 2200 Hz to the F_3 frequency for the vowel; the F_3 locus for bilabials is low compared with that for vowels, with the possible exception of /u/.

Alveolar: F_1: same as for bilabial. F_2 begins from a value close to the assumed F_2 locus of 1800 Hz. The direction of F_2 shift depends on the F_2 of the following vowel. Generally, F_2 has a rising transition for the high-front vowels /i I/, a flat transition for /ɛ/, and a falling transition for other vowels.

Velar: F_1: same as for bilabial. F_2 has at least two loci, one at a low frequency of about 1300 Hz and the other near 2300 Hz. A characteristic of velars is that the F_2 and F_3 formant frequencies are initially very close but diverge during the transition, giving the F_2 to F_3 pattern a wedge or pinch shape.

Voicing refers to the voiced-voiceless pho-

netic contrast. Stops may be voiced or voiceless, but this apparently simple binary alternation is not matched by an equivalent simplicity in acoustic cues. Many cues signal voicing for stops. The following summary is organized by position: initial, medial, and final. Most of the acoustic characteristics described here that distinguish voicing are evident in the spectrogram and sound pressure wave of Figure 5-16.

For stops in utterance-initial position, the primary acoustic cues of voicing are **voice onset time (VOT)**, F_1 cutback, and fundamental frequency. VOT is the interval between release of the stop (signaled acoustically by the release burst) and the onset of voicing (vocal fold vibrations). Voiced stops in English in initial position usually have a VOT that (1) slightly precedes release (**prevoicing**), (2) is simultaneous with release, or (3) slightly follows release (short lag). Voiceless stops in initial position usually have a long VOT (long lag). Voiced and voiceless stops in initial position also can differ in the apparent onset of F_1. Voiceless stops may have F_1 cutback or a delay in F_1 relative to the higher formants. Fundamental frequency can also be a cue: the fundamental frequency for a vowel portion of the speech waveform tends to be higher for vowels following voiceless stops than for vowels following voiced stops. The relative perceptual significance of these cues may vary with speaker and utterance. Forrest and Rockman (1988) examined the acoustic cues of voicing for children with phonological disorders and concluded that a number of different cues contribute to the listener's decisions about voicing for word-initial stops.

Stops in medial position also have multiple cues that signal voicing, including voice bar (for voiced stops), fundamental frequency (higher in vowels following voiceless stops), and closure duration for the stop (longer for voiceless stops).

SUMMARY Clearly, stop consonants are not associated with an invariant sequence of acoustic cues. Features such as silence, burst, and aspiration are variably evident in acoustic analysis. However, in general, syllable-initial stops have the following sequence of acoustic cues: silence, burst, aspiration (voiceless stops only), transition. Stops in medial position often will have the same cues but also may have another transition leading into the silence, so that the cue sequence is transition, silence, burst, aspiration, transition. Stops in final position typically have the cue

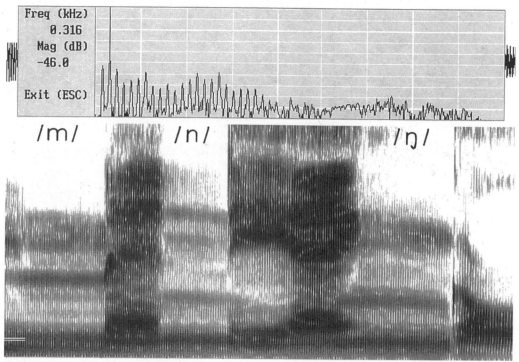

```
Freq (kHz)
   0.316
Mag (dB)
  -46.0

Exit (ESC)
```

/m/   /n/   /ŋ/

FIGURE 5-18   Nasal consonants. The spectrogram in the lower part of the figure shows /m n ŋ/ in the context of the phrase "many angles." The top of the figure shows a fast Fourier transform spectrum for the /n/.

sequence of transition, silence, burst (optional), aspiration (optional).

Nasal Consonants

Phonemes: /m n ŋ/.

  Key words: /m/—sum, /n/—sun, /ŋ/—sung.

  Phonetic features: Manner—nasal; Place—bilabial, alveolar, or velar.

  Acoustic cues: murmur and transitions.

Figure 5-18 shows a spectrogram of the three English nasal consonants as they appear in the phrase "many angles." The **fast Fourier transform (FFT)** spectrum at the top of the figure shows the frequency distribution in /n/.

Murmur, or nasal murmur, is the acoustic pattern associated with nasal radiation of acoustic energy. The spectrum of the murmur is dominated by low-frequency energy, often less than 0.5 kHz for men speakers. Although higher energy can be present, it is greatly attenuated compared with the low-frequency energy band. This is shown in the spectrum of Figure 5-18, where the spectral peak for /n/ occurs at 0.316 kHz. This band reflects the nasal formant, or the

resonance associated with the resonating cavity that extends from the larynx to the nares. Although the murmurs of the three nasal consonants are not exactly alike, the acoustic differences among them may not be perceptually distinctive for all speakers and conditions. Murmur is probably most effective as a manner cue signaling nasal resonance.

The spectrum of a murmur reflects a combination of formants and antiformants in the transfer function. In addition, the acoustic transmission tends to be heavily damped, owing to both the long distance of sound travel and the absorptive nature of the tissues lining the nasal cavities.

Transitions are the result of oral articulations for the nasal consonant. For example, if the nasal is both preceded and followed by a vowel, then both nasal + vowel and vowel + nasal formant transitions will be evident. The general shape of the transitions is very much like that for a homorganic stop. That is, the transitions are similar for the stop-nasal pairs /b/—/m/, /d/—/n/, and /g/—/ŋ/. (See the description of stops for information on formant transitions.) Formant

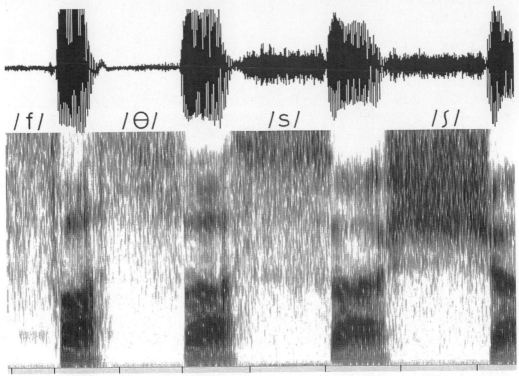

/f/   /θ/   /s/   /ʃ/

FIGURE 5-19 Waveform and spectrogram of voiceless fricatives in the context /fʌ θʌ sʌ ʃʌ/.

transitions, then, are cues for place of articulation.

Voicing is always present for nasals except in whispered speech. Therefore, voicing is the source of acoustic energy for nasals in English.

SUMMARY Nasal consonants typically are associated with a sequence of murmur and transitions. Perceptual experiments show that the murmur and transition cues are integrated in the identification of nasals.

Fricative Consonants

Phonemes: Voiced /v ð z ʒ/ and voiceless /f θ s ʃ h/.

Key words: /v/—van, /ð/—this, /z/—zip, /ʒ/—rouge, /f/—fan, /θ/—thin, /s/—sip, /ʃ/—ship, /h/—hip.

Phonetic features: Manner—fricative or frication; Place—labiodental, linguadental, linguaalveolar, linguapalatal, glottal.

Acoustic cues: Frication (noise) and transitions. Voicing also is a cue, especially in distinguishing the voiced-voiceless cognates /v f/, /ð θ/, /z s/, and /ʒ ʃ/. Figure 5-19 shows a waveform (top) and **spectrogram** (bottom) of the four

voiceless English fricatives in the context of the nonsense syllables /fʌ θʌ sʌ ʃʌ/.

Frication is noise energy. As discussed earlier, noise is generated as air is forced through a narrow constriction. Once turbulence is generated, the noise energy is subjected to filtering by the vocal tract. This filtering is imposed by the cavity in front of the constriction and in certain conditions by the cavity behind the constriction. The contribution of the back cavity depends primarily on the geometry of the vocal tract constriction. There is no single widely accepted spectral index for frication noise. One of the more frequently used descriptions is in terms of the frequency region of primary noise energy, but such descriptions do not always satisfy a reliability criterion. The following summary by place of articulation describes the salient spectral properties of the fricatives.

Labiodental: low-energy, diffuse spectrum. The front cavity is short and therefore has relatively little effect in shaping the noise energy. The second moment of the spectrum tends to be large, reflecting the diffuseness of the spectrum.

Linguadental: low-energy, diffuse spectrum. The short front cavity has relatively little shaping effect, which contributes to the overall

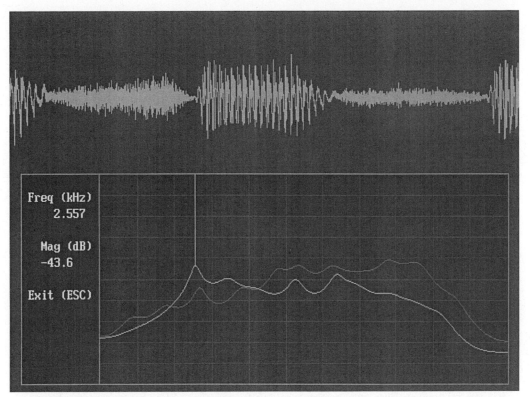

FIGURE 5-20 Waveform and contrasting spectra for the fricatives in /sʌ/ and /ʃʌ/. The vertical marker indicates the relatively low frequency peak for the linguapalatal fricative /s/. The bolder line represents the /ʃ/.

spectral flatness. The second moment tends to be large.

Linguaalveolar: intense noise with most energy in the high frequencies (above 4 kHz for adult male speakers, or above the F_4 frequency average of the speaker's vowels). The front cavity is long enough to introduce a significant resonance. With respect to spectral moments, linguaalveolars tend to have a high mean and a marked skewness, the latter reflecting the dominance of high-frequency energy.

Linguapalatal: intense noise with most energy in the mid to high frequencies (above 2 kHz, or above the F_3 frequency average of the speaker's vowels). The front cavity has a significant resonance effect. The spectral mean is lower than that for the linguaalveolar fricatives.

Glottal: low-energy diffuse noise. The vocal tract as a whole shapes the noise energy, and vowel-like formant patterns can be apparent in the radiated noise. The second spectral moment tends to be large, similar to that for labiodentals and linguadentals.

Figure 5-20 exemplifies the spectral contrast in linguaalveolar and linguapalatal fricatives. The waveform at the top of the figure shows the

sound pressure variations for /s/, followed by /ʃ/. Clearly the overall energy level is higher for /s/. In the spectra at the bottom of the figure, the lighter line shows the spectrum for /ʃ/, with the vertical marker at a relatively low frequency resonance peak (2.557 kHz). The darker line shows the spectrum for /s/, with relatively greater amplitude in the high frequencies (above 4500 Hz).

Transitions occur for fricative consonants much as they do for other consonants. Whenever the oral articulation changes, the change can be reflected as bends in the formant pattern. As with the stops and nasals discussed earlier, the formant transitions are a cue for place of articulation.

Voicing for fricatives is described phonetically in terms of a binary contrast. The expectation is that voiced fricatives will have the quasi-periodic energy of voicing in addition to the noise energy generated at the constriction. Voiceless fricatives will have the noise energy only. This simple expectation does not always conform to reality, especially for fricatives that follow vowels. The voicing cue for postvocalic fricatives can be the duration of the preceding

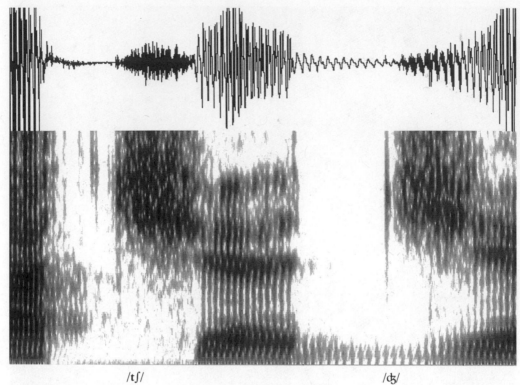

FIGURE 5-21 Waveform and spectrogram for affricates/tʃ/ and /dʒ/, in the context of the phrase "I gotcha, Jerry."

vowel, and as Denes (1955) has shown, both the voiced and voiceless fricatives in word pairs such as *use* (verb) and *use* (noun) can be acoustically voiceless. The longer duration of the vowel preceding a voiced fricative can signal the voicing feature.

SUMMARY Fricatives typically involve the acoustic cues of transition and frication, but the relative importance of the cues varies among the fricatives. The fricatives categorized as sibilants or stridents have intense noise energy, and the noise segment alone is usually sufficient for fricative identification. The fricatives categorized as nonsibilants or nonstridents have weak noise energy, which may not be sufficient for their identification. Transition information may be important for the perception of these weaker sounds. Fricatives can be either voiced or voiceless, and although the acoustic cues for voicing are not as complex as those for stops, the presence or absence of vocal fold vibration is not the only cue to be recognized. Duration of a vowel preceding a fricative can be an important and perhaps sufficient cue for fricative voicing.

Affricate Consonants

Phonemes: voiced /dʒ/ and voiceless /tʃ/.

Key words: /dʒ/—gin, /tʃ/—chin.

Phonetic features: Manner—fricative and stop; Place—linguapalatal.

Acoustic cues: Stop gap (silence or low-energy interval) and frication. Affricates are described phonetically as combination sounds because they combine the features of a stop consonant with those of a fricative. Figure 5-21 shows a waveform and spectrogram of an excerpt from the phrase "I gotcha, Jerry!" illustrating the two English affricates.

Silence, or low-energy interval, is the consequence of articulatory closure. This interval is similar to the stop gap that occurs for stop consonants. For voiceless /tʃ/, this interval may be genuinely silent in the sense that there is no radiation of acoustic energy. The voiced /dʒ/ usually will have low-frequency energy, or the so-called voice bar. This is evident in the waveform and spectrogram of the example in Figure 5-21. Depending on its position in an utterance, the affricate's stop gap may blend with preceding silences such as pauses. Therefore, the stop gap may not be

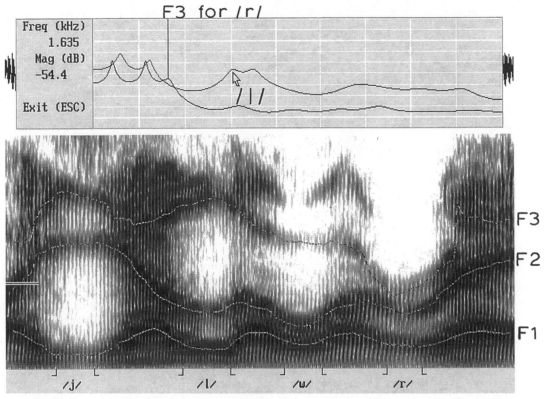

FIGURE 5-22 Spectrogram of liquids /l,r/ and glides /w,j/ in the phrase "a yellow array." The spectra at the top show differences in F₃ for /l/ (high, as indicated by the arrow) and /r/ (low, as indicated by the vertical marker). The formant tracks are highlighted for F₁, F₂, and F₃.

well defined as a discrete event in acoustic analyses.

Frication is generated in essentially the same way as for fricatives. The spectral energy for /ʤ/ and /tʃ/ is similar to that for /ʒ/ and /ʃ/. One difference may lie in the amplitude envelope of the noise energy. The affricates have been reported to have a relatively rapid increase in noise energy, or in other words, a short rise time. Fricatives have a relatively slow increase in noise energy, or a long rise time. The perceptual significance of this difference in noise rise time has been questioned (Kluender and Walsh, 1992). Because the frication interval is quite intense, noise energy is a salient feature of affricates, providing information on both place and manner of articulation. Possibly the fricatives /ʒ/ and /ʃ/ are distinguishable from the affricates /ʤ/ and /tʃ/ solely on the basis of the duration of the noise interval (Kluender and Walsh, 1992). The fricatives tend to have longer noise intervals.

Transition cues arise as the consonant articulation is released into a following sound, especially a vowel. See Table 5-1 for general information on formant loci.

SUMMARY Frication probably is the most reliable and effective cue and may be sufficient to signal both place information from noise spectrum and manner information from duration of noise. However, affricates should be understood as sounds with an essentially two-phase pattern of production. Both the stop gap and frication intervals figure into the temporal structure of affricates.

Glide Consonants

Phonemes: /j/ and /w/.

Key words: /j/—yet, /w/—wet.

Phonetic features: Manner—glide or semivowel; Place—palatal or labiovelar.

Acoustic cues: A gradual transition manifest acoustically as gliding formant transition. Although a steady-state formant pattern is possible, such an event is rare in conversational speech. Figure 5-22 presents a spectrogram showing both glides and **liquids** in the phrase "a yellow array."

Transition is the hallmark cue. The formant transitions typically have a duration of about 75

TABLE 5-3 Primary acoustic cues for various consonants in syllable-initial prevocalic position

	Bilabial	Labiodental	Linguadental
Stop	[b] [p] F_1 increases F_2 increases Burst has flat or falling spectrum		
Nasal	[m] F_1 increases F_2 increases Nasal murmur		
Fricative		[v] [f] F_1 increases F_2 increases except for some back vowels Noise segment has weak and flat spectrum	[ð] [θ] F_1 increases F_2 increases except for some back vowels Noise segment has weak and flat spectrum
Glide	[w] F_1 increases F_2 increases		

to 150 ms, compared with a duration of about 50 to 75 ms for stop transitions. Therefore, duration of transition is a distinguishing property of these two classes of sounds. For both /w/ and /j/, the first-formant frequency begins at a very low value, slightly above that typical for stops. It then rises to the first-formant frequency of the following sound (according to some phonetic descriptions of English, glides always are followed by vowels). The second- and third-formant frequencies have different onsets or loci for the two glides. For adult males /w/ has F_2 and F_3 loci of about 800 Hz and 2200 Hz, respectively. The F_2 and F_3 loci for /j/ are about 2200 Hz and 3000 Hz, respectively. Thus, the F_2 and F_3 transitions are defined by shifts in frequency toward the F_2 and F_3 values of the following vowel.

Liquid Consonants

Phonemes: Lateral /l/ and rhotic /r/.
   Key words: /l/ — lay, /r/ — ray.
   Phonetic features: Manner — lateral or rhotic; Place — linguaalveolar for /l/, palatal for /r/.
   Acoustic cues: Formant pattern, steady state and transition. The steady state is sometimes present.

Steady-state formant pattern is the set of formants (and for /l/, antiformants) that characterize a prolonged /l/ or /r/ sound. Although the steady state may not be evident in all productions of these speech sounds, it is helpful to describe it to gain an appreciation of the acoustic structures of the liquids.

Because /l/ is produced with a divided vocal tract, with radiation of sound energy on either side of the midline tongue closure, it has a complex filter function composed of formants and antiformants. The energy is primarily in the low frequencies, so much so that /l/ resembles the nasal /n/ in spectrograms. The steady-state formant values for /l/ are approximately as follows: 360 Hz for F_1, 1300 Hz for F_2, and 2700 Hz for F_3. Liquid /r/ has similar steady-state frequencies for F_1 and F_2 but a much lower F_3 frequency, about 1600 Hz. A low F_3 frequency is an important characteristic of rhotic sounds, both consonants and vowels. The spectra at the top of Figure 5-22 contrast the frequency distributions for /r/ and /l/. The arrow points to the high F_3 for /l/ (about 3 kHz). The vertical marker shows the low F_3 (1.635 kHz) for /r/.

The steady-state formant patterns can be taken as onset patterns for the liquids. The formant frequencies then change directions ac-

Linguaalveolar	Linguapalatal	Linguavelar	Glottal
[d] [t] F_1 increases F_2 decreases except for high-front vowels Burst has rising spectrum		[g] [k] F_1 increases F_2 increases or decreases Wedge-shaped F_2-F_3 Burst has mid- frequency spectrum	[ʔ] Little formant change
[n] F_1 increases F_2 decreases except for high-front vowels Nasal murmur		[ŋ] F_1 increases F_2 increases or decreases Nasal murmur	
[z] [s] F_1 increases F_2 decreases except for high-front vowels Noise segment has intense, high- frequency (above 4 kHz) spectrum	[ʒ] [ʃ] F_1 increases F_2 increases or decreases Noise segment has intense, high- frequency (above 3 kHz) spectrum		[h] Little formant change Noise segment has weak and flat spectrum
	[j] F_1 increases F_2 decreases		

Formant transitions are described as increasing or decreasing in frequency during the consonant-to-vowel transition.

cording to the following sound. The formant transitions often are shorter for /l/ than /r/, especially for F_1. Productions of /r/ are often conspicuous in spectrograms by virtue of the marked changes in F_3 frequency between /r/ segments and neighboring sounds.

Summary of Place Cues for Consonants

Table 5-3 summarizes the major cues for place of consonant articulation by manner of articulation categories.

SUPRASEGMENTAL FEATURES OF SPEECH

In Chapter 6 Lehiste describes **suprasegmental features**, or prosody, of speech as properties of speech sounds or their sequences that are simultaneous with and that modify the segmental, or phonetic, features in a manner that does not change the distinctive phonetic quality but that may change the meaning of the utterance.

Kent and Read (1992, p. 152) indicate that prosody is

. . . not merely the melodic and rhythmic

decoration of language . . . prosody might be regarded as the fabric of speech, within which segments are the individual stitches or fibers. Prosodic patterns span the linguistic levels, holding together the many influences that make up the rich tapestry of language in context. Prosody serves essential, if sometimes subtle, functions in communication, and its acoustic foundations are no less important in the speech signal than those which distinguish segments.

Thus, suprasegmental or prosodic features are not confined to phonetic segments but instead are frequently described in terms of larger units overlaid or superimposed on syllables, words, phrases, and sentences. The suprasegmental features of a language can reveal speakers' feelings and attitudes in a manner that **segmental features** alone cannot achieve.

The suprasegmental features of English are conveyed by the acoustic parameters of fundamental frequency (perceived as pitch), intensity (perceived as loudness), and duration. Among the suprasegmentals to be discussed here are intonation, stress, and quantity. (For a more detailed discussion of suprasegmentals, see Chapter 6.)

Intonation

Intonation (i.e., changes in vocal fundamental frequency, or f_o, perceived as the intonation contour or pitch pattern of a phrase or sentence) can be used to express differences in the speaker's meaning. It is "... the linguistically significant functioning of fundamental frequency at the sentence level" (Lehiste, Chapter 6). For example, "It's going to rain today" spoken with a rising intonation (increasing perceived vocal pitch during the production of "today") converts a declarative statement to a question. Conversely, a grammatically constructed question can be converted to a declarative statement by means of the appropriate intonation contour (e.g., "Is he a good golfer," produced so as to convey confidence in the subject's golf game). In addition, variations in intonation can vary the meaning of a sentence (e.g., "What a great idea!") from a positive to a negative assessment (sarcasm). Intonation patterns can be imposed on a sentence, a phrase, and even a word (where it is called *tone*).

American English is characterized by a rise-fall intonation curve (i.e., a declining f_o) for declarative sentences (with the pitch rising during the first part of an utterance and falling at the end), and an end-of-utterance pitch rise for questions and incomplete sentences. Figure 5-23 illustrates rise-fall (A) and end-of-utterance pitch rise (B) intonation contours.

The physiological correlate of intonation involves the rate of vibration of the vocal folds. While this analysis is not universally accepted, a rising intonation curve is considered by some to be the result primarily of increased subglottal pressure causing the vocal folds to vibrate more rapidly. Conversely, according to this theory, a falling intonation curve results from a decreased rate of vocal fold vibration caused by a decrease in subglottal pressure characteristically present at the end of a breath group (Lieberman, 1967). In fact, decreased subglottal pressure accounts for the decrease in f_o and intensity found at the end of a declarative sentence. However, the nature of this f_o declination, also called *downdrift,* is an unresolved issue (Cohen, Collier, and 't Hart, 1982). Some consider this linear f_o declination as a universal property of spoken language, with f_o falling gradually and linearly throughout a sentence ('t Hart and Cohen, 1973; 't Hart and Collier, 1975; Maeda, 1976; Sorensen and Cooper, 1980; Vaissiere, 1983; Thorsen, 1985) . However, others disagree with this linear declination hypothesis, particularly in spontaneous speech (Lieberman, Katz, Jongman, Zimmerman, and Miller, 1985).

Evidence of this linear f_o declination as a universal property of spoken language comes from numerous studies. For example, Thorsen (1985) investigated intonation patterns in four standard Danish speakers' recordings of declarative sentences. Based on acoustic analysis of the recordings, she found that standard Danish intonation contours in declarative sentences agree with those in other languages, including English and Swedish. Each declarative sentence in a read text was found to be associated with its own declining intonation contour. Moreover, all three languages manifest a superordinate text intonation structure upon which individual sentences are superimposed. Thus, there is a more coherent, less segregated intonational structure.

An alternative theory, a breath-group theory, proposes that f_o in the nonterminal portion of a declarative sentence varies, while the terminal portion usually shows a rapid decline in f_o (Lieberman, 1967). This theory has been supported by the findings of Umeda (1982), who showed that declination of f_o depends on the speaking situation, with the f_o pattern becoming more complex as the contextual information increases in complexity. Further support for this view comes from evidence that f_o and intensity declination at the end of a breath group constitute an important acoustic cue for syntactic structure (Pierrehumbert, 1979; Landahl, 1980; Lieberman and Tseng, 1981; Lieberman, Katz, Jongman, Zimmerman, and Miller, 1985). For a review of these issues, see Gussenhoven and Rietveld, 1988.

In addition to marking syntactic contrasts (i.e., phrase endings and interrogative versus declarative statements) and changing linguistic meaning, intonation also conveys nonlinguistic meanings; that is, it is used to convey attitudes and feelings. Affect (attitude, mood, emotion) can strongly affect intonation. States of excitement are commonly accompanied by large intonation shifts, and calm, subdued states manifest a narrow range of intonation variation.

Stress

Stress is the degree of force of an utterance. It is a complex feature that may involve several interacting phenomena. Moreover, there is no one physiological mechanism to which the

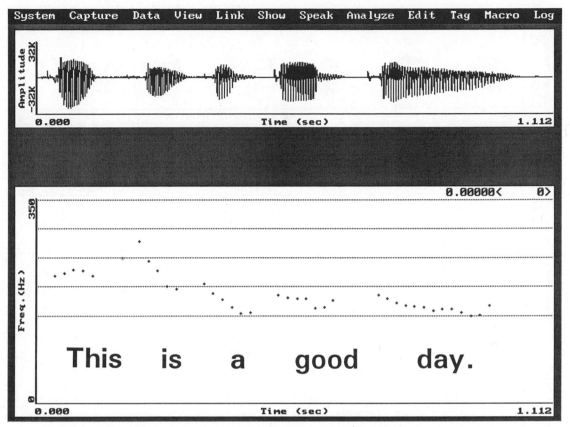

FIGURE 5-23   *A*, Waveform (upper illustration) and fundamental frequency contour (lower illustration) showing the rise-fall intonation contour for a declarative sentence, produced by a young adult female speaker (Kay Elemetrics Corp. Communication Science Lab Model 4300).

production of stress can be attributed as, for example, f_o can be attributed to the rate of vocal fold vibration. Whether lexical or contrastive, stress involves all three acoustic parameters of intensity, duration, and fundamental frequency. However, there is no one-to-one correspondence between stress and any single acoustic parameter (Beckman, 1986; Terken, 1991).

The acoustic characteristics associated with stressed syllables are increases in vocal f_o, duration, and intensity (Table 5-4) (Fry, 1955, 1958; Lieberman, 1960; Lehiste, 1970), while a change in f_o is the most reliable cue for prosodic stress (Bolinger, 1958; Currie, 1980, 1981; Cooper, Eady, and Mueller, 1985). The higher f_o is a result of increased tension on the vocal folds. The increased laryngeal effort may be accompanied by increased respiratory effort, which will raise subglottal pressure, hence f_o. In addition, it will displace the vocal folds farther from their rest position, leading to a rise in vocal intensity

that is often associated with stressed syllables. Furthermore, the longer duration of stressed syllables indicates that more muscular effort, particularly articulatory effort, is involved in stressed than unstressed syllables. This increase in duration allows the articulators more time to reach their target positions in the oral cavity for vowels in stressed syllables, as indicated by the formant frequencies of stressed vowels. Segments in stressed syllables usually manifest larger articulatory movements than segments in unstressed syllables and an acoustically distinctive formant pattern resembling the target pattern for a vowel produced in isolation (i.e., articulatory achievement of target position). This acoustic distinctiveness decreases in vowels in unstressed syllables that manifest the effects of not reaching their target positions, a phenomenon called **articulatory undershooting.** Thus, stress also alters segmental properties such as consonantal and vowel articulation (Kent and Netsell, 1971; de Jong, 1991).

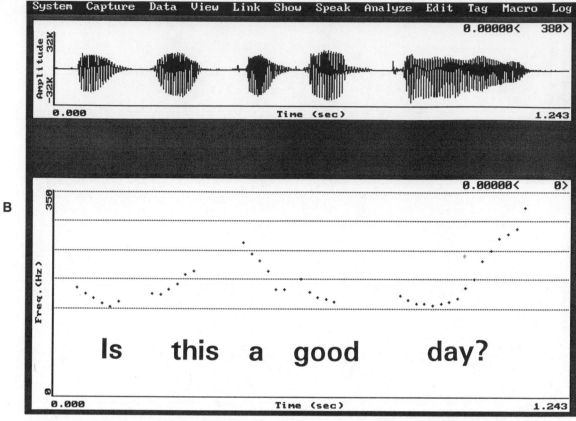

FIGURE 5-23   *B*, Waveform (upper illustration) and fundamental frequency contour (lower illustration) showing the end-of-utterance pitch rise intonation contour for a question produced by a young adult female speaker. (Kay Elemetrics Corp. Communication Science Lab Model 4300).

TABLE 5-4   Vowel durations and intensities of 12 speakers' productions of the word "object" produced with: (*A*) stress on the first syllable and (*B*) stress on the second syllable. (From Fry, 1955).

Vowel Durations				Vowel Intensities			
A		B		A		B	
OBject		obJECT		OBject		obJECT	
V1	V2	V1	V2	V1	V2	V1	V2
(seconds)		(seconds)		(decibels)		(decibels)	
0.12	0.09	0.05	0.16	15	9	5	12
0.14	0.13	0.07	0.13	20	12	6	11
0.16	0.15	0.07	0.16	16	8	7	12
0.17	0.10	0.05	0.19	16	11	9	13
0.13	0.11	0.04	0.20	15	3	3	9
0.13	0.09	0.06	0.14	18	14	6	12
0.14	0.15	0.09	0.18	18	15	11	16
0.15	0.08	0.05	0.19	15	6	3	15
0.19	0.12	0.02	0.19	18	11	4	15
0.18	0.15	0.06	0.18	14	4	12	15
0.17	0.14	0.06	0.18	12	6	15	18
0.16	0.15	0.07	0.16	13	7	12	12

Stress also functions at the word level as a pointer to contrast lexical meaning by highlighting the most important syllables. For two-syllable orthographically identical words in English, verbs and nouns are differentiated primarily by the placement of stress. For example, the word "con'·vict," with stress on the first syllable, is a noun referring to a person who has been found guilty of a crime, while the word "con·vict'," with stress on the second syllable, is a verb describing the process of finding one guilty of a crime. For polysyllabic words there is a tendency to include a secondary stress for verbs (pre'·di·cate') but to abandon the secondary stress for nouns (pre'·di·cate).

In addition to lexical stress, contrastive stress can occur in English on almost any word, phrase, or clause that the speaker intends to contrast with another, either stated or implied. For example, "This is *her* house" is uttered when the speaker may believe that the listener incorrectly said or thinks that the house belongs to someone else.

Stress appears to be judged in terms of effort. Greater effort will produce more perceived stress, provided all other factors are kept constant (see Chapter 6). The more stress intended for a syllable, the more effort will be expended in producing the syllable. In addition, stress involves knowledge of the language in which the utterance is spoken and presupposes a certain amount of learning (see Chapter 6). Experiments have shown that the perception of stress does not have simple and direct representations in the acoustic signal, and while fundamental frequency, intensity, and duration all contribute to stress perception, they do not do so equally (Bolinger, 1958; Fry, 1958), nor is this differential effect true for all languages (Bertinetto, 1980; Eek, 1987; Lehiste and Fox, 1992).

In a series of experiments on the perception of stress, Fry (1958) synthesized speech stimuli in which the parameters of f_o, intensity, and duration could be controlled and varied over a considerable range for the construction of listening tests. He found that (1) both duration and intensity are cues in stress judgments and (2) the direction of a step change of f_o had a strong effect on stress judgments, but the magnitude of the f_o change had no such effect.

Quantity

Quantity is the contrastive function of duration within a phonological system. An understanding of this prosodic feature rests on an understanding of the intrinsic duration of segments as well as the effect of preceding and following phonemes on segmental duration. Spectrographic analyses have shown that speech sounds vary in their intrinsic duration. For example, diphthongs have longer durations than vowels, and continuant consonants (fricatives, semivowels, and nasals) are longer than stop plosives. Furthermore, the duration of vowels correlates with the height of the tongue in the oral cavity. In English, other variables being equal, low vowels have longer duration than high vowels (Peterson and Lehiste, 1960). The intrinsic duration of consonants is affected by their place as well as manner of production. For example, voiceless fricatives are longer than other consonants (Crystal and House, 1988).

Contextual effects also influence duration. For example, while the influence of a preceding consonant on vowel duration is negligible, the nature of the consonant that follows a vowel can strongly influence the vowel's duration. Thus, in English the duration of a vowel that precedes a voiced consonant (e.g., "seed", "leave") is approximately 1.5 times that of the same vowel preceding a voiceless consonant (e.g., "seat", "leaf") (Peterson and Lehiste, 1960; Kluender, Diehl, and Wright, 1988) (Fig. 5-24). Moreover, vowels are longer in duration when they appear before continuants (e.g., "sieve") than before stop plosives (e.g., "seap"). These differences in duration before voiced and voiceless consonants, while present in different languages, appear to be especially pronounced in English, suggesting a learned phenomenon in addition to physiologically based conditioning.

Although these intrinsic durational variations are not contrastive in English, they can be cues for the identification of particular sounds. For example, the duration of one segment can signal the presence or absence of a feature (e.g., voicing) in another segment (see Chapter 6).

The function of the prosodic feature of quantity at the sentence level is considerably different from its function at the word level. While changes in the relative durations of linguistic units in words can change their meaning, durational changes of linguistic units within a sentence (i.e., considerable changes in the tempo of speech from a neutral rate of articulation) can be used to convey information about the speaker's mood or about the circumstances surrounding the utterance (see Chapter 6).

Quantity interacts with other suprasegmental

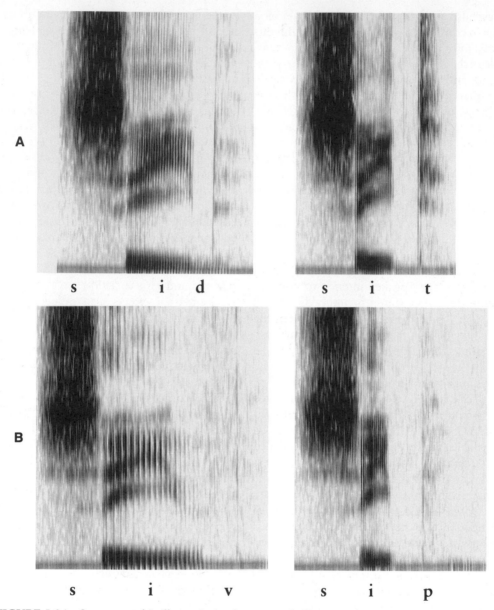

FIGURE 5-24 Spectrographic illustrations of contextual effects on phoneme durations. *A,* The duration of a vowel that precedes a voiced consonant (as in *seed)* is greater than the duration of the same vowel preceding a voiceless consonant (as in *seat*). *B,* Vowels are longer in duration when they appear before continuants as in *sieve* than before stop plosives (as in *seap*).

features of speech in various ways. For example, duration and f_o cue stress in English. In addition, duration is one of the mechanisms used to signal word boundaries. As Lehiste (1960) has shown in minimal word pairs with essentially identical segmental sequences (e.g., "white shoes–why choose"), duration is the most important phonetic cue signaling the word boundary. The diphthong [aI] in the first word of "white shoes" is relatively short because it is followed by a voiceless consonant ([t]) within the same syllable; the first word in "why choose" has no

final consonant and instead ends in a diphthong, making the diphthong in "why" much longer than the same diphthong in "white."

Duration also signals phrase and sentence boundaries (Lehiste, 1980). Spectrographic analysis of sentences reveals that the last syllable of a word or the last word of a phrase or sentence is longer in duration than the same syllable or word in other than final position (Fig. 5-25).

Quantity also is important at the syntactic level, as illustrated in phrase-final lengthening in

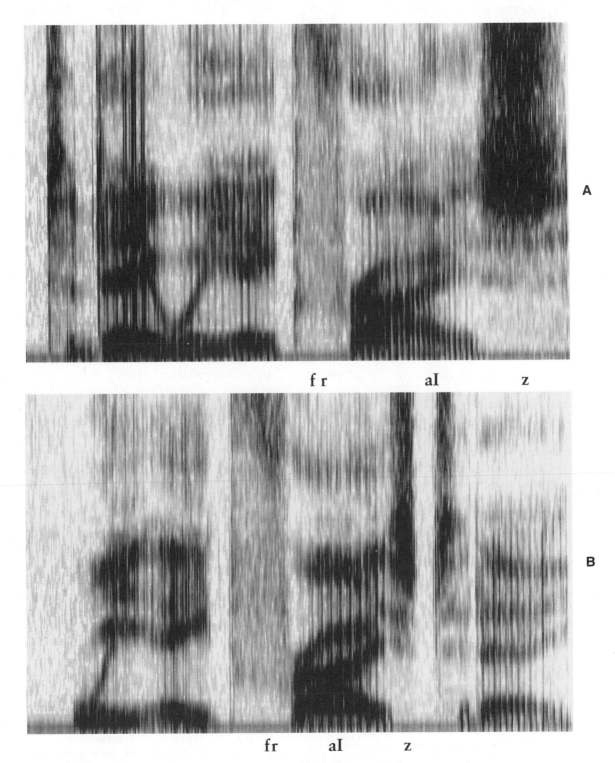

FIGURE 5-25   Spectrographic illustrations of the effect of position of words in phrases and sentences on their duration. The word *fries* is longer in duration in *A*, "Today we ate fries" than in *B*, "We ate fries today."

which the last stressable syllable in a phrase or clause is lengthened. For example:

"Hot dogs, popcorn, and peanuts are sold at baseball games"

"Peanuts, popcorn, and hot dogs are sold at baseball games"

The first syllable of "peanuts" will be longer in the first than in the second sentence because in the first sentence this word is at the end of the subject noun phrase. (Note: although "peanuts" has two syllables, only the first one can be stressed.) In addition, the word "games" will be longer in duration in both sentences than if it appeared in the middle of a phrase (Klatt, 1976). It has been shown that listeners use phrase-final lengthening to recognize the structure of spoken sentences (Read and Schreiber, 1982).

Juncture, a prosodic feature related to duration, is concerned with the manner in which sounds are joined to or separated from each other. Junctural variations affect lexical meanings in English. For example, the distinction between "I'm eating" and "I'm meeting" is junctural. If the speaker articulates so that the [m] is more closely linked to the preceding diphthong [aɪ] than to the following vowel [i], then "I'm eating" will be produced and perceived. However, "I'm meeting" will result if the [m] is joined to the [i] and disjoined from the preceding diphthong.

In summary, acoustic and perceptual studies of speech have revealed the importance of f_o, intensity, and duration in conveying the suprasegmental (prosodic) features of English. However, although intonation, stress, and quantity are perceived principally by contrasts and variations in pitch, loudness, and/or length, which are determined by the acoustic parameters of f_o, intensity, and duration, respectively, there is a need to distinguish between the perception of these suprasegmental features and their acoustic parameters because they do not have direct linear representations in the acoustic signal but rather rely on the degree of variation and covariation of a number of acoustic variables. As Kent and Read (1992, p. 152) conclude:

> When one contemplates the possible interactions of all . . . sources of prosodic variation, one cannot wonder that prosody is generally less well understood than segment structure. We can describe quite well . . . the formant structure of the vowel [a], but we have scarcely begun to describe the prosodic differences between using that vowel as an exclamation of sudden discovery ("Ah!") and

as listener's interjection, warning the speaker that something controversial or offensive is about to be said.

UNRESOLVED ISSUES

Swift progress in the acoustic analysis of speech has resulted in the development of high-quality speech synthesis, machine speech recognition, and analyses of speech produced by normal adult talkers, children who are acquiring speech, and some individuals who have speech, hearing, or language disorders. Unresolved issues include some very old problems as well as some new problems associated with advances in acoustic analysis and its applications. Some of these issues are as follows:

Speaker (vocal tract) **normalization,** or the adjustment of acoustic data to cancel differences associated with vocal tract size, remains a challenge. Although a variety of algorithms have been proposed, no one of them rivals the capability of the human listener to recognize sounds produced by different speakers.

Automatic speech recognition, or the ability to build machines that understand speech, has been an area of dramatic progress. However, much work remains before speech recognition systems will be as robust as the ordinary human in perceiving speech. Some researchers question whether machines will ever come close to humans in this respect.

Acoustic description of different voices, including vocal pathologies, entails the use of acoustic methods to derive quantitative descriptions of normal or disordered voices. Only limited success has been attained in the effort to develop acoustic profiles that capture the differences among voices. On a larger scale, the same problem pertains to the acoustic description of different *speech* (voice plus articulation) patterns, including dialects and speech disorders. Clinical specialists would benefit from an analysis system that provided automatic derivation or an efficient set of speech and voice descriptors.

Inference of the articulatory patterns underlying acoustic signals of speech has as its goal the derivation of physiological information from analyses of the acoustic signal, particularly a portrayal of the vocal tract configurations that correspond to major segments in the acoustic pattern. This difficult problem has not yet been solved with sufficient generality to permit widespread application.

Reconciling differences in acoustic patterns for speech sounds produced in different conditions addresses the fact that speech sounds perceived to be the same phonetically are often quite variable in their acoustic representation. Differences arise because of variations in phonetic context, speaking rate, stress, emotional character of the utterance, and the effort that the speaker gives to an individual production.

Integrating segmental and suprasegmental information requires that acoustic characteristics for these two aspects of speech organization be combined into a systematic framework. Research has identified some basic principles, but the knowledge in this area is far from complete.

Expanding the acoustic database to include information on children and women is an area of recent progress. However, more data are needed on women speakers and children of both genders. Acoustic theories of speech may need to be revised to take these new data into account.

For further discussion of these unresolved issues, see Chapters 7, 11, and 13 of this volume, as well as Pickett (1980), Fujimura (1990), and Kent and Read (1992).

SUMMARY

The study of the acoustic signal of speech has yielded a large amount of information. Only some of the most general aspects of this knowledge have been summarized in this chapter. The discussion has included two major topics: (1) the acoustic theory of speech production and (2) the acoustic characteristics of the sounds in American English. A general understanding of these two topics is the key to more detailed information and to more sophisticated applications of the acoustic method. A large number of factors can influence the acoustic characteristics of a given sound, but the basic descriptions given in this chapter should be useful for the broad categorization of sounds into the phonemes of American English.

Review Questions

1. A young child, a woman, and a man all produce a vowel that listeners agree is the same vowel phonetically, for example, the vowel /i/ in *"he"*. Describe how the acoustic characteristics of this vowel are expected to vary among the three speakers. Consider especially the fundamental frequency and the formant frequencies.

2. Draw a sketch of the vocal tract and use this drawing to explain the acoustic theory of speech production described in this chapter.

3. Describe the source of energy for each of the following sounds: vowels, voiceless stops, and voiceless fricatives.

4. How is the acoustic theory of speech production for nonnasalized vowels modified to account for nasalized sounds?

5. What are the primary acoustic cues for the identification of stop consonants? Discuss how these cues relate to decisions about manner of production, place of articulation, and voicing.

6. How does a spectrogram represent the acoustic signal of speech? Draw some simple sketches to show the general spectrographic appearance of a vowel sound, an isolated fricative like /s/ in *see,* and a stop + vowel sequence in a word such as *bee.*

7. List distinguishing acoustic properties for the following classes of sounds: stops, fricatives, affricates, nasals, and liquids.

8. What are the primary acoustic parameters associated with the suprasegmental features of intonation, stress, and quantity in English?

References

Beckman, M. E. (1986). *Stress and non-stress accent.* Riverton, USA: Foris.

von Békésy, G. (1960). *Experiments in hearing.* New York: McGraw-Hill.

Bertinetto, P. M. (1980). The perception of stress by Italian speakers. *Journal of Phonetics, 8,* 385-395.

Bladon, A. (1983). Two-formant models of vowel perception: Shortcomings and enhancements. *Speech Communication, 2,* 305-313.

Blumstein, S. E., & Stevens, K. N. (1979). Acoustic invariance in speech production: Evidence from measurements of the spectral characteristics of stop consonants. *Journal of the Acoustical Society of America, 66,* 1001-1017.

Bolinger, D. L. (1958). A theory of pitch accent in English. *Word, 14,* 109-149.

Carlson, R., Fant, G., & Granstrom, B. (1975). Two-formant models, pitch and vowel perception. In Fant, G., & Tatham, M.A.A. (Eds.), *Auditory Analysis and Perception of Speech.* London: Academic Press (pp. 55-82).

Cohen, A., Collier, R., & 't Hart, J. (1982). Declination: Construct or intrinsic feature of speech pitch? *Phonetica, 39,* 254-273.

Cooper, W. E., Eady, S. J., & Mueller, P. R. (1985). Acoustical aspects of contrastive stress in question-answer contexts. *Journal of the Acoustical Society of America, 77,* 2142-2156.

Crystal, T. H., & House, A. S. (1988). A note on the durations of fricatives in American English. *Journal of the Acoustical Society of America, 84,* 1932-1935.

Currie, K. L. (1980). An initial search for tonics. *Language and Speech, 23,* 329-350.

Currie, K.L. (1981). Further experiments in 'search for tonics.' *Language and Speech, 24,* 1-28.

Denes, P. (1955). Effect of duration on the perception of voicing. *Journal of the Acoustical Society of America, 27,* 761-764.

Eek, A. (1987). The perception of word stress: A comparison of Estonian and Russian. In Channon, R., & Shockey, L. (Eds.), *In honor of Ilse Lehiste.* Providence: Foris (pp. 19-32).

Fant, G. (1960). *Acoustic theory of speech production.* The Hague: Mouton.

Fant, G. (1973). *Speech sounds and features.* Cambridge, MA: MIT Press.

Fant, G. (1986). Glottal flow: Models and interactions. *Journal of Phonetics, 14,* 393-399.

Forrest, K., & Rockman, B. K. (1988). Acoustic and perceptual analyses of word-initial stop consonants in phonologically disordered children. *Journal of Speech and Hearing Research, 31,* 449-459.

Forrest, K., Weismer, G., Milenkovic, P., & Dougall, R. N. (1988). Statistical analysis of word-initial voiceless obstruents: Preliminary data. *Journal of the Acoustical Society of America, 84,* 115-123.

Fry, D. B. (1955). Duration and intensity as physical correlates of linguistic stress. *Journal of the Acoustical Society of America, 23,* 765-769.

Fry, D. B. (1958). Experiments in the perception of stress. *Language and Speech, 1,* 126-152.

Fujimura, O. (1961). Bilabial stop and nasal consonants: A motion picture study and its implications. *Journal of Speech and Hearing Research, 4,* 233-247.

Fujimura, O. (1990). Methods and goals of speech production research. *Language and Speech, 33,* 195-258.

Gussenhoven, C., & Rietveld, A. C. M. (1988). Fundamental frequency declincation in Dutch: Testing three hypotheses. *Journal of Phonetics, 16,* 355-369.

Halle, M., Hughes, G.W., & Radley, J.P. (1957). Acoustic properties of stop consonants. *Journal of the Acoustical Society of America, 29,* 107-116.

't Hart, J., & Cohen, A. (1973). Intonation by rule: A perceptual quest. *Journal of Phonetics, 1,* 309-327.

't Hart, J., & Collier, R. (1975). Integrating different levels of intonation analysis. *Journal of Phonetics, 3,* 235-256.

Heinz, J. M., & Stevens, K. N. (1961). On the properties of voiceless fricative consonants. *Journal of the Acoustical Society of America, 33,* 589-596.

de Jong, K. J. (1991). The oral articulation of English stress accent. Unpublished doctoral dissertation, Ohio State University.

Kent, R. D. (1993). Vocal tract acoustics. *Journal of Voice, 7,* 97-117.

Kent, R. D., & Netsell, R. (1971). Effects of stress contrasts on certain articulatory parameters. *Phonetica, 24,* 23-44.

Kent, R.D., & Read, C. (1992). *The acoustic analysis of speech.* San Diego: Singular.

Klatt, D. H. (1975). Voice onset time, frication and aspiration in word-initial consonant clusters. *Journal of Speech and Hearing Research, 18,* 686-706.

Klatt, D.H. (1976). Linguistic uses of segmental duration in English: Acoustic and perceptual evidence. *Journal of the Acoustical Society of America, 59,* 1208-1221.

Kluender, K.R., Diehl, R.L., & Wright, B.A. (1988). Vowel-length differences before voiced and voiceless consonants: An auditory explanation. *Journal of Phonetics, 16,* 153-169.

Kluender, K. R., & Walsh, M. A. (1992). Amplitude rise time and the perception of the voiceless affricate/fricative distinction. *Perception and Psychophysics, 51,* 328-333.

Landahl, K.H. (1980). Language-universal aspects of intonation to children's first sentences. *Journal of the Acoustical Society of America, 67* (Supplement 1), S63.

Lehiste, I. (1960). An acoustic-phonetic study of internal open juncture. *Phonetica, 5,* (Suppl.), 1-54.

Lehiste, I. (1970). *Suprasegmentals.* Cambridge, MA: MIT Press.

Lehiste, I. (1980). Phonetic manifestation of syntactic structure in English. *Annual Bulletin, Research Institute of Logopedics and Phoniatrics, University of Tokyo, 14,* 1-27.

Lehiste, I., & Fox, R. A. (1992). Perception of prominence by Estonian and English listeners. *Language and Speech, 35,* 419-434.

Lieberman, P. (1960). Some acoustic correlates of

word stress in American English. *Journal of the Acoustical Society of America, 22,* 451-454.

Lieberman, P. (1967). *Intonation, perception, and language.* Cambridge, MA: MIT Press.

Lieberman, P., Katz, W., Jongman, A., Zimmerman, R., & Miller, M. (1985). Measures of the sentence intonation of read and spontaneous speech in American English. *Journal of the Acoustical Society of America, 77,* 649-657.

Lieberman, P., & Tseng, C. Y. (1981). On the fall of the declination theory: Breath-group versus "declination" as the base form for intonation. *Journal of the Acoustical Society of America, 67,* (Suppl.), S63.

Maeda, S. (1976). *A characterization of American English intonation.* Cambridge, MA: MIT Press.

Peterson, G. E., & Lehiste, I. (1960). Duration of syllable nuclei in English. *Journal of the Acoustical Society of America, 24,* 693-703.

Pickett, J. M. (1980). *The sounds of speech communication.* Baltimore: University Park Press.

Pierrehumbert, J. B. (1979). The perception of F_o declination. *Journal of the Acoustical Society of America, 66,* 363-369.

Read, C., Buder, E. H., & Kent, R. D. (1992). Speech analysis systems: An evaluation. *Journal of Speech and Hearing Research, 35,* 314-332.

Read, C., & Schreiber, P.A. (1982). Why short subjects are harder to find than long ones. In Wanner, E., & Gleitman, L. (Eds.), *Language acquisition: The state of the art.* Cambridge, UK: Cambridge University Press.

Sander, E. K. (1972). When are speech sounds learned? *Journal of Speech and Hearing Disorders, 37,* 55-63.

Scully, C. (1990). Articulatory synthesis. In Hardcastle, W.J., & Marchal, A. (Eds.), *Speech production and speech modelling.* Dordrecht, Netherlands: Kluwer (pp. 151-186).

Shadle, C. H. (1990). Articulatory-acoustic relationships in fricative consonants. In Hardcastle, W.J., and Marchal, A. (Eds.), *Speech production and speech modelling.* Dordrecht, Netherlands: Kluwer (pp. 187-209).

Sondhi, M.M. (1986). Resonances of a bent vocal tract. *Journal of the Acoustical Society of America, 79,* 1113-1116.

Sorensen, J. M., & Cooper, W. E. (1980). Syntactic coding of fundamental frequency in speech production. In Cole, R.A. (Ed.), *Perception and production of fluent speech.* Hillsdale, NJ: Erlbaum.

Stevens, K. N. (1989). On the quantal nature of speech. *Journal of Phonetics, 17,* 3-45.

Stevens, K. N., & Blumstein, S. E. (1978). Invariant cues for place of articulation in stop consonants. *Journal of the Acoustical Society of America, 64,* 1358-1368.

Strange, W. (1987). Evolving theories of vowel perception. *Journal of the Acoustical Society of America, 85,* 2081-2087.

Syrdal, A. K., & Gopal, H. S. (1986). A perceptual model of vowel recognition based on the auditory representation of American English vowels. *Journal of the Acoustical Society of America, 79,* 1086-1100.

Terken, J. (1991). Fundamental frequency and perceived prominence of accented syllables. *Journal of the Acoustical Society of America, 89,* 1768-1776.

Thorsen, N. G. (1985). Intonation and text in standard Danish. *Journal of the Acoustical Society of America, 77,* 1205-1216.

Umeda, N. (1982). Fundamental frequency decline is situation dependent. *Journal of Phonetics, 10,* 279-290.

Vaissiere, J. (1983). Language-independent prosodic features. In Cutler, A., & Ladd, D. R. (Eds.), *Prosody: Models and measurements.* New York: Springer-Verlag (pp. 53-66).

Westbury, J. (1983). Enlargement of the supraglottal cavity and its relation to stop consonant voicing. *Journal of the Acoustical Society of America, 73,* 1322-1336.

Suggested Readings

General Readings on Speech Acoustics

Fant, G. (1960). *Acoustic theory of speech production.* The Hague: Mouton.

Kent, R. D., & Read, W. C. (1992). *The acoustic analysis of speech.* San Diego: Singular.

Olive, J. P., Greenwood, A., & Coleman, J. (1993). Acoustics of American English speech: A dynamic approach. New York: Springer-Verlag.

Vowel Acoustics

Assman, P., Nearey, T., & Hogan, J. (1982). Vowel identification: Orthographic, perceptual, and acoustic aspects. *Journal of the Acoustical Society of America, 71,* 975-989.

Lindblom, B. E. F. (1963). Spectrographic study of vowel reduction. *Journal of the Acoustical Society of America, 35,* 1773-1781.

Miller, J. D. (1989). Auditory-perceptual interpretation of the vowel. *Journal of the Acoustical Society of America, 85,* 2114-2134.

Nearey, T. M. (1989). Static, dynamic, and relational properties in vowel perception. *Journal of the Acoustical Society of America, 85,* 2088-2113.

Peterson, G. E., & Barney, H. E. (1952). Control methods used in a study of vowels. *Journal of the Acoustical Society of America, 24,* 175-184.

Stevens, K. N., & House, A. S. (1961). An acoustical theory of vowel production and some of its implications. *Journal of Speech and Hearing Research, 4,* 303-320.

Strange, W. (1987). Evolving theories of vowel perception. *Journal of the Acoustical Society of America, 85,* 2081-2087.

Syrdal, A. K., & Gopal, H. S. (1986). A perceptual model of vowel recognition based on the auditory representation of American English vowels. *Journal of the Acoustical Society of America, 79,* 1086-1100.

Teager, H., & Teager, S. (1985). A phenomenological model for vowel production in the vocal tract. In Daniloff, R. (Ed.), *Speech science: Recent advances.* San Diego: College-Hill Press (pp. 73-101).

Obstruent Consonants: Stops, Fricatives, and Affricates

Blumstein, S. E., & Stevens, K. N. (1979). Acoustic invariance in speech production: Evidence from measurements of the spectral characteristics of stop consonants. *Journal of the Acoustical Soceity of America, 66,* 1001-1017.

Cooper, F. S., Delattre, P. C., Liberman, A. M., Borst, J. N., & Gerstman, L. J. (1952). Some experiments on the perception of synthetic speech sounds. *Journal of the Acoustical Society of America, 24,* 597-606.

Delattre, P., Liberman, A. M., & Cooper, F. S. (1955). Acoustic loci and transitional cues for consonants. *Journal of the Acoustical Society of America, 27,* 769-774.

Halle, M., Hughes, G. W., & Radley, J. P. (1957). Acoustic properties of stop consonants. *Journal of the Acoustical Society of America, 29,* 107-116.

Heinz, J. M., & Stevens, K. N. (1961). On the properties of voiceless fricative consonants. *Journal of the Acoustical Society of America, 33,* 589-596.

Hughes, G. W., & Halle, M. (1956). Spectral properties of fricative consonants. *Journal of the Acoustical Society of America, 28,* 303-310.

Kewley-Port, D., Pisoni, D. B., & Studdert-Kennedy, M. (1983). Perception of static and dynamic acoustic cues to place of articulation in initial stop consonants. *Journal of the Acoustical Society of America, 73,* 1779-1793.

Repp, B. H., Liberman, A. M., Eccardt, T., &

Pesetsky, D. (1978). Perceptual integration of acoustic cues for stop, fricative, and affricate manner. *Journal of Experimental Psychology: Human Perception and Performance, 4,* 621-637.

Shadle, C. H. (1990). Articulatory-acoustic relationships in fricative consonants. In Hardcastle, W. J., & Marchal, A. (Eds.), *Speech production and speech modelling.* Dordrecht, Netherlands: Kluwer (pp. 187-209).

Stevens, K. N. (1989). On the quantal nature of speech. *Journal of Phonetics, 17,* 3-45.

Strevens, P. (1960). Spectra of fricative noise in human speech. *Language and Speech, 3,* 32-49.

Consonant Voicing

Abramson, A. S. (1977). Laryngeal timing in consonant distinctions. *Phonetica, 34,* 295-303.

Barry, W. (1979). Complex encoding in word-final voiced and voiceless stops. *Phonetica, 36,* 361-372.

Chen, M. (1970). Vowel length variation as a function of the voicing of the consonant environment. *Phonetica, 22,* 129-159.

Hogan, J. T., & Rozsypal, A. J. (1980). Evaluation of vowel duration as a cue for the voicing distinction in the following word-final consonant. *Journal of the Acoustical Society of America, 67,* 1764-1771.

Klatt, D. H. (1975). Voice onset time, frication and aspiration in word-initial consonant clusters. *Journal of Speech and Hearing Research, 18,* 686-706.

Lisker, L., & Abramson, A. S. (1964). A cross-language study of voicing in initial stops: Acoustical measurements. *Word, 20,* 384-422.

Port, R. F., & Dalby, J. (1982). Consonant/vowel ratio as a cue for voicing in English. *Perception and Psychophysics, 32,* 141-152.

Raphael, L. (1972). Preceding vowel duration as a cue to the perception of the voicing characteristic of word-final consonants in English. *Journal of the Acoustical Society of America, 51,* 1296-1303.

Slis, I. H., & Cohen, A. (1969). On the complex regulating the voiced-voiceless distinction. I. *Language and Speech, 1,* 80-102.

Wardrip-Fruin, C. (1982). On the status of phonetic cues to phonetic categories: Preceding vowel duration as a cue to voicing in final stop consonants. *Journal of the Acoustical Society of America, 71,* 187-195.

Weismer, G. (1979). Sensitivity of voice-onset time (VOT) to certain segmental features in speech production. *Journal of Phonetics, 7,* 197-204.

Sonorant Consonants: Liquids, Glides, and Nasals

Cooper, F. S., Delattre, P. C., Liberman, A. M., Borst, J. N., & Gerstman, L. J. (1952). Some experiments on the perception of synthetic speech sounds. *Journal of the Acoustical Society of America, 24,* 597-606.

Dalston, R. (1975). Acoustic characteristics of English

/w,r,l/ spoken correctly by young children and adults. *Journal of the Acoustical Society of America, 57,* 462-469.

Delattre, P., Liberman, A. M., & Cooper, F. S. (1955). Acoustic loci and transitional cues for consonants. *Journal of the Acoustical Society of America, 27,* 769-774.

Fujimura, O. (1962). Analysis of nasal consonants. *Journal of the Acoustical Society of America, 34,* 1865-1875.

Kurowski, K., & Blumstein, S. E. (1984). Perceptual integration of the murmur and formant transitions for place of articulation in nasal consonants. *Journal of the Acoustical Society of America, 76,* 383-390.

Liberman, A. M., Cooper, F. S., Shankweiler, D. S., & Studdert-Kennedy, M. (1967). Perception of the speech code. *Psychological Review, 74,* 431-461.

Liberman, A. M., Delattre, P. C., Cooper, F. S., & Gerstman, L. J. (1956). Tempo of frequency change as a cue for distinguishing classes of speech sounds. *Journal of Experimental Psychology, 52,* 127-137.

O'Conner, J. D., Gerstman, L. J., Liberman, A. M., Delattre, P. C., & Cooper, F. S. (1957). Acoustic cues for the perception of initial /w,j,r,l/ in English. *Word, 13,* 24-43.

Suprasegmental Features of Speech: Intonation, Stress, Quantity

Beckman, M. E. (1986). *Stress and non-stress accent.* Riverton, USA: Foris.

Cutler, A., & Ladd, D. R. (Eds.), (1983). *Prosody: models and measurements.* New York: Springer-Verlag.

Fry, D. B. (1970). Prosodic phenomena. In Malmberg, B. (Ed.), *Manual of phonetics.* Amsterdam: North-Holland (pp. 365-410).

Lehiste, I. (1960). An acoustic-phonetic study of internal open juncture. *Phonetica, 5,* (Suppl.), 1-54.

Lehiste, I. (1970). *Suprasegmentals.* Cambridge, MA: MIT Press.

Lieberman, P., Katz, W., Jongman, A., Zimmerman, R., & Miller, M. (1985). Measures of the sentence intonation of read and spontaneous speech in American English. *Journal of the Acoustical Society of America, 77,* 649-657.

Maeda, S. (1976). *A Characterization of American English intonation.* Cambridge, MA: MIT Press.

Pierrehumbert, J. B. (1979). The perception of F$_o$ declination. *Journal of the Acoustical Society of America, 66,* 363-369.

Sorensen, J. M., & Cooper, W. E. (1980). Syntactic coding of fundamental frequency in speech production. In Cole, R. A. (Ed.), *Perception and production of fluent speech.* Hillsdale, NJ: Erlbaum.

Terken, J. (1991). Fundamental frequency and perceived prominence of accented syllables. *Journal of the Acoustical Society of America, 89,* 1768-1776.

Chapter 6

Suprasegmental Features of Speech

Ilse Lehiste

INTRODUCTION

The term "**suprasegmental features**" refers to phenomena that used to be included under *prosody*. The new term arose when linguists needed to emphasize the difference between prosodic features and segmental features. In plain language, segmental features characterize speech sounds, and suprasegmental features are properties of speech sounds or their sequences that are simultaneously present, that do not change the distinctive phonetic quality of the speech sounds, but do modify the sounds in a way that may change the meaning of the utterance.

Suprasegmental features are usually considered either as the set of pitch, **stress**, and **quantity** (contrastive duration) or as features whose domain extends over more than one segment. Neither definition is adequate. If suprasegmentals are to be defined with reference to their domain, then pitch, stress, and quantity would not qualify as suprasegmentals when they happen to be manifested over a single segment. On the other hand, there are other features whose domain can be larger than a single segment and that do not function as do the suprasegmentals (for example, the palatalization of a consonant cluster in such a manner that the palatalization extends over all segments constituting the cluster). If stress, pitch, and quantity behave in ways that set them apart from features determining segmental phonetic quality, the definition should be revised.

It appears that suprasegmental features relate to segmental features by constituting an overlaid function of the inherent segmental features. The term *suprasegmental* is appropriate, referring to features superimposed on segments. Inherent features of a segment can be defined with reference to a segment itself and identified by inspection of the segment. A consonant may be voiced or voiceless; a vowel is usually voiced. The fundamental frequency of an inherently voiced segment, besides characterizing the segment as voiced, may also signal a tonal or intonational pattern. To be recognizable as a segment, every segment must have a certain duration. At the same time, that duration may be contrastive, for example, characterizing the segment as being distinctively short rather than long. (Contrastive duration is referred to as *quantity*.) Every segment also has a certain amount of intensity;

whatever the acoustic and physiological correlates of stress, they consist of intensifying phonetic factors already present in a lesser degree.

Furthermore, in contrast to segmental features, suprasegmental features are established by a comparison of items in sequence, whereas segmental features are identifiable by inspection of the segment itself. For example, the rounding of a vowel in a sequence of rounded vowels can be established without reference to preceding or following vowels; however, the stressedness of a vowel cannot be established without reference to other vowels that carry relatively weaker stress. Thus, the differences between suprasegmental features and segmental features are simultaneously differences of both kind and degree.

DURATION AND QUANTITY

The first suprasegmental feature considered in this chapter is quantity, a linguistic term referring to the contractive function of duration within a phonological system or relative duration. Control over quantity presupposes control over the duration of articulatory gestures. Various models have been developed to explain ways in which temporal control over articulatory gestures can be achieved. There is some evidence (Sternberg et al., 1988) that before an utterance starts, the speaker organizes the sequence of articulatory movements as a highly complex cortical program. As Fujimura (1990) has shown, to a certain extent articulatory organs appear to organize their movement patterns freely; interactions among different events within each articulatory dimension may affect the temporal course of its own dimension but not necessarily events in other dimensions simultaneously. While articulatory gestures are continuous, they are executed so that the resulting acoustic signal contains discontinuities that make it possible to establish the duration of units of spoken language such as segmental sounds, syllables, and words.

Given that the duration of both segments and sequences of segments can be controlled with considerable precision, it appears natural that languages make use of temporal distinctions within their phonological systems. For a feature to serve as an element in a phonological system, it must be independently controllable. To estab-

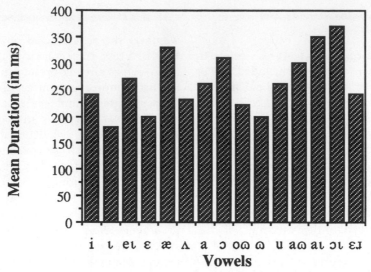

FIGURE 6-1   Intrinsic duration of English syllable nuclei. (From Peterson, G.E., & Lehiste, I. [1960]. Duration of syllable nuclei in English. *Journal of the Acoustical Society of America, 32,* 693-703.)

lish whether this is so, it is necessary to describe (and thus eliminate from consideration) all conditioned variation in the duration of segments and segment sequences. These conditioning factors include the phonetic nature of the segment itself (its **intrinsic duration**), preceding and following sounds, other suprasegmental features, and position of the segment within a higher-level phonological unit.

The duration of vowels appears to be correlated with tongue height: other factors being equal, a high vowel is shorter than a low vowel. Evidence for this has emerged from experimental studies of many and diverse languages, including English, German, Danish, Swedish, Thai, Lapp, and Spanish. In an early study, Peterson and Lehiste (1960) found that in English, the average duration of the syllable nucleus of a large number of productions of the word *"bead"* was 206 ms, while the average duration of the vowel of *"bad"* was 280 ms. Detailed information about various characteristics of American English vowels is given in Crystal and House (1988); for comparable data for German vowels, see Antoniadis and Strube (1981). Figure 6-1 presents the average duration of English syllable nuclei derived from a set of 1263 monosyllabic words pronounced in an identical frame by the same speaker.

The influence of preceding consonants on the duration of vowels following them appears to be negligible; however, the phonetic nature of the following consonant may exert considerable influence on the duration of a preceding vowel. In English, for example, the duration of a vowel preceding a voiced consonant is approximately 1.5 times greater than that of the same vowel preceding a voiceless consonant. Peterson and Lehiste (1960) found that in 118 minimal pairs such as *beat-bead, sight-side,* the average duration of the syllable nucleus before the voiceless member of the consonant pair was 197 ms, while the duration before the voiced member was 297 ms, yielding an approximate ratio of 2:3. This is a characteristic of English; the effect of voicing is much smaller in other languages, although it may be present. For an overview and an attempt to explain vowel-length differences before voiced and voiceless consonants, see Kluender, Diehl, and Wright (1988). For a recent comparison of English and French voicing-conditioned vowel duration, see Laeufer (1992). Figure 6-2 illustrates the effect of final consonant voicing on the duration of a preceding syllable nucleus.

The point of articulation of a following consonant may likewise influence the duration of a preceding vowel: vowel duration tends to increase as the point of articulation of the postvocalic consonant shifts farther back in the mouth. However, this depends largely on the language, as does the influence of the manner of articulation upon the duration of a preceding vowel. In English, vowels are shortest before voiceless stops, and their duration increases when they precede voiceless fricatives, nasals, voiced stops, and voiced fricatives. Peterson and

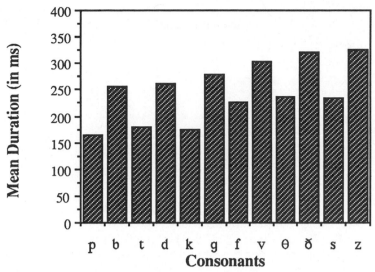

FIGURE 6-2 **Influence of final consonant voicing on the duration of the syllable nucleus (all syllable nuclei combined).** (From Peterson, G.E., & Lehiste, I. [1960]. Duration of syllable nuclei in English. *Journal of the Acoustical Society of America, 32,* 693-703.)

Lehiste (1960) found that the average duration of vowels was 147 ms before /t/, 199 ms before /s/, 216 ms before /n/, 206 ms before /d/, and 262 ms before /z/.

The intrinsic duration of consonants is influenced both by their point of articulation and by the manner of articulation. There is general agreement that labials are longer than alveolars and velars, other factors being kept constant (Fischer-Jørgensen, 1964). Unvoiced fricatives tend to be longer than other consonants; taps and flaps are the shortest. A **tap** is a very rapid articulation of a stop closure; in a **flap,** one articulator strikes another in passing while on its way back to its rest position (Ladefoged, 1982.)

Differences in vowel length frequently are accompanied by equally noticeable quality differences. In many languages long vowels tend to be articulated with a more extreme articulatory position; short vowels tend to be articulated closer to the center of the articulatory vowel space. However, languages differ with respect to the extent and kind of influence of the length of a vowel on its quality, and this is not a universal property of vowel systems.

Such kinds of intrinsic durational differences are not contrastive in a given language, but they can serve as cues for the identification of a particular sound. As mentioned above, in English the syllable nucleus preceding a voiceless consonant is shorter than the same syllable nucleus preceding a voiced consonant. Perceptual tests with synthetic stimuli have shown that

vowel duration is a sufficient cue for determining the perception of voicing of a final consonant: if one synthesizes a sequence like [jus], with a voiceless /s/, and lengthens the duration of the vowel, English-speaking listeners will begin to hear [juz], even though the fricative is voiceless. The function of duration here is quite complex: the duration of one segment signals the presence or absence of a feature — voicing — of another segment.

One of the problems in the study of suprasegmentals is their tendency to co-occur, so that it is difficult to determine which is the independent variable. In many languages, stress is one of the factors that conditions the duration of a sound or a sequence of sounds. Correspondingly, duration may be considered as one of the phonetic manifestations of stress. In some languages, including English, a stressed syllable is regularly longer than an unstressed syllable, other factors being constant. In other languages (for example, Czech) stress seems to be manifested to a greater extent by other phonetic features and an increase in duration is minimal.

The last of the factors influencing the duration of a sound to be considered here is its position within a higher-level phonological unit, such as a word or phrase. This phenomenon has been observed in many languages, including English. The duration of the syllable nucleus of a stem decreases as the duration of the word is increased by suffixes (Lehiste, 1972a). Representative average values for one

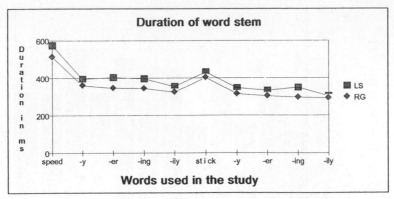

FIGURE 6-3 Duration of the monosyllabic words *speed* and *stick* and the duration of that word stem in words where suffixes have been added to the stem. Data are presented for two speakers, LS and RG. (From Lehiste, I. [1972a]. The timing of utterances and linguistic boundaries. *Journal of the Acoustical Society of America, 51,* 2018-2024.)

subject and one set of test words were as follows: duration of /i/ in "speed", 266 ms; "speedy", 150.5 ms; "speeder", 141.5 ms; "speeding", 136 ms; "speedily", 120 ms; "speediness", 115.5 ms. Figure 6-3 shows the effect of an added syllable on the duration of the word to which the syllable was added; here the base words were *speed* and *stick*. Both subjects show the same pattern.

More generally, the duration of a stressed syllable nucleus in languages like English depends on the number of syllables in a word; if the word contains other syllables in addition to the stressed syllable, the duration of the stressed syllable is shortened. But the process is nonlinear; the difference between the effects of adding a single unstressed syllable and two unstressed syllables is minimal (Lehiste, 1975). This has implications for the hierarchical analysis of spoken language: the next higher unit is composed of syllables, but its duration is not a simple addition of building blocks with fixed duration.

Inclusion in a higher-level unit is one factor that influences the duration of segments and syllables. Another factor is the use of lengthening to indicate the termination of an utterance, or more generally, to signal various syntactic boundaries (Lehiste, 1980; Gussenhoven and Rietveld, 1992).

Assuming that all conditioned variation has been identified and accounted for, further durational features in a language may be considered as independent variables. The term *quantity* is applied to duration when it functions as an independent variable in the phonological system of a language. The simplest example is a language in which vowels can be contrastively long or short, as with Czech and Finnish. The domain of quantity in these cases appears to be the segment. Quantity manifested over a single segment can be analyzed linguistically in diverse ways. It can be treated as a prosodic distinctive feature, [+long], being included in the list of features characterizing a contrastively long segment. Another way to handle the fact that there are long and short sounds in a language is to list long and short vowels and/or consonants in the phonemic inventory of the language. However, this doubles the number of units in the inventory. If the system is symmetrical, it is more economical to extract length from the system and treat it as a **prosodeme** of length (i.e., a prosodic distinctive feature) (Lehiste, 1970).

In many languages it is appropriate to treat long sounds as clusters of two identical sounds, particularly for example, if the language contains diphthongs and if long vowels and diphthongs occupy similar positions in the phonology. With long consonants, a complicating factor enters the discussion: the possible treatment of long consonants as geminates (Lehiste, Morton, and Tatham, 1973; Lahiri and Hankamer, 1988). If a language has consonant clusters that function in the same manner as long consonants, it may be useful to analyze them as clusters of identical consonants, whether or not it is possible to phonetically demonstrate their geminate nature.

In some languages the quantity of a given segment must be related to the quantity of other

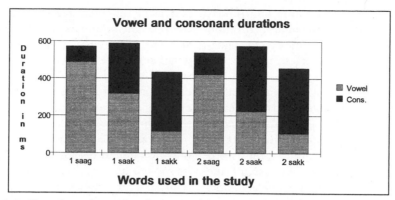

FIGURE 6-4   Duration of vowel and postvocalic consonant in three minimally contrastive monosyllabic Estonian words, produced by two speakers. (From Lehiste, I. [1972b]. Temporal compensation in a quantity language. *Proceedings of the Seventh Internaional Congress of Phonetic Sciences.* The Hague: Mouton, pp. 929-939.)

segments in the sequence. For example, Icelandic, Norwegian, and Swedish have an inverse relationship between the quantity of a vowel and that of the following consonant, so that a short vowel is followed by a long consonant and a long vowel by a short consonant. These contrasts can occur in monosyllabic words, so the domain of the placement of quantity patterns appears to be the syllable.

Similar patterns can be observed in other Germanic languages. German, for example, has such minimal pairs as *raten–Ratten* ("to advise"–"rats", nom. pl. masc.), *baden–baten* ("to bathe"–"they requested"). Kohler (1980) has shown that in such word pairs, the duration of the vowel + plosive sequence remains approximately constant. That is, in a word like *baten,* the vowel is shorter and the consonant is longer, while in words like *baden,* the relationship is reversed; a longer vowel is followed by a shorter consonant. The domain of the quantity patterns here appears to be the disyllabic word.

In Estonian there are three contrastive durations, which are manifested likewise in a complex way. It has monosyllabic words consisting of the same segmental sounds, but the different ratio between the durations of the syllable nucleus and the final consonant results in three different meanings. The minimal triple *saag–saak–sakk* ("saw"–"harvest"–"jag, notch"), given here in conventional spelling, consists of identical segments (the letter *g* is used to indicate a short voiceless velar plosive), and the duration of the whole monosyllabic word remains more or less the same; the three-way contrast is achieved by changing the relative durations of

the segments within the word. In *saag,* the vowel is longest and the final consonant shortest. In *saak,* both have intermediate duration. In *sakk,* [a] is shortest and [k] is longest (Lehiste, 1972b). Figure 6-4 gives measurements of the duration of the syllable nucleus and the final consonant closure in these three minimally contrastive monosyllabic words, produced by two speakers in an identical sentence frame.

In disyllabic words it is not just segmental duration that differentiates between such minimal triples as *vilu–viilu–vii:lu* ("cool"–"slice" gen. sing–"slice" partitive sing). The overlength of the vowel /i/ is indicated by the colon. Such words have an inverse relationship between the durations of the two syllables so that their ratios are approximately 2:3 for words in short quantity, 3:2 for words in long quantity, and 2:1 in words with overlength. The fundamental frequency pattern applied to the whole sequence also plays a significant role, distinguishing between the two long quantities and providing a characteristic identificatory feature for overlength (Lehiste, 1989).

The function of duration at the sentence level is quite different from its function at the word level. Changes in the relative durations of linguistic units within a sentence do not change the meanings of individual words, as they may do when quantity functions at the word level. However, significant changes in tempo — changes from a neutral rate of articulation — may convey something about the mood of the speaker or about the circumstances under which the utterance is made.

Duration interacts with the other prosodic

features in various ways. Duration and fundamental frequency serve as stress cues. Duration also is one of the prosodic means to signal various boundaries and the syntactic structure of a sentence.

Duration is intimately involved in signaling the boundaries of individual words. An early study (Lehiste, 1960) of minimal pairs like *white shoes–why choose*, showed that duration was the most significant phonetic cue to the word boundary. For example, in *white shoes* the diphthong of the first word is relatively short because it is followed by a voiceless consonant within the same syllable. In *why choose* there is no final consonant, and the diphthong of *why* is much longer than the diphthong of *white*.

Duration also signals phrase and sentence boundaries through **preboundary lengthening.** The last syllable of a word, or the last word of a phrase, is produced with greater duration than the same syllable or word in other positions. Preboundary lengthening occurs naturally before syntactic boundaries and thus can be used to signal the presence of a boundary in English (Lehiste, 1980), German (Kohler, 1983), and French (Vaissière, 1992).

An earlier study (Lehiste, 1973), consisted of both production and perception tests of sentences that consist of the same words but whose meanings depend on the position of a phrase boundary. For example, "the old men and women stayed at home" can mean either that both the men and women were old or that only the men were old: "the old // men and women stayed at home" versus "the old men // and women stayed at home". That paper reported the results of an investigation involving 15 such ambiguous sentences produced by four speakers and heard by 30 listeners. The speakers first read the sentences from a randomized list. Then the ambiguities were pointed out, and the speakers were asked which of the two possible meanings they had in mind. The sentences were recorded twice again, the speaker making a conscious effort to convey one or the other meaning. The sentences were analyzed acoustically and the phonetic means that had been used to achieve disambiguation were established.

Of particular interest were cases in which the spontaneous version received a random score in the listening test but the consciously disambiguated versions were correctly identified. In every case, disambiguation was successful when the speakers had manipulated the time dimension by

increasing the interstress interval that contained the relevant boundary. The speakers used several means to achieve the same aim, namely, lengthening the interstress interval; the most straightforward was the insertion of a pause, but equally successful were other means, like lengthening one or more segmental sounds preceding the boundary.

O'Malley, Kloker, and Dara-Abrams (1973) obtained similar results in a study of parentheses in spoken algebraic expressions. They located their boundary signals at given points in a linear sequence without relating them to the general rhythmic structure of the utterances. Pauses, the primary cue, were accompanied by segmental lengthening and pitch changes.

Lehiste, Olive, and Streeter (1976) showed that an increase in the interstress interval is a sufficient boundary signal, even without intonation and specific segmental lengthening. Lehiste (1973) processed 10 sentences through an analysis-resynthesis program, changed the fundamental frequency to monotone, and systematically manipulated the duration of interstress intervals. No preboundary lengthening was introduced, but the interstress intervals were increased by increasing the duration of each sampling period by the same factor. The durational relationships of the segments to each other remained unchanged. A listening test of 30 subjects showed that disambiguation was achieved when the relevant interval reached a certain duration, the particular value of which depended on the given sentence.

These results apply to English and possibly to other languages characterized by stress timing — if indeed languages can be classified by temporal organization into stress-timed and syllable-timed languages. (See Wenk and Wioland [1982] and Dauer [1983] for reviews of earlier literature and discussions of the issues.) Speech rhythm and its linguistic functions are under intensive study (Cutler, 1991; Fant, Kruckenberg, and Nord, 1991). Since all spoken language is physically realized in time, the study of the time dimension of speech remains at the heart of phonetic science.

TONE AND INTONATION

The prosodic feature considered in this section is commonly referred to by such terms as **pitch, tone,** and **intonation.** Here, *pitch* is the perceptual correlate of frequency, *tone* is the feature used distinctively at the word level, and *intonation* is the feature when it functions at the sentence level.

The physiological correlate of tone and intonation is the vibration of the vocal folds in phonation. For the anatomy and physiology of the larynx, see Chapter 4 and Ohala (1978). Two basic mechanisms produce changes in the rate of vibration of the vocal folds. One is an increase in the rate of airflow through the glottis (caused by increased activity of the respiratory muscles producing increased subglottal pressure); the other is an increase in the tension of the laryngeal musculature itself, especially the vocalis muscle. Decreases in the rate of vibration of the vocal folds may be brought about by decreasing the rate of airflow and/or by relaxing the laryngeal musculature. There is some evidence that some extrinsic laryngeal muscles may act to lower the rate of vibration of the vocal folds (Honda and Fujimura, 1991).

The acoustic correlate of vocal fold vibration is the fundamental frequency of the sound wave generated at the glottis. The perceptual correlate of fundamental frequency is pitch. The nonlinear nature of pitch is well known. The fact that pitch perception is nonlinear acquires linguistic importance because the normal speaking frequencies of individuals may vary a great deal, ranging from very high frequencies used by children and some women to very low frequencies used by some men. Pitch perception operates by intervals rather than by absolute frequencies, so a difference between 200 and 100 Hz is considered perceptually equivalent to a difference between 300 and 150 Hz or to other differences in which the ratio is likewise 2:1. Tone and intonational signals used by different speakers may differ in absolute frequencies but customarily involve similar ratios.

The absolute differential threshold for fundamental frequency varies with frequency. Subjective pitch increases less rapidly as the stimulus frequency rises linearly and more rapidly as the stimulus frequency rises logarithmically. The just-noticeable differences in pitch depend on a number of factors and may fluctuate for the same subjects. In the linguistic study of tone and intonation, it is necessary and adequate to measure fundamental frequency in steps of about ± 1 Hz in the octave range of 80 to 160 Hz, the range usually employed by adult male speakers.

Phonetic conditioning factors of the funda-

mental frequency at which a syllable nucleus is realized include **intrinsic pitch,** preceding and following sounds, and other suprasegmental features, especially stress. Intrinsic pitch is the pitch determined by the phonetic quality of a vowel. There is a connection between vowel quality and the relative height of the average fundamental frequency associated with it: other factors being constant, higher vowels have higher fundamental frequency. Lehiste and Peterson (1961) found that the average fundamental frequencies of high and low vowels in 1263 test words produced by and averaged over five speakers at the peak of the intonation contour were 183 Hz for /i/, 182 Hz for /u/, and 163 Hz for /a/. Similar results have been obtained for other languages (Hombert, 1978; Antoniadis and Strube, 1981; Ladd and Silverman, 1984). Honda (1983) has proposed a physiological explanation for intrinsic pitch differences between high and low vowels, demonstrating that tongue gestures inherent in vowel articulation have an effect on laryngeal positions that affect fundamental frequency in the observed directions (Fig. 6-5).

While preceding consonants seemed to have little influence on the duration of following vowels, there is no doubt that they influence the fundamental frequency of following syllable nuclei (Hombert, 1978). Higher fundamental frequencies are associated with voiceless initial consonants. The influence of an initial consonant may counterbalance intrinsic pitch. Thus, Lehiste and Peterson (1961) found that the average for /ka/ sequences was 172 Hz and that of /gi/ sequences was 170 Hz (recall that the intrinsic pitch of /i/ was 183 Hz and that of /a/ was 163 Hz). The difference in average peak value due to the voicelessness or voicing of an initial consonant usually is accompanied by a different distribution of the fundamental frequency movement over the studied word. After a voiceless consonant, especially a fricative, the highest peak will occur immediately after the consonant. However, after a voiced consonant, especially a resonant, the fundamental frequency will tend to rise slowly, and the peak may be expected approximately in the middle of the test word.

Final consonants appear to have but little influence on the fundamental frequency of syllable nuclei, except for the fact that a tonal movement may continue during a following voiced resonant. In that respect, sequences

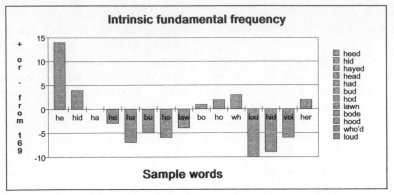

FIGURE 6-5 Intrinsic fundamental frequencies (in Hz) of English syllable nuclei averaged from a set of productions by six speakers expressed as the difference from the overall average **(169 Hz).** (From Lehiste, I., & Peterson, G. E. [1961]. Some basic considerations in the analysis of intonation. *Journal of the Acoustical Society of America, 33,* 419-425.)

consisting of vowels and postvocalic resonants may function as complex syllable nuclei, with a tonal contour distributed over the complete sequence. This is the case in some tone languages (e.g., Lithuanian).

Fundamental frequency may also be influenced by other suprasegmental features, especially stress. Quantity appears to have no influence on fundamental frequency, except that long vowels may be articulated with more extreme targets and long high vowels may thus have higher intrinsic pitch. Stress, however, is frequently associated with higher fundamental frequency. Increased rate of airflow raises the rate of vocal fold vibration. Since stress is associated with increased subglottal pressure, the increase in vocal fold vibration may be considered automatic. If no increase is registered, it must be assumed that other adjustments are made (for example, in the tension of the vocal folds) to counteract the influence of the airflow.

Tonal features may condition other tonal features in two ways. Either the occurrence of tone on a syllable (or word) or its phonetic realization may be influenced by the presence or type of tone on an adjacent syllable (or word). This phenomenon is referred to in linguistic literature as **tone sandhi.** The other phenomenon involves fundamental frequency functioning at word and sentence level and consists of the fact that the realization of tones in a tone language may be influenced by intonation applied to the sentence as a whole. This is analogous to the influence of tempo on quantity.

Contrastive fundamental frequency at word

level is *tone; intonation* is the linguistically significant functioning of fundamental frequency at the sentence level. In some languages—for example, Chinese—contrastive tone is associated with differences in the meaning of roots and stems; this is *lexical tone.* In other languages, differences in tone may signal different case forms of nouns or different forms within the verbal paradigm.

The smallest possible domain of tone is a single syllabic sound; however, it has been argued persuasively that the proper domain of tones is a syllable (Wang, 1967; Howie, 1974). In addition, in some languages, including Swedish, Norwegian, and Serbo-Croatian, a tonal pattern may be realized over a sequence of two or more syllables. Languages with syllabic tone have been divided into *register tone* and *contour tone* languages (Pike, 1948; Maddieson, 1974; Anderson, 1978). The first type includes systems composed largely of level tones: tones that are realized in such a manner that within the limits of perception the pitch of a syllable does not rise or fall during its production. The contrastive levels are sometimes called *registers.* The second type contains gliding tones. Some languages contain elements of both systems.

Figure 6-6 shows fundamental frequency contours in disyllabic and trisyllabic Serbo-Croatian words differing in duration and tone (Lehiste and Ivić, 1963). The top three diagrams show accentual contrasts in disyllabic words, and the bottom three represent trisyllabic words. All words bear the **accent** on the first syllable. \\, Short falling accent. \, Short rising accent. ⌢, Long falling accent. ╱, Long rising

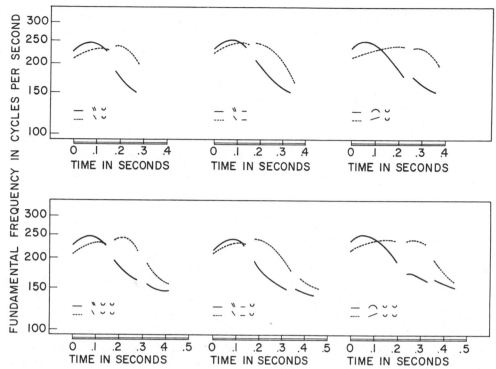

FIGURE 6-6 Fundamental frequency contours in minimally contrastive Serbo-Croatian words. (From Lehiste, I., & Ivić, P. [1963]. *Accent in Serbo-Croatian: An experimental study.* Michigan Slavic Materials 4. Ann Arbor: University of Michigan.)

accent. ——, Unaccented length. ˇ, Unaccented short syllables. ——, Show fundamental frequency contours associated with falling accents. ----, Rising accents. Contrastive length appears both in accented and in unaccented syllables, and the contrastive fundamental frequency pattern is distributed over two syllables.

Intonation includes the use of tonal features to carry linguistic information at the sentence level, as well as nonlinguistic meanings. In this respect it is analogous to tempo; that is, duration is used at the sentence level to reflect the attitudes of the speaker and the urgency of the message. Attempts to separate the linguistic and paralinguistic aspects of intonation have not always been successful. Intonation does not change the meaning of lexical items, but constitutes part of the meaning of the whole sentence. Certain changes in intonation may be accompanied by changes in the function of the utterance, signaling, for example, a difference between a statement and a question.

A phonetic characteristic of declarative sentences in many languages is **frequency declination, or downdrift** — the tendency of peak values of **accents** to drop (Pike, 1945; Gussenhoven and Rietveld, 1988). Cohen, Collier, and t'Hart

(1982) raised the question of whether declination is a theoretical construct to account for the interpretation of acoustic fundamental frequency recordings or an intrinsic feature of speech pitch. Noninitial accent peaks are successively lower than preceding peaks. Pierrehumbert (1979) showed that for two accent peaks to sound equal in pitch height, the fundamental frequency of the second peak must be lower than that of the first.

In a series of experiments Gussenhoven and Rietveld (1988) tested three possible explanations for the declination effect. The three hypotheses assumed that the declination effect was the result of (1) a uniform, time-dependent downslope of the contour, (2) a drop in the final portion of the contour only, and (3) a time-independent peak-by-peak drop. Their results confirmed (for Dutch) that listeners take the declination effect into account when judging the prominence of accent peaks and thus judge later peaks to be more prominent than earlier peaks when the fundamental frequency is equal. They found no evidence for a peak-by-peak lowering function and concluded that the declination effect is due to both time-dependent downsloping and final lowering.

Vaissière (1983) proposed several physiological explanations for declination: decline in transglottal pressure toward the end of the utterance, trachea pull, or a laziness principle, the rise supposedly being more difficult to produce than the falls. Pierrehumbert (1979) proposed that declination is a by-product of the perceptual system. Vaissière suggests that the rate of declination contributes to the perception of a sentence spoken in the declarative mode as an acoustic whole; it is a factor in the contrast between declarative and interrogative sentences in a number of languages. She concludes that the natural tendency for fundamental frequency to decline has been integrated into the linguistic code in the form of controlling or entirely suppressing the fundamental frequency decline. Baselines are naturally reset after a pause; thus, resetting can be used as a boundary marker, and the degree of resetting indicates the importance of the boundary. Fundamental frequency, together with stress and duration, also signals sentence-level phenomena such as sentence stress, focus, and **emphasis.**

An integrated analysis of sentence-level prosody in English has been developed by several groups of researchers interested in establishing an agreed system for prosodic transcription of large speech corpora (Silverman et al., 1992). The system comprises four parallel tiers: (1) orthographic, (2) tone, (3) break-index, and (4) miscellaneous. Of primary importance in the present context are the tone and the break-index tiers.

The break-index tier has five possible values: 0 for clear phonetic marks of clitic groups (indicators that two words are fused into one, as when a sequence like "did you" is pronounced with a medial affricate); 1 for most phrase-medial word boundaries; 2 for a boundary either marked by a pause with no tonal marks or weaker than a clear phrase boundary; 3 for an intermediate intonation phrase boundary; and 4 for a full intonation phrase boundary marked by a final boundary tone.

The tonal tier handles pitch events associated with both intonational boundaries and accented syllables (pitch accents). Boundary tones mark the beginning and end of a phrase. Pitch accent tones are marked at every accented syllable; there are five types of pitch accents using "high" and "low" tones within the speaker's range. The system also allows for downstepped pitch accents and phrase accents. However, the resulting

prosodic transcription does not automatically relate the prosody of the sentence to its syntactic structure.

STRESS AND EMPHASIS

Of the three suprasegmental features considered in this chapter, stress for a long time has been the most elusive. There is no single mechanism to which stress can be attributed in the same manner as the generation of fundamental frequency can be attributed to the vibration of the vocal folds. Furthermore, in defining stress the points of view of the speaker and the listener are often confused. When the point of view is the speaker's, stress may be defined in terms of greater effort that enters into the production of a stressed syllable as compared to an unstressed syllable. From a listener's standpoint, stressed syllables may be considered louder than unstressed syllables. Loudness can be tested through psychoacoustic techniques, but until recently, it has been practically impossible to measure effort. Furthermore, other suprasegmental features affect stress, which makes it difficult to isolate the stress feature from the other simultaneously occurring characteristics.

It is also necessary to distinguish stress from accent and from **prominence** in order to understand discussions of stress in phonetic and linguistic literature. Fischer-Jørgensen (1983, p. 81) uses *accent* as a general term covering stress and tone:

> Stress is used to indicate culminative accent, by which one syllable is made more prominent than other syllables in the given unit, whereas tone or tonal accent characterizes a syllable or part of a syllable or a word without giving special prominence to it. It is inherent in the idea of prominence that something stands out compared with the surroundings. Thus stress is a concept of relations in the speech chain.

Fischer-Jørgensen does not specify how a stressed syllable is made more prominent; her definition also seems to exclude the possibility that in a tone language, a syllable might be simultaneously stressed and carry a contrastive tone.

Beckman (1986, p. 1), on the other hand, defines accent thus:

> ...a system of syntagmatic contrasts used to construct prosodic patterns which divide an utterance into a succession of shorter phrases and to specify

relationships among these patterns which organize them into larger phrasal groupings. And "stress" means a phonologically delimitable type of accent in which the pitch shape of the accentual pattern cannot be specified in the lexicon but rather is chosen for a specific utterance from an inventory of shapes provided by the intonation system.

Languages may differ with respect to whether accentual prominence is achieved by fundamental frequency or intensity (*pitch accent* or *stress accent*). For a discussion of the terminology of stress and accent, see Cutler and Ladd (1983, Chapter 11). *Stress* is used here to mean perceived relative prominence that has a strong intensity component due to increased physical effort. Stress may function contrastively at the word level, distinguishing lexical meaning. At the sentence level, stress may function to identify a word as being in focus or emphasized. *Accent* here means prosodic prominence of more than one of the three prosodic features. Thus, Serbo-Croatian is called an accent rather than a tone language, even though it has contrastive rising and falling tones, since all three prosodic features—stress placement, contrastive duration, and distinctions based on fundamental frequency contours—are involved in the phonological system.

There is no one-to-one correspondence between stress and any single acoustic parameter (Beckman, 1986; Terken, 1991). Thus, there is also no automatic way to identify stressed syllables. Although subglottal pressure peaks may be associated with sentence stress and emphasis, neither electromyography nor measurements of subglottal pressure yield unambiguous evidence for the location of stress within word-level units unless the word receives sentence stress or emphasis.

Nevertheless, some evidence suggests that stress is judged in terms of effort. If all other factors are kept constant, greater effort will produce a higher degree of perceived stress. The force exerted by respiratory muscles is directly transmitted to the air inside the lungs, and this effort is reflected in subglottal pressure. The subglottal pressure in the lungs produces an airstream that passes through the glottis with a volume velocity proportional to the subglottal pressure. In the production of voiced sounds, the airstream sets the vocal folds into vibration, and the kinetic energy of the airflow is transduced into acoustic energy. Acoustic energy is related to effective sound pressure. As a first approxi-

mation, peak subglottal pressure is proportional to the 0.6 power of the peak effective sound pressure. Sound intensity is proportional to the square of the pressure variations of the sound wave.

The smallest amount of pressure that produces an audible sound is approximately 0.0002 dynes/cm^2. The threshold of audibility varies a great deal from individual to individual and may vary for the same person under different conditions. Moreover, the sensitivity of the ear differs a great deal in the different frequency regions. The ear is most sensitive to frequencies between 1000 and 6000 Hz. If that range is taken as reference and the intensity of the just-noticeable sound is assigned a value of 0 dB at that frequency, then a just-audible tone at 100 Hz must have an intensity that is 40 dB higher. At 10,000 Hz, a tone must be about 10 dB more intense than the reference intensity to be just audible. The minimum intensity change that normal listeners can detect for 1000 Hz at 30 dB sensation level of the reference tone is approximately 1 dB.

Intensity is a physical characteristic of a sound, and loudness is the subjective property of a sound that is most directly related to intensity. Sounds with greater intensity are perceived as louder, other factors being constant. However, loudness also depends on fundamental frequency, spectral characteristics, and duration of the sound. All of these relationships have been studied extensively. As in most psychophysical studies, the stimuli used in these experiments have been primarily pure tones and noises. Such studies usually reveal more about the capacities of the organs of perception than about the function of the perceived differences in speech. When loudness judgments are made about real speech, the results differ a great deal from judgments made about psychoacoustic stimuli.

Furthermore, stress seems to be perceived quite differently from loudness. It presupposes a speech setting as well as a certain amount of learning. Jones (1940) stated explicitly that stress perception also involves knowledge of the language in which the utterance is spoken and distinguished between stress and prominence. According to Jones, the prominence of a syllable is its general degree of distinctness—the combined effect of the timbre, length, stress, and (if voiced) intonation of the syllabic sound. Stress is the degree of force of utterance only; it is independent of length and intonation, although

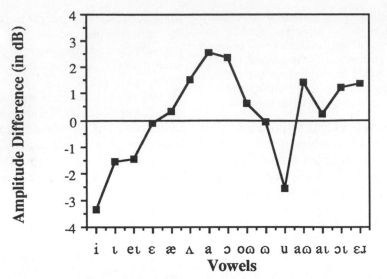

FIGURE 6-7 Intrinsic amplitudes of English syllable nuclei produced by one speaker, expressed in decibels relative to the average amplitude of all productions. (From Lehiste, I. & Peterson, G.E. [1959]. Vowel amplitude and phonemic stress in American English. *Journal of the Acoustical Society of America, 31,* 428-435.)

it may be combined with them. Prominence is a perceptual quantity that may be decreased or increased by means of any of the sound attributes, such as length, stress, pitch, or timbre; stress is an articulatory gesture. Jones anticipated the motor theory of speech perception (Liberman et al., 1963) when he suggested that a person familiar with a language perceives the sound from the physical stimulus subjectively: the sounds call to mind the manner of making them, and immediate *inner speech* reveals where the stress is. Although Jones distinguishes between stress and prominence, he does not make clear which of them has linguistic function or whether or not they may have different linguistic functions.

The problem of the phonetic correlates of stress is an intricate one. The intensity of a sound depends largely on its manner of articulation; different configurations of the vocal tract give rise to sounds of differing intensity, even if the input intensity (the effort employed in the production of the sounds) is the same. **Intrinsic intensity** is intensity considered in relation to phonetic quality. Lehiste and Peterson (1959) showed that the average intensities of low vowels were considerably higher than those of high vowels. In a set of 1263 test words produced by five speakers, the average for /i/ was 71.3 dB; for /a/, 79.5 dB (Fig. 6-7). Intrinsic intensities have been established for a number of other languages; for example, in Hungarian, a range of 12 dB was found between the intensities

of long /a/ and long /u/. These differences should certainly be above the perceptual threshold. Hierarchies of intrinsic intensity have also been established for consonants.

Thus, the intrinsic intensity of speech sounds due to their phonetic quality is one factor that must be taken into consideration in the interpretation of intensity data. Another factor is the interaction between fundamental frequency and formant frequency. The spacing of the harmonics generated at the glottis is independent of the center frequencies of the resonances of the vocal tract. If the articulatory configuration of the vocal tract remains fixed and the fundamental frequency of the voice is changed, extensive changes in overall level will occur. The amplitude will increase if a harmonic coincides with the frequency of one of the lower formants, especially the first formant, since most of the energy of the vowel is contained in the first formant. These differences may be of the order of several decibels. Although the differences in intrinsic intensity and those due to interaction between fundamental frequency and formant frequency may have magnitudes that would be above the perceptual threshold if the experiment were conducted with pure tones, it appears that listeners discount such differences when listening in a speech mode and making judgments about stress.

One of the main problems in the interpretation of the physiological and acoustic correlates of stress is the ambiguous role of intensity in the perception of stress. One reason for this ambiguity is that output intensity changes with the articulatory configuration of the vocal tract. Another reason is that subglottal pressure is also one of the physiological factors that influences the rate of vocal fold vibration, so stress is connected intimately with frequency. Unless the tension of the vocal folds is adjusted, increased subglottal pressure results automatically in an increased rate of vocal fold vibration. Therefore, in many languages, higher fundamental frequency provides a strong cue for the presence of stress.

While an increase in respiratory effort is an obvious physiological cause for increases in intensity and in the rate of vocal fold vibration, no such reason is apparent for a frequent third phonetic correlate of stressedness: greater duration. In many languages a stressed syllable is longer than an unstressed one. However, this is by no means a universal correlate of stress; Finnish, for example, carries fixed word-level stress on the first syllable of a word but has contrastive length oppositions in any syllable, resulting in possible word types with stressed short syllables and unstressed long syllables.

The relative importance of intensity, fundamental frequency, and duration in the perception of stress has been studied in several languages. For English, the order of importance appears to be thus: duration is more important than intensity, and sentence intonation is an overriding factor in determining the perception of stress; in this sense the fundamental frequency cue may outweigh the duration cue. The order of importance of the various parameters may differ for languages with a different phonological structure.

In a study of the perception of stress by Italian speakers, Bertinetto (1980) found that duration provided the most effective prominence cue. Eek (1987) compared word stress perception in Estonian and Russian and found that the stress judgments of Estonians were mostly associated with fundamental frequency patterns; a considerable difference in fundamental frequency failed to be the determining factor only if the corresponding syllable duration pattern did not occur in Estonian words. For Russians, however, duration was the leading parameter, the effect of a higher fundamental frequency becoming noticeable only if the two syllables under comparison were of equal duration. Duration is, of course, contrastive in Estonian and thus is not available as a stress cue to the same extent as in

Russian. Intensity played a negligible role for listeners with either language background.

Lehiste and Fox (1992) tested perception of prominence in Estonian and English with monotone speechlike signals and with noise tokens. Listeners heard sequences of four tokens in which one token could be lengthened and/or increased in intensity, the two changes being independent of each other. Listeners were required to indicate which token was more prominent. Listening tests were given to 24 native speakers of English in Columbus, Ohio, and to 38 native speakers of Estonian in Tallinn. The responses showed that for English listeners, intensity cues overrode duration, but Estonian listeners were more responsive to duration cues. Such results support Sorin (1981), who conducted an extensive investigation of intensity and concluded that its linguistic functions remain to be clarified.

In considering the linguistic function of stress, it is useful to separate the questions of type and position. In traditional phonetics, stress frequently was divided into *dynamic* (or *expiratory*) stress and *musical* (or *melodic*) stress. Other phoneticians have maintained that in word stress, both dynamic and musical factors are always present but that one may predominate. This view appears satisfactory for treating languages with no independent tonal contrasts; that is, languages in which pitch contrasts are always associated with a stressed syllable.

Insistence on the independence of stress and pitch became strong among American linguists who worked with tone languages in which every syllable could carry contrastive tone, regardless of stress. Indeed, there is no automatic direct correlation between intensity and fundamental frequency; thus one has to assume the possibility of independent control of the two mechanisms. There is valid evidence, however, of various dependence relationships between them. Just as increases in subglottal pressure produce an increase in the rate of vibration of the vocal folds unless there is some compensatory adjustment in their tension, increases in subglottal pressure also result in greater amplitude of the sound wave even if fundamental frequency is kept constant by the just-postulated compensatory adjustment of the vocal folds. This means that each individual pulse produced by the vocal folds contains a greater amount of acoustic energy. Increases in the amplitude of the sound wave normally produce an impression of greater loudness, since more energy reaches the ear in a given unit of time. However, from what is known about the integrating time constant of the ear, it seems that the same effect should be achieved by a greater number of pulses reaching the ear per unit of time. Thus, higher frequency should produce impressions not only of higher pitch but also of greater loudness. At the frequencies of the human vocal range, the ear is also increasingly sensitive to higher frequencies. An increase in perceived loudness can be caused both by greater amplitude of the individual pulses (produced by increased subglottal pressure) and by a greater number of these pulses reaching the ear per unit of time (as a secondary result of higher subglottal pressure or as a primary result of increased tension of the vocal folds). It is not surprising, then, that the listener may attribute both types of increase to the same underlying cause and call them by the same name: stress.

There is no evidence that the listener can distinguish between increases of fundamental frequency that are caused by the two possible physiological mechanisms. However, it is probable that the speaker can distinguish between them, since the two mechanisms involve different and widely separated organs. The speaker knows which syllable he has stressed; the listener uses knowledge of the language and the phonetic cues in the sound wave to determine which syllable was stressed. This analysis-by-synthesis approach was anticipated by Jones (1940), who also discussed the problems of identifying the location of stress of unknown languages and the pitfalls of interpreting prominence achieved by other means as being due to stress.

Stress may function linguistically at word level and at sentence level. The minimum size of the unit of stress placement is the syllable; however, stressed and unstressed monosyllabic words can be distinguished only within a larger utterance. Thus the minimal unit of contrastive stress placement is a sequence of two syllables. If the placement of stress on one syllable of the word is not predictable by distributional, morphological, or lexical criteria, it is said that stress occupies an independent position in the phonology of the language; the term *phonemic stress,* or **free stress** is applied to this kind of linguistically significant stress. Languages in which stress distinguishes between otherwise identical words include, among others, Russian and English. The functional yield of stress in English is much smaller than in Russian. English

has very few pairs of words distinguished solely by stress; noun-verb pairs like *per'mit—permit',* *con'duct—conduct'* are the usual examples. However, the place of stress is fairly firmly fixed in English and serves an identificational feature: placement of stress on a different syllable changes a word into a nonword. In Russian stress is essentially free; it may occur on any syllable of a word. And in both English and Russian, unstressed syllables are reduced, so that an unreduced syllable nucleus constitutes an additional segmental cue for the presence and location of stress.

In a number of languages, the placement of stress on a certain syllable is determined wih the reference to the word; conversely, the position of stress identifies the word as a phonological unit. In languages with such *bound stress,* there is no opposition between stressed and unstressed syllables within word-level phonology, although there is an obvious phonetic difference between them. Bound stress may occur on the first syllable of a word, as in Czech and Hungarian; on the last syllable of a phonological phrase, as in French; or on the penultimate (next to last) syllable, as in Polish. Bound stress also may follow more complicated rules, as in Latin, in which stress is placed on the penultimate syllable if it is long and on the antepenultimate (third from last) if the penultimate syllable is short.

Another problem to be considered within word-level phonology is degrees of stress. It has been widely believed that there are four distinctive degrees of stress in English; however, the phonetic reality behind these degrees has been widely questioned. There exists no phonetic evidence for differences in degree of expiratory stress. Nevertheless, many linguists claim that between strong and weak stress, there are several intermediate degrees of stress that have a certain kind of subjective reality.

Word-level stress is probably an abstract quality, a potential for being stressed. It is the capacity of a syllable within a word to receive sentence stress when the word is realized as part of the sentence. The degrees of stress of other syllables within the word are usually predictable by rules and are therefore noncontrastive. Not all syllables that are perceived as stressed are associated with peaks of subglottal pressure; this supports the idea that what is realized phonetically is sentence-level rather than word-level stress. In other words, our knowledge of the structure of the language informs us which syllables have the potential to be stressed; we "hear" the underlying phonological form.

Stress at the sentence level does not change the meaning of any lexical item, but it increases the relative prominence of one of the lexical items. Each sentence has a *primary stress* (non-emphatic sentence stress). *Contrastive stress* occurs in sentences with parallel constituents filled with different morphemes. In other words, contrastive stress is used to distinguish a particular morpheme from other morphemes in the same position. *Emphatic stress* is used to call special attention to a word. Occasionally it is phonetically indistinguishable from contrastive stress, but in some instances and languages the two are different. Stress is also used with other prosodic features to identify a word or phrase as the focus of the sentence.

Phonetic evidence suggests that emphasized words are associated with subglottal pressure peaks; emphasis thus has a first-order phonetic correlate that word stress does not seem to have. As with stress in general, emphasis may be reflected in phonetic parameters other than, or in addition to, increased intensity.

SUMMARY AND OUTLOOK

This chapter surveys the suprasegmental features of duration, pitch, and stress and their role in spoken language. For each feature, production, acoustic manifestation, perception, and linguistic function have been considered. Of necessity, not all aspects have received equally thorough treatment; in particular, the function of suprasegmental features at levels higher than a sentence have been omitted. The discussion focuses on linguistic functions; each of the discussed parameters also has nonlinguistic communicative functions, such as signaling (or betraying) the speaker's attitude toward what is being communicated and degree of urgency. Voice quality, as distinct from vocal quality, is likewise used for paralinguistic purposes not addressed in this chapter.

An attempt has been made to separate the general from the language-specific. All humans share the same basic vocal tracts and sensory capacities. A search for language universals is still in progress; each language shares in the universal characteristics of language and uses a special subset of the available features and processes. Nevertheless, there is danger in assuming that what is specific for one's native language is universal. A phonetic study of genetically unrelated and typologically different languages will make it possible to separate the general from the specific (Fox and Lehiste, 1989; Lehiste and Fox, 1992). However, a study of phonetics without a parallel study of linguistics is unlikely to lead to real understanding of the ways spoken language functions.

While relatively more is known about duration and pitch, our knowledge of the phonetic manifestation of stress is still incomplete. This is an avenue for further research. All three prosodic features interact in the manifestation of stress, and there are interactions between the production and perception of duration and pitch. The relational nature of all prosodic features should be emphasized and studied: To what extent can the same message be conveyed with different phonetic means? What are the possibilities for compensatory substitutions? There are explanations to be found, reasons to be discovered, generalizations to be drawn, models to be built, hypotheses to be proposed, and theories to be established. The field is open for practically unlimited possibilities of future research.

Review Questions

1. Describe and discuss the notions of intrinsic duration, intrinsic pitch, and intrinsic intensity.

2. What is the influence of preceding and following segments on the duration and pitch of a segmental sound?

3. What is contrastive duration (linguistic quantity)?

4. What is contrastive fundamental frequency at the word level?

5. What is the relationship between tone and intonation?

6. What is the role of duration as a boundary signal?

7. What is the phonetic manifestation of stress?

8. Discuss the functions of stress at word level and sentence level.

References

Anderson, S. R. (1978). Tone features. In Fromkin, V. A. (Ed.), *Tone: A linguistic survey*. New York: Academic Press (pp. 133-175).

Antoniadis, Z., & Strube, H. W. (1981). Untersuchungen zum "intrinsic pitch" deutscher Vokale. *Phonetica, 38*, 277-290.

Beckman, M. E. (1986). *Stress and non-stress accent*. Dordrecht-Holland/Riverton-USA, Riverton, N.J.: Foris Publications.

Bertinetto, P. M. (1980). The perception of stress by Italian speakers. *Journal of Phonetics, 8*, 385-395.

Cohen, A., Collier, R., & 't Hart, J. (1982). Declination: Construct or intrinsic feature of speech pitch? *Phonetica 39*, 254-273.

Crystal, T. H., and House, A. S. (1988). The duration of American-English vowels: An overview. *Journal of Phonetics, 16*, 263-284.

Cutler, A. (1991). Linguistic rhythm and speech segmentation. In Sundberg, J. Nord, L., & Carlson, R. (Eds.), *Music, language, speech, and brain*. Houndmills and London: MacMillan.

Cutler, A., & Ladd, D. R. (Eds.). (1983). *Prosody: Models and measurements*. New York: Springer-Verlag.

Dauer, R. M. (1983). Stress-timing and syllable-timing reanalyzed. *Journal of Phonetics, 11*, 51-62.

Eek, A. (1987). The perception of word stress: A comparison of Estonian and Russian. In Channon, R., & Shockey, L. (Eds.), *In honor of Ilse Lehiste*. Providence, RI: Foris (pp. 19-32).

Fant, G., Kruckenberg, A., & Nord, L. (1991). Durational correlates of stress in Swedish, French and English. *Journal of Phonetics 19* (3/4), 351-365.

Fischer--Jørgensen, E. (1964). Sound duration and place of articulation. *Zeitschrift für Sprachwissenschaft und Kommunikationsforschung, 17*, 175-207.

Fischer-Jørgensen, E. (1983). The acoustic manifestation of stress in Danish with particular reference to the reduction of stress in compounds. In van den Broecke, M., van Heuven, V., & Zonneveld, W. (Eds.), *Studies for antonie cohen: Sound structures*. Cinnaminson, NJ: Foris (pp. 81-104).

Fox, R. A., & Lehiste, I. (1989). Discrimination of duration ratios in bisyllabic tokens by native English and Estonian listeners. *Journal of Phonetics 17* (3), 167-174.

Fujimura, O. (1990). Articulatory perspectives of speech organization. In Hardcastle W. J., & Marchal, A. (Eds.), *Speech production and speech modelling*. The Netherlands: Kluwer Academic Publishers (pp. 323-342).

Gussenhoven, C., & Rietveld, A. C. M. (1988). Fundamental frequency declination in Dutch: Testing three hypotheses. *Journal of Phonetics, 16*, 355-369.

Gussenhoven, C., & Rietveld, A. C. M. (1992). Intonation contours, prosodic structure and pre-boundary lengthening. *Journal of Phonetics 20* (3), 283-303.

Hombert, J.-M. (1978). Consonant types, vowel quality, and tone. In Fromkin, V. A. (Ed.), *Tone: A linguistic survey*. New York: Academic Press (pp. 77-111).

Honda, K. (1983). Relationship between pitch control and vowel articulation. In Bless, D. M., & Abbs, J. H. (Eds.), *Vocal fold physiology*. San Diego: College Hill Press (pp. 286-299).

Honda, K., & Fujimura, O. (1991). Intrinsic vowel F_o and phrase-final F_0 lowering: Phonological versus biological explanations. In Gauffin, J., and Hammarberg, B. (Eds.), *Phonatory mechanisms: Physiology, acoustics, and assessment*. San Diego: Singular Publishing Group (pp. 149-157).

Howie, J. M. (1974). On the domain of tone in Mandarin. *Phonetica, 30*, 129-148.

Jones, D. (1940). *An outline of English phonetics*, (6th ed.). New York: Dutton.

Kluender, K. R., Diehl, R. L., & Wright, B. A. (1988). Vowel-length differences before voiced and voiceless consonants: An auditory explanation. *Journal of Phonetics, 16*, 153-169.

Kohler, K. J. (1980). Timing of articulatory control in the production of plosives. *Phonetica 38*, 116-125.

Kohler, K. J. (1983). Prosodic boundary signals in German. *Phonetica 40*, 89-134.

Ladd, D. R., & Silverman, K. E. A. (1984). Vowel intrinsic pitch in connected speech. *Phonetica, 41*, 31-40.

Ladefoged, P. (1982). *A course in phonetics*. San Diego: Harcourt Brace Jovanovich.

Laeufer, C. (1992). Patterns of voicing-conditioned vowel duration in French and English. *Journal of Phonetics 20* (4), 411-440.

Lahiri, A., & Hankamer, J. (1988). The timing of geminate consonants. *Journal of Phonetics, 16*, 327-338.

Lehiste, I. (1960). An acoustic-phonetic study of internal open juncture. *Supplement to Phonetica 5*, 1-54.

Lehiste, I. (1970). *Suprasegmentals*. Cambridge, MA: MIT Press.

Lehiste, I. (1972a). The timing of utterances and linguistic boundaries. *Journal of the Acoustical Society of America, 51*, 2018-2024.

Lehiste, I. (1972b). Temporal compensation in a quantity language. In Rigault, A., & Charbonneau, R. (Eds.), *Proceedings of the Seventh International Congress of Phonetic Sciences*. The Hague: Mouton (pp. 929-939.)

Lehiste, I. (1973). Phonetic disambiguation of syntactic ambiguity. *Glossa 7*, 107-122.

Lehiste, I. (1975). Some factors affecting the duration of syllable nuclei in English. *Salzburger Beiträge zur Linguistik, 1,* 81-104.

Lehiste, I. (1980). Phonetic manifestation of syntactic structure in English. *Annual Bulletin, Research Institute of Logopedics and Phoniatrics, University of Tokyo, 14,* 1-27.

Lehiste, I. (1989). Current debates concerning Estonian quantity. *Proceedings of the Sixth Annual Meeting of the Finno-Ugric Studies Association of Canada.* Lanham, MD: University Press of America, 77-86.

Lehiste, I., & Fox, R.A. (1992). Perception of prominence by Estonian and English listeners. *Language and Speech 35* (4), 419-434.

Lehiste, I., & Ivić, P. (1963). *Accent in Serbocroatian: An experimental study.* Michigan Slavic Materials 4. Ann Arbor: University of Michigan.

Lehiste, I., Olive, J. P., & Streeter, L. A. (1976). Role of duration in disambiguating syntactically ambiguous sentences. *Journal of the Acoustical Society of America, 60,* 1199-1202.

Lehiste, I., & Peterson, G.E. (1959). Vowel amplitude and phonemic stress in American English. *Journal of the Acoustical Society of America, 31,* 428-435.

Lehiste, I., & Peterson, G.E. (1961). Some basic considerations in the analysis of intonation. *Journal of the Acoustical Society of America, 33,* 419-425.

Lehiste, I., Morton, K., & Tatham, M. (1973). An instrumental study of consonant gemination. *Journal of Phonetics, 1,* 131-148.

Liberman, A.M., Cooper, F.S., Harris, K.S., & MacNeilage, P.F. (1963). Motor theory of speech perception. Paper D 3 in *Stockholm Speech Communication Seminar,* Vol. 2. Stockholm: Speech Transmission Laboratory, Royal Institute of Technology.

Maddieson, I. (Ed.). (1974). An annotated bibliography of tone. *UCLA Working Papers in Phonetics, 28,* 1-78.

Ohala, J. J. (1978). Production of tone. In Fromkin, V. A. (Ed.), *Tone: A linguistic survey.* New York: Academic Press (pp. 5-39).

O'Malley, M.H., Kloker, D.R., & Dara-Abrams, B. (1973). Recovering parentheses from spoken algebraic expressions. *IEEE Transactions on Audio and Electro-acoustics, AU-21,* 217-220.

Peterson, G.E., & Lehiste, I. (1960). Duration of syllable nuclei in English. *Journal of the Acoustical Society of America, 32,* 693-703.

Pierrehumbert, J.B. (1979). The perception of F_o declination. *Journal of the Acoustical Society of America, 66,* 363-369.

Pike, K.L. (1945). *The intonation of American English.* Ann Arbor: University of Michigan Press.

Pike, K.L. (1948). *Tone Languages.* Ann Arbor: University of Michigan Press.

Silverman, K., Beckman, M., Pitrelli, J., Ostendorf, M., Wightman, C., Price, P., Pierrehumbert, J., & Hirschberg, J. (1992). *TOBI: A standard for labeling English prosody.* In Ohala, J. J., Nearey, T. M., Derwing, B. L., Hodge, M. M., & Wiebe, G. E. (Eds.), *ICSLP 92 Proceedings. 1992 International Conference on Spoken Language Processing.* Edmonton: University of Alberta (pp. 867-870).

Sorin, C. (1981). Functions, roles and treatments of intensity in speech. *Journal of Phonetics, 9,* 359-374.

Sternberg, S., Knoll, R. L., Monsell, S., & Wright, E. C. (1988). Motor programs and hierarchical organization in the control of rapid speech. *Phonetica, 45,* 175-197.

Terken, J. (1991). Fundamental frequency and perceived prominence of accented syllables. *Journal of the Acoustical Society of America, 89,* 1768-1776.

Vaissière, J. (1983). Language-independent prosodic features. In Cutler, A., & Ladd, D.R. (Eds.), *Prosody: Models and measurements.* New York: Springer-Verlag (pp. 53-66).

Wang, W. S.-Y. (1967). Phonological features of tone. *International Journal of American Linguistics, 33,* 93-105.

Wenk, B. J., & Wioland, F. (1982). Is French really syllable-timed? *Journal of Phonetics, 10,* 193-216.

Suggested Readings

General

Couper-Kuhlen, E. (1986). *An introduction to English prosody.* Baltimore: Edward Arnold.

Denes, P.B., & Pinson, E.N. (1993). *The speech chain: The physics and biology of spoken language.* New York: W.H. Freeman.

Dickson, D. R., & Maue-Dickson, W. (1982). *Anatomical and physiological bases of speech.* Boston: Little, Brown.

Kent, R. D., Atal, B. S., & Miller, J. L. (Eds.). (1991). *Papers in speech communication: Speech production.* Woodbury, New York: Acoustical Society of America.

Kohler, K. J. (Ed.). (1986). Prosodic cues for segments. *Phonetica 43,* 1-154.

Lehiste, I. (1970). *Suprasegmentals.* Cambridge, MA: MIT Press.

Miller, J. L., Kent, R. D., & Atal, B. S. (Eds.). (1991). *Papers in Speech Communication: Speech Perception.* Woodbury, New York: Acoustical Society of America.

Ohala, J. J., & Jaeger, J. J. (Eds.). (1986). *Experimental phonology.* Orlando, FL: Academic Press.

Sundberg, J. (1991). *The science of musical sounds.* San Diego, CA: Academic Press.

Duration and Quantity

Klatt, D. H. (1976). Linguistic uses of segmental duration in English: Acoustic and perceptual evidence. *Journal of the Acoustical Society of America, 59,* 1208-1221.

Kohler, K. J. (Ed.). (1981). Temporal aspects of speech production and perception. *Phonetica, 38,* 1-212.

Tone and Intonation

Fromkin, V. A. (Ed.). (1978). *Tone: A linguistic survey.* New York: Academic Press.

Kohler, K. J. (Ed.). (1982). Pitch analysis. *Phonetica, 39,* 185-336.

Pierrehumbert, J. B., & Beckman, M. E. (1988). *Japanese tone structure.* Cambridge, MA: MIT Press.

Stress and Emphasis

Beckman, M. E. (1986). *Stress and non-stress accent.* Dordrecht-Holland/Riverton-USA, Riverton, N.J.: Foris.

Napoli, D. J. (Ed.). (1978). *Elements of tone, stress, and intonation.* Washington, DC: Georgetown University Press.

Chapter 7

Speech Analysis and Synthesis

Hector R. Javkin

Chapter Outline

Key Terms

INTRODUCTION

This chapter discusses both analysis and synthesis but puts less emphasis on analysis because it is discussed in detail in Chapter 13. This chapter addresses areas of analysis not covered in Chapter 13 and those most relevant to synthesis. It also treats basic tools such as sampling, time analysis of the waveform, and the settings and results of Fourier analysis. Synthesis is addressed with particular emphasis on its most challenging and useful aspects, *synthesis by rule* and *text-to-speech*. Text-to-speech is viewed as both a practical application and a research goal.

The analysis and synthesis of speech are related in many ways, but they are distinct processes. Some methods for the transmission of speech explicitly combine the two processes, but there is a broader-based if less direct link: the knowledge gained by improving methods of analysis has significantly influenced progress in synthesis. Furthermore, certain methods of analysis have been refined and reduced to practice because they were needed for the development of synthetic speech.

Speech analysis consists of making the acoustic speech signal easier to understand, most often by breaking it into its constituent frequencies. Since speech varies over time, it must be broken down over intervals. It is typical to take a portion of speech 2 to 3 seconds long—a time that may well encompass a sentence—and analyze it in 10-ms intervals, although some instruments can depict the entire sentence at once.

Speech **synthesis** consists of bringing together elements of sound to create an acoustic signal that sounds more or less like human speech. It is typical to create a sound similar to that produced by the vocal folds and to filter it to produce synthetic speech. If the filters do not vary, only certain speech sounds, such as vowels or fricative consonants, can be produced. However, varying the elements allows the synthesis of words and sentences. A type of synthesis that has attained considerable importance is text-to-speech, which automatically converts typed material into speech.

SPEECH ANALYSIS

The purpose of speech analysis is to represent the speech signal in a way that permits an understanding of some aspect of speech. Although this rather broad goal has remained constant, the practice of analysis has changed greatly in recent years with advances in computers. Some methods are possible only with computers because of the large number of repetitive calculations that they require. A few methods have remained essentially the same, becoming only more convenient and somewhat more accurate with the advance of technology.

The vast majority of analysis methods take the time waveform, the variations in pressure over time that make up sound, and produce a spectral representation, a breakdown of the energy into the different frequencies found at particular times. However, before most analyses the signal has to be entered into a computer.

Preliminaries: Sampling

So much acoustic analysis is performed computationally that normally the first step is to input speech to a computer. Even the sound **spectrograph**, once the most frequently used nondigital speech analysis instrument, is now usually a specialized computer, so any speech it analyzes first must be moved into its memory. How the input is done has important consequences for the analysis. The continuously varying pressure wave that is speech is put into a computer-usable form by converting the voltage from a microphone into numbers through a process of measuring it, or **sampling** it, at regular intervals (Figure 7-1).

The voltage is measured in this case (used only for illustration) once per millisecond and converted to integer form in the computer. The integers will retain the relative values that were sampled, but often not the actual voltage. However, this is not a concern; the voltage will be affected by the strength of the amplifier and the speaker's distance from the microphone. Within certain bounds these factors do not affect the essential information in speech. It is important that the gain of the amplifier and microphone not change during the sampling of the speech segment to be analyzed, so that the values that are sampled maintain their relation to each other.

The typical sampling rate, or sampling frequency, for speech is 8000 to 40,000 Hz. The sampling rate will determine, among other aspects of the analysis, how high a frequency can be measured in a computer analysis. For an undistorted representation, the sampling rate must be at least twice the frequency of any components present in the signal. Any components that are higher than half the sampling frequency will cause distortion that cannot be removed by subsequent processes; the only solution is to sample once again. The distortion caused by having components that are higher than half the sampling rate is **aliasing.** Half the sampling rate is the *Nyquist rate.* Nyquist (1924), is generally credited with proving that any energy over half the sampling frequency will lead to distortion. To avoid such distortions, prior to sampling the signal must be filtered to remove frequency components above the Nyquist frequency.

Fourier Analysis

Speech is a complex wave consisting of a number of frequency components, and most analyses consist of separating speech into individual components. One variation of Fourier analysis is the most commonly used method for this purpose. It is based on the theorem of Jean Baptiste Fourier (Bloomfield, 1976) who showed that any complex wave can be broken down into sine waves. Although Fourier analysis can provide information not only about the **magnitude spectrum** (the magnitude of each of the components by frequency) but also about *phase* (the relative timing of each of the components) it is very common in speech research to discard the phase information and retain only the magnitude spectrum. This is largely because humans are considerably more sensitive to the magnitude spectrum of a speech sound than they are to the phase relation of its components (Patterson, 1973). The analysis, a **transformation,** takes data in the time domain and transforms them to frequencies. Since computers process information in discrete samples in time, a variation of this analysis, called the *discrete Fourier transform,* or DFT, was developed for computation. A version of DFT, the *fast Fourier transform,* or FFT (Cooley and Tukey, 1965), was developed to make computation faster. It requires that the speech

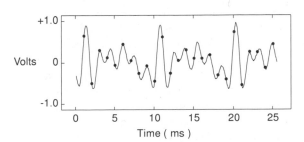

FIGURE 7-1 A sound waveform from which samples have been measured. The dots represent the samples, one per millisecond.

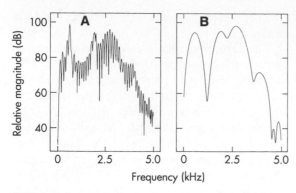

FIGURE 7-2 Comparison of *A*, a 256-point FFT, and *B*, a 32-point FT.

sample to be analyzed have a length in sample points that is a power of two (for example, a 256-point FFT). Another more important reason the length of the sample is often reported is that it affects the **resolution,** or fineness of detail, of the analysis. Figure 7-2 shows the difference between an FFT performed with 256 points and with 32 points. The sample rate for the speech data was 10 KHz.

The 256-point analysis provides much more resolution than the 32-point analysis. To calculate the resolution, divide the sample rate (10 KHz in this case) by the number of sample points. The 256-point analysis thus gives approximately 40 Hz resolution, and the 32-point analysis, about 300 Hz. The trade-off is that a 32-point analysis gives information about a much shorter moment, and hence permits the observation of fast-changing acoustic events such as the release burst of stop consonants. This trade-off between temporal and frequency resolution is an important characteristic of all acoustic analyses and is particularly significant in spectrograms, which are discussed in Chapter 13 and also briefly in the next section.

Zero padding is sometimes used to bring an analysis window up to a number of sample points of a power of two. In zero padding, a short piece of waveform is selected and zeros are added to the end to extend it. For example, a 100-point window can have 28 points with zeros added to make it a window with 128 points. This procedure will make the faster FFT procedure usable but cannot increase the frequency resolution of an analysis (Kay, 1988). Zero padding will neither harm the analysis nor add any resolution. In other words, the analysis of a 100-point section of waveform that has been padded to 128 points will still give the frequency resolution of a 100-point analysis.

The fact that the frequency resolution is determined by dividing the sample rate over the number of points in the FFT analysis means that for many analyses it is not necessary to make the sampling rate as high as possible. Increasing the number of points in the analysis to raise the frequency resolution requires more computer time, and many computer analysis programs have an upper limit to the number of points. Since most of the information in vowels lies below 4000 Hz, a relatively low sample rate, about 8000 to 10,000 Hz, can be used for vowels. Therefore, if the speech is initially sampled into the computer only for analyzing vowels, a low sample rate can be used. If the speech is sampled for a variety of purposes, some of which require a high sample rate, a *down-sampled* copy can be made for vowel analysis. **Downsampling** is taking samples from a signal that has already been sampled into the computer. It is frequently used with analyses designed to recover **fundamental frequency,** since the higher-frequency information is not needed. Prior to downsampling, the signal must be filtered, as in the original sampling, to avoid aliasing.

Spectrographic Analysis

Speech can be described in terms of three variables: *magnitude, frequency,* and *time*. The sound spectrograph presents these three variables on a two-dimensional display, with magnitude shown as darkness. The contemporary spectrograph is a specially adapted computer. A sample of sound 2 to 5 seconds long is introduced via a microphone or by playing a recording. The resulting display is shown on a computer screen, where it can be examined and possibly selected for printing. Since the variations in amplitude are given by the darkness of the display, it is standard to use a gray-scale printer to observe differences in amplitude. In practice much detail is lost, and only the higher-amplitude components are visible. Nevertheless, these higher-amplitude components are most important in speech, and combining the three acoustic variables on a single page has made the spectrograph an important tool for viewing the speech signal. Particularly useful is the fact that changes in the spectrum over time are noticed easily. Figure 7-3 shows a sentence, "We owe you a yoyo," often used in the early days of spectrographic analysis. The large move-

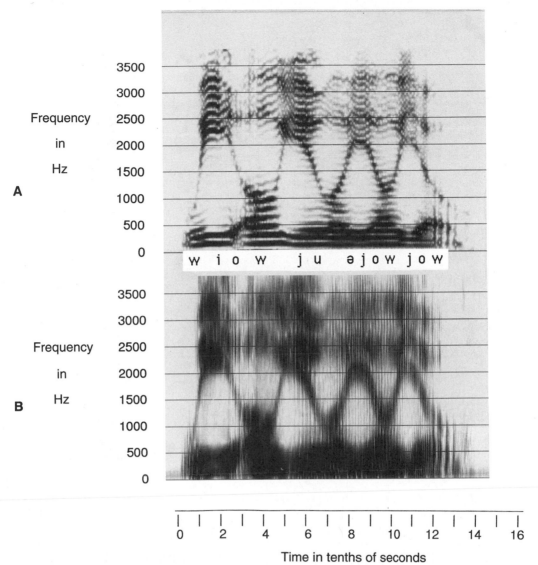

FIGURE 7-3   Narrowband *(A)* and wideband *(B)* spectrograms of the utterance, "We owe you a yoyo," spoken by a 22-year-old male.

ments of the second formant start around 700 Hz at 80 ms, go up to about 2400 Hz at 170 ms, and continue rising and falling. Note the thin horizontal lines providing frequency reference. The spectrograph is also used for the analysis of many other sounds, including music, environmental noise, engine vibration, medically significant sounds such as heart murmurs, and underwater sounds produced by marine mammals.

This trade-off between temporal and frequency resolution is clearly visible in the sound spectrograph. Narrowband **spectrograms** (high frequency resolution, low temporal resolution) have been used primarily to determine fundamental frequency, and wideband spectrograms (low frequency resolution, high temporal reso-

lution) were used for most other speech analyses because they give a useful image of formant movements, stop bursts, and other features. It is now uncommon to use spectrograms for fundamental frequency extraction because faster and usually more accurate computer-based methods are available. Nevertheless, narrowband spectrograms are sometimes used with wideband spectrograms of the same speech sample to determine formant values, particularly when two formants appear as a single dark area on wideband spectrograms.

Figure 7-4 shows the name "Harry" extracted from the phrase "Tom, Dick, Harry" at about 1250 to 1400 ms. Formant movements in the wideband spectrogram are difficult to see in

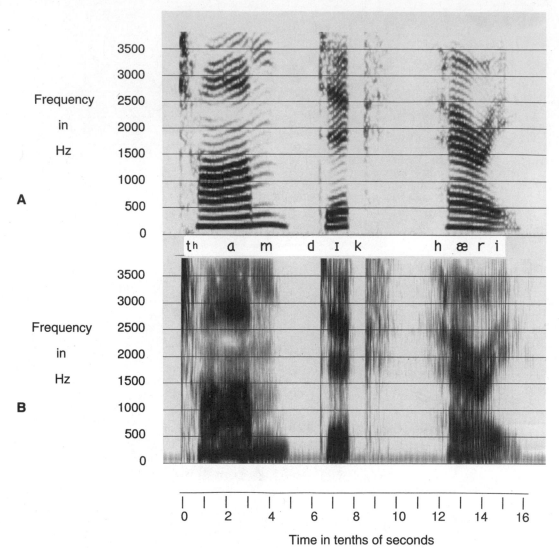

FIGURE 7-4   Narrowband *(A)* and wideband *(B)* spectrograms of the utterance, "Tom, Dick, Harry," spoken by a 22-year-old male.

the narrowband version. However, the separation between formants at about 1000 Hz is easier to see in the narrowband version. The dark horizontal lines in the narrow band show the **harmonics** of the voice. They can give a false sense of accuracy because harmonics often do not coincide with the center of a formant. Thus, even a carefully measured formant value on a narrowband spectrogram can be inexact.

Visual Analysis of the Time Waveform of Speech

A commonly neglected type of analysis is a direct observation of the time waveform of speech. It cannot be used for any large amount of data

because it is very time-consuming, but it can be essential if there is reason to suspect that something is wrong with another analysis method; it should be checked. Figure 7-5 shows the waveform of an unknown vowel. The vertical axis indicates pressure as measured by the diaphragm of a microphone, and the horizontal axis shows time.

This waveform reveals the approximate fundamental frequency, the frequency at which the waveform more or less repeats itself. This particular waveform has some major upward vertical deflections that can be used as a reference to determine the time of the repetition. Begin counting from the deflection at about 4 ms. The beginning of the next repetition is at

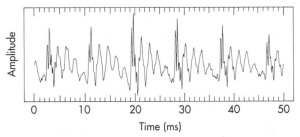

FIGURE 7-5   The waveform of an unknown vowel.

about 11 ms, so that the period of the waveform is about 7 ms. If the period stays the same, in 1 second there will be 1000/7 or 143 cycles. (Note that the period actually changes after the first cycle, so the frequency should be calculated again.) This visual analysis can be very accurate for determining fundamental frequency if the analyst displays the waveform on a computer screen and uses a cursor to locate the points to be measured. However, its main usefulness is its reliability: the duration of the signal will yield a reasonable estimate of fundamental frequency, which can be compared with the results of the method being tested.

Additional information can be extracted from the waveform. The first formant will often be very visible as oscillations that follow the major deflections, so that its frequency can also be estimated. In this waveform the spacing of the oscillations is such that about five fit into a fundamental frequency cycle, so that the frequency is approximately 5 × 143, or about 715 Hz. Here the measurement is inherently an estimate because it is more difficult to determine the exact end of the oscillation. In addition some caution is necessary with formant estimates, because two formants can be very close together and interact so as to give the appearance of a single formant at a given frequency.

Direct observation of the waveform can also suggest undesired **clipping** of the signal. Clipping occurs when amplitude exceeds the range of the equipment. When the maximum allowable amplitude for an amplifier or a computer is exceeded, the signal will be distorted, although sometimes the distortion is not noticed. Unfortunately, it is not possible to distinguish between a signal at the maximum (which is acceptable) and one beyond the maximum (which is distorted). The only safe procedure is to rerecord at a lower level any signal that shows values at the maximum. To avoid clipping, measure the signal level with a meter connected to the input circuit

and allow some **headroom** between the highest signal observed and the meter's indication of the maximum level that the computer can accept.

Time Analysis of the Glottal Waveform

Time analysis is sometimes the indicated method of analyzing the glottal waveform, in part because the time waveform is the easiest way to relate the acoustic signal to the movements of the vocal folds. The waveform of airflow through the vocal folds, the *airflow volume velocity,* or *glottal volume velocity,* reflects quite closely the pattern of physical opening and closing of the vocal folds. The time waveform is useful for synthesized speech, which is more nearly natural-sounding if its source waveform is similar to the human glottal waveform.

The human glottal waveform cannot be viewed directly. The output of the **glottis** passes through the vocal tract, whose **resonances** introduce formants, and changes again as it leaves the vocal tract and radiates from the lips. The **radiation** of this wave through the lips raises the amplitude of the high frequencies of the waveform. This is often called *raising the spectral tilt.* To examine the glottal waveform, it is necessary to remove both the radiation's effects on the spectral tilt and the formants introduced by the vocal tract. This can be done by means of an **inverse filter** (Rothenberg, 1973). Since the vocal tract filters the glottal signal, the inverse of the vocal tract filter will remove its effect. Similarly, a filter that lowers the amplitude of the higher frequencies (called an **integrator** because it performs a mathematical **integration** on the waveform) can be used to lower the spectral tilt (Fig. 7-6).

Inverse filtering to recover the source signal is a complex process. Although the integrator (which restores the original spectral tilt) stays constant, the frequency and **bandwidth** of the formants vary, and the inverse filter settings have

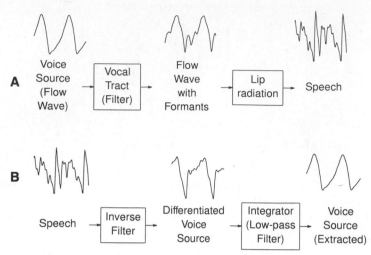

FIGURE 7-6 *A,* A voice source filtered by the vocal tract and lips. *B,* A speech wave filtered to recover the voice source.

to vary in precisely the same way to avoid erroneous output. It is particularly difficult to measure bandwidths; sometimes the only way to do it is to examine the waveform, try different filtering values, and observe when the formants are removed. This time-consuming process is worthwhile for the development of speech synthesis because it yields a thorough knowledge of the acoustic characteristics of the glottal volume velocity waveform.

Future Directions in the Analysis of Speech

Computer speech analysis will continue to become easier as computers with very large memories get faster and cheaper. In addition, analysis programs will become easier to use, which is likely to have negative as well as positive effects. Early speech analysis programs required considerable patience and knowledge of speech analysis. However, the ease of use of many contemporary computer programs may allow users to perform analyses without understanding their limitations. For example, fundamental frequency extraction algorithms sometimes momentarily mistake the second harmonic for the fundamental frequency and therefore display an apparent sudden shift in the fundamental to twice its value. Although such shifts can occur in speech, the possibility of error from a fundamental frequency extraction algorithm should be explored by testing with an alternate analysis method, possibly including direct observation of

the acoustic waveform. Therefore, it is important, even with apparently user-friendly analysis programs, to be alert to possible errors.

A promising direction is shown by analyses that mimic aspects of human perception. In particular, analyses that model the human listener's frequency and temporal resolutions are likely to be improved and used more in the future. The decreasing frequency sensitivity of the human ear with increasing frequency can be represented with a *Mel scale* (Stevens, Volkman, and Newman, 1937), but this phenomenon does not represent the interaction between different frequency components that occur in hearing.

Some analyses reflect the fact that the human auditory system acts somewhat like a set of overlapping filters, each tuned to a different frequency, as established by Wegel and Lane (1924) and Fletcher (1940). Surrounding a given frequency there is a range of frequencies, or **critical band,** that is most effective in masking the energy of that frequency. The width of the critical bands increases at higher frequencies, and the term *Bark* describes the width of the critical band at any frequency. The estimates of its frequencies have varied (Greenwood, 1961; Zwicker, 1961; Greenwood, 1974; Houtgast, 1977). Recent analyses using critical band data and other characteristics of human audition as a starting point (Ghitza, 1988, 1992; Seneff, 1988; Shamma, 1988) not only clarify how speech is perceived but also improve the automatic recognition of speech. On the assumption that speech has evolved at least to some extent to use the characteristics of human audition, a model of human audition may be the most effective way to analyze speech. These models emulate the auditory apparatus in that they use true filters with narrow bandwidths for lower frequencies and increasingly wider bandwidths for higher frequencies.

Other analyses create a similar effect by simply converting the output of an FFT into a scale with narrow bandwidths at the low frequencies and wide bandwidths at the high frequencies. Although this will represent the frequency resolution of human hearing, it fails to represent the increasing temporal resolution in the higher frequencies. This is another complication of the trade-off between frequency resolution and temporal resolution. The ear's decreasing frequency sensitivity with increasing frequency is accompanied by an increased temporal resolution. This pattern can be modeled when filters are used to provide the critical band scale spacing. When an FFT is used, the frequency and temporal resolutions are the same all along the spectrum. Converting an FFT analysis to Bark frequency spacing does not change the temporal resolution because the maximum temporal resolution is determined by the number of points used for the FFT.

One of the characteristics of human perception is that a change in a parameter can be more salient than a steady-state value. Analyses that model this characteristic by measuring the slopes of speech parameters, such as those of Furui (1986) and Hanson and Applebaum (1990), are likely to be of increasing importance in the future. Performing analysis at places in the waveform where the results are best is another promising future direction. Childers and Lee (1991) used this method to improve the inverse filtering analysis of the glottal waveform. The formants and bandwidth are easiest to measure when the vocal folds are closed; Childers and Lee made their measurements at those times.

SPEECH SYNTHESIS

In speech synthesis, a machine or computer is used to create, not merely reproduce, sound that can be recognized as speech. The difference between synthesis and playing speech from a tape recorder or a computer functioning as a tape recorder is that components of speech are joined to create speech that need not have been previously spoken by a human. Analyzing speech into components and resynthesizing those components into the same utterance is *speech coding*. Coding is usually used to decrease the amount of data necessary to transmit or store speech. Although it is a form of synthesis and an interesting engineering problem, coding will not be addressed in this chapter, which treats methods to generate new utterances.

Speech synthesis has shown its usefulness in research both as a means of preparing perceptual experiments and as a test of knowledge of speech. Synthetic speech has the advantage over edited natural speech for perceptual experiments in that all the variables can be precisely controlled. As a model of knowledge, synthesis has an incomparable advantage over many scientific models; unlike many simulations, the output of a speech synthesizer is inherently available to the ears. However, sound quality is not the only test. The internal workings of the model must be evaluated along with the sound to determine what knowledge is being tested.

Various forms of synthesized speech are used in man-machine communication. The synthesized speech used in automobiles and some other machines to provide a limited number of stored messages is usually coded. The quality of such speech can be excellent, depending on the coding method, and can lead listeners to conclude that the research issues in speech synthesis have been resolved. Listening to the mechanical quality of text-to-speech can therefore be a disappointment. The reason that text-to-speech is more difficult to develop stems from the highly complex way the sounds of human speech are joined to make words and sentences. Nevertheless, text-to-speech synthesis has reached a quality sufficient to make it a useful tool for many people. Reading machines for the blind that combine an optical character reader, a computer controller, and a text-to-speech system can free visually impaired persons from the need for human readers (Kurzweil, 1976). A variation of this is reading material for the blind in a computer-readable form, which can be accessed by a text-to-speech system (van Bezooijen and Jongenburger, 1993). The advantages of this method over a reading machine are that no errors are introduced by the optical scanning and that sometimes the material can be edited to optimize it for a spoken rather than a visual form. Text-to-speech can allow the use of an ordinary telephone to access computer databases containing medical information, bank balances, telephone numbers, and so on. The accuracy of proofreading of material that has been typed into a computer can sometimes be improved by having it read aloud by a synthesizer.

First Attempts

The first interesting speech synthesizer was built in the nineteenth century by Wilhelm von Kempelen, who earlier in his career built a "chess-playing machine" by hiding a small, legless man who was an excellent player inside an impressive-looking box. Its "mechanism" was eventually discovered. In contrast, von Kempelen's speech synthesizer (Dudley and Tarnoczy, 1950) was a well-considered system: bellows substituted for lungs, a vibrating reed substituted for the vocal folds, and a malleable leather resonator substituted for the vocal tract. Two outlets served as nostrils, and a whistle was used to generate some fricatives.

Von Kempelen's machine is particularly notable in that he used mechanisms that are principled analogs to human speech production. Bellows, like the lungs, are air containers that can be compressed to produce airflow. A vibrating reed (unlike, for example, a motor-driven siren) works on the same principle as the human vocal cords: they are alternatively closed and opened by a combination of pressure and **Bernoulli forces** generated by the airstream (van den Berg, 1958). Von Kempelen's malleable leather resonator, like the human vocal tract, varied in shape to create different resonating cavities, producing different formants. Creating a second cavity for the nasals with additional outlets uses the same general principle as human nasal sounds, although his nasal outlets appear to have been smaller than would be needed for an adequate resonance. A whistle normally creates periodic sounds, but a whistle with its constriction increased will, like a vocal tract shaped for a fricative, produce aperiodic sound by creating turbulence.

Determining to what extent a model is a good analogy to what is being modeled can be important. If a model (1) is related in a principled way to what is modeled, and (2) is more convenient to manipulate than the phenomenon that is modeled, it can lead to increased knowledge. In von Kempelen's synthesizer, for example, the addition of some mass to the reed representing the vocal folds while holding other parameters constant will lower fundamental frequency. By comparison, certain musical instruments can imitate certain speech sounds while functioning in a very different way; one can imitate the sound of the release of a stop consonant such as /t/ by using metal brushes on a snare drum. However, manipulating the sound produced by a snare drum will teach us little about the production of speech.

Methods of Synthesis

With the invention of the telephone and the development of electronic circuitry, speech synthesizers began to be developed as electric analogs and eventually as computational analogs to speech production.

The separation of speech into a source and a filter has been fundamental for speech synthesis. The source of speech can be the vibration of the vocal folds, the **frication** resulting from a constriction in the vocal tract, or the explosion resulting from the sudden opening of closure in the vocal tract after a pressure difference has built up. The filter is the vocal tract, whose shape and properties of sound absorption and radiation determine its resonating properties. The absorption and radiation essentially do not change. Changing the vocal tract shape changes the resonances, producing different sounds. The source and filter in speech production are relatively independent. When the source consists of vocal fold vibration, it is for the most part unaffected by the resonances of the vocal tract. In other words, fundamental frequency essentially does not change when the vocal tract position alters to form another vowel. Similarly, the resonances of the vocal tract are mostly unaffected by changes in the vocal fold vibration, although there are small interaction effects. Since the vocal folds are at one end of the vocal tract, the resonances of the vocal tract are affected by whether the vocal folds are open or not, even though the opening is relatively small. When they are vibrating, the effects of the difference between an open and a closed position take place at the rate of vibration. Since many analysis methods take a time slice that includes one or more whole cycles, these effects are usually obscured.

The resonances of the vocal tract also slightly affect vocal fold vibration. Resonances favor certain frequencies. When the vocal tract is positioned so that the frequency of the first resonance is close to the fundamental frequency, the resonance will have a tendency to pull the

TABLE 7-1   Measurements of the cross-sectional area for Russian vowels converted to diameters

Distance from Lips (cm)	a *diameter* (cm)	e *diameter* (cm)	i *diameter* (cm)	o *diameter* (cm)	u *diameter* (cm)
0	2.52	3.19	2.26	2.02	0.91
1	2.52	2.52	2.02	2.02	0.64
2	2.88	2.26	1.29	2.88	1.60
3	3.19	1.60	0.91	4.07	3.66
4	3.19	1.82	0.91	4.07	4.07
5	3.19	2.26	0.91	3.66	4.07
6	3.19	2.26	0.91	3.19	3.19
7	2.52	2.52	1.82	2.88	2.52
8	2.02	3.19	2.88	2.52	1.82
9	1.82	3.19	3.19	2.02	1.60
10	1.60	3.66	3.66	1.43	1.43
11	1.29	3.66	3.66	1.29	1.60
12	0.91	3.19	3.66	0.91	1.13
13	0.91	2.88	3.66	1.13	1.13
14	1.43	2.88	3.19	1.43	1.43
15	2.26	1.29	1.60	2.02	2.52
16	1.29	1.60	1.82	2.52	3.19
17	1.82			1.29	3.66
18				1.43	1.60
19					1.82

(Adapted from Fant, G. [1960]. *Acoustic theory of speech production*. The Hague: Mouton.)

fundamental frequency toward the frequency of the first resonance.

Most speech synthesis systems are based on the separation of the filter in the vocal tract, which determines the resonances through which a signal passes from the original signal. Not only does this separation reflect what is occurring in the human speech signal, it also allows the separation of an extremely complicated process into two parts that are somewhat more manageable.

Vocal Tract Models

One way to implement source-filter theory in a speech synthesizer is to create a source waveform and to pass it through a model that simulates the reflections and output characteristics of the vocal tract. Such models can be physical resonators having the same dimensions as the human vocal tract or electronic or computer simulations.

HOW TO BUILD A VOWEL SYNTHESIZER WITH PLASTICINE   Chiba and Kajiama (1941) described plasticine models of vocal tract shapes for Japanese vowels. Such models can be useful for illustration purposes, and it is easy to build one with similar interior dimensions to the measurements of Fant (1960), which are very well known.

Table 7-1 shows Fant's measurements converted into diameters so that they can be measured more easily with a ruler. Furthermore, although Fant gave his measurements at 0.5-cm intervals, 1-cm intervals are adequate for this purpose. First make a set of rings of plasticine having the correct internal cross-sectional area. Roll the plasticine into a dowel slightly more than 1 cm thick to allow for some pressing together of the rings when they are joined into a tube. To determine approximately how long the dowel that will make the ring for each section should be, multiply the diameter by 3.25, or slightly more than π because some of the interior diameter will be reduced as the plasticine is formed into a ring. Join the ends of the plasticine dowels to make each ring. Then join the rings, taking care not to reduce the length of vocal tract that they represent. It is probably a good idea to measure the diameter of each ring and its thickness as each ring is added. A plaster of paris reinforcement of the outside can be very useful to keep the model's shape. A sound source for the model can be improvised by using the lips as if playing a trumpet (essentially a tight labial trill). Several such models, each shaped to represent a different vowel, will permit surprisingly good vowel identification.

Electronic and computer models are a more

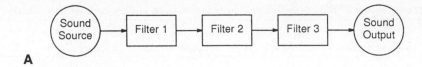

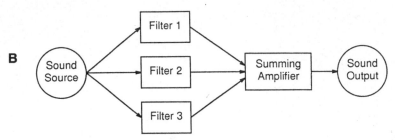

FIGURE 7-7   *A,* Filters arranged in cascade. *B,* Filters arranged in parallel.

sophisticated way of modeling the vocal tract, although the user of such models might envy the way the plasticine model mimics the losses through and within the walls of the vocal tract. Fant (1960) carefully developed an analytic model of the vocal tract based on electrical simulation. It considers the vocal tract as a series of discrete sections of varying cross-sectional areas. Electric circuits represent each cross-sectional area. As the signal passes from one section to another, the changes in area cause changes in the signal. The accumulated changes yield a signal that evidences the resonances of the vocal tract. Computer models of the vocal tract follow essentially the same procedure, considering the vocal tract as a series of sections of varying cross-sectional areas. Both electric and computer models have been used to confirm the source-filter theory (Fant, 1960), to predict the sound output that results from a particular vocal tract configuration (Fant, 1960; Wakita, 1972), and to determine the effect of coupling a nasal cavity to the oral cavity as a result of nasalization (Wright, 1980).

Some vocal tract models have been used with models of the timing of vocal gestures that control the shape of the vocal tract in an attempt to shed light on the dynamics of speech production. This work is discussed later in this chapter.

Cascade and Parallel Formant Synthesizers

Another way to design a synthesizer is to model only the filtering effects of resonances in *formant synthesis.* Resonances are the characteris-

tics of electric circuits or vocal tracts that cause them to favor certain frequencies, and **formants** are the concentrations of energy themselves.

For several reasons it is easier to synthesize formants than to model the cross-sectional area. First, the circuitry or computer simulation is simpler; five resonant circuits are normally sufficient for the formants of a male voice with a frequency response of up to 5000 Hz. Secondly, and more important, the formants can be found by looking at the energy distribution with an acoustic analysis, while the cross-sectional areas of the vocal tract have to be determined by measurements. Although Wakita (1972) shows that it is possible to derive vocal tract area functions from formants, using the formants directly is easier. Therefore, formant synthesis has been used more extensively unless there are research reasons to model the tract.

A major division in the types of transfer functions used in speech synthesis is between **cascade** and **parallel** designs, which differ in the way the formant filters are arranged. The two types of synthesizer design are illustrated in Figure 7-7.

Filter cascades consist of a series of filters arranged so that the output of the first filter becomes the input of the second, the output of the second becomes the input of the third, until the last filter's output reflects the characteristics of all of the filters. The term *cascade* stems from the similarity of this process to a series of waterfalls. A characteristic of this design is that the frequency and bandwidth of each formant can be controlled independently, but the gain, or amplification, is controllable only for the entire cascade. Other things being equal, an increase in the bandwidth of a formant will reduce the peak amplitude of that formant, so that the amplitude of individual formants can be controlled indirectly through their bandwidth. Such a scheme essentially models one of the conditions in the human vocal tract, where the increase in bandwidth resulting from nasalization and other factors is associated with reduced amplitude. If the formant frequencies and bandwidths are correct for a particular vowel, the relative amplitudes of the different formants will be those of a vocal tract model (Fant, 1956). This makes it easier to maintain generated sounds within the range of the possible sounds produced by humans.

In parallel designs, the sound source is passed to a set of different filters whose output is summed. This permits the independent setting of frequency, bandwidth, and gain. However, since either bandwidth or gain can be used to control formant amplitude, many synthesizer designers set one of these to a constant and vary the other. Most often the bandwidth is set to a constant for each formant and the amplitude is varied. The advantage of this arrangement is that bandwidth can be time-consuming to extract. The amplitude at a given frequency is easier to determine.

While the synthesis of vowels, nasals, and other **continuant** sounds permits a relatively straightforward application of a cascade model, this is not true for fricatives and stop bursts. In the case of vowels and continuant consonants, the constraints of a cascade synthesizer limit the values of formants and bandwidths to humanly possible combinations. This is not the case with consonants. While the sounds of vowels and continuant consonants all arise at the vocal cords, those of consonants arise at the place of maximum constriction or closure, which can vary greatly. For example, the burst of noise that follows the release of the stop consonants /p/ and /t/ essentially does not pass through a front resonating cavity, but the burst that follows /k/ does. All three consonants, /p/, /t/ and /k/, are affected by the resonating cavities between the place of articulation and the vocal cords. These *back cavities* are one cause of *antiresonances,* also found in nasal consonants and /l/, which are *inverse resonances* in that they diminish sound energy at their characteristic frequencies and bandwidths. Voiced fricatives combine a sound source at the vocal cords with a frication source at the place of articulation. Voiced stops and fricatives have two sources, one at the vocal cords and one at the place of articulation.

As a result, stops and fricatives are probably best synthesized by examining the spectral characteristics found in the magnitude spectrum and attempting to match them without reference to the interaction between amplitude and bandwidth inherent in the cascade model. Using a noise source with a flat spectrum, a set of parallel formants can be adjusted to produce a very good match, as was shown by Holmes (1961). The fact that such a method does not include the zeros in the spectrum is not a fatal limitation. Zeros per se appear not to have a very strong perceptual effect except in their interaction with formants. The amplitude of formants can therefore be adjusted to mimic the effect of zeros. This is more easily done with a parallel system, using a noise source with a flat spectrum and adjusting the frequency and amplitude of several parallel formants. In a text-to-speech system, the spectral characteristics are implemented in parameters and rules.

Since there are clear advantages to parallel synthesis for stops and fricatives and certain advantages to a cascade design for vowels and other continuants, one solution is a **hybrid** design that uses one or the other depending on a switch setting, as in Klatt's well-known system (Klatt, 1980). Klatt's system contains both a parallel and a cascade. The outputs of the two synthesizers, or synthesizer branches, are summed. This system allows a user to select whichever method will work best.

Sound Source Generation

The three types of sound sources relevant to speech are necessary for speech synthesis. They are the source of the voice, the noise source for fricatives, and the impulse source for bursts. The source of the voice has received the most attention.

THE VOICE SOURCE The quality of the voice source not only affects the naturalness of synthetic speech; it can also affect whether the speech is understood. Languages such as Hindi and Korean use differences in the type of voicing to produce differences in meaning. In Hindi sounds transliterated in English as "b" and "bh" differentiate between **murmured** and normal

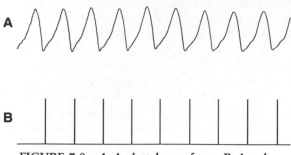

FIGURE 7-8   *A,* A glottal waveform, *B,* A pulse train, as used in some synthesizers.

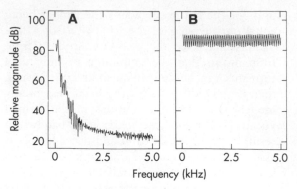

FIGURE 7-9   A comparison of the spectra of *(A)* a glottal waveform and *(B)* a pulse train.

voice following the consonant, which is used to make meaning distinctions.

The synthesizer constructed by von Kempelen used a vibrating reed for the voice source. Because this source worked on the same principle as the human vocal folds, it probably produced a closer representation of vocal fold output than was used in the early electronic speech synthesizers, which used a series of pulses, a *pulse train.* The human vocal cords open relatively gradually and normally produce most of their output toward the end of the closing part of the cycle. Figures 7-8 and 7-9 show a close approximation to the pattern of opening and closing of the vocal folds extracted from inverse filtering compared with a pulse train. Both signals have the same fundamental frequency, about 94 Hz.

A pulse train has characteristics that differ from the source of the human voice in both temporal pattern and in its spectrum. The illustrations show that the pulse train has an essentially flat spectrum, but the human voice has much less energy in the higher frequencies, dropping off at about 12 dB per octave. Since the effect of speech radiating into the air from the vocal tract raises the spectrum by about 6 dB per octave, the overall effect is a drop-off at a net 6 dB per octave. Filtering can be used to change the spectrum of a pulse train to approximate that of the human voice (e.g., Klatt, 1980).

Filtering a pulse train is particularly successful in parallel synthesizer designs because the independent control of each formant filter permits the correction of its differences from the human voice. A different approach has been taken in several synthesizers with cascade or hybrid designs, in which a model consisting of one or more equations is used to generate a waveform that looks very much like the human voice

source. Parameters in the models are varied to produce different characteristics. This approach produces more natural-sounding speech for these synthesizers, and if the parameters are well-chosen, they can clarify the acoustic and perceptual effects of different voice source characteristics.

Klatt and Klatt (1990) described a voice source model that uses an equation to generate the overall wave shape (Fig. 7-10). In effect, the equation first models the relatively smooth rise and fall of airflow through the vocal folds, corresponding to the opening and then closing of the vocal folds, and then completes the fall of airflow very abruptly, as if the vocal folds had closed rather violently. This abrupt end to the airflow, if unmodified, would create more high-frequency energy than is found in the human voice source. Therefore, a low-pass filter is used to lower the high-frequency energy, effectively smoothing the abrupt end of airflow. The frequency and sharpness of cutoff of this filter determine how much smoothing will take place.

The waveform of airflow through the vocal folds does not have a direct relationship to some of the more important parameters of speech synthesis. In particular, the amplitude is related not to the maximum airflow but to the deceleration of airflow. To put it another way, in human speech it is the degree of abruptness of the vocal folds coming together rather than the extent of their movement that determines how much amplitude will be created. The radiation of sound out of the vocal tract into the air parallels the velocity at which airflow is changing. Mathematically, it is equivalent to differentiating, or taking the slopes of, the airflow signal.

Fant, Liljencrants, and Lin (1985) described a model of the voice source that generates a wave

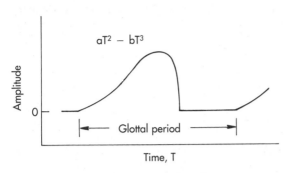

$$aT^2 - bT^3$$

a, b = coefficients controlling shape
of the voice pulse

FIGURE 7-10   A voice source model. (From Klatt, D. H., & Klatt, L. C. [1990]. Analysis, synthesis and the perception of voice quality variations among female and male talkers. *Journal of the Acoustical Society of America, 87,* 820-857.)

incorporating the differentiation of the signal. Carlson, Granstrom, and Karlsson (1991), working with this model, showed a close approximation to natural voice source signals. A different approach is to take one or more cycles of a human voice source, modify its amplitude and frequency, and use it as the source for a text-to-speech system (Pearson et al., 1990). Although this method somewhat distorts the quality of the human voice source as it is stretched or compressed, it captures some of the small details of voice quality that are difficult to include in a mathematical model.

Concatenation of Speech

Newcomers to speech synthesis sometimes wonder why one cannot simply record all the sounds of a language, spoken by a human with a pleasant voice, and then synthesize speech by concatenating the appropriate sounds. This approach is more difficult than it might seem. Speech sounds vary greatly with their context (coarticulatory effects), even when the contextual influence is not immediately adjacent (Öhman, 1966). In addition, since varying situations call for many different fundamental frequencies of any sound, a very large number of sounds have to be stored. Furthermore, discontinuities in an acoustic signal, which occur when two speech sounds are simply abutted, are very jarring to listeners.

Concatenation is relatively successful when it is possible to concatenate a small number of individual words separated by pauses. An example is telephone directory information. A telephone operator finds the number the customer is seeking and passes the task of saying the number to the concatenation device. The device selects from a recording: "The number is ... five ... five ... five ... three ... one ... nine ... four." Without pauses or normal coarticulatory effects the speech is not only unpleasant but also unintelligible. The method works in part because there are relatively few words to be produced and because the intonational pattern that people use for lists of words separated by pauses is relatively flat until the last word or two. Although the intonation pattern at the end of the concatenated string is not optimal, the message is clear. This method of synthesis is useful for its limited purpose, but it is not particularly interesting for research and not very flexible. Research to make concatenation more general is being conducted. The **coarticulation** between speech sounds can be dealt with to an extent by amassing a very large number of sounds, so that the environment surrounding the sound in the synthesized string is as close as possible to the environment of the original sound. The discontinuities in the signal can be made less jarring by overlap-add techniques, which blend one sound into the next. Another method of dealing with the discontinuities and the problem of variation in fundamental frequency due to intonation is to concatenate parameters describing the speech signal rather than the speech signal itself. One set of parameters that may be particularly suitable for concatenation are those from linear predictive coding (LPC) (Atal and Hanauer, 1971).

Synthesis Based on Linear Predictive Coding

LPC-based analysis and resynthesis first require the LPC analysis described in Chapter 13. LPC extracts a series of coefficients essentially characterizing the vocal tract transfer function and a **residue,** or **error,** signal. Typically this residue is dominated by the voicing source signal. The inverse process can be used to resynthesize the signal analyzed by LPC. In this case analysis and synthesis are essentially a coding method that can be used to transmit speech more economically than the unanalyzed signal. It is also possible to store the LPC coefficients that produce different sounds and use them in synthesizing previously unspoken speech. The source signal can be taken from LPC analysis or produced separately. The source must be controlled as to its fundamental frequency and intensity, as with formant synthesis. The LPC coefficients for each segment can be concatenated while the source signal is supplied according to intonational rules as in formant synthesis. Regenerating the speech from LPC parameters can overcome the discontinuities in the signal. LPC-based synthesis can produce reasonably understandable speech and has been widely used. It is perhaps best known in the relatively inexpensive device Speak-n-Spell from Texas Instruments.

Synthetic Speech in Research

Speech synthesis can be used as a research tool, as a model of some aspect of speech, or to determine the perceptually relevant cues in the speech signal. When it is used as a model, it is crucial to determine what aspect of speech is being modeled. For example, using a parallel formant synthesizer, it is possible to model knowledge about the formant frequencies and amplitudes in speech but not about speech production. When synthesis is used for perception research, what matters is precise control of the acoustic output so that the acoustic cues that signal speech can be discovered.

Early Experiments

Synthetic speech came to be used heavily in the 1950s to discover the perceptually relevant cues used by listeners to distinguish different sounds. It was used to establish the **difference limen** (just-noticeable differences) for vowel formant frequency (Flanagan, 1955), vowel formant amplitude (Flanagan, 1957a), and fundamental frequency (Flanagan, 1957b). Although the conclusions from this early work have been somewhat refined by later studies (Bernstein, 1977, 1981; Nord and Sventelius, 1979), they essentially remain valid and continue to be the basic reference. A great deal of work on the acoustic cues for consonants was conducted at Haskins Laboratories using a device called the pattern-playback. The pattern-playback machine permitted researchers to draw schematic spectrograph-like patterns on a transparent sheet in order to synthesize speech. This greatly facilitated the process of preparing experiments. A researcher could observe a pattern on a spectrograph, trace a possibly relevant pattern, and put the traced pattern into the synthesizer for testing. This research led to a series of conclu-sions about the role of stop releases and **consonant transitions** in the identification of stops. The Haskins researchers showed that the acoustic cues for the place of articulation of stops were found both in the burst following the release of the stops and in the formant transitions out of preceding vowels and into following vowels (Cooper et al., 1952; Liberman et al., 1954; Delattre, Liberman, and Cooper, 1955; Liberman, 1957). These researchers developed the theory that each place of articulation for stops has a unique locus for the transition of the second formant that identified the place of articulation. Although this early theory was later shown to be in need of modification (Öhman, 1966), it formed the basis for understanding how stop consonants are perceived and showed the way to the beginning of speech synthesis by rule.

Some current research in synthesis is directed toward understanding the speech production process. Articulatory synthesis, in which the researcher controls the vocal tract configurations rather than the acoustic parameters, models the speech production process. By constructing the model to reflect articulatory movements, or gestures, researchers can study the coordination of vocal tract movements, called **orchestration.** Correcting the structure and processes of the model when they differ from human speech can yield fundamental insights. Fant's (1960) work on essentially steady-state sounds, in which he used electric circuits to model the articulatory-acoustic relations in the vocal tract, was a fundamental advance. Stevens (1972) suggested why sounds are produced in certain parts of the vocal tract much more than in other parts. He found that in some parts of the vocal tract relatively little precision is required for producing a sound, but in other parts high precision is required.

Current Research

While much current work on speech synthesis is devoted to the development of text-to-speech, discussed later in this chapter, there has been considerable work in modeling the articulation of speech. This modeling is in some sense a continuation of the modeling of the vocal tract, although here the task is modeling the dynamics of vocal tract gestures (Browman and Goldstein, 1989, 1990). This work aims to develop a model of the way humans control the vocal tract to produce speech.

The model converts discrete articulatory

specifications to the continuous movements characteristic of human articulation, while taking into account the timing constraints of the system (Fig. 7-11).

Viewing speech production in this way allows the testing of hypotheses about the coordination of vocal tract gestures. To what extent are they independent of one another? To what extent do they overlap? What general organization of gestures is responsible for how speech is produced? These kinds of questions are under study in work using articulatory synthesis as a model, supported by data from x-ray and magnetic resonance imaging (MRI) of articulatory movements.

Speech Synthesis by Rule and Text-to-Speech

The most challenging task in speech synthesis, and the one with the greatest variety of applications, is to produce synthetic speech automatically, using rules to perform the conversion from phonemes (synthesis by rule) (Holmes, Mattingly, and Shearme, 1964) or from written text (text-to-speech system) (Coker, Umeda, and Browman, 1973). The ability to take any text typed in or stored on a computer file and turn it into speech requires

knowledge about language as well as about the acoustics of speech.

Work on text-to-speech was first defined as *synthesis by rule,* in which a phoneme string was used as input and the system produced speech. This terminology distinguished it from trial-and-error work aided by experimenters' intuitions as to what might work to synthesize a particular utterance, which was called *synthesis by art.* Today, synthesis by rule, since it excludes the conversion of written language into a phonemic string, forms a portion of *text-to-speech synthesis,* described in the next section.

Elements of a Text-to-Speech System

TEXT NORMALIZATION The initial input to a text-to-speech system is generally expected to consist of fully spelled words. A text **normalizer** thus converts any abbreviations and mathematical equations, to the extent possible, into words. Unrecognized abbreviations are converted into letters to be spelled out, any uninterpretable input, such as binary code, which cannot be converted to characters, is discarded.

Text-to-speech has developed to the point that it is relatively intelligible, particularly if users have a little experience with it. In effect, this means that it is usable by persons who need

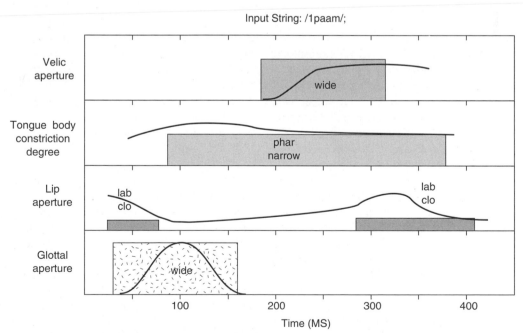

FIGURE 7-11 **Gestural score for the word *"palm"*. The boxes indicate the activation of gestures, and the curves indicate the generated vocal tract movements.** (From Browman, C. P., & Goldstein, L. [1990]. Gestural specifications using dynamically defined articulatory structures. *Journal of Phonetics, 18,* 299-320.)

to use it repeatedly but impractical if many people will encounter it for the first time. For example, using it for telephone information is not yet feasible; too many people will misunderstand. However, using it to provide spoken computer output for someone with a visual disability is feasible; a person can learn to comprehend it very quickly. Still, the need to adapt is not desirable, so perfecting text-to-speech output is important.

MORPHOLOGICAL DECOMPOSITION, LETTER-TO-SOUND RULES, AND THE LEXICON   Turning written text into spoken speech via a text-to-speech computer program has problems similar to those facing a person reading out loud. If the text contains an unknown word in an alphabetic language, letter-to-sound correspondences can be used to pronounce the word. However, most languages written with an alphabet do not have a fully predictable relationship between spelling and pronunciation. English, which has received the most attention from researchers in text-to-speech, presents particular difficulties, in part because there is no single authority periodically conducting spelling reform. English borrows a large number of words from other languages (e.g., "quiche," "machismo," "cafe") and typically pronounces them contrary to its rules for non-borrowed words. In addition, for reasons having to do with the history of the language, frequently used words in English are pronounced with different rules from words less frequently used. This is the case, for example, in words beginning with "th", which is a voiced consonant in a limited set of words including "the," "though," and "them," but voiceless in words such as "think" and "thistle." The letter combination "gh" is even less predictable; consider "ghost," "cough," "dough," and "hiccough" (one of two acceptable spellings).

These irregularities, or exceptions to the most frequently invoked rules of a language, can be dealt with in two ways. One solution is to include the exceptionally pronounced words in a lexicon, or dictionary. The dictionary can never be complete because words are continually coming into the language. Therefore, a text-to-speech system needs both a set of rules converting letters to a representation of sounds and a lexicon to cover exceptions to those rules. Such a dictionary can be made both more compact and more productive if it is structured so that its entries can be morphs (meaningful word components) rather than words. In this way, not only can words such as "philosophical" and "magical" share morphs and reduce the number of entries, but words coming into the language can be handled much more easily (e.g., adding "fax" automatically adds "faxing," "faxed"). The rules that handle the joining of morphs can also be used to handle words formed by the compounding of complete words (e.g., "blackboard"). Since the lexicon can be used not only to provide the pronunciation for a word but also its grammatical content (part of speech, etc.) for syntactic analysis, a number of morphs that are not pronouncing exceptions but that appear in large numbers of words are also included.

When a word input is received, it is first compared with the entries in the exceptions dictionary. The search proceeds from the largest possible morph to the smallest. Words such as "pothole" have to be included whole, rather than as part of two separate entries, because the combination "th" is ambiguous. If no match is found between the word and the morph lexicon, it is assigned a pronunciation by the letter-to-sound rules. This is the approach used in the MITalk system developed at the Massachusetts Institute of Technology (Allen, Hunnicutt, and Klatt, 1987), the basis of a number of other text-to-speech systems.

It is possible to do without an exceptions dictionary, as did Hertz (1982). By formulating the exceptions as rules sufficiently specific as to apply perhaps to a single word, it is possible to deal with exceptions without an explicit separate dictionary. An exaggerated example is to have a special rule for the letters "gh" followed by word boundary and preceded by the letters "c," "o," and "u" and a different rule for other environments, such as "gh" preceded by "t," "h," "o," and "u."

PARSING   For a text-to-speech system to produce appropriate segment durations and fundamental frequency contours, the structure of the text has to be determined. Determining this structure, usually in sentence or phrase-sized units, is *parsing*. The requirements for a parser for text-to-speech are less comprehensive than for many other applications (e.g., a translation system). The parser must (1) divide the text into phrases to be spoken without an internal pause, and (2) determine what words are to be emphasized. One absolute requirement is that the parser provide a single, unambiguous parse, even if the input stream is itself ambiguous. An example of this occurs when the text-to-speech system receives a series of isolated words. A number of words in English are pronounced in a different way according to their grammatical use, which cannot be determined from a single word. Thus, depending on whether they are nouns or verbs, "extract" will differ in stress placement, and "use" will differ in the voicing of the final consonant and the duration of the vowel (Denes, 1955). Although the parser cannot determine the intended reading of these words when they are supplied in isolation, it must have a mechanism for giving a single interpretation as to what they are, so that the steps that follow in the generation of speech do not have to deal with a grammatical ambiguity.

The mechanism for parsing incorporates two components: a grammar, which contains a representation of the rules of the language, and a parser per se, a mechanism for forming the structure of the text to be spoken on the basis of the grammatical rules. The rules are supplied to the parser so that an incoming group of words can be assigned a structure.

A widely used parsing method is the augmented transition network (ATN), developed by Woods (1970). An ATN consists of a set of transitions between states. A *state* is a condition. A *transition* is a change from one state to another. Transitions between states are graphically represented by arcs, and it is common to call the connections between states arcs. The words to be spoken go into the network in left-to-right order, where they typically encounter three types of arcs. *Part-of-speech* arcs are invoked when a particular part of speech is identified. These increment the word counter; that is, they *consume* the current word and go on to the next word. *Jump* arcs go to another part of the network to test a new possibility for the current word. *Pop* arcs create a node; that is, they create a structure out of the words (or nodes) processed since the last time a pop occurred.

In processing the sentence, a parser such as that used in Allen, Hunnicutt, and Klatt (1987) will try to find the longest noun or verb group in the sentence, and if unsuccessful, will look for the longest verb or noun group. Words that do not fall within a verb or noun group are identified; the programs that use the parser's outputs are set up to handle these cases as well.

Parses in which words cannot be assigned as

forming part of noun or verb groups are only one of many ways parses for text-to-speech can be incomplete or inaccurate. Parsers almost invariably analyze sentences in isolation, without the paragraph or situational context that would allow the interpretation of ambiguous sentences. Even a text-to-speech system that takes previous sentences into account will not correctly analyze a context easily understood by humans. Let us take the three-word sentence "They can fish." In a context describing how a group of people can amuse themselves on the water, the word "can" has the meaning "are able to." In a context describing what different workers do at a food-packing plant, the word "can" has the meaning "put things in sealable containers." In most dialects of American English, these yield two different pronunciations of the word "can." A person reading this sentence out loud in context will provide the proper pronunciation. However, parsers that incorporate knowledge about the world are beyond present-day capabilities. A text-to-speech system literally does not know what it is talking about. It does not know what is intended to be emphasized and what is not, since the writing system does not provide that information. The lack of a fully defined parse is most often a problem in assigning fundamental frequency and duration. These topics are discussed next.

GENERATING FUNDAMENTAL FREQUENCY Assigning fundamental frequency to sentences is one of the difficult tasks of a text-to-speech system because parsers cannot provide all the information necessary for fundamental frequency to be properly selected. Pierrehumbert (1981) pointed out that because a synthesis system will make errors as a result of this underspecification, it may be more important to minimize the abrasiveness of the errors than to try to achieve the closest match to the fundamental frequency of human speech.

There are four influences on fundamental frequency in speech: (1) The prosodic pattern of a sentence determines the large-scale falls and rises in fundamental frequency, depending on what words are emphasized, whether the sentence is a statement or a question, and so on. (2) The fundamental frequency within a word is affected by either its lexical tone in languages such as Chinese or by the location of the prominent syllables in languages such as English. (3) Individual speech sounds alter fundamental frequency over relatively short duration by manipulating the articulatory and aerodynamic conditions that affect vocal fold vibration. (4) Individual differences between speakers, including gender and age differences, bring about large differences in overall range as well as in intonation and phrasing.

The first two of these influences have received the most attention in work on text-to-speech because they have the strongest influence in making synthetic speech sound like speech. With very few exceptions as noted by Pike and Wistram in an unpublished manuscript, the vast majority of languages, including English, exhibit an overall falling fundamental frequency pattern for declarative sentences (Cruttenden, 1986) and for some types of interrogative sentences. The range of variation also decreases toward the end of a sentence. In English, questions that can be answered with a yes or no are produced with a final rising fundamental frequency pattern. Question intonation tends to have a final rising pattern. The overall slope of the sentence is its **declination.** This overall slope can be created explicitly, as in Pierrehumbert (1981) and in Hirose and Fujisaki (1982), or it can be the result of a set of rules that in each part of the sentence lower fundamental frequency more than they raise it, as in Kohler (1991). Emphasized words can also be assigned fundamental frequency variations in a number of ways.

Perhaps a more accurate term than sentence is *intonation group* (Cruttenden, 1986), a group of words spoken with no intervening pause. To use such a unit is more accurate because pauses often occur within a sentence and reset the falling fundamental frequency pattern. As Cruttenden (p. 35) points out, many other terms have been used for this unit: "sense group, breath group, tone-group, tone-unit, phonological phrase, phonological clauses or intonational phrases."

Within the intonation group momentary fundamental frequency changes are associated with words that receive accent. In English, this is typically a rise followed by a fall. In line with the diminishing fundamental frequency range, these rise-falls become smaller toward the end of a sentence. The fundamental frequency typically continues to have an overall fall between the syllables that receive accent. Pierrehumbert (1981) uses a "sagging transition" to handle the fundamental frequency pattern between accents.

The effects of speech segments on fundamental frequency have been examined by a number of researchers (Lehiste and Peterson, 1961; Mohr 1971; Lea 1973; Hombert, Ohala, and Ewan, 1979). Other things being equal, high vowels such as /i/ and /u/ raise fundamental frequency, and low vowels such as /a/ lower it. Voiceless stops bring about a relatively high fundamental frequency on the portion of the vowel immediately following, and voiced stops lower the fundamental frequency on the portion of the vowel immediately following. These effects typically last about 100 ms into the following vowel (Hombert, 1975). It is difficult to know how to deal with a glottal stop (the sound in the middle of "oh-oh") in speech synthesis. It has been associated with both lowering (Pierrehumbert, 1981) and raising (Hombert, 1978) the fundamental frequency. Mohr (1971) reports no effect on fundamental frequency, although apparently this is a result of his averaging it with the effects of /h/ which, like breathy voice quality, lowers fundamental frequency (Hombert, 1978). The differences in fundamental frequency associated with different vowels are comparatively small, about 4 to 25 Hz (Ohala, 1987). Although they can influence the perception of segments (Haggard, Ambler, and Callow, 1970) and may yet contribute to the kind of detail that helps make synthetic speech natural, they have not received much attention because researchers in text-to-speech for the most part have concentrated on the prosodic effects (but see Kohler, 1991).

Differences in intonation between adult female and male talkers have been examined in a review by Henton (1989). Female speakers tend to have a larger fundamental frequency range as measured in Hertz, although Henton argues that the range is actually similar in proportion to the average fundamental frequency of adult male and female talkers. Karlsson (1991) notes that this a controversial view.

DURATION In a number of languages, such as Italian, duration is distinctive, so that the duration of a segment signals the difference between two different meanings (e.g., *polo* meaning "ball" and *pollo* meaning "chicken"). In these languages, assigning the correct duration not only affects the naturalness of synthetic speech but whether it is understood. Even English, which is not considered to have distinctive duration, requires proper duration for the identification of many sounds. Denes (1955) showed that if the relatively long vowel in "use" (verb) is spliced away and attached to the voiceless final consonant in "use" (noun), the percept will be as if the final consonant were voiced, so that the listener will hear the verb. Lisker (1957) showed that altering the silence gap in "rupee" will bring about the percept of "ruby", as if the medial consonant were voiced. Lisker and Abramson (1964) showed that the distinctive difference between so-called voiced stops written with b, d, or g and so-called voiceless stops written with p, t, or k was in fact the duration of the aspiration following the stop release. Furthermore, they found that the duration of aspiration depends on the place of articulation of the stop. Durations of speech sounds in American English can range from about 300 ms, in the case of the vowel in the word "bat" (/æ/) spoken in isolation, to the duration of the second consonant in the word "kitty," in which "tt" is a *tap*, taking only about 30 ms.

These durational effects coexist and interact with the location of a word within a sentence and with syntactic function (Klatt, 1975). One approach to this problem is to set upper and lower limits on the duration of each phoneme and to construct a set of rules, most of which altered duration by percentages (Allen, Hunnicutt, and Klatt, 1987). This approach has been relatively successful in producing segment durations similar to those of natural speech. The upper and lower limits for each phoneme are stored in tables, and the rules modify the durations for each phoneme according to where in an utterance it occurs and what phonemes are in its vicinity. A new table, containing the rule-adjusted durations to be used in the utterance, is passed to the parameter generation program.

GENERATING PARAMETERS Once the phonetic segments, fundamental frequency contours, and durations have been calculated, it is possible to convert a phonetic transcription to a set of time-varying parameters. A typical text-to-speech system contains an inventory of phonetic segments with a set of target parameters for each segment. Parameter tables specify for each segment the beginning and ending formant values, bandwidths, voicing amplitudes, and other features.

What the parameters should be and how the parameters associated with each segment should be joined is one of the difficult questions of speech synthesis by rule and text-to-speech. The work of Lindblom (1963), Stevens and House

(1963), Öhman (1966), Stevens, House, and Paul (1966) and others shows that speech contains great variability. Consonants are altered by the surrounding vowels, and vowels are altered by the surrounding consonants and other vowels. The degree to which the surrounding consonants affect vowels is determined partly by speech rate. Even sounds not immediately adjacent to each other affect each other (Öhman, 1966). Developers of text-to-speech systems found it necessary to determine the acoustic characteristics of each segment by examining the characteristics of several prior and following segments within an utterance. The interaction between segments requires that text-to-speech systems have a large set of rules to vary target values and transition times according to what segments are being joined.

Consider the generation of formants one, two, and three in the synthesis of "kitty". Table 7-2 shows formant target values for some steady vowels.

Even voiceless stop consonants, which are silent during closure, are assigned formant targets. The motion of the vocal organs from a vowel to a stop consonant or from a consonant toward a vowel affects the vowel formants, particularly immediately adjacent to the consonant. Different stop consonants have a different effect on the formants, so stop consonant formant targets must be specified. Table 7-3 shows formant targets for some stops.

Notice that in addition to /k/, palatal /k/ is listed with different values. The /k/ sound in English shows considerable variety in its position in the vocal tract, and consequently in its

TABLE 7-2 Formant target frequencies for two vowels of American English

Vowel	F1	F2	F3
/i/	290	2250	2790
/I/	390	2000	2610

TABLE 7-3 Formant target frequencies for some American English voiceless stops

Phoneme	Formant 1	Formant 2	Formant 3
/p/	280	850	2160
/t/	280	1530	2820
/k/	320	1700	1940
palatal /k/	280	2300	2850

TABLE 7-4 The frequencies (in Hz) and durations (on ms) of the segments in the word "kitty"

Phoneme	Palatal-k Closure	Palatal-k Release	I	t Closure	t Release	i
Duration	100	90	70	30	20	130
Formant 1	280	—	390	280	—	290
Formant 2	2200	—	1900	1530	—	2250
Formant 3	3010	—	2610	2820	—	2950

formant targets, depending on the surrounding vowels. With vowels such as /ɑ/, /ɔ/, and /o/, it produces the so-called standard /k/. In proximity to many other vowels, such as /i/ and /I/, it is produced toward the front of the mouth, in the palatal region, and consequently has a different set of targets.

Given the stored target values for the vowels and the voiceless stop consonants, Table 7-4 is constructed from the duration information supplied by duration rules of the formants and durations in "kitty". In the table the formant values during the release portions are not assigned, but they are later interpolated between the existing values and adjusted by rules to bring about the desired formant pattern. Stops such as /k/ have both a closure portion, which is silent, and a release portion, which contains considerable energy. The /t/ in this position is a tap; the tongue closes against the palate and immediately releases. It has a very short duration and release segment.

Because speaking humans do not jump from one static position to another, formant values change continuously during each phoneme. Rules are used in the text-to-speech system to bring about formant values such as those shown in Figure 7-12.

Other parameters such as the presence or absence of voicing, the bandwidths of the formants, and the amount of frication or aspiration noise to include also must be specified. Once all the parameters are specified, they are passed to a computer *synthesizer program,* or algorithms, to be turned into an acoustic waveform (Klatt, 1980).

Using phonemes as the basic unit is only one way of producing text-to-speech. It is possible to use syllables joined according to rules. Another method is to use **demisyllables,** or half-syllables (Browman, 1980). Demisyllables consist of a section of speech starting in the final portion of a stop consonant and running halfway through the following vowel, hence including the transitions from consonants to vowels. Since so much of the effort in creating text-to-speech goes into

producing transitions, this can be a fruitful approach.

Text-to-Speech for Nonalphabetical Languages

There is a particular problem for languages such as Chinese, written with characters that represent words instead of with an alphabet or syllabary. Such languages force a text-to-speech system to store the phonetic transcription for each word that the system is expected to produce. In one sense this makes the task easier because it requires less analysis of the language to enter a complete phonetic dictionary than it does to determine the letter-to-sound rules. However, the analysis of a limited sample of the words of a language can yield a surprisingly comprehensive set of letter-to-sound rules, especially if a small dictionary takes care of any exceptions. Furthermore, including every word in the lexicon produces a system that cannot handle new words. It also uses a great deal of computer memory, although this is becoming less important as computer technology advances.

Present-Day Systems

Text-to-speech systems are showing relatively good intelligibility under good listening conditions, approaching but not quite matching human speech. The output of text-to-speech still requires some perceptual adjustment, and it appears to be more tiring for listeners. An important part of improving speech quality is evaluation.

Evaluation of Text-to-Speech

Anyone who listens to present-day synthetic speech can distinguish it from human speech. It is more difficult to quantify the difference, to determine its causes, and to compare different text-to-speech systems accurately. Tests such as the modified rhyme test (House et al., 1965) for words spoken in isolation, often for the testing

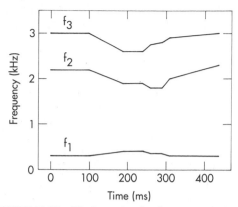

FIGURE 7-12   Trajectories for formants 1, 2, and 3 as generated by a text-to-speech system for "kitty".

of persons with speech impairments, have been used in various forms on synthetic speech. Nye and Gaitenby (1974) and Kalikow, Stevens, and Elliot (1977) developed tests for words spoken in context.

As text-to-speech systems became more generally available, comparisons between different systems became important. A comparison test for segmental intelligibility was conducted by Logan, Greene, and Pisoni (1986), who evaluated 10 voices from nine text-to-speech systems plus a human voice. They found that several systems had intelligibility close to that of human speech and that there was a wide range of intelligibility scores among the different systems. On the basis of work by Yuchtman, Nusbaum, and Pisoni (1985) they cautioned that under conditions of noise the text-to-speech systems would suffer more degradation of intelligibility than does human speech. Multiple synthesizer tests were also conducted by Mirenda and Beukelman (1990), examining text-to-speech systems commonly used in augmentative communication for persons with disabilities. They found some text-to-speech systems to have sentence intelligibility close to that of human speech for adult listeners but not for children.

Among the more interesting tests were those conducted for comprehension of synthesized paragraphs rather than words (Bernstein and Pisoni, 1980; Pisoni and Hunnicutt, 1980; Pisoni, Manous, and Dedina, 1986). While words in isolation or within a sentence measure intelligibility in a highly controlled way, they may give less information as to how well a text-to-speech system is providing information to listeners. Such testing takes into account factors such as intonation.

Silverman (1990) hypothesized that tests in which listeners simply identify words (particularly in closed-set, forced-choice tests) may not indicate how acceptable a given text-to-speech system is. In particular, a system that gets high scores might nevertheless require a great deal of concentration on the part of listeners. He therefore obtained listeners' responses to synthetic speech while they were performing a distracting second task. The difficulty of the distractor was adjusted for each listener so that he performed similarly on it. The assumption was that a similar level of performance indicated a similar level of difficulty in the distractor task, so that presumably listeners were distracted to a similar degree as they heard the synthetic speech. Text-to-speech systems that performed best with no distractions did not always perform best when a distractor task was presented simultaneously. This provided an empirical measure of how easy it was to listen to each text-to-speech system. This is important because it affects the ability of listeners to use a system for extended periods as well as the willingness of people to accept text-to-speech.

Pols (1992) reviewed text-to-speech quality assessment and noted some of the problems with text-to-speech. Among his many observations was that written text is prepared for reading, not for speaking, and that we do not yet know how best to prepare texts for speaking machines. He added that semantic and pragmatic information is not used in present-day systems. Pols mentioned problems with intonation, segments, voice quality, and overarticulation. It is clear from this assessment, which Klatt (1987) and the present author share, that much work remains in text-to-speech.

Applications of Synthesis and Future Directions

The potential and actual applications of synthetic speech have increased along with advances in computers. Perhaps the most common ones use text-to-speech to provide information stored on computers. Such applications include voice computer mail, bank account information and stock quotations over the telephone, as well as the supply of medical databases to users without a terminal. In conjunction with relatively inexpensive computers, text-to-speech systems can be extremely useful to persons with certain disabilities. Those who are unable to talk but can type are obvious candidates for the use of text-to-speech. In conjunction with an optical character reader and some mediating computer programs, a text-to-speech system can read to the blind, providing a much higher measure of independence than relying on specially prepared tapes or human readers. Interestingly, blind users of such synthesizers prefer very fast speech, much faster than normal human speech, more closely resembling the rates at which many people read. Blind users learn to use such speech, which is not intelligible to unpracticed listeners. Although human speech can be computationally compressed to increase its speed, it is likely that synthetic speech can be made more intelligible than compressed speech at very high rates, because the synthetic speech can be designed to optimize its high-speech-rate intelligibility. A possible application is an output for automatic translation systems. At present automatic translation is successful only if the realm of discourse can be severely limited, but improvements can be expected.

The goals of research on synthetic speech are clear. First, the best text-to-speech is nearly as intelligible as human speech, but it sounds unnatural to the extent that it usually requires less than a sentence for a listener to know that it is not human. The only synthetic speech that sounds natural is speech that has been synthesized by art, by speech researchers who have painstakingly adjusted the parameters of short passages. The lack of naturalness of text-to-speech is both an intellectual challenge for researchers and an impediment to its use for commercial purposes. Second, the ability to synthesize female voices lags behind work on male voices. Given that both female and male voices are desired for a number of applications, much attention is turning to female speech. Third, since natural-sounding voices necessarily have an individual quality, there is a growing interest in producing a variety of voices. Fourth, speech synthesis is likely to be used increasingly in research on speech production.

What Makes Speech Sound Natural?

Synthetic speech usually sounds machine-made to an extent that many listeners consider it unpleasant. Much effort has gone into improving the naturalness of synthetic speech, both to make it more acceptable and as part of learning about speech by producing it. The few instances in which synthetic speech sounds natural can be divided into several categories: (1) The "synthetic" speech is in fact human speech that has been stored in a computer. The computer is merely a recording instrument, and there is nothing special about the naturalness of the sound. (2) Synthetic speech by art, in which a researcher painstakingly adjusts the parameters controlling a synthesized utterance and uses trial and error to match a recorded human voice. Holmes (1961) achieved excellent results with this method. Often called *copy synthesis,* it is interesting because the parameters manipulated to produce speech are the same ones controlled by a set of rules in synthesis-by-rule or text-to-speech. This suggests that with the proper rules, natural-sounding synthetic speech could be produced automatically. One difficulty in writing the proper rules is that the perception of naturalness is affected by numerous small details. The task of producing such details by rule has thus far proved overwhelming. The development of the kind of detailed rules necessary for improving naturalness may be helped in the future by methods that automate the rule development process, as Hertz, Kadin, and Karplus (1985) have done for present-day systems.

The characteristics of the voice source signal have an important effect on naturalness. When a recorded human voice was modified to control its fundamental frequency and amplitude and introduced into a text-to-speech system, it improved somewhat the naturalness of the resulting synthesized speech (Pearson et al., 1990). The work described in the section on the voice signal is aimed at improving the naturalness of synthesized speech by improving the source signal. This may be particularly important in formant synthesizers with cascade designs that are relatively constrained compared with parallel synthesizers. Parallel synthesizers, although they provide so much flexibility that they can complicate the writing of rules, may compensate somewhat for an unnatural voice source with an opposite filtering effect. This is undoubtedly why Holmes (1961), working with a source signal inferior to those available today, was able to produce high-quality synthesis by art. Researchers today are working with both parallel and cascade designs.

Male and Female Synthesized Speech

Much early work on synthetic speech has been done for male voices, and the quality of synthetic speech still is higher for male voices. This is unfortunate, because some instances call for high-quality female speech. For example, for synthetic speech to replace natural speech for a person with a speech impairment, it is desirable to have the speech match the person's gender.

There is more data in the literature describing male speech than female speech, but this is not the entire reason for the superior quality of male speech. Female speech is breathier than male speech. Henton and Bladon (1985) address this, although their reasons have been disputed by Javkin, Hanson, and Kaun (1990). Male voice has a greater *modal voice* component; that is, most of the energy comes from the closing of the vocal folds. When the vocal folds reduce velocity as they approximate each other in midline, the modal energy component is diminished, so that more of the voice energy will come from the friction of the air passing through the vocal folds. This friction will be modulated by the vocal fold vibration in that it will vary as the open area between the vocal folds varies, although not necessarily as a simple function of the open area. It is likely that one of the characteristics not yet successfully modeled in producing female synthetic speech is the modulation of the noise component.

Karlsson (1991) suggests that part of the explanation for the greater difficulty in synthesizing female speech is that the formants do not appear as easily in acoustic analyses. The female voice, because it is higher in vocal fundamental frequency than the male voice, contains more widely spaced harmonics. This means that the formants will more frequently fall between the harmonics, so that more errors will be made in measuring them. With less breathiness, a male voice can be modeled with a simpler source function than can a female voice. Karlsson also notes that there is less knowledge about female voices but adds that such knowledge is growing, so that an improvement in the quality of female synthetic speech can be expected.

CONCLUSION

It is clear that analysis and synthesis of speech are very broad areas, with many choices to be made when attempting to analyze or synthesize speech. Perhaps the most important part of either process from the point of view of the researcher is the selection of method. It is important to match the method to the purpose. Plasticine models are completely appropriate for determining whether a certain set of vocal tract cross-sections will produce formants at certain frequencies. In analysis, a breakdown by frequency is most commonly needed, but a time analysis can be more useful when working with the voice source signal. Selection of a method, together with an understanding of its limitations, is key to both the analysis and synthesis of speech.

Review Questions

1. What speech parameters can be determined from the time waveform of a speech utterance?

2. What happens to the temporal resolution of an analysis that is altered to increase the frequency resolution?

3. What precautions should be taken in the sampling of speech into a computer in order to avoid errors in the signal?

4. What is the process of extracting the voice source from a speech signal?

5. What are the relationships between von Kempelen's synthesizer and human speech production?

6. What are the advantages of parallel designs in speech synthesis? Of cascade designs?

7. What are some of the difficulties in synthesizing speech by concatenation? Can they be overcome?

8. What are some of the differences between female and male voice that have to be taken into consideration in speech synthesis?

9. What are some of the reasons why the rules that convert from spelling to pronunciation have exceptions?

10. Why will text-to-speech systems always have difficulties in synthesizing sentences taken out of context?

11. How is text-to-speech different for alphabetical languages such as English versus non-alphabetical languages such as Chinese?

References

Allen, J. A., Hunnicutt, M. S., & Klatt, D. H. (1987). *From text to speech: The MITalk system.* Cambridge, UK: Cambridge University Press.

Atal, B. S., & Hanauer, S. L. (1971). Speech analysis and synthesis by linear prediction of the speech wave, *Journal of the Acoustical Society of America, 50*, 637-655.

Bernstein, J. C. (1977). *Vocoid psychoacoustics, articulation, and vowel phonology.* Unpublished doctoral dissertation, University of Michigan.

Bernstein, J. (1981). Formant-based representation of auditory similarity among vowel-like sounds, *Journal of the Acoustical Society of America, 69*, 1132-1144.

Bernstein, J., & Pisoni, D. (1980). Unlimited text-to-speech device: Description and evaluation of a microprocessor-based system. *The 1980 IEEE International Conference Record on Acoustics, Speech and Signal Processing*, 576-579.

van Bezooijen, R., & Jongenburger, W. (1993). Evaluation of an electronic newspaper for the blind in the Netherlands. *Speech and Language Technology for Disabled Persons: Proceedings of an ESCA Workshop*, Stockholm, Sweden.

Bloomfield, P. (1976). *Fourier analysis of time series: An introduction.* New York: Wiley.

Browman, C. P. (1980). Rules for demisyllable synthesis using lingua, a language interpreter. *Proceedings of the IEEE International Conference on Acoustics, Speech and Signal Processing, 561*, 564.

Browman, C. P., & Goldstein, L. (1989). Gestural structures and temporal patterns. *Haskins Laboratories Status Report on Speech Research SR 97/98*, 1, 24.

Browman, C. P., & Goldstein, L. (1990). Gestural specification using dynamically-defined articulatory structures. *Journal of Phonetics, 18*, 299-320.

Carlson, R., Granstrom, B., & Karlsson, I. (1991). Experiments with voice modeling in speech synthesis. *Speech Communication, 10*, 481-489.

Chiba, T., & Kajiyama, M. (1941). *The vowel, its nature and structure.* Tokyo: Kaiseikan.

Childers, D. G., & Lee, C. K. (1991). Vocal quality factors: Analysis, synthesis, and perception. *Journal of the Acoustical Society of America, 90*, 2394-2410.

Coker, C. H., Umeda, N., & Browman, C. P. (1973). Automatic synthesis from ordinary English text. *IEEE Transactions on Audio and Electroacoustics, AU-21*, 293-298.

Cooley, J. W., & Tukey, J. (1965). An algorithm for the machine calculation of complex Fourier series. *Mathematics of Computers, 19*, 297-301.

Cooper, F. S., Delattre, P. C., Liberman, A. M., Borst, J. M., & Gerstman, L. J. (1952). Some experiments on the perception of synthetic speech sounds. *Journal of the Acoustical Society of America, 24*, 597-606.

Cruttenden, A. (1986). *Intonation.* Cambridge UK: Cambridge University Press.

Delattre, P., Liberman, A. M., & Cooper, F. S. (1955). Acoustic loci and transitional cues for consonants. *Journal of the Acoustical Society of America, 27*, 769-774.

Denes, P. (1955). Effect of duration on the perception of voicing. *Journal of the Acoustical Society of America, 27*, 761-764.

Dudley, H., & Tarnoczy, T. H. (1950). The speaking machine of Wolfgang von Kempelen. *Journal of the Acoustical Society of America, 22*, 151-166.

Fant, G. (1956). On the predictability of formant and spectrum envelopes from formant frequencies. In Halle, M., Lunt, H., & McLean, H., (Eds.), *For Roman Jakobson.* Mouton: The Hague (pp. 109-120).

Fant, G. (1960). *Acoustic theory of speech production.* The Hague: Mouton.

Fant, G., Liljencrants, J., & Lin, Q. (1985). A four parameter model of glottal flow. *Speech Transmission Laboratory,* Quarterly Progress and Status Report 4, 1-13.

Flanagan, J. L. (1955). A difference limen for vowel formant frequency. *Journal of the Acoustical Society of America, 27*, 603-617.

Flanagan, J. L. (1957a). Difference limen for formant amplitude. *Journal of Speech and Hearing Disorders, 22*, 205-212.

Flanagan, J. L. (1957b). Estimates of the maximum precision necessary in quantizing certain dimensions of vowel sounds. *Journal of the Acoustical Society of America, 29*, 533-534.

Fletcher, H. (1940). Auditory patterns. *Review of Modern Physics, 12*, 47-65.

Furui, S. (1986). Speaker independent isolated word recognition using dynamic features of the speech spectrum. *ASSP, 34*, 52-59.

Ghitza, O. (1988). Temporal non-place information in the auditory-nerve firing patterns as a front-end for speech recognition in a noisy environment. *Journal of Phonetics, 16*, 109-123.

Ghitza, O. (1992). Auditory nerve representation as a basis for speech processing. In Furui, S., & Sondhi, M. M. (Eds.), *Advances in speech signal processing* New York: Marcel Dekker (pp. 453-485).

Greenwood, D. D. (1961). Critical bandwidth and the frequency coordinates of the basilar membrane. *Journal of the Acoustical Society of America, 33*, 1344-1356.

Greenwood, D. D. (1974). Critical bandwidth in man and some other species in relation to the traveling wave envelope. In Moskowitz, H. R., Scharf, B., & Stevens, J. C.(Eds.), *Sensation and measurement*, Reidel (pp. 231-239).

Haggard, M., Ambler, S., & Callow, M. (1970). Pitch as a voicing cue. *Journal of the Acoustical Society of America*, 613-617.

Hanson, B. A., & Applebaum, T. H. (1990). Features for noise-robust speaker-independent word recognition. *Proceedings of the ICSLP International Conference on Spoken Language Processing*, 1117-1120.

Henton, C. G. (1989). Fact and fiction in the description of female and male speech. *Language and Communication, 9*, 299-311.

Henton, C. G., & Bladon, R. A. W. (1985). Breathiness in normal female speech: Inefficiency versus desirability. *Language and Communication, 5*, 221-227.

Hertz, S. R. (1982). From text to speech with SRS. *Journal of the Acoustical Society of America, 72*, 1155-1170.

Hertz, S. R., Kadin, J., & Karplus, K. (1985). The delta rule development system for speech synthesis from text. *Proceedings IEEE Special Issue on Man-Machine Speech Communication*, 1589-1601.

Hirose, K., & Fujisaki, H. (1982). Analysis and synthesis of voice fundamental frequency contours of spoken sentences. *Proceedings of the IEEE International Conference on Acoustics, Speech, and Signal Processing*, 950-953.

Holmes, J. N. (1961). Research on speech synthesis carried out during a visit to the Royal Institute of Technology, Stockholm, from November 1960 to March 1961. *Joint Speech Research Unit Report JU 11.4,* Eastcote, UK: British Post Office.

Holmes, J. N., Mattingly, I. G., & Shearme, H. N. (1964). Speech synthesis by rule. *Language and Speech, 7*, 127-143.

Hombert, J. M. (1975). *Towards a theory of tonogenesis: An empirical, physiological and perceptually-based account of the development of tonal contrasts in languages.* Unpublished doctural dissertation, University of California, Berkeley.

Hombert, J. M. (1978). Consonant types, vowel quality, and tone. In Fromkin, V. (Ed.), *Tone: A linguistic survey.* New York: Academic Press (pp. 77-111).

Hombert, J. M., Ohala, J. J., & Ewan, W. G. (1979). Phonetic explanations for the development of tones. *Language, 55*, 37-58.

House, A. S., Williams, C. E., Hecker, M. H., & Kryter, K. D. (1965). Articulation testing methods: Consonantal differentiation with a closed-response set. *Journal of the Acoustical Society of America, 37*, 158-166.

Houtgast, T. (1977). Auditory filter characteristics derived from direct-masking data and pulsation-threshold data with a rippled noise masker. *Journal of the Acoustical Society of America, 62*, 409-415.

Javkin, H., Hanson, B., & Kaun, A. (1991). The effects of breathy voice on intelligibility. *Speech Communication, 10*, 539-543.

Kalikow, D. N., Stevens, K. N., and Elliott, L. L. (1977). Development of a test of speech intelligibility in noise using sentence materials with controlled word predictability. *Journal of the Acoustical Society of America, 61*, 1337-1351.

Karlsson, I. (1991). Female voices in speech synthesis. *Journal of Phonetics, 19*, 111-120.

Kay, S. M. (1988). *Modern spectral estimation: Theory and application.* Englewood Cliffs, NJ: Prentice-Hall.

Klatt, D. H. (1975). Vowel lengthening is syntactically determined in connected discourse. *Journal of Phonetics, 3*, 129-140.

Klatt, D. H. (1980). Software for a cascade/parallel formant synthesizer. *Journal of the Acoustical Society of America, 67*, 971-995.

Klatt, D. H. (1987). Review of text-to-speech conversion for English. *Journal of the Acoustical Society of America, 82*, 737-793.

Klatt, D. H., & Klatt, L. C. (1990). Analysis, synthesis and the perception of voice quality variations among female and male talkers. *Journal of the Acoustical Society of America, 87*, 820-857.

Kohler, K. J. (1991). Prosody in speech synthesis: The interplay between basic research and TTS application. *Journal of Phonetics, 19*, 121-138.

Kurzweil, R. (1976). The Kurzweil reading machine: A technical overview. Redden, M. R., & Schwandt, W. (Eds.), *Science, technology and the handicapped.* American Association for the Advancement of Science, Report 76-R-11, Washington, DC (pp. 3-11).

Lea, W. (1973). Segmental and suprasegmental influences on fundamental frequency contours. In L. Hyman (Ed.), *Consonant types and tone.* Southern California Occasional Papers in Linguistics, University of Southern California, Los Angeles.

Lehiste, I., & Peterson, G. E. (1961). Some basic considerations in the analysis of intonation. *Journal of the Acoustical Society of America, 33*, 419-425.

Liberman, A. M. (1957). Some results of research on speech perception. *Journal of the Acoustical Society of America, 29*, 117-123.

Liberman, A. M., Delattre, P., Cooper, F. S., & Gerstman, L. J. (1954). The role of consonant-vowel transitions in the perception of the stop and nasal consonants. *Psychological Monographs, 68*, 1-13.

Liberman, A. M., Ingemann, F., Lisker, L., Delattre, P., & Cooper, F. S. (1959). Minimal rules for synthesizing speech. *Journal of the Acoustical Society of America, 31*, 1490-1499.

Lindblom, B. (1963). Spectrographic study of vowel reduction. *Journal of the Acoustical Society of America, 35*, 1773-1781.

Lisker, L. (1957). Closure duration and intervocalic voiced-voiceless distinction in English. *Language, 33*, 42-49.

Lisker, L., & Abramson, A. S. (1964). A cross-language study of voicing in initial stops: Acoustical measurements. *Word, 20,* 384-422.

Logan, J. S., Greene, B. G., & Pisoni, D. B. (1986). Segmental intelligibility of synthetic speech produced by rule. *Journal of the Acoustical Society of America, 86,* 566-581.

Mirenda, P., & Beukelman, D. R. (1990). A comparison of speech synthesis intelligibility among natural speech and seven speech synthesizers with listeners from three age groups. *Augmentative and Alternative Communication, 6,* 61-68.

Mohr, B. (1971). Intrinsic variations in the speech signal. *Phonetica, 29,* 65-93.

Nord, L., & Sventelius, E. (1979). Analysis and perception of difference limen data for formant frequencies. *Speech Transmission Laboratory Quarterly Status Progress Report,* 3-4, 60-72.

Nye, P. W., & Gaitenby, J. (1974). The intelligibility of synthetic monosyllabic words in short, syntactically normal sentences. *Haskins Laboratories Status Report on Speech Research, 38,* 169-190.

Nyquist, J. (1924). Certain factors affecting telegraph speed. *Bell System Technical Journal, 3,* 324.

Ohala, J. J. (1987). Explaining the intrinsic pitch of vowels. In Channon, R., & Shockey, L. (Eds.), *In honor of Ilse Lehiste.* Dordrecht: Foris (pp. 207-215).

Öhman, S. E. G. (1966). Coarticulation in VCV utterances: Spectrographic measurements. *Journal of the Acoustical Society of America, 39,* 151-158.

Patterson, R. D. (1973). The effects of relative phase and the number of components on residue pitch. *Journal of the Acoustical Society of America, 53,* 1565-1572.

Pearson, S. D., Javkin, H. R., Matsui, K., & Kamai, T. (1990). Text-to-speech synthesis using a natural voice source. *Proceedings of the International Conference on Spoken Language Processing, 1,* 193-196.

Pierrehumbert, J. (1981). Synthesizing intonation. *Journal of the Acoustical Society of America, 70,* 985-994.

Pike, E., & Wistram, K. *Terrace level tones in Acatlan Mixtec.* Unpublished manuscript, Summer Institute in Linguistics.

Pisoni, D. B., & Hunnicutt, M. S. (1980). Perceptile evaluation of MITalk: The MIT unrestricted text-to-speech system. *The 1980 IEEE International Conference Record on Acoustics, Speech and Signal Processing,* 572-575.

Pisoni, D. B., Manous, L. M., & Dedina, M. J. (1986). Comprehension of natural and synthetic speech: 2. Effects of predictability on the verification of sentences controlled for intelligibility. *Research on Speech Perception Progress Report No. 12,* Indiana University, Bloomington.

Pols, L. C. W. (1992). Quality assessment of text-to-speech synthesis by rule. In Furui, S., & Sondhi, M. M. (Eds.), *Advances in speech signal processing* New York: Marcel Dekker (pp. 387-416).

Rothenberg, M. (1973). A new inverse-filtering technique for deriving the glottal air flow waveform during voicing. *Journal of the Acoustical Society of America, 53,* 1632-1645.

Seneff, S. (1988). A joint synchrony/mean-rate model of auditory speech processing. *Journal of Phonetics, 16,* 55-76.

Shamma, S. (1988). The acoustic features of speech sounds in a model of auditory processing: Vowels and voiceless fricatives. *Journal of Phonetics, 16,* 77-91.

Silverman, K. (1990, November). Evaluating synthesizer performance: Is segmental intelligibility enough? *Proceedings of the International Conference on Spoken Language Processing,* 981-984.

Stevens, K. N. (1972). The quantal nature of speech: evidence from articulatory-acoustic data. In David, E. E., & Denes, P. B. (Eds.), *Human Communication, a Unified View.* New York: McGraw-Hill.

Stevens, K. N., & House, A. S. (1963). Perturbation of vowel articulation by consonantal context: An acoustical study. *Journal of Speech and Hearing Research, 6,* 111-128.

Stevens, K. N., House, A. S., & Paul, A. P. (1966). Acoustical description of syllable nuclei: An interpretation in terms of a dynamic model of articulation. *Journal of the Acoustical Society of America, 40,* 123-132.

Stevens, S. S., Volkman, J., & Newman, E. B. (1937). A scale for measurement of the psychological magnitude of pitch. *Journal of the Acoustical Society of America, 8,* 185-190.

Van den Berg, J. (1958). Myoelastic-aerodynamic theory of voice production. *Journal of Speech and Hearing Research, 1,* 227-244.

Wakita, H. (1972). Estimation of the vocal tract shape by optimal inverse filtering and acoustic/articulatory conversion methods. *Speech Communication Research Laboratory Monographs, 9,* Speech Communications Research Laboratory, Santa Barbara, CA.

Wegel, R. L., & Lane, C. E. (1924). The auditory masking of a pure tone by another and its probable relation to the dynamics of the inner ear. *Physical Review, 23,* 266-285.

Woods, W. A. (1970). Transition network grammars for natural language analysis. *Communications of the Association of Computing Machinery, 13,* 591-606.

Wright, J. (1980). The behavior of nasalized vowels in the perceptual vowel space. *Report of the Phonology Laboratory, 5,* Department of Linguistics, University of California, Berkeley, Berkeley, CA, 127-163.

Yuchtman, M., Nusbaum, H. C., & Pisoni, D. B. (1985). Consonant confusions and perceptual spaces for natural and synthetic speech. *Journal of the Acoustical Society of America, 78,* (Suppl. 1), 83.

Zwicker, E. (1961). Subdivision of the audible frequency range into critical bands. *Journal of the Acoustical Society of America, 33,* 248-249.

Suggested Readings

Speech Analysis

Cooke, M., Beet, S., & Crawford, M. (Eds.). (1983). *Visual representation of speech signals.* New York: Wiley.

Fant, G. (1973). *Speech sounds and features.* Cambridge, Massachusetts: MIT Press.

Flanagan, J. (1972). *Speech analysis, synthesis and perception.* Berlin, Heidelberg, New York: Springer-Verlag.

Furui, S., & Sondhi, M.M. (Eds.). (1992). *Advances in speech signal processing.* New York: Marcel Dekker.

Kraniauskas, P. (1994). A plain man's guide to the FFT. *IEEE Signal Processing Magazine,* 11 (No. 2), 24-50.

Ladefoged, P. (1962). *Elements of acoustic phonetics.* Chicago: University of Chicago Press.

Rothenberg, M. (1973). A new inverse-filtering technique for deriving the glottal air flow waveform during voicing. *Journal of the Acoustical Society of America, 53,* 1632-1645.

Foundations for Speech Synthesis

Bailly, G., & Benoit, C. (1992). *Talking machines—theories, models, and designs.* Amsterdam: North-Holland.

Cooper, F.S., Delattre, P.C., Liberman, A.M., Borst, J.M., & Gerstman, L.J. (1952). Some experiments on the perception of synthetic speech sounds. *Journal of the Acoustical Society of America, 24,* 597-606.

Fant, G. (1960). *Acoustic theory of speech production.* The Hague: Mouton.

House, A.S., Williams, C.E., Hecker, M.H., & Kryter, K.D. (1965). Articulation testing methods: Consonantal differentiation with a closed-response set. *Journal of the Acoustical Society of America, 37,* 158-166.

Lindblom, B. (1963). Spectrographic study of vowel reduction. *Journal of the Acoustical Society of America, 35,* 1773-1781.

Lisker, L. (1957). Closure duration and intervocalic voiced-voiceless distinction in English. *Language,* 33, 42-49.

Lisker, L., & Abramson, A.S. (1964). A cross-language study of voicing in initial stops: acoustical measurements. *Word,* 20, 384-422.

Öhman, S.E.G. (1966). Coarticulation in VCV utterances: spectrographic measurements. *Journal of the Acoustical Society of America, 39,* 151-158.

Speech Synthesis by Rule and Text-to-Speech

Allen, J.A., Hunnicutt, M.S., & Klatt, D.H. (1987). *From text to speech: the MITalk system.* Cambridge, England: Cambridge University Press.

Cruttenden, Alan. (1986). *Intonatio.* Cambridge, England: Cambridge University Press.

Klatt, D.H. (1987). Review of text-to-speech conversion for English. *Journal of the Acoustical Society of America, 82,* 737-793.

Kohler, K.J. (1991). Prosody in speech synthesis: the interplay between basic research and TTS application. *Journal of Phonetics,* 19, 121-138.

Liberman, A.M., Ingemann, F., Lisker, L., Delattre, P., & Cooper, F.S. (1959). Minimal rules for synthesizing speech. *Journal of the Acoustical Society of America, 31,* 1490-1499.

Pierrehumbert, J. (1981). Synthesizing intonation. *Journal of the Acoustical Society of America, 70,* 985-994.

van Heuven, V., & Pols, L.C.W. (Eds.). (1993). *Analysis and Synthesis of Speech—Strategic Research Towards High-Quality Text-to-Speech Generation.* Berlin: Mouton de Gruyter.

The Synthesis of Female and Male Voices

Karlsson, I. (1991). Female voices in speech synthesis. *Journal of Phonetics,* 19, 111-120.

Klatt, D.H., & Klatt, L.C. (1990). Analysis, synthesis and the perception of voice quality variations among female and male talkers. *Journal of the Acoustical Society of America, 87,* 820-857.

Part III

Speech Perception

Chapter 8

Speech Perception and Spoken Word Recognition:
Research and Theory

Stephen D. Goldinger, David B. Pisoni, Paul A. Luce

Chapter Outline

Key Terms

INTRODUCTION

The study of speech perception is concerned with the listener's ability to perceive the acoustic waveform produced by a speaker as a string of meaningful words and ideas. By this definition, speech perception has been researched since at least the turn of the century, when one of the earliest empirical studies was published by Bagley (1900-1901; see Cole and Rudnicky, 1983). Bagley's experiments addressed a surprisingly wide variety of topics that have since been rediscovered, including phonemic restoration, semantic priming, importance of word-initial information, and sentence context effects on word recognition. A common theme of Bagley's experiments was their focus on the influence of semantic and lexical knowledge on the perception of distorted words. As Cole and Rudnicky (1983) observed, Bagley anticipated many empirical phenomena and theoretical accounts of speech perception and spoken word recognition that remain central to discussions today.

If Bagley's results and arguments were presented today, they would most likely be considered relevant to language perception rather than to speech perception per se. *Speech perception* has, for a variety of reasons, come to refer more specifically to phoneme perception than to the perception of words or phrases. Unlike a process such as visual perception, in which the recognition of objects or motion is available to the observer, speech perception as the researcher defines it is a process of which we are generally unaware. As Darwin (1976, p. 175) comments, "Our conscious perceptual world is composed of greetings, warnings, questions, and statements; while their vehicle, the segments of speech, goes largely unnoticed and words are subordinated to the framework of the phrase or sentence." Despite the truth of Darwin's observation, the majority of research on speech perception in the past three decades has focused only on the unnoticed vehicle, phonetic perception. This rather myopic approach has resulted in a large theoretical body of literature that is somewhat divorced from more general theories of perception and mainstream cognitive psychology. For example, only recently have serious efforts been applied to model the process of speech perception not as an end in itself but as subservient to word recognition (Pisoni and Luce, 1987). This chapter considers the effects

of this segregated research and theorizing on our understanding of speech as the front end of language.

Numerous papers and chapters review the theories and data in speech perception (Studdert-Kennedy, 1974, 1976; Darwin, 1976; Cutting and Pisoni, 1978; Pisoni, 1978; Pisoni and Luce, 1986; Luce and Pisoni, 1987; Miller, 1990). In large part, the fundamental issues in speech perception and the data relevant to those issues have remained unchanged over the past several years. Accordingly, although this chapter will address several fundamental issues in speech perception, it is not a comprehensive review of the empirical literature in the field. Nevertheless, this chapter is fairly eclectic, and we hope to address a sufficiently wide range of topics. We do not marshal evidence for one particular theory or class of theories at the expense of all others; instead, we examine and evaluate a wide range of theories. Finally, throughout the chapter we examine how research and theory in speech perception have or have not developed over the years with respect to the fundamental "problems" of speech. The next section begins with a review of several of the long-standing basic issues in speech perception.

BASIC ISSUES IN SPEECH PERCEPTION

Linearity, Lack of Acoustic-Phonetic Invariance, and the Segmentation Problem

Since the mid-1950s no finding has influenced speech research and theory more profoundly than the failures of the speech signal to satisfy the linearity and invariance conditions. The *linearity* condition assumes that for each perceived phoneme, there must be a particular corresponding stretch of sound in the utterance (Chomsky and Miller, 1963). For example, if the listener perceives that phoneme X occurs before phoneme Y, the stretch of sound associated with phoneme X must precede the stretch of sound associated with phoneme Y in the physical signal. The *invariance* condition assumes that for each phoneme X, a specific set of acoustic correlates must occur in all phonetic contexts. Under these conditions, recognition of phoneme X implies that the features for X occurred in the speech signal in a discrete time window and that

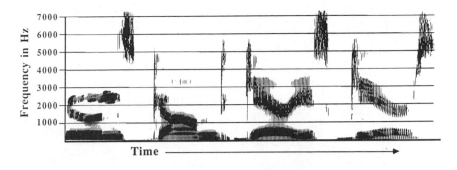

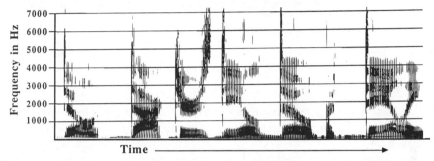

FIGURE 8-1   Spectrograms showing acoustic-phonetic invariance for the word-initial consonants /g/ and /d/. The upper spectrogram shows the sentence, "Goons gummed Gary's gears."
The lower spectrogram shows the sentence, "Don't doctors deal dope daily?"

no other features or temporal distributions of features could have occurred.

Neither the linearity nor the invariance condition is met in natural speech, primarily because of the way speech is produced: the speech articulators move continuously in production so that the shape of the vocal tract for each intended phoneme is influenced by the shapes for the preceding and following phonemes. Coarticulation results in overlapping features, *smearing*, among neighboring phonemes. Hockett (1955) likens the relation between intended phonemes and the physical speech signal to a series of Easter eggs that are pushed through a wringer. The effect of the speaker's coarticulatory wringer is to create a speech signal in which there is rarely a stretch of sound that corresponds uniquely to a given phoneme. Instead, the cues overlap in time, resulting in what Liberman et al. (1967) termed the "encoded nature of speech." Coarticulation produces complex mappings between acoustic cues and perceived phonemes. Acoustic features for phonemes vary widely as a function of varying phonetic contexts, speaking rates, and other factors. Figure 8-1 shows the variations in the acoustic forms of second-formant transitions for the phonemes /d/ and /g/ as a function of varying vowel contexts (Liberman et al., 1954; Delattre,

Liberman, and Cooper, 1955). Comparison of the various physical manifestations of the /d/s and /g/s demonstrates acoustic-phonetic variability. Although the second-formant transitions provide the cues for place of articulation necessary to recognize these phonemes, the acoustic realizations of transitions are clearly not invariant.

The failure of the speech signal to satisfy the linearity and invariance conditions is perhaps the most important puzzle in speech perception. It constitutes what Studdert-Kennedy (1983) calls the "animorphism paradox"—the invariant units of perception do not correspond to invariant acoustic segments in the signal. Indeed, the problems of **acoustic-phonetic invariance** have guided speech research since its beginning, and many researchers are working on these problems today. While some researchers have continued the quest for invariant aspects of the acoustic signal (Stevens and Blumstein, 1978, 1981; Kewley-Port, 1982, 1983; Kewley-Port and Luce, 1984; Sussman, 1989, 1991; Sussman, McCaffrey, and Matthews, 1991; Sussman, Hoemeke, and Ahmed, 1993; Fowler, 1994), and others have addressed the problems of invariance via theoretical innovation (Liberman and Mattingly,

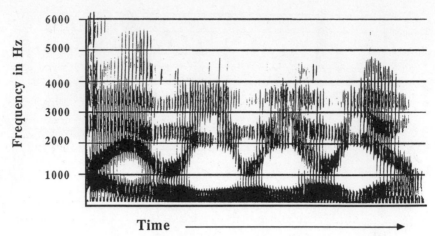

FIGURE 8-2   Spectrogram of the utterance, "I owe you a yo-yo," demonstrating that perceptual segmentation is not clearly reflected in acoustic segmentation.

1985; McClelland and Elman, 1986), the problem of contextual variability in speech remains central in research.

Coarticulation poses another problem for research, namely the lack of clear segmentation in the speech signal. Although listeners perceive speech as a series of discrete phonemes and words, physical temporal boundaries between phonemes are not reliably found in the spoken utterance. Although the sentence in Figure 8-2 displays almost no physical landmarks on which to base segmentation, it does not pose any special difficulty for listeners. The rate of information transmission in speech is enormous, clearly requiring that listeners somehow convert the continuous waveform into discrete, abstract units for cognitive processing (Liberman et al., 1967; Neisser, 1967). However, the speech signal does not lend itself to simple segmental analysis. Although it is possible to segment speech according to purely acoustic criteria (Fant, 1962), the segmentation provided by such algorithms typically does not correspond to the segmented representation that a listener would perceive. The importance and the difficulty of segmentation become immediately apparent when considering recent attempts to develop speech recognition devices; lack of segmentation, linearity, and invariance have been intractable problems.

Units of Analysis in Speech Perception

Nonlinearity, the lack of acoustic-phonetic invariance, and the nonsegmental nature of speech create another problem, the selection of a minimal unit of perceptual analysis. Given the information-rich speech waveform and limited channel capacities of the auditory system and auditory memory, it is clear that raw sensory information must be encoded into some scheme that can be efficiently processed (Broadbent, 1965; Liberman et al., 1967). Consider the estimate of Liberman, Mattingly, and Turvey (1972) that the conversion of speech sounds into phonemes reduces the information transfer rate of speech from approximately 40,000 bits per second to 40 bits per second. The conversion of phonemes into higher units of linguistic analysis further reduces the bit rate.

Figure 8-3 shows several possible units of analysis. The question for theories of speech perception has typically concerned selection of the "best" or most natural coding unit; claims of primacy have been made for phonetic features, phonemes, syllables, and words. Researchers in generative linguistic theory have even proposed units as large as the clause or sentence (Miller, 1962; Bever, Lackner, and Kirk, 1969).

Debates concerning the primacy of various units were prevalent in the literature for several years. A long-standing debate in the 1970s that has returned to prominence recently (see Pitt and Samuel, 1993) centered on claims that the syllable is a more basic perceptual unit than the phoneme (Savin and Bever, 1970; Massaro, 1972). Massaro (1972) argued that syllables are more discretely represented in the speech signal than phonemes, so selection of the syllable as the primary unit of perception resolves the

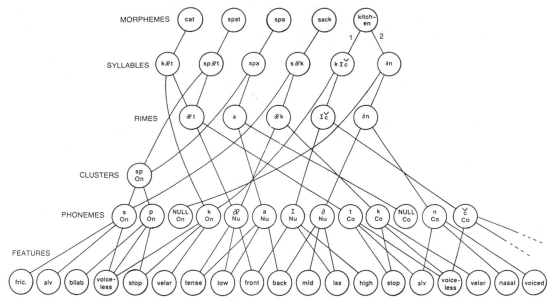

FIGURE 8-3 A section of a speech processing network containing numerous units of analysis, including morphemes, syllables, syllable rimes, consonant clusters, phonemes, and phonetic features. (From Dell, G. [1986]. A spreading activation theory of retrieval in sentence production. *Psychological Review, 93*, 283-321.)

problems of segmentation and invariance quite easily. Unfortunately, invariance is no more tractable with syllable-sized units than with phoneme-sized units. Furthermore, the information conveyed by syllables may depend on retrieval of their segmental constituents, so the issue of primary units is not resolved (Hawles and Jenkins, 1971; Pisoni, 1978).

Recent theories in speech perception imply that during comprehension of fluent speech, the primacy of any particular unit of speech may be less important than the obligatory units of speech and their interactions (McClelland and Elman, 1986). Although problems of coarticulation have discouraged researchers from positing the phoneme as an obligatory unit, numerous alternatives have been proposed. Examples include syllables (Cole and Scott, 1974a, 1974b; Studdert-Kennedy, 1974, 1980; Massaro and Oden, 1980; Segui, 1984), context-sensitive allophones (Wickelgren, 1969, 1976), and context-sensitive spectra (Klatt, 1979). All of these approaches have attempted to alleviate the problem of acoustic-phonetic invariance via the proposal of units that are relatively invariant in continuous speech. Although there is still ample reason to consider the importance of segmental representations in speech perception and word recognition (Pisoni and Luce, 1987), other context-sensitive perceptual units incorporate

contextual variability directly in their representations and may therefore prove more robust to the problems of coarticulated speech.

These four fundamental problems have shaped speech perception research and theory for nearly four decades and will no doubt figure prominently in future work as well. Although other issues have characterized speech research in recent years, these issues capture the essence of the problem of speech perception: how does the listener convert the continuously varying speech waveform into a series of discrete representations for linguistic analysis? Any reasonable theory of speech perception must address this fundamental question. The next section addresses other issues that have been less focal but no less interesting. These include the specialization of speech, the problem of perceptual constancy, and the importance of suprasegmental and source information in speech.

FURTHER ISSUES IN SPEECH PERCEPTION

Specialization of Speech Perception

For many years, Liberman and his colleagues at Haskins Laboratories have proposed a view of speech perception as a specialized process requiring specialized neural mechanisms unique to humans (Studdert-Kennedy, 1980; Mattingly and Liberman, 1988; Liberman and Mattingly, 1989). Early support for the claim that speech is special came from a well-known study by Liberman et al. (1957), who generated a synthetic continuum of consonant-vowel (CV) syllables ranging from /b/ to /d/ to /g/ by changing the second-formant transitions in graded steps. Although the physical changes between adjacent stimuli were small, subjects' identification responses were sharply discontinuous. Despite the graded steps in the continuum, subjects' perception of the syllables shifted abruptly, falling into natural categories for the phonemes /b/, /d/, and /g/. Moreover, when subjects were asked to discriminate among tokens from the stimulus continuum, their discrimination of tokens from different phonemic categories was nearly perfect, but their discrimination of tokens within the same phonemic category was nearly at chance. The phenomenon of discontinuous, categorical perception for speech sounds was markedly different from typical results of psychophysical experiments employing nonspeech stimuli such as pure tones. Nonspeech continua are perceived continuously, resulting in discrimination functions that are monotonic with respect to the physical scale. These differences between speech and nonspeech perception led researchers to propose that speech perception is subserved by specialized mechanisms distinct from mechanisms for general audition (see Repp [1983a] for a comprehensive review of the categorical perception literature).

A number of other phenomena have been purported to demonstrate the specialized nature of speech. These include findings of phonetic discrimination in infants, the rigidity of adult phonetic categories, cross-modal cue integration, cue trading relations, and duplex perception. These phenomena are considered in this chapter. However, for the development of speech perception, see Aslin and Pisoni, 1980; Eimas, et al., 1971; Walley, Pisoni, and Aslin, 1981; and Chapter 9 of this volume.

Perception of Speech and Nonspeech Signals

Some of the earliest empirical support for the claims of specialization for speech came from the categorical perception of speech stimuli compared with the continuous perception of nonspeech stimuli. The explanation for these differences offered by Liberman (1970a, 1970b),

Liberman et al. (1967), and Studdert-Kennedy and Shankweiler (1970) was based on the **motor theory** of speech perception, in which speech perception is assumed to be mediated by knowledge of articulation. Considering the stimulus continuum examined by Liberman et al. (1957), although the physical scale was composed of many graded steps of second formant transitions, production of /b/, /d/, and /g/ corresponds to three discrete, discontinuous places of articulation. Listeners' perception of these sounds does not follow the continuous physical attributes of the signal but seems to follow the abstract, discontinuous places of articulation. The fact that nonspeech signals are continuously perceived was taken as further support that at least for stop consonants, speech perception entails a specialized **speech mode of perception.**

The motor theory account of categorical perception, and the generality of the data themselves, were challenged by researchers who believed that the same phenomena could be explained via general principles of auditory perception (Massaro, 1972, 1987; Cutting, 1978; Schouten, 1980; Pastore, 1981). A problem with using the basic psychophysical studies as the contrast to the speech perception studies was that neither the nonspeech stimuli nor nonspeech categorization tasks were adequately matched to their speech counterparts (Pisoni, 1991). More recently, a number of experiments using analogs of speech have demonstrated that subjects can perceive continuously varying stimuli categorically even though they reportedly hear the stimuli as nonspeech events such as tones or beeps. Such demonstrations of categorical perception for nonspeech signals imply that generic psychophysical principles may account for categorical perception; perception may be discontinuous, ostensibly without reference to articulatory knowledge. Accordingly, these researchers have attempted to account for categorical perception of speech stimuli via general auditory processing of acoustic stimuli, whether speech or nonspeech.

Lisker and Abramson (1964, 1967) demonstrated that categorical perception between voiced and voiceless stops (/b/ versus /p/, /d/ versus /t/, /g/ versus /k/) is determined by voice onset time. VOT is the silent interval between the burst release at the articulators and the onset of voicing. In voiceless stops, there is typically a long lag between the burst release and voicing; in voiced stops, the lag is shorter and may even be negative (voicing begins before the stop is released). The finding that the temporal coordination of articulatory gestures determines categorical perception is consistent with an articulation-based mode of speech perception. However, similar findings have been obtained in experiments using nonspeech materials. Miller et al. (1976) created nonspeech VOT analogs by generating stimuli that contained aperiodic noise bursts followed by periodic buzzing. The interval between the noise burst and the buzz was varied in small steps, following Lisker and Abramson's earlier VOT experiments. Subjects asked to classify the stimuli according to "noise" vs. "no noise" showed categorical perception and discrimination very similar to those found with speech stimuli. Similarly, Pisoni (1977) employed stimuli that were even less speechlike than those used by Miller et al. (1976) and still observed categorical perception. Pisoni presented stimuli composed of only two tones, one at 500 Hz and one at 1500 Hz. The low tone either preceded or followed the high tone by as much as 50 ms, with graded steps in between. Categorical identification and discrimination closely resembled those obtained by Lisker and Abramson (1967). In addition, Jusczyk et al. (1980) found that infants perceive the two-tone stimuli categorically, just as they perceive speech stimuli (Eimas et al., 1971).

Comparison of the perception of speech and nonspeech signals reveals that other phenomena believed to demonstrate specialized speech processing can be explained by general auditory mechanisms. In a study of the effect of perceived speaking rate on phonetic classification, Miller and Liberman (1979) generated a series of synthetic speech stimuli ranging from /ba/ to /wa/ by gradually changing the duration of the formant transitions leading into the steady-state vowel formants. The most important manipulation was varying the duration of the syllables, hence the perceived speaking rate of the syllables. Miller and Liberman found that, as perceived speaking rate increased, subjects' category boundaries shifted toward /wa/, implying that at faster speaking rates, listeners accept shorter transitions as /w/. Miller and Liberman accounted for these data by proposing that specialized perceptual mechanisms compensate for changes in speaking rate in the perception of stops versus glides (see also Miller and Wayland, 1993). Eimas and Miller (1980) demonstrated the same compensatory phenomenon with in-

fant subjects, implying that the specialized mechanism is innate.

However, it was later found that the compensation for speaking rate could be obtained using nonspeech analogs of speech. Pisoni, Carrell and Gans (1983) generated nonspeech analogs (three component tones) of the Miller and Liberman (1979) stimuli. Subjects categorized these stimuli as either "gradual onset" or "abrupt onset" and displayed a category boundary shift dependent upon duration that bore a striking resemblance to the speech data (Fig. 8-4). From these data Pisoni, Carrell, and Gans (1983, p. 320) suggested that postulation of specialized, rate-sensitive mechanisms for speech may be unwarranted. Instead, they argued that "context effects in discrimination may simply reflect the operation of fairly general auditory processing capacities." Indeed, Oller, Eilers, and Ozdamar (1990) proposed a simple psychophysical model based on linear regression to account for the rate compensation effect. Finally, Jusczyk et al. (1983) replicated the Pisoni, Carrell, and Gans (1983) experiments, showing that 2-month-old infants exhibit the boundary shift for nonspeech as well as speech.

These speech-nonspeech comparison studies suggest that the proposal of specialized mechanisms for speech perception may be unwarranted. However, despite the studies demonstrating the similarities of speech and nonspeech perception, important differences have also been observed (Pisoni, 1991). A number of studies have shown that when listeners are induced to process nonspeech auditory signals in a speech mode (for instance, when told they will hear poor-quality synthetic speech and should label the stimuli using phonetic categories), their perception changes markedly. Such demonstrations are typically provided by between-subjects experiments using a common pool of perceptually ambiguous stimuli that can be heard as either speech or nonspeech, according to the listener's expectations. In one condition subjects are told that they will hear synthetic speech, and in the other they are told that they will hear beeps or tones. After some performance measure is collected from subjects, they are typically queried to ensure that they actually thought the stimuli sounded like either speech or tones, depending upon their assigned group.

When subjects were presented with the **sine wave speech** sentence "Where were you a year ago?" Remez et al. (1981) found that simply

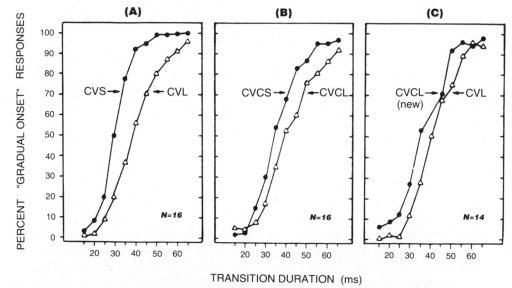

FIGURE 8-4   *A* shows categorization functions for synthetic speech stimuli (Miller and Liberman, 1979). *B* shows similar categorization functions for nonspeech stimuli that subjects heard as tones. (Adapted from Pisoni, D. B., Carrell, T. D., & Gans, S. J. [1983]. Perception of the duration of rapid spectrum changes in speech and nonspeech signals. *Perception & Psychophysics, 34,* 314-322.)

informing subjects that the signal was speech changed subjects' perception from a series of whistles and beeps to a correctly transcribed sentence (see also Bailey, Summerfield, and Dorman, 1977; Grunke and Pisoni, 1982; Tomiak, Mullennix, and Sawusch, 1987). Of course, the Remez et al. (1981) results may have been due to either a qualitative change in perception or any number of changes in response biases. In an experiment that left less room for a bias interpretation, Schwab (1981) found substantial backward masking and upward spread of masking for sine wave stimuli heard as tones. However, all masking was eliminated when subjects heard the stimuli as speech.

The major difference between perception in the speech and nonspeech modes for ambiguous stimuli appears to be the difference between holistic and componential analysis. It seems that listeners in the speech mode spontaneously forego detailed spectral analysis of the stimuli and make their speech categorizations based on entire, complex configurations of cues.* Conversely, subjects in a nonspeech mode behave more analytically, actually hearing the component parts of the stimuli individually. Further evidence of this was provided by Tomiak, Mullennix, and Sawusch (1987) in an experiment using the Garner (1974) speeded classification task. When told that they would classify nonspeech patterns, subjects separately processed the component dimensions of noise-tone analogs of fricative-vowel syllables. Irrelevant variation in the noise spectra did not affect reaction times for classifying tones. However, when subjects were told that the stimuli were synthetic fricative-vowel syllables, the components were processed integrally so that irrelevant variation in either dimension increased reaction times to classify stimuli along the other dimension. Finally, in an experiment reported by Grunke and Pisoni (1982), subjects were asked to identify ambiguous stimuli with either phonetic or acoustic labels, depending on their assignment to conditions. The stimuli were composed of either one, two, or three component tones. In the one- and two-tone conditions, subjects who used the acoustic categories "rising" and "falling" performed better than subjects who used phonetic categories. However, when a third tone was added, acoustic classifi-

cations were greatly impaired and phonetic classifications were substantially improved. Apparently the third tone made the signal more speechlike to listeners in the speech mode and noisier to listeners in the nonspeech mode.

Given these and similar findings, it is apparent that speech and nonspeech modes of perception differ in fundamental, qualitative respects (see Fowler [1990] for a different view). However, the basis of these differences remains to be explained. Are the differences due to the selective operation of different perceptual modules, response strategies, or attentional capacities? This question carries great theoretical importance and merits deeper investigation.

In sum, studies comparing speech and nonspeech perception have repeatedly called into question the strong claims regarding the specialized nature of speech perception. However, the evidence and arguments on both sides are equivocal, and the implications of these studies are subject to interpretation. To appreciate the degree to which the meaning of these studies is in the eye of the beholder, compare the conclusions from two reviews of the speech-nonspeech literature on categorical perception:

> The nonspeech studies to this point do more than just refute the view that categorical perception is specific to speech. They demonstrate that there are certain important similarities in the ways certain classes of speech and nonspeech sounds are perceived. (Jusczyk, 1986, p. 43).

> In summary, despite a few suggestive results, there is no conclusive evidence so far for any significant parallelism in the perception of speech and nonspeech. (Repp, 1983a, p. 50).

Duplex Perception

Duplex perception is a phenomenon discovered by Rand (1974) and recently cited as strong evidence for a dissociation of phonetic perception from general auditory perception (Liberman, 1982; Repp, 1982; Studdert-Kennedy, 1982; Liberman and Mattingly, 1985, 1989). The general procedure for eliciting the duplex percept is simple. A listener is presented with two simultaneous, dichotic stimuli. One ear hears an isolated third-formant transition that sounds like a nonspeech chirp. At the same time the other ear receives a base syllable. This base syllable consists of the first two formants, complete with transitions, and the third formant without a transition. Typically, the transition presented in isolation completes the syllable to

---

*Another interpretation may be that subjects in a speech mode process components of the signal separately but in accordance with well-learned combinations.

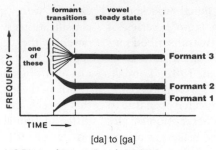

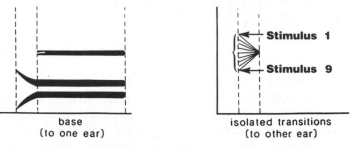

FIGURE 8-5 Stimuli used in a duplex perception experiment. The upper panel shows a synthetic speech syllable with a range of third formant transitions. When presented binaurally, these syllables range from /da/ to /ga/. The lower left panel shows the constant syllable base that is always presented in the dichotic listening task. The lower right panel shows a series of third-formant transitions, ranging from /ga/ to da/, which are combined with the syllable base. (From Mann, V. A., & Liberman, A. M. [1983]. Some differences between phonetic and auditory modes of perception. *Cognition, 14,* 211-235.)

create a /da/ or /ga/, sometimes in graded steps along a continuum (Fig. 8-5). When the base and the transition are presented dichotically, the listener's percept is duplex; that is, the completed syllable is perceived and the nonspeech chirp is heard at the same time. Liberman and Mattingly (1989) argue that the phonetic module and a separate general auditory module each respond to different aspects of the stimuli, thus creating the duplex percept.

Several further findings support the claim that segregated modes of processing are responsible for the separate percepts. For example, in one study, Mann et al. (1981; reported in Liberman, 1981) presented a series of different third-formant transitions such that upon fusion the entire syllables consisted of a continuum from /da/ to /ga/. When subjects attended to the nonspeech side of the percept, continuous discrimination functions typical of nonspeech were obtained. When subjects attended to the speech percept, categorical discrimination functions were obtained, implying that the separate percepts are subserved by separate processing systems. Other experiments have demonstrated

that various stimulus or procedural manipulations can affect the speech or nonspeech percept independently, again implicating separate processors (Isenberg and Liberman, 1978; Bentin and Mann, 1990; Nygaard and Eimas, 1990; Nygaard, 1993).

Taken together, these findings on duplex perception support the claim of an independent and specialized phonetic recognition system. As Repp (1982, p. 102) concludes:

Duplex perception phenomena provide evidence for the distinction between auditory and phonetic modes of perception. They show that, in the duplex situation, the auditory mode can gain access to the input from the individual ears, whereas the phonetic mode operates on the combined input from both ears. The "phonological fusion" discovered by Day (1968)—two dichotic utterances such as "banket" and "lanket" yield the percept "blanket"—is yet another example of the abstract, nonauditory level of integration that characterizes the phonetic mode.

Similarly, Whalen and Liberman (1987, p. 171) describe the phenomenon of duplex perception as evidence for the preemptiveness of speech, arguing that the speech module gets the first crack at interpreting an auditory signal: "The phonetic mode takes precedence in processing the transitions, using them for its special linguistic purposes until, having appropriated its share, it passes the remainder to be perceived by the nonspeech system as auditory whistles."

These interpretations of duplex perception are not universal; several lines of counterevidence have been offered. Pastore et al. (1983) observed duplex perception for musical chords (two notes in one ear, a third note in the other), casting doubt on the claim that duplex perception is a solely speech-based phenomenon. In addition, Nusbaum, Schwab, and Sawusch (1983) demonstrated that listeners use the information in the third-formant transition independently of the base, casting doubt on the claim that the transition in isolation is a true nonspeech signal (see, however, Nusbaum, 1984, and Repp, 1984). This finding by Nusbaum, Schwab, and Sawusch (1983) implies that subjects in the studies reported earlier could have generated their phonetic decisions without any process of auditory fusion between the ears.

An especially strong challenge to the speech module interpretation of duplex perception comes from Fowler and Rosenblum (1990, 1991). Borrowing language and ideas from Gibson's (1966) event perception, Fowler and Rosenblum argue that duplex perception may demonstrate not the preemptiveness of speech per se but simply the preemptiveness of any meaningful event. The argument is that human sensory systems have evolved to recognize important objects and events around us ("affordances," in Gibson's [1979] terminology). Therefore, our perceptual and cognitive systems are naturally attuned to perceive meaning from any stimulation. Accordingly, Fowler and Rosenblum predicted that duplex perception would occur whenever two acoustic fragments, when integrated, specify a natural event and when one of the fragments has any unnatural quality. Fowler and Rosenblum (1991, pp. 51, 52) write, "Under these conditions, the integrated event should be preemptive and the intense fragment should be duplexed regardless of the type of natural sound-producing event that is involved, whether it is speech or nonspeech, and whether it is profoundly biologically significant or biologically trivial."

To demonstrate duplex perception for a

biologically trivial event, Fowler and Rosenblum dichotically presented a low-pass filtered recording of a slamming metal door to one ear and the remaining high-frequency noise to the other ear. Alone, the base sounded like a wooden door slamming, and the chirp sounded to the authors like a can of rice being shaken (recall that we are biased to perceive sounds as events). When the stimuli were played together with the chirp at a higher amplitude than the base, most subjects reported the duplex perception of metal door + chirp. This demonstration of duplex perception for such a completely nonspeech signal calls into question both the relevance of duplex perception to speech research and the specialized nature of speech perception (see Hall and Pastore [1992] for a similar demonstration of duplex perception using musical chords). Findings such as Fowler and Rosenblum's clearly underscore the need for deeper investigation into duplex perception before it is too richly interpreted.

Trading Relations and Integration of Cues

A third class of findings cited as evidence for the specialization of speech perception comes from studies of cue trading and cue integration (see Repp, 1982). The speech signal is replete with cues to phonetic contrasts, and several different cues may indicate a single contrast (Delattre et al., 1952; Denes, 1955; Harris, et al., 1958; Hoffman, 1958; Repp, 1982). This makes it possible that when the utility of one cue is reduced, another cue becomes primary. It is assumed that trading relations occur because the cues are phonetically equivalent with respect to the contrast in question. The cues may trade in importance when necessary or may integrate to provide robust contrasts when all cues are provided equally. Examples of cue trading have been provided by Denes (1955) and Fitch et al. (1980), who demonstrated the perceptual equivalence of closure durations and first-formant transitions in signaling the contrast between minimal pairs such as *slit–split* (Repp, 1982). In Figure 8-6 the phonetic trading relation of closure duration and formant transition is clearly evident.

Phonetic trading relations have been cited as evidence of a speech mode of perception for two main reasons: First, trading relations can occur between both spectral and temporal cues distributed over relatively long intervals. Repp (1982) argues that it is difficult to imagine that such cues

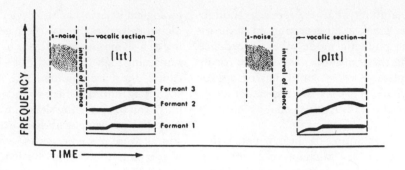

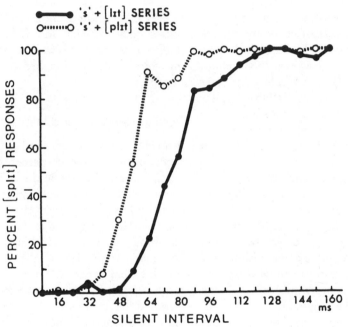

FIGURE 8-6   Examples of stimulus materials and typical data displaying a phonetic trading relation. The upper panel shows synthetic stimuli for the syllables "slit" and "split"; the duration of the silent closure intervals varies along a continuum during a perceptual experiment. The lower panel shows identification data for both syllables as a function of closure duration. When proper transitions are present, a short closure duration is sufficient to perceive "split"; when transitions are absent, a longer duration is sufficient to perceive "split". (From Fitch, H. L., Hawles, T., Erickson, D. M., & Liberman, A. M. [1980]. Perceptual equivalence of two acoustic cues for stop-consonant manner. *Perception and Psychophysics, 27,* 343-350.

would be integrated into a single percept unless some speech-specific system were mediating perception. Repp argues further that listeners must possess abstract articulatory knowledge to integrate such disparate cues (see also Liberman and Mattingly, 1985). Repp (1982, p. 95) suggests that:

Trading relations may occur because listeners perceive speech in terms of the underlying articu-

lation and resolve inconsistencies in the acoustic formation by perceiving the most plausible articulatory act. This explanation requires that the listener have at least a general model of human vocal tracts and of their ways of action.

The second reason that trading relations have been cited as evidence for the speech mode of perception comes again from comparisons of speech and nonspeech perception. Best, Morrongiello, and Robson (1981) reported two experiments using sine wave speech, which may be heard as either speech or nonspeech, depending primarily upon the listener's expectation. They found that listeners in a speech mode exhibit cue trading and integration, but listeners in a nonspeech mode do not. They considered these findings proof that the integration and perceptual equivalence of multiple cues are specific to speech.

Their conclusion has been challenged. For example, Massaro and Oden (1980) have presented a model of speech perception that accounts for trading relations while making no assumptions of specialized processing (see also Massaro, 1972, 1987, 1989; Massaro and Cohen, 1976, 1977; Oden and Massaro, 1978; and Derr and Massaro, 1980). Massaro and Oden argue that multiple features corresponding to a single phonetic contrast are extracted independently from the speech waveform and are integrated multiplicatively into a unitary percept. The weight given to each feature in this integration is determined by the strength, or certainty, of the feature's presence. By this account, speech perception reduces to a "prototypical instance of pattern recognition" (Massaro and Oden, 1980, p. 131).

Repp (1983b, p. 132) arrived at a conclusion similar to that of Massaro and Oden, stating that trading relations ". . . are not special because, once the prototypical patterns are known in any perceptual domain, trading relations follow as the inevitable product of a general pattern matching operation. Thus, speech perception is the application of general perceptual principles to very special patterns."

In short, as in the earlier debates regarding speech versus nonspeech perception and duplex perception, the evidence provided by trading relations is ambiguous with respect to claims of a specialized speech mode of processing.

Cross-Modal Cue Integration (The McGurk Effect)

Another recent finding in speech perception attributed to specialized mechanisms is *cross-modal cue integration,* or the McGurk effect (MacDonald, 1976; MacDonald and McGurk, 1978; Summerfield, 1979, 1983; Roberts and Summerfield, 1981). The phenomenon is a perceptual illusion, demonstrated as follows: A subject is presented with a video display of a talker (or synthesized face; see Massaro and

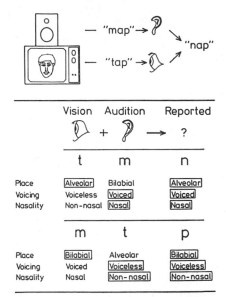

FIGURE 8-7   The procedure used to elicit the McGurk illusion. The video displays a face articulating the syllable /tap/ and the audio channel outputs the syllable /map/. Audiovisual integration leads the subject to perceive the syllable /nap/. (From Summerfield, Q. [1983]. Audio-visual speech perception, lipreading and artificial stimulation. In Lutman, M. E., & Haggam, M. P. (Eds.), *Hearing Science and Hearing Disorders.* London: Academic Press.)

Cohen, 1990) articulating simple CV syllables and hears spoken syllables synchronized with the visual display. The McGurk effect occurs when the visual and auditory syllables are incongruous. The listener typically reports hearing neither the spoken syllable nor the lip-read syllable, but something in between. For example, when presented with a face that articulates /ma/ and an auditory syllable /ta/, most subjects report hearing /na/ (Fig. 8-7).

According to subjective reports of the McGurk illusion, the effect is quite striking. Liberman (1982) points out that the procedure affects listeners' experience of hearing the syllable as an integrated event, to an extent that listeners cannot determine the degree to which their perception of syllable identity is due to either source of information. For example, Repp (1982, p. 102) reports,

> I have experienced this effect myself (together with a number of my colleagues at Haskins) and can confirm that it is a true perceptual phenomenon and not some kind of inference or bias in the face of conflicting information. The observer really believes that he or she hears what, in fact, he or she only sees on the screen; there is little awareness of anything odd happening.

The McGurk illusion has been interpreted as particularly strong evidence for a specialized speech perceptual system that makes reference to articulatory gestures. Fowler and Rosenblum (1991, p. 37) speculate, "Why does integration occur? One answer is that both sources of information, the optical and the acoustic, provide information about the same event of talking, and they do so by providing information about the talker's phonetic gestures." However, there are detractors to this position. Massaro and Cohen (1983, 1990, 1993) have shown that their fuzzy logical model of perception provides precise accounts of the McGurk and MacDonald data without postulation of any speech-specific mechanisms. In addition, the generality of the phenomenon is limited. Easton and Basala (1982) found that the illusion is not invoked if whole words are used instead of syllables (although Dekle, Fowler, and Funnell, 1992, reported otherwise). This finding and Massaro's model suggest that the illusion is the product of general perceptual biases that are revealed only by highly ambiguous stimuli. Finally, one of the principal assumptions of cognitive psychology is that humans routinely perform intricate information processing that may involve any number of stages, computations, heuristics, or biases without any awareness of the operations they perform. Accordingly, despite the impressions of listeners regarding the illusion, the fact that a phenomenon seems truly perceptual does not allow us to conclude by fiat that the results cannot be due to biases (Neisser, 1967; Cutting, 1987).

Two further findings related to cross-modal integration do seem to tip the scales back in favor of a specialized-processing account. Miller (1990) cites 4- and 5-month-old infants' sensitivity to auditory-articulatory correspondence as strong evidence for innately specified perceptual mechanisms (Kuhl and Meltzoff, 1982; MacKain et al., 1983). Kuhl and Meltzoff (1982) found that infants prefer to watch a display of an articulating face if the accompanying spoken syllables match the articulation rather than incongruent audiovisual displays. Furthermore, Roberts and Summerfield (1981) used the McGurk phenomenon in a clever test of selective adaptation (see Eimas and Corbit, 1973). They presented subjects with an auditory syllable /bɛ/ and visual syllable /gɛ/, producing the percept of /dɛ/. However, on a test of adaptation, the perceived audiovisual syllable had the same effects as a purely auditory /bɛ/ on a /bɛ/–/dɛ/

series; subjects' phonetic perception of the stimulus as /dɛ/ was not reflected in their adaptation data. Studdert-Kennedy (1982, p. 7) considers this finding a powerful indication of the dissociation of general auditory and phonetic perception:

> I take [the procedure of] audio-visual adaptation to demonstrate unequivocally the on-line dissociation of auditory and phonetic perception. Moreover, following Summerfield (1979), I take the results of the audio-visual adaptation study to demonstrate that the support for phonetic perception is information about the common source of acoustic and optical information, namely, articulatory dynamics.

Studdert-Kennedy may be correct. Alternatively, we may assume, as in an information-processing model of speech perception (Cutting and Pisoni, 1978), that the pathway from audition to phonetic perception is composed of processing stages (see also Studdert-Kennedy, 1974, 1976). The locus of the phonetic perception of the McGurk paradigm and the locus of the adaptation effect could be separated so that the adaptation manipulation affects some stage of processing that precedes the audiovisual integration. This seems likely. Presumably the integration of information from vision and audition occurs somewhat late in the speech perception process. If so, the Roberts and Summerfield (1981) data may not imply a strict auditory versus phonetic dissociation; the adaptation stimulus may simply affect precategorical phonetic perception, an explanation that would be compatible with either a motor theory or an auditory theory. Perhaps the only firm conclusion is that the McGurk effect, like duplex perception, may eventually constitute compelling evidence for specialized speech perception based on articulatory gestures. For the present, however, more complete investigation of these phenomena is clearly necessary.

Role of Linguistic Experience in Speech Perception

An important but neglected issue relevant to the question of specialization concerns the role of linguistic experience on adult speech perception (see Studdert-Kennedy et al., 1970). It has long been known that infants can categorically discriminate among the phonemes of their native language and among many other nonnative phonemes. With continued linguistic experi-

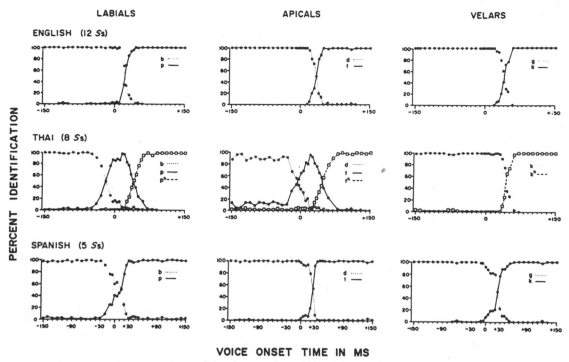

FIGURE 8-8   Cross-language identification data for labial, apical, and velar stops ranging in voice onset time from −150 to +150 msec. Categorization is clearly affected by the linguistic background of the listener. (Adapted from Pisoni, D. B., Aslin, R. N., Perey, A. J., & Hennessy, B. L. [1982]. Some effects of laboratory training on identification and discrimination of voicing contrasts in stop consonants. *Journal of Experimental Psychology: Human Perception and Performance, 8*, 297-314.)

ence, the listener's ability to discriminate between speech sounds not phonemically contrastive in the native tongue seems to be virtually lost (Strange and Jenkins, 1978; Aslin and Pisoni, 1980; Aslin, 1985; Logan, Lively, and Pisoni, 1991; Pisoni, Logan, and Lively, 1994). Maturation appears to pare down the set of all possible contrasts (or at least most; see Best, MacRoberts, and Sithole, 1988) that listeners can originally discriminate to only the set required for the native language (see Polka, 1992; Best, 1994; Polka and Werker, 1994). Evidence for the language-specific discrimination abilities of adults was first provided by Lisker and Abramson (1964, 1967; see also Abramson and Lisker, 1967). They investigated the abilities of speakers of varying languages to perceive three sets of synthetic speech stimuli that formed continua along the dimension of VOT that corresponded to labial, velar, and palatal sounds. The results of their experiments demonstrated that, in general, subjects from different linguistic backgrounds identified and discriminated the stimuli according to the contrastive phonological categories of their languages. The cross-language identification functions obtained by Lisker and Abramson (1967), shown in Figure 8-8, demonstrate the influence of the native language on perceptual classification.

Beyond the influence of the native phonemic repertoire on the typical identification of speech sounds, many studies have demonstrated the inflexibility of the adult listener's phonemic categories. Training an adult speaker of one language to discriminate reliably between phonemes of another language is very difficult and requires extensive training to obtain even small improvements (Strange, 1972; Vinegrad, 1972; Strange and Jenkins, 1978; Strange and Dittmann, 1984). Therefore, it was argued that the development of phonetic categories may require a plastic neural substrate that becomes less flexible after a critical period (Eimas, 1975). This view of the nature and development of phonetic categories is clearly compatible with the assumption, recently defended by Liberman and Mattingly (1989), that speech perception is modular. Fodor (1983) describes perceptual modules as innately specified, neurally hardwired and nonmodifiable. Fodor's modularity is therefore compatible with the view that speech perception is subserved by perceptual and memory systems that are flexible only in infancy, becoming autonomous and impenetrable as early as possible.

More recent research, however, has demonstrated that significant improvements in discrimination of nonnative phonetic contrasts can be obtained using laboratory training procedures. In one experiment, Pisoni et al. (1982) trained English-speaking subjects to perceive three categories along a VOT continuum where only two categories naturally exist. A more recent example comes from training procedures employed by Logan, Lively, and Pisoni (1991; see also Pisoni, Logan, and Lively, 1994) to teach Japanese listeners to discriminate /r/ from /l/. Previous research showed that training Japanese listeners to distinguish these phonemes is extremely difficult and usually produces only marginal results (Goto, 1971; MacKain, Best, and Strange, 1981; Mochizuki, 1981; Strange and Dittmann, 1984). However, Logan, Lively, and Pisoni argued that neither the stimulus materials nor the training procedures employed in most of these studies were ideal for teaching listeners the intended contrast. For example, Strange and Dittmann (1984) used laboratory training procedures. Their methods failed and they concluded that training procedures are ineffective in modifying the phonetic categories of adult listeners. However, several aspects of their methodology call this global conclusion into question. First of all, the stimuli were synthetic tokens of "rock" and "lock", and no other stimuli were used. In addition, the procedure was a standard same-different discrimination task with limited feedback.

Logan, Lively, and Pisoni used natural tokens of minimal pairs contrasting /r/ and /l/. Furthermore, to provide listeners with more robust categories, they presented tokens produced by a variety of talkers. In addition, the target phonemes occurred in a variety of phonetic environments. Clearly, these natural and variable tokens contain far more cues and more ecological validity than the synthetic tokens employed in earlier studies. Using these varied materials and extensive feedback, Logan, Lively, and Pisoni observed substantial improvements in discrimination for all of their subjects. Similar preliminary results have been reported by Pruitt et al. (1990) in training English listeners to distinguish Hindi retroflex-dental consonants. Findings such as these, as well as a large body of developmental data (Aslin and Pisoni, 1980; and Chapter 9 of this volume) have prompted several researchers (e.g., Jusczyk, 1985, 1986) to propose that phonological categories develop and are maintained by general attention and categorization mechanisms. These theories assume that the phonological inventory for any given language can be derived by selectively attending to relevant contrastive dimensions while selectively ignoring variation along irrelevant dimensions. Nosofsky (1986, 1987) has shown that this kind of selective attention strategy applied in simple category learning tasks can account for a wide variety of findings in the literature on categorization, perceptual identification, and the nature of psychological similarity. Logan, Lively, and Pisoni (1991) also refer to these attentional mechanisms to explain their learning data and to account for the learning failures of earlier studies. These proposals imply that the processes of speech perception rely on general cognitive principles of pattern recognition, attention, and categorization rather than highly specialized mechanisms unique to speech perception. However, we cannot determine whether these training procedures affect early phonetic perceptual processes or some later decisional processes. Clearly, we are still a long way from complete understanding of these issues, especially the developmental aspects of phonetic perception. For the present, however, we can maintain that adult phonetic categories are not rigid, as has been suggested, and that their flexibility is consistent with a view of speech perception based on general cognitive mechanisms.

Studies of Speech Perception in Nonhumans

One final area of research that merits consideration in this discussion is speech perception by nonhuman animals. The logic that motivates such research is simple: When strong claims were made that categorical perception was a speech-specific phenomenon, researchers attempted to demonstrate categorical perception of nonspeech signals. Similarly, when claims were made that categorical perception was uniquely human and speech-specific, researchers attempted to demonstrate that nonhuman animals with auditory systems roughly analogous to the human auditory system could also perceive speech sounds categorically. Clearly, animals do not derive phonetic content from human speech, so any discrimination or categorization data provided by the animals must reflect general auditory and classification processes.

In studies of speech discrimination by monkeys, Morse and Snowdon (1975) and Waters and Wilson (1976) found preliminary evidence that monkeys perceive place of articulation categorically. More convincing evidence was provided in experiments conducted by Kuhl and Miller (1975, 1978) on perception of speech by chinchillas. In experiments on categorization (as indicated in an avoidance-conditioning task), it was demonstrated that, for stimulus continua varying VOT, chinchillas' categorization boundaries were remarkably similar to those for English-speaking listeners (Fig. 8-9). Moreover, Kluender, Diehl, and Killeen (1987) demonstrated that Japanese quail can learn apparently robust phonetic categories for stop consonants /b/, /d/, and /g/. The quail learned the stops in CV syllables followed by four different vowels and later could discriminate the three stops in the context of eight novel vowels; this generalization implies some form of abstraction of the category.

What are we to make of this? The results are certainly suggestive: If nothing else, they imply that given an auditory system similar to the human and a rudimentary ability to distinguish between stimuli, animals tend to respond differentially to speech signals that correspond to human phonetic categories. This implies that we need not hypothesize specialized, articulatory-based perceptual mechanisms to account for human speech perception. Unfortunately, the results of the animal studies can be taken only as suggestive. There is no reason to assume, for instance, that human languages would have evolved phonetic contrasts that were especially difficult for our auditory systems to discriminate (Stevens, 1972). The animal data may simply illustrate that phonetic categories are evolutionarily well conceived. Furthermore, since we have no access to the animals' experience, we have no basis for assuming that anything speechlike is perceived at all. In short, examining their behavior is rather like examining the behavior of a Turing machine—it may resemble human performance, but that does not mean it derives from the same underlying mechanisms (see also Repp, 1983a).

Finally, what are we to conclude about the entire debate concerning the specialization of

speech perception? There are viable arguments on both sides of the issue. This debate has been fruitful for the sake of continuing research—more data have been generated and energy devoted to its resolution than to any other issue in speech perception. At the same time, the specialization hypothesis may be empirically unassailable. This may be true especially now that the specialization mechanism has been described in terms of the modularity hypothesis. Fodor (1985) describes three necessary characteristics of any experiment considered a bona fide counterexample to the modularity of a perceptual system: (1) The experiment must demonstrate the influence of background information (higher cognitive processes) on perceptual output. (2) This influence must clearly involve the perceptual system; it cannot reflect postperceptual processing or a decisional criterion shift. (3) The cognitively penetrated system must be the usual system for natural perception in the given domain, not involving some backup systems that are required only in special circumstances, such as in perceiving degraded stimuli. Consider, for example, the finding that mere instructions change the percept of sine wave speech from a sequence of tones into a sentence (Remez et al., 1981). At first glance, this appears to violate the impenetrable nature of the phonetic module, whose operations are supposed to be impervious to the listener's beliefs and expectations. (Fodor's preferred examples are optical illusions, such as the Mueller-Lyer illusion, which persists even when the observer knows that the lines are of equal length.) Clearly the sine wave speech demonstration satisfies the first condition, but the second and third are questionable. Furthermore, almost any experiment aimed at demonstrating the nonspecialized nature of phonetic perception may fail to satisfy at least one of these criteria. The challenge for future research is to address the relevant issues while circumventing these pitfalls.

Normalization Problems in Speech Perception

The problems posed for theories of speech perception by the inherent nonlinearity, variability, and nonsegmental nature of the speech signal arise from the basic assumption that listeners must somehow map distorted information in the speech signal onto canonical linguistic representations in memory. Typically, researchers in

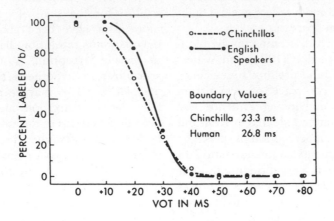

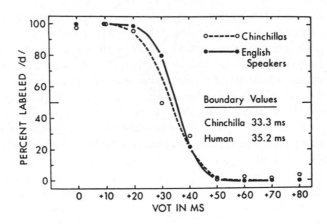

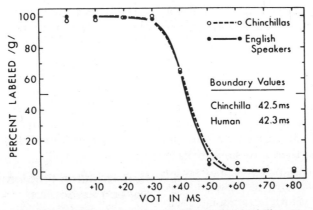

FIGURE 8-9   Phonetic categorization data for humans and chinchillas. Upper panel, /b/-/p/ continuum; middle panel, /d/-/t/ continuum; lower panel, /g/-/k/ continuum. In all three cases, the phonetic boundaries of humans and chinchillas are quite similar. (Adapted from Kuhl, P. K., & Miller, J. D. [1978]. Speech perception by the chinchilla: Identification functions for synthetic VOT stimuli. *Journal of the Acoustical Society of America, 63,* 905-917.)

speech perception have limited their study of variability to the effects of different phonetic contexts. However, many factors beyond phonetic context influence the acoustic realizations of phonetic contrasts. Collectively, perceptual accommodations to variations in speech patterns to recover canonical linguistic units fall into the category of *perceptual normalization*. Recent research on normalization focuses on sources of variation such as talkers' vocal tract differences and speaking rate differences (although the problem of perceptual constancy is also introduced by a speaker with a mouthful of food, a singing voice, etc.).

Individuals differ in the sizes and shapes of their vocal tracts (Joos, 1948; Peterson and Barney, 1952; Fant, 1973), glottal characteristics (Carr and Trill, 1964; Monsen and Engebretson, 1977; Carrell, 1984), their idiosyncratic articulatory strategies for producing speech (Ladefoged, 1980; Johnson, Ladefoged, and Landau, 1993), and the dialects of their native regions (Abercrombie, 1967). This produces wide variability in production of the same words and phrases across individuals. Nevertheless, human listeners accurately perceive speech across virtually all (reasonably intelligible) speakers without any apparent difficulty. At present, little is known about the perceptual processes responsible for the implied perceptual compensations, nor is it known whether perceptual compensation occurs at all.

A related matter is time and rate normalization. Speech is a temporally distributed signal. Accordingly, the cues to individual phonetic contrasts in speech are distributed in time and are substantially influenced by changes in speaking rate. Moreover, the acoustic durations of phonetic segments are influenced by the locations of syntactic boundaries in fluent speech, by syllabic stress, and by the component features of adjacent segments (Gaitenby, 1965; Lehiste, 1970; Klatt, 1975, 1976, 1979). Segmental durations are modified further by contextual factors in speech. For example, vowels of words spoken in sentences are approximately half the duration of vowels of the same words spoken in isolation (Luce and Pisoni, 1987). In sum, phonetic contrasts in conversational fluent speech are characterized by widespread durational variation. Furthermore, it is well known that some durational variation in speech carries important information about numerous phonetic contrasts, word boundaries, and so on. In

English, numerous phonetic contrasts are distinguished by durational cues. Thus, the listener must attend to and use durational cues to stress, phonemic contrasts, and pragmatics while ignoring irrelevant durational variations due to particular talkers or circumstances (Port, 1977; Miller, 1980).

Indexical Information in Speech

The human voice conveys information about a speaker's age and gender, as well as more cultural information such as regional origin, temperament, and social group membership. Such aspects of speech, known as **indexical information** (Abercrombie, 1967), do not, in general, relate directly to processes of phonetic perception (other than adding still more variability) but are heavily used in linguistic communication nonetheless. For example, most of us are reasonably expert at discriminating a New England accent from a Japanese accent, just as we are reasonably expert at discriminating the speech patterns of children from those of adults. Indexical information also alerts the listener to the speaker's identity and to important changes in the physical or emotional state of the speaker. Ladefoged and Broadbent (1957) call these aspects of the voice "personal information."

The use of indexical information in everyday communication is pervasive, as when we infer quite extensive information about a speaker's origin and background; in many societies speech patterns are commonly associated with social status (Abercrombie, 1967). Aside from cultural speech patterns, speech patterns of an individual speaker are richly informative. We are remarkably sensitive to the emotional or physical state of a speaker within our own culture, and we can readily identify people we know from their voice alone (Van Lancker, Kreiman, and Emmorey, 1985; Van Lancker, Kreiman, and Wickens, 1985). We also recognize signature voices; for instance, most of us can identify even a poor impersonation of W. C. Fields or Porky Pig. Finally, the entire realm of changes we call "tone of voice" is pervasive in communication and is readily perceived as anger, depression, or joy. Occasionally, tone of voice modifies the semantic content of an utterance, as in a sarcastic comment. Finally, research has demonstrated that listeners incidentally store detailed information about speakers' voices and implied connotative states when listening to speech

(Geiselman and Bellezza, 1977; Geiselman and Crawley, 1983).

These facts raise two apparently contradictory questions in consideration of variability among talkers. The first concerns the listener's ability to recognize the segments of the language despite the idiosyncratic variability introduced by each new voice. The second concerns the listener's ability to exploit such variability to perceive the characteristics of the talker and the communicative situation.

Talker Variability in Speech Perception and Word Recognition

Although Joos (1948) described the problem of talker variability, one of the first empirical demonstrations of its effects was provided by Ladefoged and Broadbent (1957; see also Peters, 1955a, 1955b). Ladefoged and Broadbent presented listeners with the synthesized sentence "Please say what this word is:" followed by "bit", "bet", "bat", or "but". The carrier phrase was altered in different conditions by raising (by 30%) or lowering (by 25%) either the first or second formant or both. This manipulation changed the perceived dimensions of the talker's vocal tract. Ladefoged and Broadbent observed reliable changes in subjects' identification of the target syllables according to the perceived talker. The authors concluded that the carrier phrase allowed the listener to calibrate the vowel space for the talker and to adjust interpretations of the target vowels accordingly (see also Gerstman, 1968). Following this early demonstration, a number of studies sought to investigate and explain the relative constancy of natural vowel perception across talkers (see Shankweiler, Strange, and Verbrugge, 1977; Johnson, 1990). The guiding notion for all such studies was the idea that listeners must somehow extrapolate the entire vowel space of any given talker from a small speech sample (Joos, 1948; Lieberman, Crelin, and Klatt, 1972).

In further research, however, Verbrugge et al. (1976; see also Shankweiler, Strange, and Verbrugge 1977) questioned the premise of this approach. They noted that despite talker variability, listeners' error rates in vowel identification tasks are low (only 4% in Peterson and Barney's 1952 experiments). Verbrugge et al. reexamined vowel identification across talkers and found that accuracy is generally quite high despite talker variability. They also found that providing examples of a speaker's point vowels did not improve listeners' performance, contrary to the notion of calibration. Finally, they found that listeners adjust their criteria according to perceived rate of articulation much more than to perceived length of vocal tract. Verbrugge et al. (1976) concluded that talker normalization either requires very little prior information or does not occur in speech perception at all (see also Strange et al., 1976). Instead they suggested that adjustment to talkers may have more to do with tracking articulatory dynamics than with frequency-based calibration (see also Green, Stevens, and Kuhl, 1994). Verbrugge and Rakerd (1986) presented listeners with /bVd/ syllables spoken by males and females. The syllables had the middle 60% removed, leaving only the beginning and ending transitions with silence in between. Their results showed that considerable vowel identity information is contained in the transitions and that this information is independent of the talker. Verbrugge and Rakerd (1986, p. 56) concluded, "This strongly suggests that a dialect's vowels can be characterized by higher-order variables (patterns of articulatory and spectral *change*) that are independent of a specific talker's vocal tract dimensions."

The fundamental claim of these reports— that talker normalization involves recovery of underlying articulatory dynamics—is familiar. These findings imply that variability introduced from individual talker characteristics may be resolved in the same manner as all other acoustic-phonetic variability. This treatment of perceptual normalization finds support from studies of development as well. Experiments conducted by Kuhl (1979) and by Kuhl and Miller (1982) demonstrated that 6-month-old infants could accurately discriminate vowels produced by three different talkers; the infants did not attend to the changing voice characteristics of the stimuli but focused on vowel identity instead. Holmberg, Morgan, and Kuhl (1977) obtained similar results, finding that infants' discrimination of fricatives was not affected by talker variability (however, see Carrell, Smith, and Pisoni, 1981). Finally, Jusczyk, Pisoni, and Mullennix (1992) examined the effects of talker variability on infants' discrimination of CVC syllables. They found that infants could discriminate syllables, such as /bug/ and /dug/, equally well in single-talker and multiple-talker conditions. All of these findings are consistent with a notion that some specialized system, perhaps a phonetic module sensitive to articulatory gestures, is involved in talker normalization, just as hypothesized with regard to more general problems of perceptual constancy in speech (e.g., Liberman and Mattingly, 1985, 1989).

Nonetheless, the data pertaining to effects of talker variability are equivocal. Essentially, the claims of noneffects of talker variability come from tasks of perceptual identification or discrimination with few attentional or time constraints. Despite these demonstrations of the listener's remarkable accuracy in perceiving speech from varying talkers, several experiments have shown reliable effects of talker variability on speech perception and word recognition. Creelman (1957) investigated the effects of talker variability on the recognition of phonetically balanced words that were presented in lists of tokens spoken by 1, 2, 4, 8, or 16 talkers. Perceptual identification of these words in noise showed that words in lists produced by 2 or more talkers were recognized slightly less accurately (differences on the order of 7% to 10%) than words in the single-talker list.

Later experiments with larger sets of stimulus materials have shown larger effects of talker variability. Summerfield and Haggard (1973; see also Summerfield, 1975) observed slower reaction times to recognize spoken words in multiple-talker blocks than in single-talker blocks. Mullennix, Pisoni, and Martin (1989) investigated the effects of talker variability on word recognition using a large sample of CVC monosyllables. Words were presented in lists spoken by either one talker or by 15 talkers, and subjects performed either perceptual identification of words in noise or auditory naming of nondegraded words. Mullennix, Pisoni, and Martin observed large and reliable effects of talker variability. Word recognition was slower and less accurate with multiple talkers than within single talkers. Moreover, as shown in Figure 8-10, talker variability was a more robust effect and was less sensitive to changes in task demands than other variables known to affect word recognition, such as **word frequency** and neighborhood density (see Luce, 1986; Luce, Pisoni, and Goldinger, 1990). Finally, Mullennix, Pisoni, and Martin also found that talker variability interacted with signal degradation, implying that noise and talker variability affect a common stage of processing. From these data

they suggested that talker variability affects early stages of speech perception responsible for immediate phonetic perception.

Talker Variability in Memory and Attention

Recent experiments in memory and attention provide further insights into the nature of talker variability effects. Martin et al. (1989) investigated serial recall of 10-item word lists spoken by either a single talker or by 10 different talkers and found that recall of multiple-talker lists was less accurate than recall of single-talker lists, but only for items in early list positions. Moreover, they found that recall of digits visually presented before the spoken lists was less accurate if the subsequent lists were multiple-talker lists than if they were single-talker lists. Finally, they found that the differences in recall between single- and multiple-talker lists were unaffected by a post-perceptual distractor task (following Peterson and Peterson, 1959). From these converging lines of evidence, Martin et al. suggested that word lists produced by multiple talkers require greater attention for rehearsal in working memory than the same lists produced by a single talker.

Further evidence of the attention-demanding nature of talker variability was provided by Goldinger, Pisoni, and Logan (1991), who presented for serial recall single-talker and multiple-talker lists at varying speeds. They found that talker variability interacted strongly with presentation rate, whereas other stimulus variables, such as word frequency, did not (Fig. 8-11). At relatively fast presentation rates, recall of single-talker lists was superior to recall of multiple-talker lists, as in the Martin et al. experiments. At very slow rates, however, recall of multiple-talker lists was more accurate than recall of single-talker lists, suggesting that voice information is retained in long-term memory (see Schacter and Church, 1992; Palmeri, Goldinger, and Pisoni, 1993; Church and Schacter, 1994). The rate manipulation has long been assumed to affect the rehearsal processes of the recall task (Murdock, 1962; Rundus, 1971), so this result suggests that talker variability taxes these attention-demanding stages of processing. Another interesting finding reported by Lightfoot (1989) was that subjects' familiarity with the talkers' voices also modifies the differences in recall of single- and multiple-talker lists. When subjects were trained to recognize the voices of

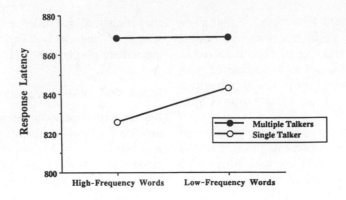

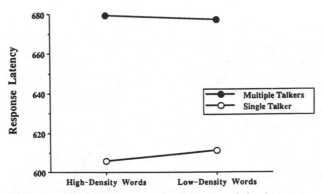

FIGURE 8-10 Auditory word naming data. The upper panel displays mean naming latencies for words from single- and multiple-talker stimulus sets as a function of word frequency. The lower panel displays mean naming latencies for words from single- and multiple-talker stimulus sets as a function of similarity neighborhood density. The effects of talker variability are more robust than the effects of either of the other stimulus variables. (From Mullennix, J. W., Pisoni, D. B., & Martin, C. S. [1989]. Some effects of talker variability on spoken word recognition. *Journal of the Acoustical Society of America, 85,* 365-378.)

the various talkers and associate them with fictional names (Brad, Mary, Jane, Sam, etc.), multiple-talker lists were recalled better than single-talker lists, even at relatively fast presentation rates. Recently, Nygaard, Sommers, and Pisoni (1994) used the same procedure to show that familiarity with a speaker's voice improves recognition of novel words produced by the speaker.

Jusczyk, Pisoni, and Mullennix (1992) further elucidated the effects of talker variability on memory. They observed, as Kuhl and her colleagues reported earlier (Holmberg, Morgan, and Kuhl, 1977; Kuhl, 1979; Kuhl and Miller, 1982), that infants recognize phonemic constancy very well despite variation of the stimulus voices. However, Jusczyk, Pisoni, and Mullennix also employed a variation of the high-

amplitude sucking (HAS) procedure (Eimas et al., 1971) that included a 2-minute delay between the habituation to one syllable and the presentation of a new syllable. This manipulation let them assess the effects of talker variability on infants' ability to encode and remember phonetic structure. They found that infants who heard speech from a single talker were able to detect a phonetic change across the 2-minute delay but the infants who heard speech from multiple talkers were not. These results, taken together with the adult data, suggest that maintaining perceptual constancy across talkers requires extra attention.

Mullennix and Pisoni (1990) demonstrated the influence of talker variability on selective attention. They employed the Garner (1974) speeded classification procedure to investigate

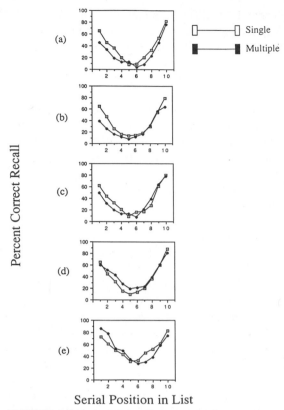

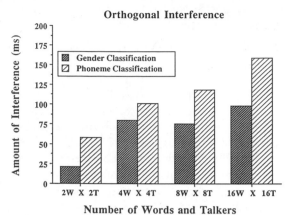

FIGURE 8-12 Garner speeded classification data. The dark bars show the amount of interference that phonetic variability caused in gender classification; light bars show the amount of interference that talker variability caused in phonetic classification. Across all stimulus sets, the dimensions of voice and phoneme were perceived integrally. (Adapted from Mullennix, J. W., & Pisoni, D. B. [1990]. Stimulus variability and processing dependencies in speech perception. *Perception & Psychophysics, 47, 379-390.*)

FIGURE 8-11 Serial recall data. The five panels display recall of single- and multiple-talker word lists presented at five different rates. One word was spoken every (a) 250 ms, (b) 500 ms, (c) 1000 ms, (d) 2000 ms, or (e) 4000 ms. The single-talker advantage in primacy recall is reversed at the slower ISIs. (From Goldinger, S. D., Pisoni, D. B., & Logan, J. S. [1991]. The nature of talker variability effects on recall of spoken word lists. *Journal of Experimental Psychology: Learning, Memory, and Cognition, 17, 152-162.*)

processing dependencies between phonetic variability and talker variability. Subjects classified monosyllabic words according to either the voicing of the initial phoneme (/b/ versus /p/) or the gender of the talker. They found that irrelevant variations in phonetic constitution or voice could not be ignored; variation along either dimension slowed classification along the other dimension. However, a large asymmetry was observed, showing that variability along the voice dimension impaired classification along the phonetic dimension more than vice versa. These data, shown in Figure 8-12, suggest that the processing of voice information and phonetic information are qualitatively different but also depend on one another, sharing a limited-capacity cognitive system (see Cutting and Pisoni,

1978). Mullennix and Pisoni suggest that both indexical information and phonetic information are processed in a mandatory fashion, following Fodor (1983; for a similar suggestion see Miller, 1987). However, the implied modules may function as a cascade system (McClelland, 1979), such that the output of the phonetic module is more strongly affected by the output of the voice module than vice versa (see also Nusbaum and Morin, 1992).

In summary, the available data on the effects of talker variability in speech perception, word recognition, attention, and memory all indicate that indexical information deserves more thorough consideration in theoretical discussions of speech perception than it has traditionally received. Talker-related information affects perception of speech and memory of spoken material, attracts selective attention, and is routinely encoded in parallel with linguistic information (Geiselman and Bellezza, 1976, 1977; Palmeri et al., 1993). The traditional approach to the study of speech perception has considered only abstract linguistic units without regard to the media that carry them. Further investigation into the generality and nature of normalization effects in speech should provide valuable insights into speech perception and perhaps the architecture of general perceptual systems as well.

Prosody and Timing in Speech Perception

Another neglected topic is the role of prosodic information in language perception. *Prosody* is the melody, timing, rhythm, and amplitude of fluent speech, and it is typically thought of as changes in the acoustic correlates of stress, such as fundamental frequency and vowel duration (Lehiste, 1970; Huggins, 1972). Most of the emphasis in speech perception research and theory has been on the segmental analysis of phonemes, whereas **suprasegmental information** has received only cursory consideration. Although the role of prosody has been researched more vigorously in recent years, a wide gap remains between research on the perception of isolated segments and features and on sentences with full prosody and natural rhythm (see Cohen and Nooteboom, 1975). However, it is becoming apparent that prosodic factors may link phonetic segments, features, and words to grammatical processes at higher levels of analysis. Moreover, prosody seems to provide useful information about the lexical, syntactic, and semantic content of the spoken utterance. We briefly review several findings that illustrate the importance of prosodic information in the perception of connected speech (Huggins, 1972; Darwin, 1975; Nooteboom, Brokx, and de Rooij, 1978; Studdert-Kennedy, 1980).

Differences in fundamental frequency can provide important cues to the proper parsing of speech into constituents for syntactic analysis. In acoustic analyses of connected speech, Lea (1973) found that a drop in fundamental frequency usually occurred at the end of each major syntactic constituent of a sentence, and a rise in fundamental frequency occurred in the beginning of the following constituent. In more detailed analyses, Cooper and Sorenson (1977) found reliable rise-fall patterns at the boundaries between the main clauses of a sentence, between main and embedded clauses, and between major phrases. Lindblom and Svensson (1973; see also Svensson, 1974) have shown that listeners can parse speech that is devoid of segmental cues but maintains prosodic integrity (see also Nakatani and Schaffer, 1978). These findings and others (Collier and t'Hart, 1975; Klatt and Cooper, 1975; Cooper, 1976; Klatt, 1976) demonstrate the importance of prosody as a cue to phrasal grouping.

Another function of prosody is the maintenance of perceptual coherence (Studdert-Kennedy, 1980). As an example, Darwin (1975) had listeners shadow a sentence played to one ear while another sentence was presented to the other ear. At some point the prosodic contours of the sentences were switched, but their lexical, syntactic, and semantic content remained unchanged. Shadowing often spontaneously followed the prosodic contour across ears rather than the syntax or semantics of the message to which subjects were originally attending. Nooteboom, Brokx, and de Rooij (1978) suggest that prosodic contours maintain the "perceptual integrity" of the signal and provide evidence that the continuity of fundamental frequency and formant frequencies underlies this integrity (see Bregman, 1978 and 1990; Remez et al., 1994).

Cutler and her colleagues (1976, 1977, 1979, 1981) demonstrated yet another important function of prosody in speech perception. Cutler has shown that prosodic contours enable listeners to predict where sentence stress will fall. Because sentence stress is usually placed on words of primary semantic importance, the ability to predict stress placement presumably guides attention to the most important words in the sentence. Thus, prosody appears to guide attention to high-information stretches of fluent speech. To demonstrate that attention follows the predicted sentence stress, Cutler and her colleagues demonstrated faster phoneme-monitoring reaction times for words predicted by prosodic contour to receive stress, regardless of the word's actual acoustic realization or form class. A word in a sentence position of predicted stress is responded to faster than the same recorded token in another sentence position.

These demonstrations of the role of prosody in guiding attention have led Cutler and others to propose accounts of word recognition in which prosody is considered a primary source of information rather than marginally relevant variability (see Cutler, 1976, 1989; Grosjean and Gee, 1987). These approaches all emphasize the prominence of strong syllables in fluent speech and suggest that such syllables may focus attention and initiate segmental analysis and lexical access. This approach, recently dubbed the *metrical segmentation strategy* (Cutler and Butterfield, 1992; Cutler et al., 1992; McQueen, Norris and Cutler, 1994), contrasts with more temporally constrained left-to-right models of speech perception and word recognition such as cohort theory (Marslen-Wilson and Welsh, 1978; Marslen-Wilson and Tyler, 1980; Marslen-Wilson, 1987) , that assume word beginnings are necessarily processed first. As Cutler (1989), p. 354) says:

> The major problem for lexical access in natural speech situations is that word starting points are *not* specified. The evidence presented here has shown how prosodic structure, in particular metrical prosodic structure, can offer a way out of this dilemma. Where do we start with lexical access? In the absence of any better information, we can start with any strong syllable.

Finally, all of these useful prosodic cues make acoustic-phonetic invariance far more problematic. The durations of phonetic segments vary widely across stressed and unstressed syllables and in varying syntactic environments (Oller, 1973; Klatt, 1974, 1975; Luce and Charles-Luce, 1985). Spoken stress also entails wide spectral variations in formant frequencies and fundamental frequency (Lehiste, 1970). The durational variations of speech timing provide useful cues to lexical identity and syntactic structure, but at the cost of further removing anything resembling canonic phonemes from the signal. This potentially contradictory nature of prosodic information underscores the necessity of some theoretically sound resolution of the problem of invariance—apparently, as more meaningful variation is added to the signal, perception is improved rather than impaired.

This chapter has identified and discussed many of the long-standing issues in speech perception as well as several issues that researchers have recently explored. We now focus on individual theories and models of speech perception. We briefly introduce and comment on only a few models in the literature (see Klatt [1989] for a more extensive review), some of the most important and influential classes of theories, particularly those that should figure prominently in future research.

THEORETICAL APPROACHES TO SPEECH PERCEPTION

The perception of spoken language, encompassing all processes from peripheral auditory coding of the speech signal to comprehension of the message, is very complex. Many sources of knowledge and multiple levels of representation interact in myriad combinations. To date, the complexity of language has precluded the formulation of theories of language perception that are both global and empirically testable. Therefore, the situation in language perception research is similar to other areas of cognitive science: most investigators have examined only the details of specific phenomena and paradigms rather than more complex or integrative issues (Newell, 1973).

The remaining sections of this chapter illustrate this situation by their unfortunate dichotomy. In this section we review several models of speech perception, and in the following section, several models of spoken word recognition. This segregation is largely due to the orientations of the models themselves. Although there are a few notable exceptions (e.g., Klatt's LAFS model and the TRACE model), most of these models were formulated to explain either the identification of phonemes in the speech signal or the mapping of phonemic strings onto lexical representations in memory. Very few models specify the integrated processes of speech perception and word recognition (Pisoni and Luce, 1987). One trend, especially in the connectionist movement, is toward grouping these processes into unitary models. Another trend is toward justifying the segregation of processes considered in different models by arguing that the processes are segregated in perception. The concept of the phonetic module (Liberman and Mattingly, 1985, 1989) clearly justifies narrow consideration of phonetic perception without regard to the mapping of speech representations onto lexical representations. Although we believe the former trend will prove more fruitful in the long run, we recognize the value of the earlier models and discuss them next, beginning with the most influential of all models of speech perception, the motor theory.

Motor Theory of Speech Perception

The original motor theory described by Liberman et al. (1967, p. 452) was based on the assumption that ". . . speech is perceived by processes that are also involved in its production." This view of speech perception was motivated by the fact that a listener is also a speaker, and a close link exists between the acoustic forms of speech sounds and their underlying articulation. Therefore, an effective and economical means of perceiving speech is to perceive the articulatory gestures that produce sounds. Advocates of the

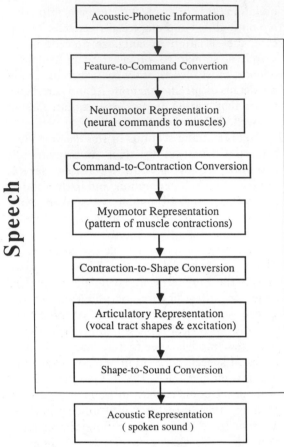

Speech

Acoustic-Phonetic Information

↓

Feature-to-Command Convertion

↓

Neuromotor Representation
(neural commands to muscles)

↓

Command-to-Contraction Conversion

↓

Myomotor Representation
(pattern of muscle contractions)

↓

Contraction-to-Shape Conversion

↓

Articulatory Representation
(vocal tract shapes & excitation)

↓

Shape-to-Sound Conversion

↓

Acoustic Representation
(spoken sound)

FIGURE 8-13   The motor theory of speech perception. The theory posits conversion of acoustic-phonetic information to a speech representation via articulatory knowledge. (From Cooper, F. S. [1972]. How is language conveyed by speech? In Kavanagh, J. F., & Mattingly, I. G. (Eds.), *Language by ear and by eye.* Cambridge, MA: MIT Press.

perception between consonants and vowels were primarily due to their differing demands on auditory short-term memory (Fujisaki and Kawashima, 1969, 1970, 1971; Pisoni, 1971, 1973, 1975). This general cognitive explanation of the continuous-categorical distinction eliminated the need to appeal to articulation for the perception of stops.

The motor theory has been revised in two key regards (Liberman and Mattingly, 1985, 1989). First, whereas the original model was based on recognition of observable gestures, the revised model is based on perception of intended gestures. Gestures are a set of movements by the articulators that result in a phonetically relevant vocal tract configuration. Each intended gesture of the language has properties that specify it uniquely, and each intended gesture is invariant, such that each segment of the language maps uniquely to a distinctive gesture. The second important modification is that gestures are perceived directly (following Gibson, 1966) by an innate phonetic module.

The revised motor theory makes four basic claims considered in turn by Klatt (1989). The first claim is that speech production and perception are linked psychologically so that they share common representations and processes. Second, the basic unit of speech perception is the underlying intended articulatory gesture associated with a phonetic segment rather than the actual physical motions implied by the acoustics. Third, perception of the intended gesture is direct, performed by a specialized module. Fourth, the model is supported by the claim that no other model can account for the the wide array of phenomena to which the motor theory has been applied over the years.

With respect to the link between production and perception, Klatt (1989) agrees that the processes must be linked in some sense (as inverses, at least), but he also notes that there is no simple way to relate the processes to make articulatory perception any easier than acoustic perception. Considering the direct perception of intended gestures, Klatt notes that while the position is attractive and would solve many problems of variability, no mechanisms described in the theory can perform this feat. Furthermore, Klatt argues that technology demonstrates the extreme difficulty of determining vocal tract shapes from speech acoustics, but the motor theory is based on faith that this transformation is possible. In contrast to the premises of Newtonian mechanics, we cannot be certain

motor theory argue that a solution to the invariance problem lies in the more reliable nature of articulatory gestures (compared with acoustic phonemes) as units of perception (Fig. 8-13).

Although, for many years, the original motor theory has held a dominant position in accounts of speech perception, the link between the theory and the data is rarely more than suggestive. As the review of evidence in the section *Specialization of Speech Perception* showed, the evidence in support of motor theory is ambiguous. For example, much of the early support for motor theory came from the finding that synthetic stop consonants were perceived categorically, whereas steady-state vowels were perceived continuously, apparently paralleling their respective articulatory origins. However, subsequent research showed that the differences in that speech is a reversible event. Finally, regarding the uniqueness of the motor theory in accounting for a wide range of phenomena, Klatt argues that the revised motor theory is so abstract that it is essentially no different from auditory theories such as LAFS, and he therefore suggests that the account is no longer unique. Klatt (1989, p. 180) concludes, "An attractive motor theory *philosophy* has been described by Liberman and Mattingly, but we are far from the specification of a motor-theory *model* of speech perception." His point is well taken; the motor theory and the revised theory are based primarily in logic, parsimony, intuitive appeal, and a measure of faith, rather than empirical support.

Direct-Realist Approach to Speech Perception

Fowler (1986, 1990) and Fowler and Rosenblum (1990, 1991) have outlined the framework for a *direct-realist* approach to speech perception. This approach assumes that, as in Gibson's (1966) view of visual perception, speech perception entails the recognition of natural phonetic events. As in the motor theory, Fowler assumes that the relevant events perceived in speech are the speaker's phonetically structured articulations. In the language of event perception, there is a fundamental distinction between the event and the informational medium. For example, an object such as a chair is an event in the world. When our eyes gaze upon the chair, we perceive it via light that is structured by the edges, contours, and colors of the chair. We do not perceive the light per se. Instead, the light is merely the medium by which the chair is perceived. The suggestion for speech perception is very similar to this example—articulatory events lend unique structure to the acoustic waveform, just as chairs lend structure to light. Accordingly, Fowler suggests that articulatory events are directly perceived via the acoustic medium.

The direct-realist approach to speech perception is similar to the motor theory in many respects. However, there are important differences. Most notably, the two theories approach the signal in different ways. Motor theory maintains that the acoustic signal is subjected to computations to retrieve underlying gestures. In contrast, the direct-realist approach maintains that no cognitive mediation whatsoever is necessary; the acoustic signal is "transparent" with respect to the underlying structure of speech (Liberman and Mattingly, 1985). Follow-

ing this difference, Fowler and Rosenblum (1991) argue that phonetic perception need not be modular, suggesting instead that general perceptual principles can be invoked to perceive the distal events of speech.

The direct-realist approach and motor theory are attractive for many of the same reasons (Studdert-Kennedy, 1986): Direct-realism has intuitive appeal, and it fares well with many of the data that the motor theory can explain. Moreover, it stems from a respected tradition of event perception theories. However, it must meet many challenges. Most important, of course, is the need for empirical support, in which regard it is similar to the motor theory (although evidence is growing; see Dekle, Fowler, and Funnell, 1992; Fowler, 1994). Forgiving the lack of critical data, many logical and theoretical challenges can be offered as well (see commentaries on Fowler's [1986] target article; Diehl and Kleunder, 1989). For example, as Remez (1986) notes, it is not clear what the proper perceptual objects in linguistic communication are. Fowler has adopted a physical perceptual object that is capable of structuring the acoustic media—the articulatory gesture — and has made its recognition the central task of speech perception. However, articulations are not ends in themselves. Unlike chairs, articulations are another medium, because language is symbolic. Strings of articulations are perceived as words and ideas, so gesture perception does not fully explain speech perception. Moreover, as noted by Diehl (1986), Porter (1986), and Remez (1986), chairs and gestures are also very different in terms of their perceptual availability. We know unambiguously when we are looking at a chair; we do not have such access to phonetic gestures. A direct-realist theory might claim that our unambiguous recognition of words and sentences implicitly demonstrates our recognition of gestures, but other less circular accounts are available (Massaro, 1986). The resolution of these and other theoretical vagaries, as well as the further collection of relevant data, will be important to the direct-realist position.

Information-Processing Theories of Speech Perception

Perhaps the polar opposite to the direct-realist perspective is the information-processing perspective. The theories and models that fall into this category are oriented toward general cog-

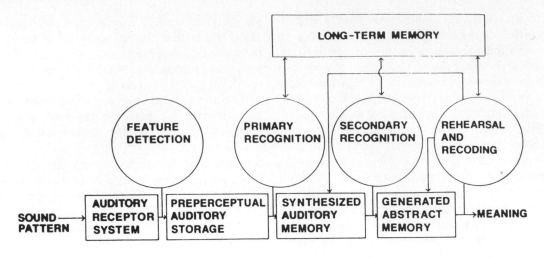

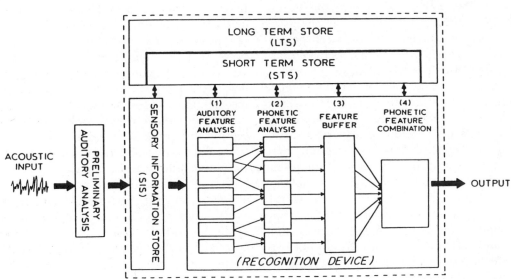

FIGURE 8-14 Two information-processing models of speech perception. Although the models differ in detail, both entail the information-processing elements of multiple stages of processing, hierarchical levels of representation, and strong interactions among perceptual buffers and memory stores. (Top panel from Oden, G. C., & Massaro, D. W. [1978]. Integration of featural information in speech perception. *Psychological Review, 85,* 172-191. Bottom panel from Pisoni, D. B., & Sawusch, J. R. [1975]. Some stages of processing in speech perception. In Cohen, A., & Nooteboom, S. G. (Eds.), *Structure and process in speech perception.* Heidelberg: Springer-Verlag [pp. 16-34].)

nition and perception. All of these models assume distinctive, hierarchically organized levels of processing. Moreover, all or most of these theories assume that limited-capacity perceptual and memory stores are intimately involved in speech analysis (Cutting and Pisoni, 1978). This view contrasts sharply with the revised motor theory and the direct-realist framework. Two

typical information-processing stage models are shown in Figure 8-14. Both exhibit multiple levels of representation and processes that interact with and depend upon memory stores and control processes. Beyond the stages of processing shown in the figure, once the information has followed the meaning or output arrow, the recognized linguistic units enter still higher stages of processing that derive syntactic and semantic content.

Studdert-Kennedy (1974, 1976) was the first to advocate an approach to speech perception based on stages of perceptual processing. He proposed four stages of speech processing: (1) auditory, (2) phonetic, (3) phonological, and (4) lexical, syntactic, and semantic (see review and discussion by Pisoni and Luce, 1986, 1987; Luce and Pisoni, 1987). As the division of Studdert-Kennedy's stages imply, this approach to speech perception synthesizes information-processing psychology and linguistic theory. An advantage of this framework is the clear division of processes of speech perception; working within such a framework provides a well-defined division of topics for investigation.

The basic appeal of stage theories is their reliance on generally accepted mechanisms of cognition and perception. As such, information-processing models introduce certain advantages over modular theories such as motor theory. For example, they can account for the effects of reduced attention or increased memory load on speech perception (Nusbaum and Schwab, 1986). Unfortunately, like many theories of speech perception, information-processing theories have typically been quite vague and not subject to direct empirical tests.

Klatt's LAFS Model

Although we introduce Klatt's lexical access from spectra (LAFS) model in this section, LAFS is a model of spoken word recognition as well. LAFS is one of the few models that successfully addresses several critical issues of speech perception along with access to the mental lexicon and the nature of lexical representations in long-term memory.

LAFS assumes direct, noninteractive access to lexical entries based on context-sensitive spectral sections (Klatt, 1979). It also assumes that adult listeners have a dictionary of all legal diphone sequences stored in memory. Associated with each diphone sequence is its proto-typical spectral representation. These spectral representations are proposed to resolve problems associated with contextual variability of individual segments. In a sense, LAFS resolves the problems of variability by precompiling coarticulatory effects directly into the representations of an input word and comparing these derived spectra to prototypes in memory. Word

recognition is accomplished when a best match is found between the input spectra and the diphone representations. In this portion of the model, word recognition is directly based on spectral representations of the sensory input, with no intermediate levels of computation corresponding to segments or phonemes.

An important aspect of LAFS is its explicit avoidance of any levels of representation corresponding to phonemes. Instead, the model assumes a precompiled, acoustic-based lexicon of words in a network of diphone power spectra. These spectral templates are assumed to be context-sensitive units, similar to "Wickel-phones," because they represent the acoustic correlates of phonemes in different phonetic environments (Wickelgren, 1969). Klatt argues that diphone concatenation is sufficient to capture much of the context-dependent variability observed for phonetic segments in spoken words (see also Marcus, 1984). Word recognition in LAFS proceeds similarly to the workings of the computerized HARPY speech recognition system, in that power spectra are computed every 10 ms and compared with the stored representations (see Klatt [1979] for details on HARPY). When finished, the best path through the diphone network is the optimal phonetic transcription of the signal. Klatt's model is an example of an extreme bottom-up recognition process and may be contrasted to more interactive models of word recognition that we consider below, such as cohort theory and TRACE.

Massaro's Fuzzy Logical Model of Perception

Massaro's fuzzy logical model of perception (FLMP) (Massaro, 1972, 1987, 1989; Massaro and Cohen, 1976, 1977, 1993; Oden and Massaro, 1978; Derr and Massaro, 1980) Massaro and Oden, 1980; was developed to account for feature integration in speech perception, regardless of the nature of the relevant features. For example, FLMP can account for the integration of multiple acoustic cues in the speech waveform as well as audiovisual integration. In this brief introduction, we restrict our attention to the recovery of phonemes from the speech signal, noting only that integration of information from other sources is possible in the model and is accomplished by processes similar to those described here.

FLMP assumes three operations in phoneme

identification. First, *feature evaluation* determines the degree to which any given acoustic-phonetic feature is present in a stretch of sound. Unlike more conventional feature detector theories, FLMP assumes that features are evaluated along a continuous scale rather than an absolute feature present-feature absent dichotomy. Features are assigned continuous, "fuzzy" values ranging from 0 to 1, indicating the degree of certainty that the feature appears in the signal (Zadeh, 1965). The second operation in FLMP is *prototype matching,* in which the feature profiles derived by the earlier operations are compared with prototypes of phonemes stored in memory. Phoneme prototypes are stored as sets of propositions that describe ideal representations of the acoustic correlates of each phoneme. The prototype-matching operation specifies the degree of correspondence between ideal phonemes and the input sets of features. The final operation, *pattern classification,* determines the best match between the candidate phonemes and the input by using goodness of fit algorithms. FLMP provides flexibility in pattern classification by using a variety of logical rules for feature integration so that perfect matches between the input and the prototypes are not required for phoneme identification.

FLMP is appealing for several reasons. First, it is a very general framework that demonstrates how acoustic information (as well as other information) can be mapped onto representations in long-term memory without the postulation of specialized speech procedures or modules. In fact, Massaro (1987, 1989) specifically rejects the notions of specialized or modular processes in speech perception. Second, the model argues that speech perception is not necessarily categorical but can be explained by integration of continuously evaluated features. The framework is therefore consistent with the data reported by Barclay (1972), Pisoni (1973), and others that continuous information remains available in speech perception, despite the categorical identification and discrimination functions obtained in typical studies (e.g., Liberman et al., 1957). Finally, FLMP is one of the only models of speech perception proposed in terms of a precise mathematical framework (Townsend, 1989). However, the quantification has been a source of criticism as well as praise. FLMP employs large numbers of free parameters to account for patterns of data, and the parameter settings do not easily transfer across exper-

imental paradigms (Jenkins, 1989; Warren, 1989). Finally, Massaro's 1987 suggestions that the FLMP framework may be extended to all forms of perception are attractive, but considerable testing and evaluation are clearly required by these claims.

THEORETICAL APPROACHES TO SPOKEN WORD RECOGNITION

The theories and models described in the previous section are models of speech perception, meaning that they primarily address phonetic perception, independent of higher-level lexical or linguistic processes (with the exception of LAFS). In this section we introduce several models of spoken word recognition, models primarily concerned with the rapid location of lexical entries in memory once the speech perception system has specified the necessary sublexical components of the input. This separation of the focus of theories is unfortunate and appears inappropriate (Pisoni and Luce, 1987), especially in light of the data on lexical effects in speech perception (Ganong, 1980; Samuel, 1986; Samuel and Ressler, 1986; Nygaard, 1993). Nevertheless, most of the models considered here assume that some input, perhaps resembling a string of phonemes, is provided by early processes of speech perception and is then compared to the mental lexicon until a best match is found. Very few models of word recognition or lexical access (except TRACE) are concerned with the entire range of processes that subserve word recognition.

The myopic nature of theories of word recognition and lexical access is primarily attributable to their origins. Most theories were designed to account for findings in *visual* word recognition, so assumptions of invariance are easily justified, although most models of visual word recognition allow for some variability. A very general assumption has been that models of visual word recognition can account for spoken word recognition as well, given rudimentary modifications to respect the temporal distribution of the speech signal (Marslen-Wilson and Tyler, 1980; Grosjean and Gee, 1987; Tyler and Frauenfelder, 1987; Cutler, 1989). While the validity of this assumption is subject to debate (Bradley and Forster, 1987), it has isolated the processes of word recognition sufficiently to allow for the development of precise, albeit simplified, theories. While ignoring questions related to the problems of early speech perception, models of word recognition focus primarily on explaining basic phenomena such as word frequency effects, context effects, types of knowledge sources brought to bear on word recognition, and the nature of representations in the mental lexicon. Indeed, these considerations largely characterize models of word recognition and are the basis of extensive experimentation and debate. Furthermore, one of the fundamental debates about models of word recognition is the distinction between modular and interactive processes (Bradley and Forster, 1987; Tanenhaus and Lucas, 1987). In this discussion we pay special attention to the models' respective approaches to all of these basic phenomena and theoretical distinctions.

In this section we briefly examine five models of word recognition:* the logogen theory, cohort theory, Forster's search theory, the neighborhood activation model, and the TRACE model. It should be noted that these are only some of the models described in the literature, but we hope this review will capture and communicate several of the key issues in spoken word recognition. We begin with one of the earliest models of word recognition, the logogen theory.

Logogen Theory

In Morton's (1969, 1979, 1982) **logogen** theory, these passive sensing devices are associated with each word in the mental lexicon. Each logogen contains all of the information about a given word, such as its meaning, possible syntactic functions, and its phonetic and orthographic structure. A logogen monitors discourse for any information indicating that its particular word is present in the signal, and once such information is encountered, the activation level of the logogen is raised. Given sufficient activation, the logogen crosses a threshold; the information about the referent word is made available to the response system and the word is recognized (Fig. 8-15).

Several important features of the logogen theory have been either strongly rejected or in-

corporated into later models. First is the emphasis on multiple interactive knowledge sources in word recognition. An important feature of the theory is that logogens monitor all possible sources of information, including higher-level semantic and syntactic information from the discourse and lower-level sensory information. (However, logogens do not "talk to each other," meaning that any given logogen is oblivious to the activity levels of other logogens.) Thus, information from several levels can combine to push the activation level of a logogen toward its threshold. In this sense, logogen theory is highly interactive, and context effects are incorporated into the early stages of word recognition. Words that are readily predicted by the semantic and syntactic context are activated and recognized more quickly than those not well predicted by context. A second important feature of the logogen theory is its portrayal of "word frequency effects." It posits that frequency differences among words produce adjustments in the recognition thresholds of their logogens. Thus, a common word has a lower threshold than a rarely used word and therefore requires less sensory or contextual input for recognition. The characterization of word frequency as a direct coding in recognition thresholds, resting activation levels, or activation functions has been adopted in many later models of word recognition (e.g., Marslen-Wilson, 1987).

Taken together, the two major assumptions of the logogen theory place the word recognition stage as the locus of both context and frequency effects. The approach is highly interactive, and its portrayal of context effects has been challenged by theorists who prefer a more modularist approach to language processing (Forster, 1979, 1990; Bradley and Forster, 1987). Likewise, the theory characterizes word frequency as an integral and automatic aspect of word recognition. However, some theorists argue that word frequency may be better characterized as a form of perceptual or response bias, as demonstrated by the task-dependent magnitude of frequency effects (Balota and Chumbley, 1984; Luce, 1986).

The details of logogen theory have changed somewhat over the years, but the basic mechanisms have remained the same. For example, Morton (1982) divided the logogen system into separate visual and auditory subsystems, but the fundamental notion of the passive threshold device that monitors information from a variety of sources has remained. Unfortunately, logogen

---

*In the remainder of this chapter, the following distinction is employed. *Word recognition* means only the recognition of an acoustic-phonetic pattern as a token of a given word held in memory. *Lexical access* is the moment when all information about the recognized word becomes available to working memory (see Morton, 1969; Pisoni and Luce, 1987).

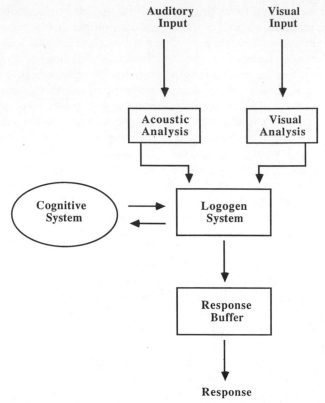

Auditory Input

Visual Input

Acoustic Analysis

Visual Analysis

Cognitive System

Logogen System

Response Buffer

Response

FIGURE 8-15 The logogen theory of word recognition. The theory emphasizes the central role of the logogen system and its interaction with the general cognitive system. The logogen system accounts for frequency effects, and the cognitive system accounts for context effects. (Adapted from Morton, J. [1979]. Word recognition. In Morton, J., & Marshall, J. D. (Eds.), *Psycholinguistics 2: Structures and processes.* Cambridge, MA: MIT Press [pp. 109-156].)

theory is rather vague. It helps us conceptualize how an interactive system works and how word frequency may operate, but it says little about precisely how acoustic-phonetic and higher-level sources of information are integrated, the time course of word recognition, or the structure of the lexicon.

Cohort Theory

Marslen-Wilson's **cohort** theory (Marslen-Wilson, 1975, 1980b, 1987; Marslen-Wilson and Tyler, 1975, 1980; Marslen-Wilson and Welsh, 1978) posits two stages in word recognition, one autonomous and one interactive. In the first autonomous stage, acoustic-phonetic information at the beginning of an input word activates all words in memory that have the same word-initial information. For example, if "slave" is presented to the system, all words beginning with /s/ are activated. The words activated on the basis of word-initial information

constitute a cohort. Activation of a cohort is autonomous in the sense that only acoustic-phonetic information can specify it. At this stage, which Marslen-Wilson (1987, 1990, 1993) calls *access,* word recognition is a completely data-driven, or bottom-up, process.

Once a cohort is activated, all possible sources of information come to bear on the selection of the appropriate word. Thus, further acoustic-phonetic information may eliminate "sight" and "save," leaving only words that begin with /sl/, such as "sling" and "slave." Note that access is based on acoustic-phonetic information and is assumed to operate in a strictly left-to-right temporal fashion. At the later integration stage of word recognition, however, higher-level knowledge may also eliminate candidates from the cohort. Thus, if "sling" is inconsistent with the available semantic or syntactic information, it will be eliminated from the cohort. At the integration stage of word recognition, the theory is highly

/s/	/l/	/e/	/v/
sight	slow	sleigh	SLAVE
safe	slip	slave	
sing	slack	•	
so	slide	•	
sound	slave		
slip	•		
store	•		
•			
•			

FIGURE 8-16   Elimination of hypothesized lexical candidates from the word-initial cohort for "slave."

interactive.* Figure 8-16 shows the elimination process: Upon isolation of a single word in the cohort, word recognition is accomplished.

An important feature of cohort theory is its sensitivity to the temporal nature of speech. It gives priority to the beginnings of words and assumes strict left-to-right processing of acoustic-phonetic information. Cohort theory also embraces the notion of optimal efficiency (Marslen-Wilson, 1980a, 1987; Tyler and Marslen-Wilson, 1982), the principle that the word recognition system selects the appropriate word candidate from the cohort at the earliest possible point (the *recognition point*). This means that the word recognition system will commit to a decision as soon as sufficient acoustic-phonetic and higher-level sources of information are consistent with a single candidate.

Although earlier discussions of cohort theory made no mention of word frequency, Marslen-Wilson (1987, 1990) suggested that frequency in cohort theory operates similarly to the logogen theory. Specifically, Marslen-Wilson proposed that word recognition may not require absolute elimination of all members of a cohort but merely a comparison of relative activation levels among candidates (following Luce, 1986), with the activation levels modified by the activation-elimination processes described

*At least to a degree. In his revisions, Marslen-Wilson (1987) suggested that the effects of top-down context on the word selection process may be limited, perhaps so that context can have only a facilitatory effect for consistent words but not an inhibitory effect for inconsistent words.

above. Word frequency is assumed to modify the individual rates of activation of the words constituting the cohort, with common words becoming active faster than rarely used words. Like the logogen theory, then, cohort theory portrays word frequency as an integral aspect of the early phases of word recognition.

Marslen-Wilson's cohort theory has attracted considerable attention for several reasons, including its relatively precise description of the word recognition process, its novel claim that all relevant words in the mental lexicon are activated in the initial stage of access, and the priority it affords to word beginnings, a popular notion in the literature (Cole and Jakimik, 1980). However, the theory is not without its shortcomings, both theoretically and empirically. First, Marslen-Wilson (1987, 1989; Warren and Marslen-Wilson, 1987) has argued that the theory requires no conventional linguistic units, such as phonemes, in order to function. He proposes that to maintain optimal efficiency the word recognition system exploits coarticulatory information that crosses phonemic boundaries (e.g., nasalization of a vowel preceding a nasal consonant) in real time, avoiding unnecessary decisional delays. Unfortunately, the data on this point are ambiguous, and the argument could be made that nasalization of a vowel is primarily a cue to phonemic rather than lexical identity. Affording priority to the lexical cue may be efficient, but it may not be correct. Nor is it clear that candidates can be efficiently eliminated from the cohort without the use of phonemic dichotomies (see Pisoni and Luce [1987] for further discussion).

Another problem with cohort theory is error recovery. For example, if "foundation" is perceived as "thoundation" due to mispronunciation or misperception, the word-initial cohort will not, according to the theory, contain the word candidate "foundation." Although Marslen-Wilson allows for some residual activation of acoustically similar word candidates in the cohort so that a second pass through the cohort structure may occur, it is still unclear how error recovery is accomplished when the intended word is not a member of the original activated cohort.

Finally, several studies have challenged some of cohort theory's stronger assumptions, especially the concept of maximally early decisions in word recognition. For example, although preliminary evidence from the gating task

(Grosjean, 1980; Tyler, 1984) supported the notion of early isolation points, later experiments showed that many words are not recognized until well after their acoustic offsets in continuous speech (Grosjean, 1985; Bard, Shillcock, and Altmann, 1988; Connine, Blasko, and Titone, 1993). Moreover, cohort theory predicts that the time it takes to decide an item is a nonword is a function of its **isolation point,** the point in the stimulus at which the item could not constitute an English word (e.g., "lotato" should be rejected faster than "potavo"). However, Goodman and Huttenlocher (1988) and Taft and Hambly (1986) have shown that lexical decisions are not reliably predicted by isolation points. Despite these problems, cohort theory is one of the most important theories in spoken word recognition, primarily because it was developed to explain spoken rather than visual word recognition, and it therefore respects the temporal nature of speech.

Forster's Autonomous Search Theory

In contrast to logogen and cohort theory, Forster's (1976, 1979) theory of word recognition and lexical access is autonomous in the strictest sense. Whereas Morton's and Marslen-Wilson's theories allow for parallel processing of information, linguistic processing in Forster's theory is completely serial. The theory posits three separate linguistic processors: lexical, syntactic, and message. The latest version of Forster's theory incorporates a fourth nonlinguistic processor, the general processing system (GPS). Forster's model may be considered the word-recognition embodiment of several of Fodor's (1983) principles of modularity in perceptual processing (see Tanenhaus and Lucas, 1987; Forster, 1989, 1990), strongly emphasizing algorithmic, noninteractive processing among separate components that are hierarchically organized.

In the first stage of Forster's model, information from peripheral perceptual systems is submitted to the lexical processor. The processor then searches for an entry in three peripheral access files: an orthographic file for visual input, a phonetic file for auditory input, and a syntactic-semantic file for either form of input. Search of the peripheral files is assumed to proceed in *frequency order,* with higher-frequency words searched before lower-frequency words. Word recognition is accomplished at the level of the peripheral access files, where the input pattern is matched to a stored

representation. Once an entry is located in these files, lexical access is accomplished by locating the entry in the master lexicon, where all other information about the word is stored (Fig. 8-17).

Upon location of an item in the master lexicon, information pointing to its location in the master list passes to the syntactic processor, which builds a syntactic structure of the discourse. Information passes from the syntactic processor to the message processor, which builds a conceptual structure of the message. Each of the three processors—lexical, syntactic, and message—can pass information to the GPS. However, the GPS cannot influence processing. Rather, it only incorporates general conceptual knowledge with the output from the linguistic processors in making a decision or response. In Fodor's terminology, the linguistic processors are vertically organized, whereas the GPS is horizontally organized, meaning that the GPS, unlike the linguistic modules, integrates information from many disparate domains.

Forster's theory postulates autonomous, nonpenetrable modules. The lexical processor is independent of the syntactic and message processors, and the syntactic processor is independent of the message processor. Furthermore, the entire linguistic system is independent of the general cognitive system, as Fodor (1983) suggests. This strictly serial and autonomous characterization of language processing means that word recognition and lexical access are not influenced in any way by higher-level knowledge sources and are exclusively bottom-up or data-driven processes. Forster (1979) attempts to explain all forms of context effects as post access, decisional or response biases. However, Forster (1990) posits that word frequency exerts an early effect on word recognition.

Forster's model is attractive because of its relative precision and the apparently testable claims it makes regarding the autonomy of processors. It also describes word recognition and lexical access in the context of sentence processing. In addition, it incorporates a specific mechanism of the word frequency effect— entries in the peripheral access files are organized according to frequency, and search proceeds from high- to low-frequency entries. This notion of the search mechanism lends itself well to empirical testing, although the majority of relevant data reported to date come from experiments in visual word recognition (Forster and Bednall, 1976; Andrews, 1989).

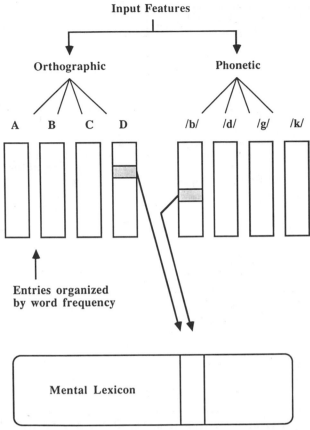

FIGURE 8-17   Forster's model of word recognition emphasizes the autonomy of the search processes and the role of a frequency-ordered search within specific access files. (Adapted from Forster, K. I. [1979]. Levels of processing and the structure of the language processor. In Cooper, W. E., & Walker, E. C. T. (Eds.), *Sentence processing: Psycholinguistic studies presented to Merrill Garrett.* Hillsdale, NJ: Erlbaum [pp. 27-86].)

Neighborhood Activation Model

The neighborhood activation model of word recognition (Luce, 1986; Goldinger, Luce, and Pisoni, 1989; Cluff and Luce, 1990; Luce, Pisoni, and Goldinger, 1990) assumes that word recognition reduces to a selection of a best match from a pool of activated word candidates and is thus similar in important respects to both Morton's logogen theory and Marslen-Wilson's cohort theory. However, the neighborhood activation model makes important assumptions about the role of competition for recognition among activated items. Central to the model is the concept of the **similarity neighborhood** (Landauer and Streeter, 1973; Coltheart et al., 1977; Luce, 1986; Andrews, 1989), a collection of words resident in the mental lexicon that are phonetically similar to each other and to any given stimulus word presented for recognition. Similarity neighborhoods are characterized by two main structural characteristics: (1) **neigh-**

borhood density, the number of words in the neighborhood and their degrees of confusability with the stimulus word, and (2) **neighborhood frequency,** the frequencies of the words in the neighborhood relative to the frequency of the stimulus word (see Fravenfeld et al., 1993).

In experiments on perceptual identification of words presented in noise, auditory lexical decision, and auditory word naming, Luce (1986) observed that these structural characteristics of similarity neighborhoods strongly affected the speed and accuracy of word recognition. Words from sparse neighborhoods were recognized faster and more accurately than words from dense neighborhoods, and words from low-frequency neighborhoods were recognized faster and more accurately than words from high-frequency neighborhoods. Indeed, neighborhood characteristics were more reliable predictors of word recognition than word frequency itself; in the auditory word-naming experiment,

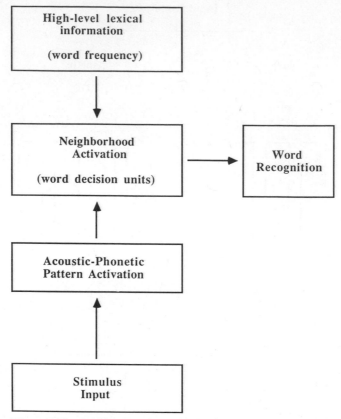

FIGURE 8-18 The neighborhood activation model of spoken word recognition. The model emphasizes the importance of similarity neighborhoods in isolating a single word candidate from the lexicon. Word frequency is assumed to bias the word decision units as they monitor activation patterns in the lexicon. (Adapted from Luce, P. A. [1986]. Neighborhoods of words in the mental lexicon. Unpublished doctoral dissertation. Indiana University.)

robust effects of neighborhood density were observed, but no effects of word frequency were evident (see Balota and Chumbley [1984, 1990] regarding the lability of word frequency effects).

In the neighborhood activation model, word recognition is much like that of both logogen theory and cohort theory, but with two basic modifications. The model (Fig. 8-18) assumes that upon stimulus input, a set of acoustic-phonetic patterns are activated in memory. The activation levels of these patterns are assumed to be a direct function of their phonetic similarity to the stimulus input. The activated phonetic patterns in turn activate a system of *word decision units,* conceptually similar to logogens. The word decision units are activated directly and autonomously from the bottom-up information provided by the signal, as in cohort theory. Once the word decision units are activated, they monitor a number of sources of information, especially the fluctuating activation levels of the acoustic-phonetic patterns. However, unlike processing in the system of logogens or the

cohort, the word decision units also monitor the overall level of activity in the decision system itself, in a manner similar to the processing units in the TRACE model. Finally, the decision units are sensitive to higher-level lexical information, including word frequency. This information biases the decisions of the units by differentially weighting the activity levels of the words to which they respond. Word recognition occurs when the system of decision units selects a best match from the activated neighborhood, at which time all information about the word is made available to working memory.

The neighborhood activation model places much of the burden of spoken word recognition on discrimination and selection among similar acoustic-phonetic patterns corresponding to words. Accordingly, it can account for effects of similarity between stimulus words and their neighbors in the lexicon. In both logogen and cohort theory, it is explicitly assumed that word recognition is independent of the number of activated candidates. Therefore, these models do not explain neighborhood density or neighborhood frequency effects. In addition, the model accounts for word frequency by assuming that frequency information biases the decisions of the word decision units. By assuming that frequency works in the late decision stage rather than in the early activation of the word units, the neighborhood activation model accounts for the common observation that word frequency effects vary across experimental tasks. Since different tasks introduce different decisional requirements, the neighborhood activation model predicts different effects of word frequency. Logogen theory, cohort theory, and Forster's search model propose that frequency is an integral and early contributor to word candidate activation or search order, and so these models are not well suited to account for experiments in which word frequency effects are attenuated or absent (e.g., Balota and Chumbley, 1984; Luce, 1986).

Despite the advantages of the neighborhood activation model over other models of word recognition, it does introduce several methodological difficulties. First, the concept of phonetic similarity among words in memory is difficult to quantify for empirical tests, and crude estimation methods, such as the N metric (Coltheart et al., 1977), are most commonly employed. Also, the concept of similarity depends on assumptions of representation. Similarity may be defined with respect to the speaker's phonetic repertoire or with respect to the listener's idealized phonetic representations, which are unavailable for inspection. Despite these difficulties, however, the concept of similarity is easily handled in theory, and the empiric effects of similarity neighborhoods are robust despite estimation. A second shortcoming of the model is the treatment of the temporal characteristics of word recognition. Unlike cohort theory, which explicitly accounts for the time course of word recognition, the neighborhood activation model offers no account of the recognition of multisyllabic words (although see Cluff and Luce, 1990).

Finally, we should mention another model to which the neighborhood activation model bears resemblance—the activation-verification model (Becker, 1976, 1979, 1980; Becker and Killion, 1977; Paap et al., 1982). In the activation verification framework, presentation of a stimulus word activates a pool of similar candidates selected by coarse sensory analysis. These candidates are subjected to *verification* in which

each candidate word is compared with the stimulus until a best match is established. The verification process is similar to the search procedure in Forster's search model; candidates are submitted for verification in descending order of word frequency. By incorporating the concept of the verification set, which is much like a similarity neighborhood, the activation-verification model can account for the effects of set size and similarity among neighbors. However, the model's assumption of the frequency-ordered verification process reduces its flexibility in predictions of word frequency effects across tasks (Dobbs, Friedman, and Lloyd, 1985).

TRACE and other Connectionist Models

The TRACE model of speech perception* (Elman and McClelland, 1986; McClelland and Elman, 1986; Elman, 1989) is a nearly completely interactive system. Coming out of the growing connectionist movement and based on the interactive-activation model of visual word recognition (McClelland and Rumelhart, 1981; Rumelhart and McClelland, 1982), TRACE advocates multiple levels of representation and rich feedforward and feedback connections between processing units. In addition, TRACE incorporates processes for both activation and inhibition of units in the network, as in the interactive-activation framework.

Figure 8-19 displays a section of a TRACE network. The functional units are simple, highly interconnected processing units called *nodes*. When information passes upward through the levels, nodes that collect sufficient confirmatory evidence to pass a threshold will fire and send activation along weighted links to their related nodes. In this manner, information consistent with the expectations of the early feature detectors is proliferated upward in the network to encourage recognition of the features' associated phonemes, and then recognition of the phonemes encourages recognition of the phonemes' associated words.

---

*Although most contemporary "models of speech perception" are clearly concerned with speech perception and most "models of word recognition" are concerned with word recognition, several models address both. LAFS is one of these. TRACE also accounts for phenomena from both the speech perception and word recognition literature. We recognize the contribution of TRACE and similar connectionist models to theories of speech perception. Our decision to discuss it in this section is simply an acknowledgment of its importance as a theory of word recognition.

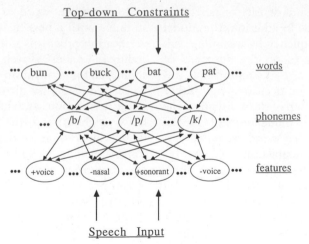

Top-down Constraints

Speech Input

FIGURE 8-19   A section of a connectionist network with TRACE architecture. The network contains nodes corresponding to phonetic features, phonemes, and words. Information is provided to the network via the speech signal and top-down knowledge. Excitatory and inhibitory links among the nodes control perception and learning in the network.

A key property of TRACE is the organization of excitatory and inhibitory links between nodes and levels. All connections from one level to another are excitatory, i.e., activation of a node on one level will increase the activity of all connected nodes on adjacent levels. As an example, if the feature detector node for voicing encounters voicing cues consistent with /k/, then the node for /k/ will be activated and in turn will activate all words in the lexicon that contain /k/. Within levels, however, all nodes are connected by inhibitory links, so the model must quickly resolve ambiguity in the signal. For example, if the features for /k/ and /g/ are encountered simultaneously, the nodes corresponding to the features and phonemes for both possibilities not only become activated but also inhibit their nearest competitors. Computationally, the end result of this process is a winner-take-all form of perceptual decision (Elman and McClelland, 1986), meaning that the node that receives the most positive activation also receives the most veto power over its competitors. A final important property of the model is its use of perceptual feedback. That is, not only do activation and the flow of information in the model proceed from the early feature detection system to the lexicon, but the expectations at the lexical and phonemic levels can bias perception on the levels below (Gamong, 1980; Nygaard, 1993).

The interactive nature of TRACE offers much to theories of speech perception and word recognition. McClelland and Elman (1986) list nearly a dozen well-known phenomena that the model can simulate, ranging from categorical perception to trading relations, as well as findings from the word recognition literature, such as earliness of word recognition. As regards speech perception, TRACE does not treat coarticulatory speech as noise imposed on an idealized string of phonemes. Instead, Elman and McClelland (1984) call contextual variability *lawful variability*, a rich source of information in TRACE. (The authors say, "You can tell a phoneme by the company it keeps.") Although the model assumes segmental representations in speech, no explicit segmentation is imposed. Instead, phones and allophones are simply assumed in the model's architecture, so segmentation falls out naturally. As regards word recognition, the inhibitive links among nodes at the lexical level allow TRACE to account for neighborhood effects. In brief, by virtue of its simple assumptions of interacting units, TRACE demonstrates many of the attributes of theories of speech perception and word recognition in an integrated system without postulating or proliferating restrictive rules or specialized mechanisms.

However, like all models, TRACE has its problems. Many of them relate to the simplifying assumptions about speech input. Others are inherent to the model. Among the most serious problems are these: (1) It has no mechanism for predicting word frequency effects (although it is easy to imagine how a set of lexical level biases could be instantiated). (2) It has no obvious way of identifying a nonword. Judging lexical status is one of the most important abilities of word recognition (Forster, 1979) and should be included in any model. TRACE could set criterial confidence values for outputs so that unfamiliar words would be judged as nonwords, but this would confound distinctions between degraded inputs and nonwords (a discrimination that human listeners make easily). (3) Perhaps the most important problem with TRACE arises from one of its most attractive features. It acknowledges and even exploits variability and coarticulation in its perceptual decisions, but it does not address other sources of variability common in natural language, such as talker idiosyncracies, changing speaking rates, stress assignments, and others. Even more troubling is the fact that TRACE demands a certain degree of invariance in its variability. It acknowledges that the cues for phonemes are not localized in specific segments, but at the same time it does require that all cues occur in a predetermined time window. While the problems of temporally distributed cues in speech are not easily resolved in the original TRACE model, it is hoped that the new breeds of *recurrent networks* (Jordan, 1986) may alleviate some of the difficulties of working with time windows in speech (for example, see Elman [1990, 1993]).

SUMMARY

This chapter identifies and elucidates several of the principal issues in research and theory on speech perception and auditory word recognition. Some are long-standing concerns in the field. Despite their long history as empirical and theoretical issues, problems such as the lack of acoustic-phonetic invariance and segmentation, the problem of perceptual normalization, and the specialization of speech perception remain vital and controversial areas of research today. And although innovative approaches to these issues have developed both in research and in theory, the fundamental complexity of speech perception continues to puzzle researchers. No comprehensive solutions to these problems are in the immediate future, but the trends are encouraging.

A particularly encouraging trend is the growing emphasis on considering speech perception and spoken word recognition as interacting stages of a unitary process. Most research on speech perception over the past 40 years has been concerned with the perception of isolated phonetic contrasts or phonemes in brief, meaningless syllables. Although the modularist approaches maintain that research and theory can proceed in a vacuum, the major current trend appears to be toward interactionism, bridging the gap that has traditionally separated the study of these different stages of speech comprehension. Already we have observed the development of several connectionist approaches to language processing, emphasizing the value of interaction between levels of representation. Perhaps the major insight of this approach has been the value of allowing models of speech perception and word recognition to constrain each other. As noted by Pisoni and Luce (1987), theorizing about one stage of language processing without regard for related stages may lead to theories that work well in artificial isolation, but if theories about one stage of processing are incompatible with our understanding of another stage, it is not clear what we have learned.

In short, we believe that the growing interest in the perception of spoken language, going beyond the level of the phoneme to the level of the word, reflects a healthful trend toward more comprehensive accounts of language perception. Of course, much research remains to be done on almost every level of spoken language understanding. The problems of speech perception and spoken word recognition, along with all aspects of language perception, promise to provide interesting and challenging research opportunities for at least another 40 years.

Acknowledgment
This work was supported by NIH Research Grant DC-00111-14 to Indiana University, Bloomington, Indiana.

Review Questions

1. What is the animorphism paradox and why has it remained a central concern in speech research?

2. Explain the problem of the information transfer rate in speech communication.

3. Discuss several possible conclusions that one might draw from studies comparing speech and nonspeech perception.

4. Why has duplex perception been cited as support for a theory of a phonetic module?

5. Does the evidence suggest that nonhuman animals perceive speech sounds in a manner similar to that of humans?

6. Explain the problem of perceptual constancy. Relate it to talker variability and changes in speaking rate.

7. What is the central claim of the motor theory of speech perception? What are the claims of information-processing models?

8. Describe three phenomena that all models of word recognition should be equipped to explain.

References

Abercrombie, D. (1967). *Elements of General Phonetics.* Chicago, IL: Aldine.

Abramson, A. S., & Lisker, L. (1967). Discriminability along the voicing continuum: Cross language tests. In B. Hála, M. Romportl, & P. Janota (Eds.), *Proceedings of the Sixth International Congress of Phonetic Sciences.* Prague: Academia (pp. 569-573).

Andrews, S. (1989). Frequency and neighborhood effects on lexical access: Activation or search? *Journal of Experimental Psychology: Learning, Memory, and Cognition, 15,* 802-814.

Aslin, R. N. (1985). Effects of experience on sensory and perceptual development: Implications for infant cognition. In Mehler, J., & Fox, R. (Eds.), *Neonate cognition: Beyond the blooming, buzzing confusion.* Hillsdale, NJ: Erlbaum (pp. 157-183).

Aslin, R. N., & Pisoni, D. B. (1980). Some developmental processes in speech perception. In Yeni-Komshian, G., Kavanagh, J. F., & Ferguson, C. A. (Eds.), *Child phonology: Perception and production.* New York: Academic Press (pp. 67-96).

Bagley, W. C. (1900-1901). The apperception of the spoken sentence: A study in the psychology of language. *American Journal of Psychology, 12,* 80-130.

Bailey, P. J., Summerfield, Q., & Dorman, M. (1977). On the identification of sine-wave analogues of certain speech sounds. *Haskins Laboratories status report on speech research SR-51/52,* 1-25.

Balota, D. A., & Chumbley, J. I. (1984). Are lexical decisions a good measure of lexical access? The role of word frequency in the neglected decision stage. *Journal of Experimental Psychology: Human Perception and Performance, 10,* 340-357.

Balota, D. A., & Chumbley, J. I. (1990). Where are the effects of frequency in visual word recognition tasks? Right where we said they were! Comment on Monsell, Doyle, and Haggard. *Journal of Experimental Psychology: General, 119,* 231-237.

Barclay, J. R. (1972). Noncategorical perception of a voiced stop: A replication. *Perception & Psychophysics, 11,* 269-273.

Bard, E. G., Shillcock, R. C., & Altmann, G. T. M. (1988). The recognition of words after their acoustic offsets in spontaneous speech: Effects of subsequent context. *Perception & Psychophysics, 44,* 395-408.

Becker, C. A. (1976). Allocation of attention during visual word recognition. *Journal of Experimental Psychology: Human Perception and Performance, 2,* 556-566.

Becker, C. A. (1979). Semantic context and word frequency effects in visual word recognition. *Journal of Experimental Psychology: Human Perception and Performance, 5,* 252-259.

Becker, C. A. (1980). Semantic context effects in visual word recognition: An analysis of semantic strategies. *Memory & Cognition, 8,* 493-512.

Becker, C. A., & Killion, T. H. (1977). Interaction of visual and cognitive effects in word recognition. *Journal of Experimental Psychology: Human Perception and Performance, 3,* 389-401.

Bentin, S., & Mann, V. (1990). Masking and stimulus intensity effects on duplex perception: A confirmation of the dissociation between speech and nonspeech modes. *Journal of the Acoustical Society of America, 88,* 64-74.

Best, C. T. (1994). The emergence of native-language phonological influences in infants: A perceptual assimilation model. In Nusbaum H. & Goodman J. (Eds.), *The development of speech perception.* Cambridge, MA: MIT Press (pp. 167-224).

Best, C. T., MacRoberts, G. W., & Sithole, N. M. (1988). Examination of the perceptual reorganization for speech contrasts: Zulu click discrimination by English-speaking adults and infants. *Journal of Experimental Psychology: Human Perception and Performance, 14,* 245-260.

Best, C. T., Morrongiello, B., & Robson, R. (1981). Perceptual equivalence of acoustic cues in speech and nonspeech perception. *Perception & Psychophysics, 29,* 191-211.

Bever, T. G., Lackner, J., & Kirk, R. (1969). The underlying structures of sentences are the primary units of immediate speech processing. *Perception & Psychophysics, 5,* 225-231.

Bradley, D. C., & Forster, K. I. (1987). A reader's view of listening. *Cognition, 25,* 103-134.

Bregman, A. S. (1978). The formation of auditory streams. In Requin, J. (Ed.), *Attention and performance VII.* Hillsdale, NJ: Erlbaum (pp. 63-75).

Bregman, A.S. (1990). *Auditory scene analysis.* Cambridge, MA: MIT Press.

Broadbent, D. E. (1965). Information processing in the nervous system. *Science, 150,* 457-462.

Carr, P. B., & Trill, D. (1964). Long-term larynx-excitation spectra. *Journal of the Acoustical Society of America, 36,* 2033-2040.

Carrell, T. D. (1984). *Contributions of fundamental frequency, formant spacing, and glottal waveform to talker identification.* Unpublished doctoral dissertation. Indiana University.

Carrell, T. D., Smith, L. B., & Pisoni, D. B. (1981). Some perceptual dependencies in speeded classification of vowel color and pitch. *Perception & Psychophysics, 29,* 1-10.

Chomsky, N., & Miller, G. A. (1963). Introduction to the formal analysis of natural language. In Luce, R. D., Bush, R., & Galanter, E. (Eds.), *Handbook of mathematical psychology,* Vol. 2. New York: Wiley (pp. 269-321).

Church, B., & Schacter, D. L. (1994). Perceptual specificity of auditory priming: Memory for voice intonation and fundamental frequency. *Journal of Experimental Psychology: Learning, Memory, and Cognition, 20,* 521-533.

Cluff, M. S., & Luce, P. A. (1990). Similarity neighborhoods of spoken two-syllable words: Retroactive effects on multiple activation. *Journal of Experimental Psychology: Human Perception and Performance, 16,* 551-563.

Cohen, A., & Nooteboom, S. G. (Eds.) (1975). *Structure and process in speech perception.* Heidelberg: Springer-Verlag.

Cole, R. A., & Jakimik, J. (1980). A model of speech perception. In Cole, R. A. (Ed.), *Perception and production of fluent speech.* Hillsdale, NJ: Erlbaum (pp. 133-163).

Cole, R. A., & Rudnicky, A. I. (1983). What's new in speech perception? The research and ideas of William Chandler Bagley, 1874-1946. *Psychological Review, 90,* 94-101.

Cole, R. A., & Scott, B. (1974a). The phantom in the phoneme: Invariant cues for stop consonants. *Perception and Psychophysics, 15,* 101-107.

Cole, R. A., & Scott, B. (1974b). Toward a theory of speech perception. *Psychological Review, 81,* 348-374.

Collier, R., & t'Hart, J. (1975). The role of intonation in speech perception. In Cohen, A., & Nooteboom, S.G. (Eds.), *Structure and process in speech perception.* Heidelberg: Springer-Verlag (pp. 107-123).

Coltheart, M., Davelaar, E., and Jonasson, J. T., & Besner, D. (1977). Access to the internal lexicon. In Dornic, S. (Ed.), *Attention and performance VI.* Hillsdale, NJ: Erlbaum (pp. 535-555).

Connine, C., Blasko, D., & Titone, D. (1993). Do the beginnings of words have a special status in auditory word recognition? *Journal of Memory and Language, 32,* 193-210.

Cooper, F. S. (1972). How is language conveyed by speech? In Kavanagh, J. F., & Mattingly, I. G. (Eds.), *Language by ear and by eye.* Cambridge, MA: MIT Press.

Cooper, W. E. (1976). Syntactic control of timing in speech production: A study of complement clauses. *Journal of Phonetics, 4,* 151-171.

Cooper, W. E., & Sorenson, J. (1977). Fundamental frequency contours at syntactic boundaries. *Journal of the Acoustical Society of America, 62,* 683-692.

Creelman, C. D. (1957). The case of the unknown talker. *Journal of the Acoustical Society of America, 29,* 655.

Cutler, A. (1976). Phoneme-monitoring reaction time as a function of preceding intonation contour. *Perception & Psychophysics, 20,* 55-60.

Cutler, A. (1989). Auditory lexical access: Where do we start? In Marslen-Wilson, W. D. (Ed.), *Lexical representation and process.* Cambridge, MA: MIT Press (pp. 342-356).

Cutler, A., & Butterfield, S. (1992). Rhythmic cues to speech segmentation: Evidence from juncture misperception. *Journal of Memory and Language, 31,* 218-236.

Cutler, A., & Darwin, C. J. (1981). Phoneme-monitoring reaction time and preceding prosody: Effects of stop closure duration and of fundamental frequency. *Perception & Psychophysics, 29,* 217-224.

Cutler, A., & Fodor, J. A. (1979). Semantic focus and sentence comprehension. *Cognition, 7,* 49-59.

Cutler, A., & Foss, D. J. (1977). On the role of sentence stress in sentence processing. *Language and Speech, 20,* 1-10.

Cutler, A., Mehler, J., Norris, D., & Segui, J. (1992). The monolingual nature of speech segmentation by bilinguals. *Cognitive Psychology, 24,* 381-410.

Cutting, J. E. (1978). There may be nothing peculiar to perceiving in a speech mode. In Requin, J. (Ed.), *Attention and performance VII.* Hillsdale, NJ: Erlbaum (pp. 229-244).

Cutting, J. E. (1987). Perception and information. *Annual Review of Psychology, 38,* 61-90.

Cutting, J. E., & Pisoni, D. B. (1978). An information-processing approach to speech perception. In Kavanagh, J. F., & Strange, W. (Eds.), *Speech and language in the laboratory, school, and clinic.* Cambridge, MA: MIT Press (pp. 38-72).

Darwin, C. J. (1975). On the dynamic use of prosody in speech perception. In Cohen, A., & Nooteboom, S. G. (Eds.), *Structure and process in speech perception.* Heidelberg: Springer-Verlag (pp. 178-194).

Darwin, C. J. (1976). The perception of speech. In Carterette, E. C. & Friedman, M. P. (Eds.), *Handbook of perception.* New York: Academic Press (pp. 175-216).

Day, R. S. (1968). Fusion in dichotic listening. Unpublished doctoral dissertation. Stanford University.

Dekle, D. J., Fowler, C. A., & Funnell, M. G. (1992). Audiovisual integration in perception of real words. *Perception & Psychophysics, 51,* 355-362.

Delattre, P. C., Liberman, A. M., & Cooper, F. S.

(1955). Acoustic loci and transitional cues for consonants. *Journal of the Acoustical Society of America, 27,* 769-773.

Delattre, P. C., Liberman, A. M., Cooper, F. S., & Gerstman, L. H. (1952). An experimental study of the acoustic determinants of vowel color: Observations of one- and two-formant vowels synthesized from spectrographic patterns. *Word, 8,* 195-210.

Dell, G. (1986). A spreading activation theory of retrieval in sentence production. *Psychological Review, 93,* 283-321.

Denes, P. (1955). Effect of duration on the perception of voicing. *Journal of the Acoustical Society of America, 27,* 761-764.

Derr, M. A., & Massaro, D. W. (1980). The contribution of vowel duration, F_O contour, and frication duration as cues to the /juz/ - /jus/ distinction. *Perception & Psychophysics, 27,* 51-59.

Diehl, R. L. (1986). Coproduction and direct perception of phonetic segments: A critique. *Journal of Phonetics, 14,* 61-66.

Diehl, R. L., & Kleunder, K. R. (1989). On the objects of speech perception. *Ecological Psychology, 1,* 121-144.

Dobbs, A. R., Friedman, A., & Lloyd, J. (1985). Frequency effects in lexical decisions: A test of the verification model. *Journal of Experimental Psychology: Human Perception and Performance, 11,* 81-92.

Easton, R. D., & Basala, M. (1982). Perceptual dominance during lipreading. *Perception and Psychophysics, 32,* 562-570.

Eimas, P. D. (1975). Auditory and phonetic coding of the cues for speech: Discrimination of the [r-l] distinction by young infants. *Perception and Psychophysics, 18,* 341-347.

Eimas, P.D., & Corbit, J. (1973). Selective adaptation of linguistic feature detectors. *Cognitive Psychology, 4,* 99-109.

Eimas, P. D., & Miller, J. L. (1980). Contextual effects in infant speech perception. *Science, 209,* 1140-1141.

Eimas, P. D., Siqueland, E. R., Jusczyk, P. W., & Vigorito, J. (1971). Speech perception in infants. *Science, 171,* 303-306.

Elman, J. L. (1989). Connectionist approaches to acoustic/phonetic processing. In Marslen-Wilson, W. D. (Ed.), *Lexical representation and process.* Cambridge, MA: MIT Press (pp. 227-260).

Elman, J. L. (1990). Finding structure in time. *Cognitive Science, 14,* 179-211.

Elman, J. L. (1993). Learning and development in neural networks: The importance of starting small. *Cognition, 48,* 71-99.

Elman, J. L., & McClelland, J. L. (1984). Speech perception as a cognitive process: The interactive activation model. In Lass, N. J. (Ed.), *Speech and Language: Advances in basic research and practice,* Vol. 102. New York: Academic Press (pp. 337-374).

Elman, J. L., & McClelland, J. L. (1986). Exploiting lawful variability in the speech waveform. In Perkell, J. S., & Klatt, D. H. (Eds.), *Invariance and variability in speech processing.* Hillsdale, NJ: Erlbaum (pp. 360-385).

Fant, G. (1962). Descriptive analysis of the acoustic aspects of speech. *Logos, 5,* 3-17.

Fant, G. (1973). *Speech sounds and features.* Cambridge, MA: MIT Press.

Fitch, H. L., Hawles, T., Erickson, D. M., & Liberman, A. M. (1980). Perceptual equivalence of two acoustic cues for stop-consonant manner. *Perception & Psychophysics, 27,* 343-350.

Fodor, J. A. (1983). *The modularity of mind.* Cambridge, MA: MIT Press.

Fodor, J. A. (1985). Précis of *The modularity of mind. The Behavioral and Brain Sciences, 8,* 1-42.

Forster, K. I. (1976). Accessing the mental lexicon. In Wales, R. J., & Walker, E.C.T. (Eds.), *New approaches to language mechanisms.* Amsterdam: North Holland (pp. 257-287).

Forster, K. I. (1979). Levels of processing and the structure of the language processor. In Cooper, W. E., & Walker, E.C.T. (Eds.), *Sentence processing: Psycholinguistic studies presented to Merrill Garrett.* Hillsdale, NJ: Erlbaum (pp. 27-86).

Forster, K. I. (1989). Basic issues in lexical processing. In Marslen-Wilson, W. D. (Ed.), *Lexical representation and process.* Cambridge, MA: MIT Press (pp. 75-107).

Forster, K. I. (1990). Lexical processing. In Osherson, D. N., & Lasnik, H. (Eds.), *An invitation to cognitive science, Vol.* 1. Cambridge, MA: MIT Press (pp. 95-131).

Forster, K. I, & Bednall, E.S. (1976). Terminating and exhaustive search in lexical access. *Memory & Cognition, 4,* 53-61.

Fowler, C. A. (1986). An event approach to the study of speech perception from a direct-realist perspective. *Journal of Phonetics, 14,* 3-28.

Fowler, C. A. (1990). Sound-producing sources as objects of perception: Rate normalization and nonspeech perception. *Journal of the Acoustical Society of America, 88,* 1236-1249.

Fowler, C. A. (1994). Invariants, specifiers, cues: An investigation of locus equations as information for place of articulation. *Perception & Psychophysics, 55,* 597-610.

Fowler, C. A., & Rosenblum, L. D. (1990). Duplex perception: A comparison of monosyllables and slamming of doors. *Journal of Experimental Psychology: Human Perception and Performance, 16,* 742-754.

Fowler, C. A., & Rosenblum, L. D. (1991). The perception of phonetic gestures. In Mattingly, I. G., & Studdert-Kennedy, M. (Eds.), *Modularity and the motor theory of speech perception.* Hillsdale, NJ: Erlbaum (pp. 33-59).

Frauenfelder, U., Baayen, R., Hellwig, F., &

Schreuder, R. (1993). Neighborhood density and frequency across languages and modalities. *Journal of Memory and Language, 32,* 781-804.

Fujisaki, H., & Kawashima, T. (1969). On the modes and mechanisms of speech perception. *Annual report of the Engineering Research Institute,* Vol. 28. Tokyo: University of Tokyo (pp. 67-73).

Fujisaki, H., & Kawashima, T. (1970). Some experiments on speech perception and a model for the perceptual mechanism. *Annual report of the Engineering Research Institute,* Vol. 29. Tokyo: University of Tokyo (pp. 207-214).

Fujisaki, H., & Kawashima, T. (1971). A model of the mechanisms for speech perception: Quantitative analysis of categorical effects in discrimination. *Annual report of the Engineering Research Institute,* Vol. 30. Tokyo: University of Tokyo (pp. 59-68).

Gaitenby, J. H. (1965). The elastic word. *Haskins Laboratories status report on speech research, SR-2,* 3.1-3.12.

Ganong, W. F. (1980). Phonetic categorization in auditory word perception. *Journal of Experimental Psychology: Human Perception and Performance, 6,* 110-125.

Garner, W. (1974). *The processing of information and structure.* Hillsdale, NJ: Erlbaum.

Geiselman, R. E., & Bellezza, F. S. (1976). Long-term memory for speaker's voice and source location. *Memory & Cognition, 4,* 483-489.

Geiselman, R. E., & Bellezza, F. S. (1977). Incidental retention of speaker's voice. *Memory & Cognition, 5,* 658-665.

Geiselman, R. E., & Crawley, J. M. (1983). Incidental processing of speaker characteristics: Voice as connotative information. *Journal of Verbal Learning and Verbal Behavior, 22,* 15-23.

Gerstman, L. H. (1968). Classification of self-normalized vowels. *IEEE Transactions on Audio and Electroacoustics, au-16,* 78-80.

Gibson, J. J. (1966). *The senses considered as perceptual systems.* Boston, MA: Houghton-Mifflin.

Gibson, J. J. (1979). *The ecological approach to visual perception.* Boston, MA: Houghton-Mifflin.

Goldinger, S. D., Luce, P. A., & Pisoni, D. B. (1989). Priming lexical neighbors of spoken words: Effects of competition and inhibition. *Journal of Memory and Language, 28,* 501-518.

Goldinger, S. D., Pisoni, D. B., & Logan, J. S. (1991). The nature of talker variability effects on recall of spoken word lists. *Journal of Experimental Psychology: Learning, Memory, and Cognition, 17,* 152-162.

Goodman, J. C., & Huttenlocher, J. (1988). Do we know how people identify spoken words? *Journal of Memory and Language, 27,* 684-698.

Goto, H. (1971). Auditory perception by normal Japanese adults of the sounds "L" and "R". *Neuropsychologica, 9,* 317-323.

Green, K. P., Stevens, E. B., & Kuhl, P. K. (1994). Talker continuity and the use of rate information during phonetic perception. *Perception & Psychophysics, 55,* 249-260.

Grosjean, F. (1980). Spoken word recognition processes and the gating paradigm. *Perception & Psychophysics, 28,* 267-283.

Grosjean, F. (1985). The recognition of words after their acoustic offset: Evidence and implications. *Perception & Psychophysics, 38,* 299-310.

Grosjean, F., & Gee, J. P. (1987). Prosodic structure and spoken word recognition. *Cognition, 25,* 135-155.

Grunke, M. E., & Pisoni, D. B. (1982). Some experiments on perceptual learning of mirror-image acoustic patterns. *Perception & Psychophysics, 31,* 210-218.

Hall, M.D., & Pastore, R. E. (1992). Musical duplex perception: Perception of figurally good chords with subliminal distinguishing tones. *Journal of Experimental Psychology: Human Perception and Performance, 18,* 752-762.

Harris, K. S., Hoffman, H. S., Liberman, A. M., Delattre, P. C., & Cooper, F. S. (1958). Effect of third formant transitions on the perception of the voiced stop consonants. *Journal of the Acoustical Society of America, 30,* 122-126.

Hawles, T., & Jenkins, J. J. (1971). Problem of serial order in behavior is not resolved by context-sensitive associative memory models. *Psychological Review, 78,* 122-129.

Hockett, C. (1955). *Manual of phonology.* Publications in Anthropology and Linguistics No. 11. Bloomington, Indiana: Indiana University Press.

Hoffman, H. S. (1958). Study of some cues in the perception of voiced stop consonants. *Journal of the Acoustical Society of America, 30,* 1035-1041.

Holmberg, T. L., Morgan, K. A., & Kuhl, P. K. (1977). Speech perception in early infancy: Discrimination of fricative consonants. *Journal of the Acoustical Society of America, 62,* S76 (Abstract).

Huggins, A. W. F. (1972). On the perception of temporal phenomena in speech. In Requin, J. (Ed.), *Attention and performance VII.* Hillsdale, NJ: Erlbaum (pp. 279-297).

Isenberg, D., & Liberman, A. M. (1978). Speech and non-speech percepts from the same sound. *Journal of the Acoustical Society of America, 64,* S20 (Abstract).

Jenkins, J. J. (1989). Is this the way to Camelot? *Contemporary Psychology, 5,* 451-452.

Johnson, K. (1990). The role of perceived speaker identity in F_0 normalization of vowels. *Journal of the Acoustical Society of America, 88,* 642-654.

Johnson, K., Ladefoged, P., & Lindau, M. (1993). Individual differences in vowel production. *Journal of the Acoustical Society of America, 94,* 701-714.

Joos, M. A. (1948). Acoustic phonetics. *Language, 24,* (Suppl. 2), 1-136.

Jordan, M. I. (1986). Serial order: A parallel distributed processing approach. *Report 8604,* Institute for Cognitive Science, University of California, San Diego.

Jusczyk, P. W. (1985). On characterizing the development of speech perception. In Mehler, J., & Fox, R. (Eds.), *Neonate cognition: Beyond the blooming, buzzing confusion.* Hillsdale, NJ: Erlbaum (pp. 199-229).

Jusczyk, P. W. (1986). A review of speech perception research. In Kaufman, L., Thomas, J., & Boff, K. (Eds.), *Handbook of perception and performance.* New York: Wiley (pp. 27-57).

Jusczyk, P. W., Pisoni, D. B., & Mullennix, J. W. (1992). Some consequences of stimulus variability on speech processing by 2-month old infants. *Cognition, 43,* 253-291.

Jusczyk, P. W., Pisoni, D. B., Reed, M. A., Fernald, A., & Myers, M. (1983). Infants' discrimination of the duration of rapid spectrum changes in nonspeech signals. *Science, 222,* 175-177.

Jusczyk, P. W., Pisoni, D. B., Walley, A. C., & Murray, J. (1980). Discrimination of relative onset time of two-component tones by infants. *Journal of the Acoustical Society of America, 67,* 262-270.

Kewley-Port, D. (1982). Measurement of formant transitions in naturally produced stop consonant-vowel syllables. *Journal of the Acoustic Society of America, 72,* 379-389.

Kewley-Port, D. (1983). Time-varying features as correlates of place of articulation in stop consonants. *Journal of the Acoustical Society of America, 73,* 322-335.

Kewley-Port, D., & Luce, P. A. (1984). Time-varying features of initial stop consonants in auditory running spectra: A first report. *Perception & Psychophysics, 35,* 353-360.

Klatt, D. H. (1974). The duration of [S] in English words. *Journal of Speech and Hearing Research, 17,* 51-63.

Klatt, D. H. (1975). Vowel lengthening is syntactically determined in connected discourse. *Journal of Phonetics, 3,* 129-140.

Klatt, D. H. (1976). Linguistic uses of segmental duration in English: Acoustic and perceptual evidence. *Journal of the Acoustical Society of America, 59,* 1208-1221.

Klatt, D. H. (1979). Speech perception: A model of acoustic-phonetic analysis and lexical access. *Journal of Phonetics, 7,* 279-312.

Klatt, D. H. (1989). Review of selected models of speech perception. In Marslen-Wilson, W. D. (Ed.), *Lexical representation and process.* Cambridge, MA: MIT Press (pp. 169-226).

Klatt, D. H., & Cooper, W. E. (1975). Perception of segment duration in sentence context. In Cohen, A., & Nooteboom, S. G. (Eds.), *Structure and process in speech perception.* Heidelberg: Springer-Verlag (pp. 69-80).

Kluender, K. R., Diehl, R. L., & Killeen, P. R. (1987). Japanese quail can learn phonetic categories. *Science, 237,* 1195-1197.

Kuhl, P. K. (1979). Speech perception in early infancy: Perceptual constancy for spectrally dissimilar vowel categories. *Journal of the Acoustical Society of America, 66,* 1668-1679.

Kuhl, P. K., & Meltzoff, A. N. (1982). The bimodal perception of speech in infancy. *Science, 218,* 1138-1141.

Kuhl, P. K., & Miller, J. D. (1975). Speech perception by the chinchilla: Voiced-voiceless distinction in alveolar plosive consonants. *Science, 190,* 69-72.

Kuhl, P. K., & Miller, J. D. (1978). Speech perception by the chinchilla: Identification functions for synthetic VOT stimuli. *Journal of the Acoustical Society of America, 63,* 905-917.

Kuhl, P. K., & Miller, J. D. (1982). Discrimination of auditory target dimensions in the presence or absence of variation in a second dimension by infants. *Perception & Psychophysics, 31,* 279-292.

Ladefoged, P. (1980). What are linguistic sounds made of? *Language, 56,* 485-502.

Ladefoged, P., & Broadbent, D. E. (1957). Information conveyed by vowels. *Journal of the Acoustical Society of America, 29,* 98-104.

Landauer, T. K., & Streeter, L. A. (1973). Structural differences between common and rare words: Failure of equivalence assumptions for theories of word recognition. *Journal of Verbal Learning and Verbal Behavior, 12,* 119-131.

Lea, W. A. (1973). An approach to syntactic recognition without phonemics. *IEEE Transactions on Audio and Electroacoustics, au-21,* 249-258.

Lehiste, I. (1970). *Suprasegmentals.* Cambridge, MA: MIT Press.

Liberman, A. M. (1970a). The grammars of speech and language. *Cognitive Psychology, 1,* 301-323.

Liberman, A. M. (1970b). Some characteristics of perception in the speech mode. In Hamburg, D. A. (Ed.), *Perception and its disorders: Proceedings of ARNMD.* Baltimore: Williams & Wilkins (pp. 238-254).

Liberman, A. M. (1982). On finding that speech is special. *American Psychologist, 37,* 148-167.

Liberman, A. M., Cooper, F. S., Shankweiler, D. P., & Studdert-Kennedy, M. (1967). Perception of the speech code. *Psychological Review, 74,* 431-461.

Liberman, A. M., Delattre, P. C., Cooper, F. S., & Gerstman, L. H. (1954). The role of consonant-vowel transitions in the perception of the stop and nasal consonants. *Psychological Monographs, 68,* 1-13.

Liberman, A. M., Harris, K. S., Hoffman, H. A., & Griffith, B. C. (1957). The discrimination of speech sounds within and across phoneme boundaries. *Journal of Experimental Psychology, 54,* 358-368.

Liberman, A. M., & Mattingly, I. G. (1985). The motor theory of speech perception revised. *Cognition, 21,* 1-36.

Liberman, A. M., & Mattingly, I. G. (1989). A specialization for speech perception. *Science, 243,* 489-494.

Liberman, A. M., Mattingly, I. G., & Turvey, M. T. (1972). Language codes and memory codes. In Melton, A. W., & Martin, E. (Eds.), *Coding processes in human memory.* New York: Winston (pp. 307-334).

Lieberman, P., Crelin, E. S., & Klatt, D. H. (1972). Phonetic ability and related anatomy of the newborn, adult human, Neanderthal man, and the chimpanzee. *American Anthropology, 74,* 287-307.

Lightfoot, N. (1989). Effects of talker familiarity on serial recall of spoken word lists. *Research on speech perception, progress report no. 15.* Indiana University.

Lindblom, B. E. F., & Svensson, S. G. (1973). Interaction between segmental and non-segmental factors in speech recognition. *IEEE Transactions on Audio and Electroacoustics, au-21,* 536-545.

Lisker, L., & Abramson, A. S. (1964). A cross language study of voicing in initial stops: Acoustical measurements. *Word, 20,* 384-422.

Lisker, L., & Abramson, A. S. (1967). The voicing dimension: Some experiments in comparative phonetics. In Proceedings of the Sixth International Congress of Phonetic Sciences. Prague: Academia.

Logan, J. S., Lively, S. E., & Pisoni, D. B. (1991). Training Japanese listeners to identify /r/ and /l/: A first report. *Journal of the Acoustical Society of America, 89,* 874-886.

Luce, P. A. (1986). *Neighborhoods of words in the mental lexicon.* Unpublished doctoral dissertation. Indiana University.

Luce, P. A., & Charles-Luce, J. (1985). Contextual effects on vowel duration, closure duration, and the consonant/vowel ratio. *Journal of the Acoustical Society of America, 78,* 1949-1957.

Luce, P. A., & Pisoni, D. B. (1987). Speech perception: New directions in research, theory, and applications. In Winitz, H. (Ed.), *Human communication and its disorders.* Norwood, NJ: Ablex (pp. 1-87).

Luce, P. A., Pisoni, D. B., & Goldinger, S. D. (1990). Similarity neighborhoods of spoken words. In Altmann, G. (Ed.), *Cognitive models of speech processing.* Cambridge, MA: MIT Press (pp. 122-147).

MacDonald, J., & McGurk, H. (1978). Visual influences on speech perception processes. *Perception & Psychophysics, 24,* 253-257.

MacKain, K. S., Best, C. T., & Strange, W. (1981). Categorical perception of English /r/ and /l/ by Japanese bilinguals. *Applied Psycholinguistics, 2,* 369-390.

MacKain, K. S., Studdert-Kennedy, M., Spieker, S., & Stern, D. (1983). Infant intermodal speech perception is a left-hemisphere function. *Science, 219,* 1347-1349.

Mann, V. A., & Liberman, A. M. (1983). Some differences between phonetic and auditory modes of perception. *Cognition, 14,* 211-235.

Mann, V. A., Madden, J., Russell, J. M., & Liberman, A. M. (1981). *Integration of time-varying cues and the effects of phonetic context.* Unpublished manuscript, Haskins Laboratories, New Haven, CT.

Marcus, S. M. (1984). Recognizing speech: On mapping from sound to meaning. In Bouma, H., & Bowhuis, D. G. (Eds.), *Attention and performance X: Control of language processes.* Hillsdale, NJ: Erlbaum (pp. 151-164).

Marslen-Wilson, W. D. (1975). Sentence perception as an interactive parallel process. *Science, 189,* 226-228.

Marslen-Wilson, W. D. (1980a). Optimal efficiency in human speech processing. Unpublished manuscript.

Marslen-Wilson, W. D. (1980b). Speech understanding as a psychological process. In Simon, J. C. (Ed.), *Spoken language generation and understanding.* Dordrecht, Holland: Reidel (pp. 39-67).

Marslen-Wilson, W. D. (1987). Functional parallelism in spoken word recognition. *Cognition, 25,* 71-102.

Marslen-Wilson, W. D. (1989). Access and integration: Projecting sound onto meaning. In Marslen-Wilson, W. D. (Ed.), *Lexical representation and process.* Cambridge, MA: MIT Press (pp. 3-24).

Marslen-Wilson, W. D. (1990). Activation, competition, and frequency in lexical access. In G.T.M. Altman (Ed.), *Cognitive Models of Speech Processing.* Cambridge, MA: MIT Press (pp. 148-172).

Marslen-Wilson, W. D. (1993). Issues of process and representation in lexical access. In Altman, G. T. M. (Ed.), *Cognitive Models of Speech Processing: The Second Sperlonga Meeting.* Cambridge, MA: MIT Press (pp. 187-210).

Marslen-Wilson, W. D., & Tyler, L. K. (1975). Processing structure of sentence perception. *Nature, 257,* 784-785.

Marslen-Wilson, W. D., & Tyler, L. K. (1980). The temporal structure of spoken language understanding. *Cognition, 8,* 1-71.

Marslen-Wilson, W. D., & Welsh, A. (1978). Processing interactions and lexical access during word recognition in continuous speech. *Cognitive Psychology, 10,* 29-63.

Martin, C. S., Mullennix, J. W., Pisoni, D. B., & Summers, W. V. (1989). Effects of talker variability on recall of spoken word lists. *Journal of Experimental Psychology: Learning, Memory, and Cognition, 15,* 676-684.

Massaro, D. W. (1972). Preperceptual images, processing time, and perceptual units in auditory perception. *Psychological Review, 79,* 124-145.

Massaro, D. W. (1986). A new perspective and old problems. *Journal of Phonetics, 14,* 69-74.

Massaro, D. W. (1987). *Speech perception by ear and eye: A paradigm for psychological inquiry.* Hillsdale, NJ: Erlbaum.

Massaro, D. W. (1989). Multiple book review of speech perception by ear and eye: A paradigm for psychological inquiry. *The Behavioral and Brain Sciences, 12,* 741-794.

Massaro, D. W., & Cohen, M. M. (1976). The contribution of fundamental frequency and voice onset time to the /zi/ - /si/ distinction. *Journal of the Acoustical Society of America, 60,* 704-717.

Massaro, D. W., & Cohen, M. M. (1977). The contribution of voice-onset time and fundamental frequency as cues to the /zi/ − /si/ distinction. *Perception & Psychophysics, 22,* 373-382.

Massaro, D. W., & Cohen, M. M. (1983). Evaluation and integration of visual and auditory information in speech perception. *Journal of Experimental Psychology: Human Perception and Performance, 9,* 753-771.

Massaro, D. W., & Cohen, M. M. (1990). Perception of synthesized audible and visible speech. *Psychological Science, 1,* 55-63.

Massaro, D. W., & Cohen, M. M. (1993). The paradigm and the fuzzy logical model of perception are alive and well. *Journal of Experimental Psychology: General, 122,* 115-124.

Massaro, D. W., & Oden, G. C. (1980). Speech perception: A framework for research and theory. In Lass, N.J. (Ed.), *Speech and language: Advances in basic research and practice,* Vol. 3. New York: Academic Press (pp. 129-165).

Mattingly, I. G., & Liberman, A. M. (1988). Specialized perceiving systems for speech and other biologically-significant sounds. In Edelman, G., Gall, W., & Cohen, W. (Eds.), *Auditory function: The neurobiological bases of hearing.* New York: Wiley (pp. 775-793).

McClelland, J. L. (1979). On the time-relations of mental processes: An examination of systems of processes in cascade. *Psychological Review, 86,* 287-330.

McClelland, J. L., & Elman, J. L. (1986). The TRACE model of speech perception. *Cognitive Psychology, 18,* 1-86.

McClelland, J. L., & Rumelhart, D. E. (1981). An interactive activation model of context effects in letter perception: Part I. An account of basic findings. *Psychological Review, 88,* 375-405.

McGurk, H., & MacDonald, J. (1976). Hearing lips and seeing voices. *Nature, 264,* 746-748.

McQueen, J. M., Norris, D., & Cutler, A. (1994). Competition in spoken word recognition: Spotting words in other words. *Journal of Experimental Psychology: Learning, Memory, and Cognition, 20,* 621-638.

Miller, G. A. (1962). Decision units in the perception of speech. *IRE transactions on information theory, IT-8,* 81-83.

Miller, J. D., Wier, C. C., Pastore, R. E., Kelley, W. J., & Dooling, R. J. (1976). Discrimination and labeling of noise-buzz sequences with varying noise-lead times: An example of categorical perception. *Journal of the Acoustical Society of America, 60,* 410-417.

Miller, J. L. (1980). The effect of speaking rate on segmental distinctions: Acoustic variation and perceptual compensation. In Eimas, P. D., & Miller, J. L. (Eds.), *Perspectives on the study of speech.* Hillsdale, NJ: Erlbaum (pp. 39-74).

Miller, J. L. (1987). Mandatory processing in speech perception. In Garfield, J. L. (Ed.), *Modularity in knowledge representation and natural-language understanding.* Cambridge, MA: MIT Press (pp. 309-322).

Miller, J. L. (1990). Speech perception. In Osherson, D. N., & Lasnik, H. (Eds.), *An invitation to cognitive science,* Vol. 1. Cambridge, MA: MIT Press (pp. 69-93).

Miller, J. L., & Liberman, A. M. (1979). Some effects of later-occurring information on the perception of stop consonant and semi-vowel. *Perception & Psychophysics, 25,* 457-465.

Miller, J. L., & Wayland, S. C. (1993). Limits on the limitations of context-conditioned effects in the perception of [b] and [w]. *Perception & Psychophysics, 54,* 205-210.

Mochizuki, M. (1981). The identification of /r/ and /l/ in natural and synthesized speech. *Journal of Phonetics, 9,* 283-303.

Monsen, R. B., & Engebretson, A. M. (1977). Study of variations in the male and female glottal wave. *Journal of the Acoustical Society of America, 62,* 981-993.

Morse, P. A., & Snowdon, C. T. (1975). An investigation of categorical speech discrimination by rhesus monkeys. *Perception & Psychophysics, 17,* 9-16.

Morton, J. (1969). Interaction of information in word recognition. *Psychological Review, 76,* 165-178.

Morton, J. (1979). Word recognition. In Morton, J., & Marshall, J. D. (Eds.), *Psycholinguistics 2: Structures and processes.* Cambridge, MA: MIT Press (pp. 109-156).

Morton, J. (1982). Disintegrating the lexicon: An information processing approach. In Mehler, J., Walker, E. C. T., & Garrett, M. (Eds.), *On mental representation.* Hillsdale, NJ: Erlbaum (pp. 89-109).

Mullennix, J. W., & Pisoni, D. B. (1990). Stimulus variability and processing dependencies in speech perception. *Perception & Psychophysics, 47,* 379-390.

Mullennix, J. W., Pisoni, D. B., & Martin, C. S. (1989). Some effects of talker variability on spoken word recognition. *Journal of the Acoustical Society of America, 85,* 365-378.

Murdock, B. B., Jr. (1962). The serial position effect in free recall. *Journal of Experimental Psychology, 64,* 482-488.

Nakatani, L. H., & Schaffer, J. A. (1978). Hearing "words" without words: Prosodic cues for word perception. *Journal of the Acoustical Society of America, 63,* 234-245.

Neisser, U. (1967). *Cognitive Psychology.* New York: Appleton-Century-Crofts.

Newell, A. (1973). You can't play 20 questions with nature and win: Projective comments on the papers of this symposium. In Chase, W. G. (Ed.), *Visual information processing.* New York: Academic Press (pp. 283-308).

Nosofsky, R. M. (1986). Attention, similarity, and the identification-categorization relationship. *Journal of Experimental Psychology: General, 115,* 39-57.

Nosofsky, R. M. (1987). Attention and learning processes in the identification and categorization of integral stimuli. *Journal of Experimental Psychology: Learning, Memory, and Cognition, 14,* 700-708.

Nooteboom, S. G., Brokx, J. P. L., & de Rooij, J. J. (1978). Contributions of prosody to speech perception. In Levelt, W. J. M., & Flores d'Arcais, G. B. (Eds.), *Studies in the perception of language.* New York: Wiley (pp. 75-107).

Nusbaum, H. C. (1984). Possible mechanisms of duplex perception: "Chirp" identification versus dichotic fusion. *Perception & Psychophysics, 35,* 94-101.

Nusbaum, H. C., & Morin, T. (1992). Paying attention to differences among talkers. In Tohkura, Y., Vatikiotis-Bateson, E. & Sagisaka, Y. (Eds.), *Speech perception, production, and linguistic structure.* Tokyo: IOS Press.

Nusbaum, H. C., & Schwab, E. C. (1986). The role of attention and active processing in speech perception. In Schwab, E. C., & Nusbaum, H. C. (Eds.), *Perception of speech and visual form: Theoretical issues, models, and research.* New York: Academic Press (pp. 113-157).

Nusbaum, H. C., Schwab, E. C., & Sawusch, J. R. (1983). The role of "chirp" identification in duplex perception. *Perception & Psychophysics, 33,* 323-332.

Nygaard, L. C. (1993). Phonetic coherence in duplex perception: Effects of acoustic differences and lexical status. *Journal of Experimental Psychology: Human Perception and Performance, 19,* 268-286.

Nygaard, L. C., & Eimas, P. D. (1990). A new version of duplex perception: Evidence for phonetic and nonphonetic fusion. *Journal of the Acoustical Society of America, 88,* 75-86.

Nygaard, L. C., Sommers, M.S., & Pisoni, D. B. (1994). Speech perception as a talker-contingent process. *Psychological Science, 5,* 42-46.

Oden, G. C., & Massaro, D. W. (1978). Integration of featural information in speech perception. *Psychological Review, 85,* 172-191.

Oller, D. K. (1973). The effect of position in utterance on speech segment duration in English. *Journal of the Acoustical Society of America, 54,* 1235-1247.

Oller, D. K., Eilers, R. E., & Ozdamar, O. (1990). A psychoacoustic model of the ba/wa boundary shift. *Journal of the Acoustical Society of America, 87,* S38 (Abstract).

Paap, K. R., Newsome, S. L., McDonald, J. E., & Schvaneveldt, R. W. (1982). An activation-verification model for letter and word recognition: The word-superiority effect. *Psychological Review, 89,* 573-594.

Palmeri, T. J., Goldinger, S. D., & Pisoni, D. B. (1993). Episodic encoding of voice attributes and recognition memory for spoken words. *Journal of Experimental Psychology: Learning, Memory, and Cognition, 19,* 309-328.

Pastore, R. E. (1981). Possible psychoacoustic factors in speech perception. In Eimas, P. D., & Miller, J. L. (Eds.), *Perspectives on the study of speech.* Hillsdale, NJ: Erlbaum (pp. 165-205).

Pastore, R. E., Schmeckler, M. A., Rosenblum, L., & Szczesiul, R. (1983). Duplex perception with musical stimuli. *Perception & Psychophysics, 33,* 469-474.

Peters, R. W. (1955a). The effect of length of exposure to speaker's voice upon listener reception. *Joint Project Report No. 44.* U.S. Naval School of Aviation Medicine, Pensacola, FL (pp. 1-8).

Peters, R. W. (1955b). The relative intelligibility of single-voice and multiple-voice messages under various conditions of noise. *Joint Project Report No. 56.* U.S. Naval School of Aviation Medicine, Pensacola, FL (pp. 1-9).

Peterson, G. E., & Barney, H. L. (1952). Control methods used in a study of the vowels. *Journal of the Acoustical Society of America, 24,* 175-184.

Peterson, L. J., & Peterson, M. J. (1959). Short-term retention of individual verbal items. *Journal of Experimental Psychology, 58,* 193-198.

Pisoni, D. B. (1971). On the nature of categorical perception of speech sounds. *Supplement to status report on speech research, SR-27.* New Haven, CT: Haskins Laboratories.

Pisoni, D. B. (1973). Auditory and phonetic memory codes in the discrimination of consonants and vowels. *Perception & Psychophysics, 13,* 253-260.

Pisoni, D. B. (1975). Auditory short-term memory and vowel perception. *Memory & Cognition, 3,* 7-18.

Pisoni, D. B. (1977). Identification and discrimination

of the relative onset of two component tones: Implications for voicing perception in stops. *Journal of the Acoustical Society of America, 61*, 1352-1361.

Pisoni, D. B. (1978). Speech perception. In Estes, W. K. (Ed.), *Handbook of learning and cognitive processes*, Vol. 6. Hillsdale, NJ: Erlbaum (pp. 167-233).

Pisoni, D. B. (1991). Modes of processing speech and nonspeech signals. In Mattingly, I. G., & Studdert-Kennedy, M. (Eds.), *Modularity and the motor theory of speech perception*. Hillsdale, NJ: Erlbaum (pp. 225-238).

Pisoni, D. B., Aslin, R. N., Perey, A. J., & Hennessy, B. L. (1982). Some effects of laboratory training on identification and discrimination of voicing contrasts in stop consonants. *Journal of Experimental Psychology: Human Perception and Performance, 8*, 297-314.

Pisoni, D. B., Carrell, T. D., & Gans, S. J. (1983). Perception of the duration of rapid spectrum changes in speech and nonspeech signals. *Perception & Psychophysics, 34*, 314-322.

Pisoni, D. B., Logan, J. S., & Lively, S. E. (1994). Perceptual learning of nonnative speech contrasts: Implications for theories of speech perception. In Nusbaum, H. C., & Goodman, J. C. (Eds.), *Development of speech perception: The transition from recognizing speech sounds to spoken words.* Cambridge, MA: MIT Press (pp. 121-166).

Pisoni, D. B., & Luce, P. A. (1986). Speech perception: Research, theory, and the principal issues. In Schwab, E. C., & Nusbaum, H. C. (Eds.), *Perception of speech and visual form: Theoretical issues, models, and research.* New York: Academic Press (pp. 1-50).

Pisoni, D. B., & Luce, P. A. (1987). Acoustic-phonetic representations in word recognition. *Cognition, 25*, 21-52.

Pisoni, D. B., & Sawusch, J. R. (1975). Some stages of processing in speech perception. In Cohen, A., & Nooteboom, S. G. (Eds.), *Structure and process in speech perception.* Heidelberg: Springer-Verlag (pp. 16-34).

Pitt, M. A., & Samuel, A. G. (1993). An empirical and meta-analytic evaluation of the phoneme identification task. *Journal of Experimental Psychology: Human Perception and Performance, 19*, 699-725.

Polka, L. (1992). Characterizing the influence of native language experience on adult speech perception. *Perception & Psychophysics, 52*, 37-52.

Polka, L., & Werker, J. F. (1994). Developmental changes in perception of nonnative vowel contrasts. *Journal of Experimental Psychology: Human Perception and Performance, 20*, 421-435.

Port, R. F. (1977). *The influence of speaking tempo on the duration of stressed vowel and medial stop in English trochu words.* Bloomington, Indiana: In-diana University Linguistics Club. Indiana University Press.

Porter, R. J., Jr. (1986). Speech messages, modulations, and motions. *Journal of Phonetics, 14*, 83-88.

Pruitt, J. S., Strange, W., Polka, L., & Aguilar, M. C. (1990). Effects of category knowledge and syllable truncation during auditory training on Americans' discrimination of Hindi retroflex-dental contrasts. *Journal of the Acoustical Society of America, 87*, S72 (Abstract).

Rand, T. C. (1974). Dichotic release from masking for speech. *Journal of the Acoustical Society of America, 55*, 678-680.

Remez, R. E. (1986) Realism, language, and another barrier. *Journal of Phonetics, 14*, 89-97.

Remez, R. E., Rubin, P. E., Berns, S. M., Pardo, J. S., & Lang, J. M. (1994). On the perceptual organization of speech. *Psychological Review, 101*, 129-156.

Remez, R. E., Rubin, P. E., Pisoni, D. B., & Carrell, T. D. (1981). Speech perception without traditional speech cues. *Science, 212*, 947-950.

Repp, B. H. (1982). Phonetic trading relations and context effects: New experimental evidence for a speech mode of perception. *Psychological Bulletin, 92*, 81-110.

Repp, B. H. (1983a). Categorical perception: Issues, methods, findings. In Lass, N. J. (Ed.), *Speech and language: Advances in basic research and practice*, Vol. 10. New York: Academic Press (pp. 243-335).

Repp, B. H. (1983b). Trading relations among acoustic cues in speech perception: Speech-specific but not special. *Haskins Laboratories status report on speech research, SR-76*, 129-132.

Repp, B. H. (1984). Against a role of "chirp" identification in duplex perception. *Perception & Psychophysics, 35*, 89-93.

Roberts, M., & Summerfield, Q. (1981). Audio-visual adaptation in speech perception. *Perception & Psychophysics, 30*, 309-314.

Rumelhart, D. E., & McClelland, J. L. (1982). An interactive activation model of context effects in letter perception: Part 2. The contextual enhancement effect and some tests and extensions of the model. *Psychological Review, 89*, 60-94.

Rundus, D. (1971). Analysis of rehearsal processes in free recall. *Journal of Experimental Psychology, 89*, 43-50.

Samuel, A. G. (1986). The role of the lexicon in speech perception. In Schwab, E. C., & Nusbaum, H. C. (Eds.), *Perception of speech and visual form: Theoretical issues, models, and research.* New York: Academic Press (pp. 89-111).

Samuel, A. G., & Ressler, W. H. (1986). Attention within auditory word perception: Insights from the phonemic restoration illusion. *Journal of Experimental Psychology: Human Perception and Performance, 12*, 70-79.

Savin, H. B., & Bever, T. G. (1970). The nonperceptual reality of the phoneme. *Journal of Verbal Learning and Verbal Behavior, 9,* 295-302.

Schacter, D. L., & Church, B. (1992). Auditory priming: Implicit and explicit memory for words and voices. *Journal of Experimental Psychology: Learning, Memory, and Cognition, 18,* 915-930.

Schouten, M. E. H. (1980). The case against a speech mode of perception. *Acta Psychologica, 44,* 71-98.

Schwab, E. C. (1981). *Auditory and phonetic processing for tone analogs of speech.* Unpublished doctoral dissertation. State University of New York at Buffalo.

Segui, J. (1984). The syllable: A basic perceptual unit in speech processing. In Bouma, H., & Bouwhis, D. G. (Eds.), *Attention and performance X: Control of language processes.* Hillsdale, NJ: Erlbaum (pp. 165-181).

Shankweiler, D. P., Strange, W., & Verbrugge, R. R. (1977). Speech and the problem of perceptual constancy. In Shaw, R., & Bransford, J. (Eds.), *Perceiving, acting, and knowing: Toward an ecological psychology.* Hillsdale, NJ: Erlbaum (pp. 315-345).

Stevens, K. N. (1972). The quantal nature of speech: Evidence from articulatory-acoustic data. In David, E. E., Jr., & Denes, P. B. (Eds.), *Human communication: A unified view.* New York: McGraw-Hill (pp. 51-66).

Stevens, K. N., & Blumstein, S. E. (1978). Invariant cues for place of articulation in stop consonants. *Journal of the Acoustical Society of America, 64,* 1358-1368.

Stevens, K. N., & Blumstein, S. E. (1981). The search for invariant acoustic correlates of phonetic features. In Eimas, P. D., & Miller, J. L. (Eds.), *Perspectives on the study of speech.* Hillsdale, NJ: Erlbaum (pp. 1-38).

Strange, W. (1972). *The effects of training on the perception of synthetic speech sounds: Voice onset time.* Unpublished doctoral dissertation. University of Minnesota.

Strange, W., & Dittmann, S. (1984). Effects of discrimination training on the perception of /r-l/ by Japanese adults learning English. *Perception & Psychophysics, 36,* 131-145.

Strange, W., & Jenkins, J. J. (1978). The role of linguistic experience in the perception of speech. In Pick, H. L., Jr., & Walk, R. D. (Eds.), *Perception and experience.* New York: Plenum (pp. 125-169).

Strange, W., Verbrugge, R. R., Shankweiler, D. P., & Edman, T. R. (1976). Consonant environment specifies vowel identity. *Journal of the Acoustical Society of America, 60,* 213-221.

Studdert-Kennedy, M. (1974). The perception of speech. In Sebeok, T. A. (Ed.), *Current trends in linguistics,* Vol. 12. The Hague: Mouton (pp. 2349-2385).

Studdert-Kennedy, M. (1976). Speech perception. In Lass, N. J. (Ed.), *Contemporary issues in experimental phonetics.* New York: Academic Press (pp. 243-293).

Studdert-Kennedy, M. (1980). Speech perception. *Language and Speech, 23,* 45-66.

Studdert-Kennedy, M. (1982). On the dissociation of auditory and phonetic perception. In Carlson, R., & Granström, B. (Eds.), *The representation of speech in the peripheral auditory system.* Amsterdam: Elsevier (pp. 3-10).

Studdert-Kennedy, M. (1983). Perceiving phonetic events. *Haskins Laboratories: Status report on speech research, SR-74/75,* 53-69.

Studdert-Kennedy, M. (1986). Two cheers for direct realism. *Journal of Phonetics, 14,* 99-104.

Studdert-Kennedy, M., Liberman, A. M., Harris, K. S., & Cooper, F. S. (1970). Motor theory of speech perception: A reply to Lane's critical review. *Psychological Review, 77,* 234-249.

Studdert-Kennedy, M., & Shankweiler, D. P. (1970). Hemispheric specialization for speech perception. *Journal of the Acoustical Society of America, 48,* 579-594.

Summerfield, Q. (1975). Acoustic and phonetic components of the influence of voice changes and identification times for CVC syllables. *Report of speech research in progress, 2(4),* Queens University of Belfast (pp. 73-98).

Summerfield, Q. (1979). Use of visual information for phonetic perception. *Phonetica, 36,* 314-331.

Summerfield, Q. (1983). Audio-visual speech perception, lipreading and artificial stimulation. In Lutman, M. E., & Haggard, M. P. (Eds.), *Hearing Science and Hearing Disorders.* London: Academic Press.

Summerfield, Q., & Haggard, M. P. (1973). Vocal tract normalization as demonstrated by reaction times. *Report of speech research in progress, 2(2),* Queens University of Belfast (pp. 12-23).

Sussman, H. M. (1989). Neural coding of relational invariance in speech: Human language analogs to the Barn Owl. *Psychological Review, 96,* 631-642.

Sussman, H. M. (1991). The representation of stop consonants in three-dimensional acoustic space. *Phonetica, 48,* 18-31.

Sussman, H. M., Hoemeke, K., & Ahmed, F. (1993). A cross-linguistic investigation of locus equations as a phonetic descriptor for place of articulation. *Journal of the Acoustical Society of America, 94,* 1256-1268.

Sussman, H. M., McCaffrey, H. A., & Matthews, S. A. (1991). An investigation of locus equations as a source of relational invariance for stop place categorization. *Journal of the Acoustical Society of America, 90,* 1309-1325.

Svensson, S. G. (1974). Prosody and grammar in speech perception. *Monographs from the Institute* of *Linguistics* No. 2. Stockholm, Sweden: University of Stockholm, Institute of Linguistics.

Taft, M., & Hambly, G. (1986). Exploring the Cohort Model of word recognition. *Cognition, 22,* 259-282.

Tanenhaus, M. K., & Lucas, M. M. (1987). Context effects in lexical processing. *Cognition, 25,* 213-234.

Tomiak, G. R., Mullennix, J. W., & Sawusch, J. R. (1987). Integral processing of phonemes: Evidence for a phonetic mode of perception. *Journal of the Acoustical Society of America, 81,* 755-764.

Townsend, J. T. (1989). Winning "20 questions" with mathematical models. *The Behavioral and Brain Sciences, 12,* 775-776.

Tyler, L. K. (1984). The structure of the initial cohort: Evidence from gating. *Perception and Psychophysics, 36,* 417-427.

Tyler, L. K., & Frauenfelder, U. H. (1987). The process of spoken word recognition: An introduction. *Cognition, 25,* 1-20.

Tyler, L. K., & Marslen-Wilson, W. D. (1982). Speech comprehension processes. In Mehler, J., Walker, E. C. T., & Garrett, M. (Eds.), *Perspectives on mental representation: Experimental and theoretical studies of cognitive processes and capacities.* Hillsdale, NJ: Erlbaum (pp. 169-184).

Van Lancker, D., Kreiman, J., & Emmorey, K. (1985). Familiar voice recognition: Patterns and parameters: Part I. Recognition of backward voices. *Journal of Phonetics, 13,* 19-38.

Van Lancker, D., Kreiman, J., & Wickens, T. D. (1985). Familiar voice recognition: Patterns and parameters. Part I: Recognition of rate-altered voices. *Journal of Phonetics, 13,* 39-52.

Verbrugge, R. R., & Rakerd, B. (1986). Evidence of talker-independent information for vowels. *Language and Speech, 29,* 39-57.

Verbrugge, R. R., Strange, W., Shankweiler, D. P., & Edman, T. R. (1976). What information enables a listener to map a talker's vowel space? *Journal of the Acoustical Society of America, 60,* 198-212.

Vinegrad, M. D. (1972). A direct magnitude scaling method to investigate categorical versus continuous modes of speech perception. *Language and Speech, 15,* 114-121.

Walley, A. C., Pisoni, D. B., & Aslin, R. N. (1981). The role of early experience in the development of speech perception. In Aslin, R. N., Alberts, J., & Peterson, M. J. (Eds.), *The development of perception: Psychobiological perspectives.* New York: Academic Press (pp. 219-255).

Warren, P., & Marslen-Wilson, W. D. (1987). Continuous uptake of acoustic cues in spoken word recognition. *Perception & Psychophysics, 41,* 262-275.

Warren, R. M. (1989). The use of mathematical models in perceptual theory. *The Behavioral and Brain Sciences, 12,* 776.

Waters, R. S., & Wilson, W. A., Jr. (1976). Speech perception by rhesus monkeys: The voicing distinction in synthesized labial and velar stop consonants. *Perception & Psychophysics, 19,* 285-289.

Whalen, D., & Liberman, A. M. (1987). Speech perception takes precedence over nonspeech perception. *Science, 237,* 169-171.

Wickelgren, W. A. (1969). Context-sensitive coding, associative memory, and serial order in (speech) behavior. *Psychological Review, 76,* 1-15.

Wickelgren, W. A. (1976). Phonetic coding and serial order. In Carterette, E. C., & Friedman, M. P. (Eds.), *Handbook of perception,* Vol. 7. New York, NY: Academic Press (pp. 227-264).

Zadeh, L. A. (1965). Fuzzy sets. *Information and Control, 8,* 338-353.

Suggested Readings

Basic Research in Speech Perception

Borden, G. J., Harris, K. S. & Raphael, L. J. (1994). *Speech Science Primer: Physiology, Acoustics, and Perception of Speech,* 3rd ed. Baltimore: Williams & Wilkins.

Cohen, A., & Nooteboom, S. G. (Eds.). (1975). *Structure and process in speech perception.* Heidelberg: Springer-Verlag.

Cole, R. A., & Rudnicky, A. I. (1983). What's new in speech perception? The research and ideas of William Chandler Bagley, 1874-1946. *Psychological Review, 90,* 94-101.

Eimas, P. D., & Miller, J. L. (Eds.). (1981). *Perspectives on the study of speech.* Hillsdale, NJ: Erlbaum.

Elman J. L., & McClelland, J. L. (1984). Speech perception as a cognitive process: The interactive activation model. In Lass, N. J. (Ed.), *Speech and language: Advances in basic research and practice* (Vol. 10). New York: Academic Press, (pp. 337-374).

Gernsbacher, M. A. (Ed.), (1994). *Handbook of Psycholinguistics.* San Diego, CA: Academic Press.

Levelt, W. J. M., & Flores d'Arcais, G. B. (Eds.). (1978). *Studies in the perception of language.* New York: Wiley.

Pisoni, D. B. (1978). Speech perception. In Estes, W. K. (Ed.), *Handbook of learning and cognitive processes,* Vol. 6. Hillsdale, NJ: Erlbaum (pp. 167-233).

Repp, B. H. (1984). Categorical perception: Issues, methods, findings. In Lass, N. J. (Ed.), *Speech and language: Advances in basic research and practice.* Vol. 10. New York: Academic Press, (pp. 243-335).

Requin, J. (Ed.). (1978). *Attention and performance VII.* Hillsdale, NJ: Erlbaum.

Specialization of Speech Perception

Garfield, J. L. (Ed.). (1987). *Modularity in knowledge representation and natural-language understanding.* Cambridge, MA: MIT Press.

Mattingly, I. G., & Studdert-Kennedy, M. (Eds.). (1991). *Modularity and the motor theory of speech perception.* Hillsdale, NJ: Erlbaum.

Variability in Speech Perception

Cole, R. A. (Ed.). (1980). *Perception and production of fluent speech.* Hillsdale, NJ: Erlbaum.

Perkell, J. S., & Klatt, D. H. (Eds.). (1986). *Invariance and variability in speech processing.* Hillsdale, NJ: Erlbaum.

Theories of Speech Perception

Altmann, G. (Ed.). (1990). *Cognitive models of speech processing.* Cambridge, MA: MIT Press.

Massaro, D. W. (1987). *Speech perception by ear and eye: A paradigm for psychological inquiry.* Hillsdale, NJ: Erlbaum.

Schwab, E. C., & Nusbaum, H. C. (Eds.). (1986). *Perception of speech and visual form: Theoretical issues, models, and research.* New York: Academic Press.

van den Broeke (Ed.). (1986). *Journal of Phonetics.* 14(1) (special issue).

Theories of Spoken Word Recognition

Bouma, H., & Bowhuis, D. G. (Eds.). (1984). *Attention and performance X: Control of language processes.* Hillsdale, NJ: Erlbaum.

Cooper, W. E., & Walker, E. C. T. (Eds.). (1979). *Sentence processing: Psycholinguistic studies presented to Merrill Garrett.* Hillsdale, NJ: Erlbaum.

Frauenfelder, U. H., & Tyler, L. K. (Eds.). (1987). *Spoken Word Recognition.* Cambridge, MA: MIT Press.

Marslen-Wilson, W. D. (Ed.). (1989). *Lexical representation and process.* Cambridge, MA: MIT Press.

Chapter 9

Developmental Speech Perception

Peter W. Jusczyk

INTRODUCTION

In a typical speech perception experiment involving 2-month-old infants, a researcher can expect to collect usable data from only 30% to 40% of the infants who come into the laboratory. The rest of the infants fail to complete testing for a variety of reasons including crying, sleeping, bowel movements, lack of interest, and other factors. Thus, to complete an experiment requiring 96 subjects, it may be necessary to test 250 infants. In addition, extra precautions and special procedures beyond those used with adults must be followed to ensure the safety of subjects. Faced with these extra demands, a researcher might be tempted to ask if everything worth knowing about speech perception could be learned simply by testing adults. Unfortunately, a drawback of using adult subjects to delineate the perceptual mechanisms underlying speech recognition is their experience with language. This presents a number of problems. First, adults may not rely solely on the acoustic information in the speech signal. Instead, they may draw upon syntax, semantics, and pragmatics. Second, if experience with the sound structure of a language influences the operation of basic perceptual capacities, there is no way of knowing in what way the sensitivity of these mechanisms has been changed by this experience. Consequently, one way of avoiding the problems of understanding how the basic perceptual capacities function in their mature state is to study them in their initial state and how they are changed as a native language is acquired.

The study of speech perception by infants began over 25 years ago. Progress before that time was impeded by inadequate methodology. One basic difficulty is finding the means of posing the experimental question so as to ensure a coherent answer. For subjects without language and with a very limited response repertoire, asking the questions in the right way is almost an art. Moreover, because infants develop so rapidly during the first year of life, methods that are effective at one age may be ineffective at another age. Most methods monitor the way infants respond to a change in auditory stimulation. Usually the infant is familiarized with a particular speech sound, and at some point a different sound is introduced. How the infant reacts to the new sound indicates whether the infant has detected a difference

between the two sounds. Other methods have been devised to investigate preferences for different types of speech materials. These often compare how long infants orient to different types of speech samples. Finally, some procedures investigate the way infants categorize speech sounds. Ideally, such procedures involve training the infants to produce one response to one category and a different response to another category (much like adults who might be asked to label sounds as /ba/ or /da/). Then as new items are introduced, the researcher would note which of the trained responses the infants make. In practice, this has been difficult to implement, so researchers have often had to resort to more indirect measures of categorization. Various methods will be discussed in more detail in conjunction with particular studies. But first, consider the kinds of issues typically addressed in studies of speech perception by infants.

Much pioneering research in infant speech perception was directed at whether infants can distinguish between different speech sounds, or whether perceiving differences between simple sounds like /ba/ and /pa/ is learned after some period of exposure to the native language (Eimas et al., 1971; Moffit, 1971; Morse, 1972; Trehub, 1973). As it became apparent that some capacity for detecting differences between speech sounds was present in the first months of life, researchers began to address a number of other issues related to discriminative capacities. One was the range of contrasts to which infants are sensitive. Are some speech contrasts more difficult for infants to perceive than others? A related question is whether infants are sensitive only to contrasts in the language spoken in their home or whether they can also discriminate foreign language contrasts. A different issue is the nature of the underlying mechanisms and whether they are specific to speech perception or operate more broadly in auditory perception.

Information about the discriminative capacities of infants provides a foundation for asking about how other elements of speech perception develop. Studies exploring the basic perceptual capacities are conducted under carefully controlled conditions with minimal possibility for distractions. Infants are often presented with only a pair of stimuli so as to determine what they can discriminate under the best of circumstances. Knowledge of these limits is important for understanding how infants function in real-world communicative situations. Knowing the perceptual limitations of the infant helps in understanding whether some communicative failure is attributable to perceptual factors or to other domains of cognitive functioning such as memory or attention. Research on how memory and attention interact with speech perception capacities is relatively new (Kuhl and Miller, 1982; Goodsitt et al., 1984; Jusczyk et al., 1990; Nozza et al., 1990). However, this area of research is important for understanding how the underlying capacities develop to support the perception of fluent speech.

One important element of fluent speech perception is being able to recognize the same word when spoken by different talkers or in different contexts. Because the acoustic characteristics of speech are a direct consequence of the shape of the vocal tracts that produce them, no two utterances will be acoustically identical. The vocal tracts of different talkers differ in many ways, so there is considerable acoustic variability in the pronunciation of a particular word. When and how infants can cope with such variability has been of great interest to researchers in speech perception. The ability to compensate for these acoustic differences and recognize the same utterance produced by different talkers, sometimes referred to as *perceptual normalization* (Kuhl, 1979), is an essential part of acquiring a native language.

The role of infant speech perception capacities in the acquisition of language is receiving considerable attention. Investigations have focused on the way such capacities help the infant to acquire a native language (Hirsh-Pasek et al., 1987; Bertoncini et al., 1988; Mehler et al., 1988; Fernald, 1989; Cooper and Aslin, 1990; Jusczyk et al., 1993). These studies explore how speech perception may help not only in acquiring the sound structure of language but also its syntactic and semantic properties. Another issue relates to how learning a native language affects speech perception capacities themselves (Werker and Tees, 1984a; Best, McRoberts and Sithole, 1988; Werker and Lalonde, 1988; Greiser and Kuhl, 1989, Kuhl, 1991). These studies trace the way sensitivity to native and nonnative contrasts changes as language is acquired. Hence, one of the more interesting developments in recent infant speech perception research has been to

tie the field more closely to general issues in the study of language acquisition.

The remainder of this chapter will briefly review the basic perceptual capacities of infants and then concentrate on attempts to examine how these capacities may be used in communication and language acquisition.

THE SPEECH PERCEPTION CAPACITIES OF INFANTS

What Infants Do with Native Language Contrasts

When Eimas et al. (1971) undertook their study of infant speech perception, it was not obvious that infants in the first few months of life could discriminate any speech contrasts. One of the major theories of speech perception, the **motor theory,** held that speech was perceived by reference to the kinds of articulatory movements used in its production (Liberman et al., 1967). Given this position, it was reasonable to suppose that the perception of speech sound differences by infants might require some experience producing speech and linking the sounds with particular articulatory movements. Because the infants in the Eimas et al. (1971) study were too young to have done much babbling (the youngest were only 1 month old), they lacked experience tying production to perception, so they might be expected not to discriminate speech contrasts. Thus, one objective of the study was to determine whether experience in producing speech is necessary to perceive differences in speech sounds. In addition, the researchers wished to explore the extent to which infants' speech perception capacities mirrored those of adults. Among adults, certain kinds of contrasts, such as stop consonant distinctions, require **categorical perception** (Liberman et al., 1967). This means that the ability to discriminate between two speech sounds is only about as good as the ability to assign them to different phoneme categories (as with [ba] and [pa]). Thus, differences between speech sounds from within the same phonemic category (two different [ba]s) are difficult for adults to detect (Fig. 9-1). Categorical perception is the exception rather than the rule for the way stimuli are perceived. In most instances the ability to discriminate differences among stimuli far exceeds the ability to label the stimuli. At the time of the Eimas et al. (1971) study there was considerable speculation about

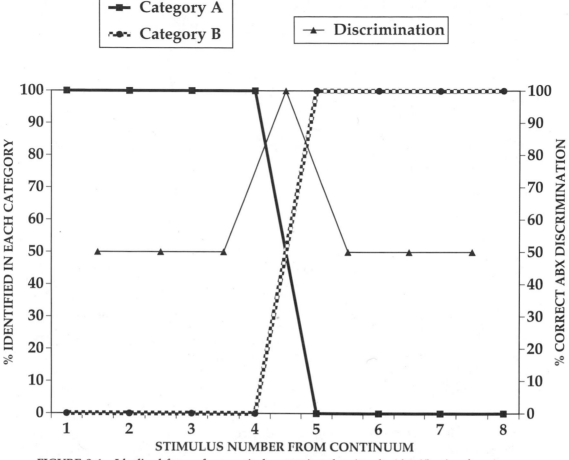

FIGURE 9-1   Idealized form of categorical perception showing the identification function (left ordinate) and the ABX discrimination function (right ordinate). (Adapted from Studdert-Kennedy, M., Liberman, A. M., Harris, K. S., & Cooper, F. S. [1970]. Motor theory of speech perception: A reply to Lane's critical review. *Psychological Review, 77,* 234-249.)

whether categorical perception was innate or learned.

Eimas et al. examined how infants respond to the voicing distinction that differentiates [ba] from [pa]. They used a version of the high-amplitude sucking (HAS) procedure developed by Siqueland and DeLucia (1969; see also Jusczyk, 1985b). In this procedure the infant is given a nonnutritive pacifier. The pacifier is connected to a pressure transducer that registers sucking responses. After a baseline measure of sucking without any auditory stimulation is taken, the familiarization period begins. At this time the presentation of a syllable is made contingent on the infant's sucking rate. The more often the infant sucks, the more often the syllables are played. Once infants have picked up the contingency, they will often suck at a high rate for several minutes, after which time they begin to habituate to the familiar syllable. Once

the sucking rate drops below a predetermined level, the test period begins. Because they were interested in not only whether infants could discriminate the voicing contrast but also whether the discriminative response was categorical, the researchers used three types of treatment conditions (Fig. 9-2). The control group continued to hear exactly the same syllable as during the familiarization period. A second group, the between categories group, heard a new syllable from the other phonemic category ([pa]) that differed in voicing characteristics from the familiar syllable ([ba]). The third group, the within categories group, also heard a new syllable that differed in voicing from the one heard during the familiarization period. However, in this case the new syllable came from the same phonemic category as the familiar syllable. The rationale behind HAS is that because infants respond to novelty, if they

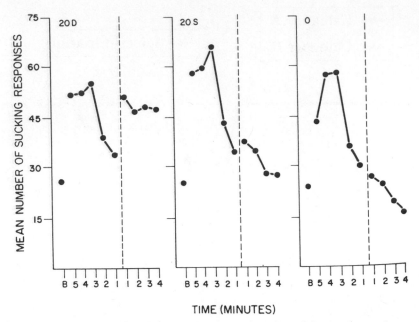

FIGURE 9-2 Mean number of sucking responses as a function of time and experimental condition for 4-month-old infants. The dashed line indicates the stimulus shift, or in the case of the control group, the time at which the shift would have occurred. Time is measured from 5 minutes before to 4 minutes after stimulus shift. B = baseline shift. 20D = between phonetic category case; 20S = within phonetic category case; 0 = no change case. (From Eimas, P. D., Siqueland, E. R., Jusczyk, P., & Vigorito, J. [1971]. Speech perception in infants. *Science, 171,* 304.)

detect a change in the syllables during the during the test period, they will show a significant increase in sucking rate. In this study this happened only for the between categories group. Hence, the infants discriminated a change from [ba] to [pa] but not among syllables from within the same phonemic category (such as two different [pa]s). Therefore, in addition to showing that infants can discriminate differences between speech sounds before they produce speech, Eimas et al. (1971) found that infants' responses followed a pattern consistent with categorical perception in adults (i.e., they discriminated pairs between categories but not pairs within categories).

This study provided the first indication that infants as young as 1 month old can perceive differences between speech sounds. Confirmation of this capacity came from several other laboratories shortly thereafter. Trehub and Rabinovitch (1972) replicated the finding by using a [ba]-[pa] contrast and extended the results by showing that infants could also distinguish a voicing contrast between [da] and [ta]. Two other studies examined a phonemic contrast differing in place of articulation ([ba] versus [ga]). Morse (1972) used a version of HAS and found that 2-month-olds discriminated

this contrast. Moffitt (1971) used an entirely different procedure, heart rate dishabituation, to test 5-month-olds and also obtained evidence of discrimination of this contrast*. Although neither Morse nor Moffitt tested whether discrimination of the place of articulation contrast followed a categorical pattern, Eimas (1974) found evidence for this in a study of the distinction between [bæ] and [dæ].

Subsequently, a number of studies were undertaken to determine the kinds of consonantal distinctions that infants are able to make. Eimas (1975) tested 2- to 3-month-olds on the distinction between [ra] and [la]. This distinction is of interest not only because it appears relatively late in the development of speech production (Templin, 1957; Strange and Broen, 1971) but also because nonnative speakers of English often have difficulty with it (Miyawaki et al., 1975). Eimas found that American infants displayed

---

*This procedure monitors the infant's heart rate response in relation to auditory stimulation. A single syllable is presented to the infant until the heart rate returns to the resting level, measured prior to the introduction of the auditory stimulus. Then a different syllable is played. A significant change in heart rate on the introduction of the new item is taken as evidence that the infant has detected the difference between the new item and the previous one.

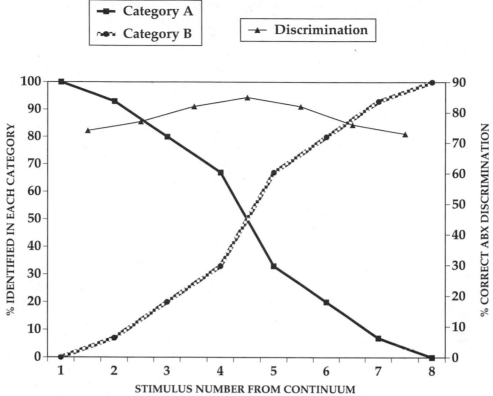

FIGURE 9-3 Idealized form of continuous perception of a vowel series showing the identification function (left ordinate) and the ABX discrimination function (right ordinate).

categorical perception of this contrast. Other kinds of manner of articulation distinctions were also investigated. Eimas and Miller (1980b) tested infants on the oral-nasal distinction for [ba] versus [ma]. Although they found that 2- to 4-month-olds discriminated this contrast, they did not find significant evidence that discrimination was categorical (i.e., the infants were also able to perceive within-category distinctions). There is also evidence from studies with 2-month-olds (Eimas and Miller, 1980a; Miller and Eimas, 1983) and with 6- to 8-month-olds (Hillenbrand, Minifie, and Edwards, 1979) that infants discriminate the stop-glide distinction between [b] and [w].

The studies mentioned thus far all used contrasts that involve at least one stop consonant. Other investigations have examined the perception of contrast within different manner of articulation classes. Eimas and Miller (1980b) found that infants could discriminate place of articulation contrasts involving nasals ([ma] versus [na]), and Jusczyk, Copan, and Thompson (1978) reported the same result for glides ([wa] versus [ja]). A number of studies have focused on fricatives (Eilers and Minifie, 1975;

Eilers, 1977; Eilers, Wilson, and Moore, 1977; Holmberg, Morgan, and Kuhl, 1977; Levitt et al., 1988). Eilers (1977) used a version of HAS and tested 3-month-olds on [s] versus [z]. She found evidence that this contrast was discriminated when it occurred syllable-finally as in [as] versus [az], but not syllable-initially as in [sa] versus [za], (but see the discussion of the latter result in Jusczyk [1981] and Aslin, Pisoni, and Jusczyk [1983]. Several place of articulation contrasts between fricatives have also been studied. Eilers and Minifie (1975) found that infants at least 2 to 4 months old discriminated a contrast between [sa] and [θa]. Similarly, Levitt et al. (1988) obtained evidence that 2-month-olds can discriminate between [fa] and [θa].

Vowel contrasts have received less attention than consonant contrasts from speech researchers who work with infants. One reason may be that vowels tend to be perceived more like nonspeech sounds — continuously rather than categorically (Fig. 9-3). That is, within-category discrimination for vowels is considerably better than chance (Fry et al., 1962; Stevens et al., 1969; Pisoni, 1973). Trehub (1973) conducted the first investigation of vowel discrimination by infants. She used HAS to present natural speech tokens of two different vowel pairs ([a] versus [i], [i] versus [u]) to 1- to 4-month-old infants. The infants discriminated both pairs of vowels. Swoboda, Morse, and Leavitt (1976) presented 2-month-olds with a contrast between [i] and [I] in their study using HAS. They tested not only for discrimination of the contrast but also whether perception was continuous or categorical. Their results indicated that infants discriminated both within-category and between-category pairs, suggesting that perception of this contrast is continuous.

These studies show that within the first 4 months of life, infants can discriminate the kinds of phonetic contrasts in their native language. The presence of these capacities during the early stages of development suggests that their basic mechanisms are innate. Consequently, further questions were raised both about the generality of these capacities (whether they are limited to native language sounds) and their specificity (whether they are specialized for speech perception).

Perception of Nonnative Language Contrasts by Infants

As evidence of infants' abilities to discriminate native language contrasts accumulated, researchers began to investigate the perception of nonnative contrasts. One question was the extent to which experience affects the way basic speech perception capacities manifest themselves. The early studies in this area presented infants with contrasts that do not occur in their native language. For example, Streeter (1976) used HAS to test Kikuyu infants on the voicing contrast between [ba] and [pa]. This distinction does not occur in Kikuyu. Nevertheless, the infants could discriminate it. Similarly, Lasky, Syrdal-Lasky, and Klein (1975) used a cardiac measure and found that 4½- to 6-month-old Guatemalan infants discriminated the English voicing contrast between [ba] and [pa], although the voicing distinction in Spanish is not the same as in English (Lisker and Abramson, 1977; Williams, 1977). Yet the infants discriminated the English voicing contrast but not the Spanish one. This finding suggests that both innate and experiential factors affect perceptual boundaries for fluent speakers of a language. The English contrast in this case maps more closely the innate perceptual boundary than does the Spanish one.

A number of studies also examined the ability of infants from English-speaking homes to perceive foreign language contrasts. The most heavily studied contrast is the prevoiced-voiced contrast in languages such as Thai (Lisker and Abramson, 1964). A number of questions surrounding methodological issues cloud the interpretation of the early studies in this area (Eimas, 1975; Eilers, Gavin, and Wilson, 1979; Eilers, Wilson, and Moore, 1979; Aslin, Pisoni, and Jusczyk, 1983). However Aslin, et al. (1981) reported evidence of discrimination of this contrast by 6-month-old American infants. They used a version of a head-turning procedure originally described by Suzuki and Ogiba (1961) and widely used today (Eilers, Wilson, and Moore 1977; Kuhl, 1979; Werker and Tees, 1984a). The infant is seated on a caregiver's lap facing an experimenter (Fig. 9-4). To one side of the experimenter are a loudspeaker and a smoked-glass box that covers an animated toy. A speech sound is played repeatedly through the loudspeaker. At various times the speech sound changes for about a 4-second period. Then the original background sound returns and plays continuously until the next sound change. If the infant looks at the loudspeaker during the change interval, the smoked-glass box lights up and the toy is animated (for a more complete description of this procedure, see Kuhl [1985]). In the Aslin et al. (1991) experiment, this procedure was combined with a computer-controlled adaptive staircase algorithm to eliminate experimenter and response biases. This made it possible to determine the smallest difference required for reliable discrimination from the repeating background stimulus. Although the differences required to discriminate the prevoiced-voiced contrast were considerably larger than for the voiced-voiceless contrast, all the infants met the criterion for discrimination.

Trehub (1976) reported a study with 1- to 4-month-old English Canadian infants listening to two other types of foreign language contrasts. One of these was oral-nasal vowel contrast ([pa] versus [pã]) that occurs in languages including Polish and French. The other contrast was between [řa] and [za], which occurs in Czech. The infants were able to discriminate each type of contrast. Other studies undertaken by Werker et al. (1981); Werker and Tees, (1984a); Werker and Lalonde (1988); and by Best and her colleagues (Best, Roberts, and Sithole, 1988; Best, 1991) have shown that 6-month-olds from

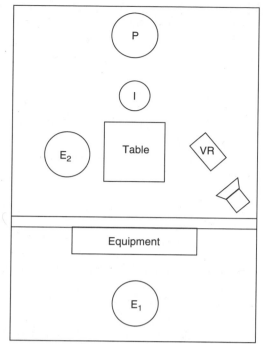

E₁- Experimenter 1
E₂- Experimenter 2
P- Parent
I- Infant
VR- Visual Reinforcer

FIGURE 9-4   The setup used in the head-turn procedure. The infant (I) has to turn the head toward the loudspeaker when the sounds change. A correct head turn is reinforced by the activation of toy animals in the box (VR). An experimenter in an adjacent room (E₁) who cannot hear the sounds presses a button that activates the toy when the infant turns following a change in sounds.

English-speaking homes can discriminate contrasts from various African, Indian, and Native American languages.

The picture that emerges from these early studies is that the capacities of infants to discriminate speech contrasts extend considerably beyond those that infants are likely to have encountered in their native environment. Thus, infants do not appear to require long exposure to speech contrasts to discriminate them. These results are often interpreted as an indication that infants are born with the capacity to discriminate phonetic contrasts that may occur in any language (Eimas, Miller, and Jusczyk, 1987). Experience appears to narrow the discrimination process to focus on contrasts in the native language.

Exploring the Nature of the Underlying Mechanisms

For many years researchers have been trying to understand the nature of the mechanisms that underlie speech processing by infants. To what extent are such mechanisms specialized adaptations for speech perception as opposed to a part of general auditory processing capacities? De-

bate in this area was initially fueled by claims that certain characteristics of speech processing, especially categorical perception, were not to be found in other realms of perceptual processing (Liberman et al., 1967). However, with the demonstration of categorical perception for nonspeech contrasts (Miller et al., 1976; Pisoni, 1977) and of nonhuman mammals apparently showing evidence of categorical perception (Kuhl and Miller, 1975, 1978), the focus has moved from categorical perception to other aspects of speech processing that are believed to be unique.

One of the first attempts to examine differences in speech and nonspeech discrimination among infants was the Eimas (1974; see also Eimas, 1975) study. Not only did Eimas test 2- to 3-month-olds' ability to discriminate contrasts between the syllables [bæ] and [dæ], but also their discrimination of nonspeech signals involving the same kinds of acoustic changes. Thus, Eimas isolated the second-formant transitions from his syllables and used these as nonspeech stimuli. The infants were able to discriminate both the speech and nonspeech contrasts. Nevertheless, discrimination was categorical

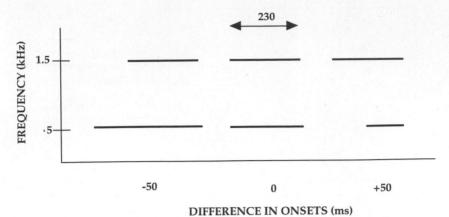

FIGURE 9-5 Schematic representations of three stimuli differing in relative onset time: leading (− 50 ms), simultaneous (0 ms), and lagging (+ 50 ms). (Adapted from Pisoni, D. B. [1977]. Identification and discrimination of the relative onset time of two-component tones: Implications for voicing perception in stops. *Journal of the Acoustical Society of America, 61,* 1352-1361.)

only for the speech contrasts. On the basis of this difference Eimas argued for specialized speech processing mechanisms. However, the speech and nonspeech sounds differed greatly in their durations and overall complexity.

Several studies have demonstrated categorical discrimination of nonspeech contrasts by infants. Jusczyk et al. (1980) used two-component tone stimuli that differed in the relative onset of one tone component to the other (Fig. 9-5). Previous work by Pisoni (1977) established that adults group these types of stimuli into three different perceptual categories. Jusczyk et al. found that, like adults, 2-month-olds could discriminate pairs of items that differed in their temporal onset characteristics and that their performance was categorical. That is, the infants detected the temporal order differences for some of the stimulus pairs but not for others. Subsequently, Jusczyk, et al. (1989) conducted a study directly comparing 2-month-olds' discrimination of voicing differences for speech sounds with their discrimination of temporal order differences in nonspeech pairs. Parallels were found in the locus of the infants' category boundaries for the speech and nonspeech pairings and it was concluded that the same general auditory processing mechanism could underlie the discrimination of the speech and nonspeech contrasts.

Other attempts to identify differences in speech and nonspeech processing by infants have focused on the way context affects perceptual boundaries. For example, in their study of

[ba] versus [wa], Eimas and Miller (1980a; Miller and Eimas, 1983) noted that changes in syllable durations corresponding to changes in speaking rate affected the way infants perceived acoustic cues that distinguish [ba] and [wa]. They argued that since a parameter like speaking rate affected perception of the contrast, the underlying mechanisms must be specific to speech. However, in a subsequent study Jusczyk et al. (1983) demonstrated comparable effects for the discrimination of nonspeech sine wave stimuli. Specifically, 2-month-olds showed systematic shifts in their category boundaries for sine wave contrasts when the overall duration of the stimuli changed. Thus, once again parallels were observed between the way speech and nonspeech contrasts are discriminated by young infants.

Although the number of studies of comparisons between speech and nonspeech processing by infants is relatively small, thus far the results appear to correspond closely. This suggests that at least in the early stages of speech processing, the underlying mechanisms are ones that function not only in speech but also in general auditory processing.

Coping with Stimulus Variability

Among the capacities of fluent speakers of a language is the ability to compensate for acoustic differences in the pronunciation of the same word by different talkers or even by the same talker on different occasions. This ability is called *perceptual normalization* (Rand, 1971; Verbrugge et al., 1976; Bladon, Henton, and Pickering, 1984). It is an important part of speech perception because it gives the listener access to the same meaning for a word despite the variations in the acoustic signal. Without some ability to perform perceptual normalization, the task of acquiring a language would be insurmountable.

The first investigations of infants' capacity for coping with variability in the signal were conducted by Kuhl (1976; Kuhl and Miller, 1982) who tested 1- to 4-month-olds using a version of HAS. In one experiment infants were exposed to two variants of [a]; one was produced with a monotone and the other with a rise-fall pitch contour. Once the habituation criterion was obtained, infants in the experimental group heard two comparable versions of [i]. The issue was whether they would discriminate the vowel change despite the irrelevant variation of pitch, and they did. Interestingly enough, on a comparable test of their ability to discriminate pitch change when vowel quality varied irrelevantly, the infants were not successful. Because the size of the pitch changes were not equated with the size of the vowel changes, it could not be determined whether infants are simply more sensitive to vowel changes than to pitch changes (Carrell, Smith, and Pisoni, 1981). In any case, infants in this age range show at least some ability to compensate for variability in the speech signal.

Much of the research in this area has been conducted with 6-month-olds using the head-turn paradigm. Kuhl (1979) expanded on her earlier work by varying both pitch contour and the voice of the talker. She first trained infants to discriminate [a] from [i] when the talker's voice and pitch contour were held constant. When infants met the discrimination criterion for the initial pairing, they were tested for their ability to compensate for changes in pitch contour and talker's voice. The variability among the vowel tokens was increased in stages. Ultimately, there were tokens of each vowel produced by three different talkers and two different pitch contours. Despite these variations, the infants maintained the discrimination between [a] and [i]. Subsequently, Kuhl (1983) tested infants on a perceptually more difficult contrast, [a] versus [ɔ]. One of the factors that makes this contrast difficult is that when productions from different talkers are used, the two vowel categories acoustically overlap. Nevertheless, once they

had passed the training stage, infants coped with the variations among the tokens produced by the different talkers. Hence these studies provide clear evidence that by 6 months of age, infants display some capacity to ignore the kinds of variations produced by changing from one talker to another.

Later Jusczyk, Pisoni, and Mullennix (1992) sought to determine not only whether 2-month-olds show evidence of perceptual normalization for the talker's voice but also whether speech processing has costs associated with normalization. HAS was used and infants were presented with tokens of the words "bug" and "dug" produced by six male and six female talkers. During the familiarization phase, infants in one test group heard all 12 tokens of one of the words, and during the test phase they heard the tokens of the other word. Infants discriminated the pair despite variations in talker's voice. In fact, they did not differ significantly from a comparable group who heard only a token of each word produced by a single talker (Fig. 9-6). To this point the results and conclusions are similar to what Kuhl observed for 6-month-olds. However, in a second experiment a 2-minute delay between the familiarization and test phases was introduced. Now, to discriminate the contrast, infants have to retain during the delay information about the identity of the word heard in the familiarization phase. Infants in the single-talker condition continued to discriminate the contrast despite the delay. However, infants in the multiple-talker condition, who heard all 12 tokens of each word, did not show evidence of discrimination following the delay. Thus, talker variability apparently interfered with the infants' retention of information about the speech sounds. Two additional experiments demonstrated that even variability among the tokens of a single talker can affect the infant's encoding and retrieval of information about speech. Specifically, a comparable series of experiments used 12 different tokens of each word produced by the same talker. The results paralleled those observed for the multiple-talker condition. Once again, when tested without delay, infants in the multiple-token condition were able to discriminate the contrast. With the delay, only infants in the single-token condition gave evidence of discrimination. Thus, the results show that although 2-month-olds compensate for variability in speech, doing so may draw upon processing resources involved in the en-

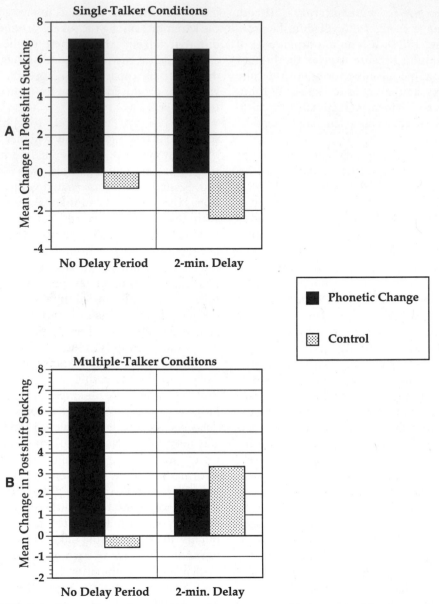

FIGURE 9-6   Mean change in postshift sucking responses for 2-month-olds. *A*, responses of infants exposed to syllables produced by a single talker with either no delay (left) or a 2-minute delay between the preshift and postshift periods. *B*, comparable data for infants exposed to syllables produced by 12 different talkers. (From Jusczyk, P. W., Pisoni, D. B., and Mullenix, J. [1992]. Some consequences of stimulus variability on speech processing by 2-month-old infants. *Cognition, 43,* 253-291.)

coding and retrieval of speech in long-term memory. Finally, there is evidence of normalization of a different sort: changes in speaking rate (Eimas and Miller, 1980a; Miller and Eimas, 1983). Thus, the dependencies observed in the way syllable duration affects the discrimination of [ba] versus [wa] by infants suggests that they can compensate for changes in speaking rate.

In summary, even in the earliest stages of development, infants show some capacity to cope with variability in speech production. They seem to compensate for variability in the signal produced by changes in talker's voice, speaking rate, and pitch contour. Nevertheless, as recent studies suggest, perceptual normalization may bear a cost to further processing of speech sounds.

SPEECH PERCEPTION AND LANGUAGE ACQUISITION

Once researchers gained some insight into the range of speech perception abilities of infants, they could begin to ask about the role of those abilities in acquiring a native language. One obvious area of interest concerns the way these capacities participate in the acquisition of the sound structure of language. Since each language has unique sound properties, the infant must learn about the regularities among the sounds in the native language. For instance, how and when do infants come to identify and order the distinctive sounds used in forming words in their language? Clearly, the basic speech perception capacities play a critical role in this process, but what exactly is the nature of their involvement? A related concern has to do with the development of a **mental lexicon** by which infants translate the acoustic signal into the appropriate set of meanings. A number of abilities related to speech perception are implicated in this process, including segmentation of the speech signal into the appropriate units, identification of the sequences of sounds in the units, and some capacity for retention of a description of the sound structure associated with a particular meaning. How, if at all, do speech perception capacities evolve to support the development of the mental lexicon?

It is much less obvious that speech perception capacities play any role in language development other than in acquiring its sound structure. Nevertheless, the acoustic signal may provide some clues to the underlying syntactic organization of the input (Gleitman and Wanner, 1982; Morgan, 1986; Hirsh-Pasek et al., 1987; Lederer and Kelly, 1991). For example, the language learner needs some means of grouping the input in ways consistent with its syntactic organization. To the extent that there are acoustic correlates of these units, speech perception capacities may help identify the syntax of the language.

This section focuses on the way research on infant speech perception is being integrated into the study of language acquisition: the way experience with language affects the underlying capacities, when elements necessary for the development of the mental lexicon are in place, and how speech perception capacities assist in acquiring important grammatical units.

How Experience Affects Speech Perception Capacities

It is well established that speakers of different native languages show differences in the way they categorize sounds along a particular phonetic dimension (Lisker and Abramson, 1964; Miyawaki et al., 1975; Williams, 1977; Werker and Tees, 1984b). Yet the cross-linguistic research reviewed earlier suggests strong similarities in the way infants from different cultures perceive particular speech contrasts. Of course, among the many developmental milestones between infancy and adulthood, the one most likely to influence the organization of speech perception capacities is the mastery of a native language.

How language acquisition affects the underlying speech perception capacities has been a subject of speculation for a long time. Aslin and Pisoni (1980) made the first serious attempt to lay out the possible ways speech perception capacities develop as a result of learning a particular language (Fig. 9-7). They identified five processes by which experience with language could modify the discriminability of sounds along phonetic dimensions. *Enhancement* occurs when stimuli in the vicinity of a perceptual category boundary become more discriminable. *Attenuation* is the reverse, when the stimuli in the category boundary region become less discriminable, such as is the case for [r] versus [l] among Japanese speakers. *Sharpening* and *broadening* are the ways stimuli in the category boundary regions become more finely or more poorly tuned respectively. Sharpening results in a more abrupt change in the identification of one category from another (as with stop consonants). Broadening leads to a more gradual transition between adjacent categories (as with vowel contrasts). In *realignment* the perceptual boundary between two phonetic categories undergoes a shift, as in the differences in the voiced-voiceless boundaries of English and Spanish speakers (Lisker and Abramson, 1964). With this framework, Aslin and Pisoni accounted for many results reported in infant and adult speech perception.

Even the earliest studies made some attempts to look at developmental changes in speech perception. For instance, Eimas et al. (1971) tested groups at 1 and 4 months of age for developmental changes in the perception of voicing contrasts during the first few months of life. How-

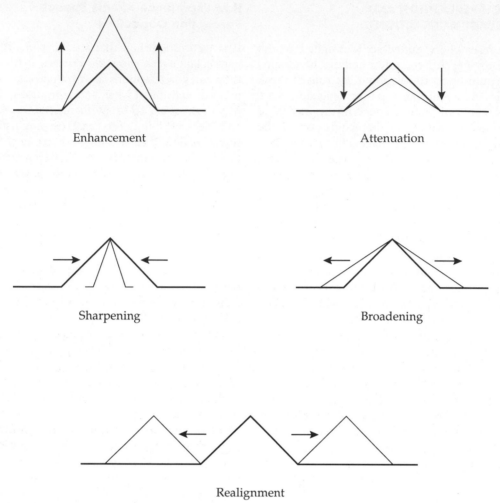

Enhancement

Attenuation

Sharpening

Broadening

Realignment

FIGURE 9-7   Five processes by which early experience in a particular language may selectively modify the relative discriminability of speech sounds based on a schematized ABX function. (Adapted from Aslin, R. N., & Pisoni, D. B. [1980]. Visual and auditory development in infancy. In Osofsky, J. D. (Ed.) *Handbook of infant development,* 2nd ed. New York: Wiley (pp. 5-97).

ever, they found no evidence of significant differences in these two age groups. In fact, until relatively recently (Bertoncini et al., 1988; Jusczyk et al., 1990), there was little indication of any developmental changes in speech perception during the first 4 months of life.

Werker and Tees (1984) provided the first evidence of important developmental changes in speech perception related to experience with a particular language. In an earlier study, Werker et al. (1981) found that 6-month-old Canadian infants could discriminate two different Hindi contrasts that do not occur in English. English-speaking Canadian adult listeners were unable to discriminate one of the contrasts and only some of them could discriminate the other one. Thus, it appeared that sensitivity to the Hindi contrasts declines for English speakers somewhere be-

tween infancy and adulthood. Werker and Tees attempted to pinpoint when the decline in sensitivity occurs. They tested Canadian infants from English-speaking homes at age 6 to 8 months, 8 to 10 months and 10 to 12 months on contrasts from Hindi, Nthlakampx (a northwest Native American language), and English. The 6- to 8-month-olds discriminated all three types of contrasts. By 8 to 10 months, only some discriminated the nonnative contrasts, and by 10 to 12 months, infants discriminated only the English contrast (Fig. 9-8). A longitudinal study using an additional group of Canadian infants verified this trend. To ensure that the poor performance by the older infants was not simply a general age-related decline in interest, they also tested several Hindi- and Nthlakampx-learning 11- to 12-month-olds. These infants

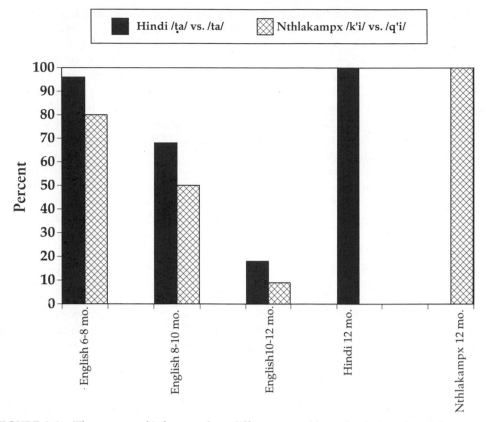

FIGURE 9-8   The percent of infants at three different ages able to discriminate English and non-English (Hindi and Nthlakampx) phonetic contrasts. (Adapted from Werker, J. F., & Tees, R. C. [1984a]. Cross language speech perception: Evidence for perceptual reorganization during the first year of life. *Infant Behavior and Development, 7,* 49-63.)

easily discriminated the contrasts from their native languages. Thus, Werker and Tees' results suggest that toward the end of the first year of life some sort of perceptual reorganization begins to occur, and sensitivity declines for contrasts not present in the native language.

Werker and Lalonde (1988) tested Canadian infants with a different, synthetically produced Hindi contrast and replicated the basic finding of a developmental decline in sensitivity to this contrast between 6 and 12 months of age. In addition, Best and McRoberts (1989), who used a different procedure, replicated the finding of a developmental decline between 6 and 12 months of age for the Nthlakampx contrast. Thus, the evidence for a developmental decline in sensitivity to nonnative contrasts appears to be fairly robust. Polka and Werker (1994) reported results of a study on cross-language vowel perception. Infants from English-speaking homes were presented with two sets of vowel contrasts from German ([U] versus [Y]

and [u:] versus [y:]) and an English vowel contrast ([a] versus [i]). Consistent with the previous work on consonant contrasts, 10- to 12-month-olds discriminated the English contrast but neither of the two German contrasts. However, in contrast to the previous studies, very few of the 6- to 8-month-olds met the criterion for discriminating either of the nonnative vowel pairs. Polka and Werker interpreted this finding as an indication that reorganization of vowel perception may occur earlier than consonant perception.

To this point, the picture that emerges from these cross-linguistic studies is that if a particular phonetic contrast does not appear in the speech input to the infant, sensitivity to this contrast will decline in the course of development. However, some data suggest that this generalization does not hold across all contrasts. Best, McRoberts, and Sithole (1988) found that English-learning infants at four ages (6 to 8, 8 to 10, 10 to 12, and 12 to 14 months of age) could discriminate a medial versus lateral **click** contrast found in Zulu but not in English. They suggested that the decline observed in previous studies may occur only when the nonnative contrasts are allophonic variants of a native language phonemic category. By comparison, sounds that fall outside the boundaries of native language, as Zulu clicks do for English, may continue to be perceived. The researchers developed a scheme for predicting which kinds of nonnative contrasts should be easy or hard to discriminate depending on how they map on categories in the native language. However, in subsequent research (Best et al., 1990; Best, 1991), 10- to 12-month-olds were significantly worse than 6- to 8-month-olds in discriminating a Zulu fricative click contrast. This contrast does map on two native language categories and therefore should be discriminated according to the model. By comparison, and in accordance with the researchers' predictions, infants in this age group discriminated another contrast between two Ethiopian ejectives that also maps onto two different English-language categories.

To summarize to this point, the results of studies investigating developmental changes in cross-linguistic perception suggest that experience in learning a particular language begins to affect underlying speech perception capacities by the end of the first year of life, if not sooner. At the same time, it is clear that not all phonetic categories are equally affected by the input that the infant receives. Some contrasts appear to be maintained despite their absence from speech input to the child. At present, it is not clear just what factors are responsible for whether a given contrast absent from the input is maintained.

Thus far, this discussion has focused on the consequences of lack of experience—that is, how perception of nonnative contrasts is affected. One can also ask about the way linguistic experience affects the way speech sounds from the native language are perceived. Kuhl (1991) and Greiser and Kuhl (1989) have reported findings suggesting that linguistic experience may affect the organization of native language vowel categories by 6 months of age. In particular, Kuhl (1991) argues that infants' vowel categories may be organized around prototypical instances. In one study using the head-turn procedure (Greiser and Kuhl, 1989), infants were exposed to either a prototypical instance (as judged by adults) or a poor instance of the vowel [i]. The particular instance was the

background stimulus, and novel instances from the category were used as test stimuli. In effect, the procedure measured the way infants generalize from the background stimulus to the novel stimuli. The results showed that when the prototypical instance was the background stimulus, the infants generalized to a significantly larger number of novel vowels. Kuhl (1991) replicated these results with a set of stimuli that provided twice the degree of acoustic variation as in the original study. In comparing the effects of the prototypical and poor instances, she found that even when the test involved the same four stimuli, generalization was much greater if the **prototype** was the background stimulus. She interprets this finding as an indication that prototypical instances form perceptual magnets that shorten perceptual distances between the center and stimuli at the edges of the category. Kuhl notes that monkeys tested with the same stimuli fail to show the same kinds of asymmetries in generalization for the prototypical and bad instances of the vowel category. Thus she speculates that the asymmetries may arise from experience in listening to a specific language.

To master the sound structure of the native language, the infant must learn something about **phones,** or the elementary sounds used in the language, and **phonotactics,** or the way they are ordered. If infants initially can perceive any phonetic distinction in any language, a good part of learning the sound structure of the language involves determining which segments are used and what constraints hold on how these segments can be ordered to form words.

From birth, infants may be sensitive to certain properties of the sound of the native language. Mehler et al. (1988) found that 4-day-olds show a preference for listening to extended passages of speech in their mothers' native language as opposed to ones from a foreign language. French infants' sucking responses were monitored while they listened to passages produced by a French and Russian bilingual talker. The infants sucked at higher rates for the French passages. Moreover, the same pattern of responding occurred when most of the phonetic information was removed by low-pass filtering the utterances. This finding suggests that the infants were responding to features in the **prosody** of speech, such as its characteristic stress patterns, intonation contours, and rhythms. This preference may be the result of prenatal experience of the mother's speech, since prosodic in-

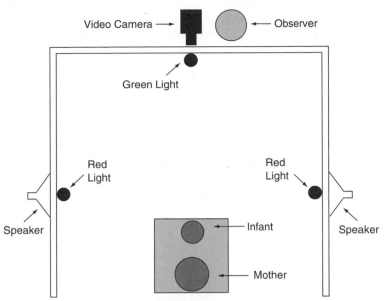

FIGURE 9-9 Layout of the testing booth used in the head-turn preference procedure. The infant is seated on the mother's lap facing the center panel. The observer behind the panel looks through holes in the pegboard to judge head turns.

formation falls within the range of frequencies transmitted through the uterus to the fetus (Vince et al., 1981). When they tested infants on comparisons of two languages neither of which the mother spoke, the infants gave no evidence of discriminating. Thus, some familiarity with the language is necessary before the infant distinguishes its prosodic characteristics from those of another language. Notwithstanding this, within the first few days of life, infants appear to be closely attuned to the prosody of the native language.

Jusczyk et al. (1993) sought to determine when infants become sensitive to more fine-grained features of the native language — its phonetic and phonotactic characteristics. This issue was explored by testing when infants begin to distinguish native from foreign words. A bilingual Dutch and English talker recorded 16 lists of low-frequency two- and three-syllable words in each language for presentation to the infants. Many of the words in each list contained phonetic segments or sequences of segments not permissible in the other language. These words were presented to infants using a version of the head-turn preference procedure (Fernald, 1985; Hirsh-Pasek et al., 1987; Kemler Nelson, Jusczyk, Mandel, Myers, Turk, and Gerken, in press). Each infant sat on a caregiver's lap in the middle of a three-sided enclosure (Fig. 9-9). The English word lists were presented from a loud-speaker on one side of the room, and the Dutch word lists were presented on the opposite side. The amount of time that infants oriented toward the loudspeaker playing each type of list was recorded and used as an index of preference. Comparable groups of Dutch and American infants were tested. At 6 months of age neither group showed significant preferences. However, at 9 months of age, both groups displayed significant preferences for their native language. To determine whether the infants were responding to the phonetic content of the utterances, a second experiment was conducted using low-pass filtered versions of the lists. With the phonetic content removed, the 9-month-olds no longer showed a significant preference for the native language lists. These results suggest that the infants were responding to the fine-grained phonetic and phonotactic features of the utterances. Hence, by 9 months of age, infants appear to have acquired considerable information about the sound properties of the native language.

To delineate when infants can use different kinds of information in the speech signal to differentiate native from nonnative language, two additional experiments were conducted using English and Norwegian, which also contrast considerably in prosody. This time it was found that 6-month-old American infants did display a consistent preference for the English word lists. Moreover, when the materials were low-pass filtered, the infants continued to show a significant preference for the English lists, suggesting that they were attentive to the prosodic characteristics that distinguish English words from Norwegian words. Thus, there appears to be a developmental progression in when infants learn characteristic features of the sound pattern of the native language. Sensitivity to the prosody of the native language appears to develop before sensitivity to phonetic and phonotactic features.

Take note of the interesting convergence between the development of sensitivity to the particular sound properties of the native language and the apparent decline in sensitivity to foreign language contrasts. Attention to fine-grained phonetic and phonotactic features develops around 9 months of age, also when discrimination of some foreign language contrasts begins to show a marked decline. Moreover, it appears that some aspects of the sound structure of the native language are acquired sooner than others. The prosody of the language is apparently noticed earlier than the finer-grained phonetic and phonotactic features. In addition, perhaps because vowels are important carriers of prosodic features, learning the vowels of the native language may precede learning the consonants.

Developments Relevant to the Formation of the Mental Lexicon

When psychologists talk about the mental lexicon, they have in mind some storehouse of information akin to a dictionary in which meanings of words are linked to their sound structures. In speech recognition, to extract meaning from the acoustic signal, the listener must segment the speech wave into the appropriate set of units (words) and use these as an entry to the lexicon. Thus, in speech recognition, the sound structure provides access to a word's meaning.

A consideration of what is required to recognize words in fluent speech suggests that the listener must discriminate one word type from another, ignore variability in the production of a particular word, and segment the speech stream into the right acoustic units. Beyond these abilities, some representation of the sound pattern of the word must be stored in long-term memory along with the meaning. This representation must be distinctive enough to allow the word to be distinguished from similar-sounding

words during speech recognition. Therefore, an important part of the recognition process depends on the encoding of the sound properties of words into long-term memory. So to understand how the mental lexicon develops, we need to know something about attentional and memory processes in infants. To which aspects of the speech signal do infants attend? What information about speech do infants retain in long-term memory?

A number of studies in the literature suggest that certain speech patterns are more apt to draw infants' attention than others. For example, infants prefer speech produced by their own mother to that of another person (Mills and Meluish, 1974; Mehler et al., 1978; DeCasper and Fifer, 1980). In addition, infants display a clear preference for **child-directed speech** over adult-directed speech (Fernald, 1985; Fernald and Kuhl, 1987; Werker and McLeod, 1989). Work by Cooper and Aslin (1990) indicates that the preference for child-directed speech is present even in newborn infants. Speech directed to infants is typically slow, high-pitched, and more modulated in frequency and amplitude (Fernald et al., 1989; Cooper and Aslin, 1990). There is some indication that infants' preference for child-directed speech is due to fundamental frequency characteristics, such as pitch height and pitch modulation (Fernald and Kuhl, 1987). However, studies demonstrating that infants attend more closely to child-directed speech are of limited use in understanding how the lexicon develops because the preference measures used in such studies provide information only about the attractiveness of a whole phrase or passage. They do not address attention to a particular word or syllable, which is required for understanding the development of the lexicon.

One objective of research in this area is to discover what information infants extract from the speech signal under normal circumstances. Studies examining the consequences of talker variability (Kuhl, 1979, 1983; Jusczyk et al., 1992) show that infants can ignore at least some irrelevant variation in talker's voice to focus on dimensions relevant for distinguishing one word from another. A different kind of approach has been to assess the consequences of embedding speech in noise (Trehub, Bull, and Schneider, 1981; Nozza et al., 1990). These studies show that infants do discriminate speech sounds under such conditions, although they require signal-to-noise ratios from 6 to 12 dB higher than do adults.

One line of research that bears a little more directly on how attentional processes affect speech perception concerns the role of **syllable stress** in discriminating phonetic contrasts. Are phonetic contrasts better discriminated by infants in stressed as opposed to unstressed syllables? Early studies with two-syllable stimuli ([daba] versus [daga]) indicated that infants were equally good at detecting a contrast in stressed and unstressed syllables (Jusczyk, Copan, and Thompson, 1978; Jusczyk and Thompson, 1978). However, Karzon (1985) used three-syllable stimuli ([malana] versus [marana]) and found that infants detected the contrast only when the critical syllables received stress characteristic of child-directed speech. When processing load is sufficiently great, exaggerating the syllable stress perhaps helps in directing attention to a phonetic contrast. Further research of this sort may yield insights about information that infants encode in their representations of words. Certainly, there are a number of suggestions in the language acquisition literature that children may attend to and imitate information in stressed syllables (Brown and Fraser, 1964; Gleitman and Wanner, 1982; Gerken, Landau, and Remez, 1989; Gerken, 1994).

An indication of the importance of attentional focus in speech perception by infants comes from a study using a modified version of HAS (Jusczyk et al., 1990). The attentional focus was manipulated by varying the perceptual similarity of their stimuli. In some conditions, infants were habituated to a set of three syllables that included perceptually similar consonants ([pa], [ta], [ka]), whereas in other conditions the set contained syllables with three very dissimilar vowels ([bi], [ba], [bu]). It was hypothesized that infants would be more apt to focus on fine distinctions among the syllables for sets of the first type but on coarser distinctions for the second type. It was predicted that when focused on fine distinctions (i.e., for items that cluster closely in perceptual similarity space), the infants would be better at detecting the addition of a new syllable to the familiarization set than when focused on coarser distinctions (i.e., for items greatly separated in perceptual similarity space). These predictions were confirmed for 4-day-old infants. When 4-day-olds were exposed to the coarse distinction set ([bi], [ba],

[bu]), they did not detect the new syllable [bʌ] which is perceptually very similar to one of the set members ([ba]). However, for familiarization sets containing some fine-grained distinctions ([pa], [ka], [ma]), the 4-day-olds detected even the addition of a perceptually very similar syllable [ta] to the set. By 2 months of age, the infants appeared more resistant to the attentional manipulation (i.e., they detected the new syllable whether they were focused on fine or coarse distinctions during the familiarization period). One possible explanation for the difference between the two age groups is that the older groups were better able to cope with the processing demands of the task. If so, increased processing demands might bring about the same pattern as found with the 4-day-olds. Alternatively, the greater experience of 2-month-olds in hearing the native language (and the kinds of fine distinctions that occur therein) may make them more resistant to the attentional focus manipulation. In any event, the results to date demonstrate how attentional focus can affect the information that infants encode from speech.

In summary, the kinds of investigations necessary to understand how infants select information from the speech signal have only begun. More detailed knowledge of what the infant attends to is required for understanding how the lexicon develops. An interesting implication of the research manipulating attentional focus is that frequently heard sound contrasts may play a major role in determining the dimensions along which the developing lexicon is organized (see Lindblom [1986] for a similar suggestion).

Thus far, the possibility has been raised that infants are selective about the information in the speech signal. Attention to some details rather than others means that these are more likely to be encoded in some auditory representation of the sound and to be stored in long-term memory. However, this conjecture assumes that the infant only attends to, encodes, and remembers a partial description of the acoustic signal. What justification is there for making such an assumption? Why should infants' representations not be as detailed as their sensory capacities allow? In fact, the available data are not sufficient to exclude the possibility that infants do store fully specified, detailed copies of speech sounds. However, evidence from studies in related domains suggests that such detailed storage is implausible. For example, studies of categorical perception show that adults are sensitive

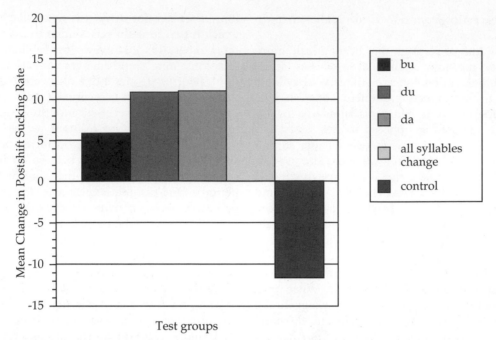

FIGURE 9-10 **Mean change in postshift sucking for 2-month-olds in various conditions.**
Scores were determined by subtracting the average sucking rates from the last 2 preshift minutes from the average of the first 2 postshift minutes. The groups are labeled according to the new syllable added during the postshift period. (From Jusczyk, P. W. and Derrah, C. [1987]. Representation of speech sounds by young infants. *Developmental Psychology, 23,* 648-654.)

to differences among tokens chosen from within the same category (Pisoni and Tash, 1974; Carney, Widin, and Veimeister, 1977; Samuel, 1977). Nevertheless, unless extraordinary measures are taken, information about these differences is not encoded during normal speech perception. Instead, only differences relevant to distinguishing among native language words appear to be encoded. Similarly, developmental studies of speech perception demonstrate that in the first few months of life infants are sensitive to distinctions that do not occur in their native language but that later on only contrasts that distinguish among native language words are encoded (Werker and Tees, 1984a; Werker and Lalonde, 1988). Thus, there is reason to believe that infants do not store everything about speech that they might.

Jusczyk and Derrah (1987) modified HAS to get a better indication of how infants represent speech sounds. Rather than presenting a single stimulus during the familiarization phase of the experiment, they used a randomized set of different stimuli. To detect a new item added to the familiar ones in the set, the infant has to do more than note whether the two successive stimuli are the same or different. Because the syllables in the familiarization set do differ from each other, the infant must encode enough distinctive information about each syllable to differentiate it from the others. Furthermore, the representations of the familiar syllables must be sufficiently distinct to discriminate each from the novel syllable that is added to the set. Therefore, by varying the similarity of the novel syllable to the familiar ones, it is possible to estimate the kind of detail that is encoded in the infants' representations.

In the Jusczyk and Perra study 2-month olds were familiarized with a randomized series of syllables that shared a common phonetic segment ([bi], [ba], [bo], [bə^]). Then a new syllable was added during the test phase. The novel syllable either shared ([bu]) or did not share ([du]) a phoneme with the other set members. It was hypothesized that if infants encode the syllables as sequences of phonetic segments, they might recognize that [bu] shared a segment with the other set members. Consequently, they might produce higher sucking rates for the more novel change, the one that did not share the common segment, [du]. The results (Fig. 9-10) showed that both types of changes were easily detected. There was no indication of increased responding to the syllable from the novel category. Hence, the study provided no evidence that 2-month-olds represent syllables as strings of phonetic segments.

A subsequent study by Bertoncini et al. (1988) replicated the basic finding for syllables with common consonant segments and demonstrated comparable results for syllables with common vowel segments ([bi], [si], [li], [mi]). In the latter case, the novel syllable added in the test phase either shared ([di]) or did not share ([da]) the same vowel. Another finding is also pertinent; it concerns a developmental difference that the researchers found between 4-day-old and 2-month-old infants. The 4-day-olds did not differentiate among the syllables if only the consonant was changed, but the 2-month-olds did. By comparison, when the change involved vowel differences, the 4-day-olds performed like the 2-month-olds. Although the researchers originally concluded that vowels might be more salient for the younger infants than consonants, an alternative explanation based on attentional factors seems more likely. Because very distinctive consonants were included in the familiarization set, the 4-day-olds may have focused on coarse distinctions and overlooked the finer distinction between [bi] and [di]. Recall the study on attentional factors (Jusczyk et al., 1990). When the familiarization set for the 4-day-olds included highly similar consonants, the infants could detect consonantal changes. In any case, the data from the Bertoncini et al. study suggest that 2-month-olds are apt to have more detailed representations of speech sounds than do 4-day-olds.

Developing a mental lexicon requires long-term memory of the sound pattern of each word. Thus, any immediate representation of speech sounds must eventually be encoded in long-term memory. To learn more about what information infants encode into representations stored in long-term memory, Jusczyk, Kennedy, and Jusczyk (1995) introduced a delay period filled with distracting visual materials between familiarization and test phases of the modified HAS procedure. For example, one group of 2-month-olds was familiarized with a randomized series consisting of [bi], [ba] and [bu] and then tested after the delay on a randomized series of [di], [da] and [du]. Had the infants' representations of the original series not contained sufficiently precise information about the nature of the syllables, the slight change that occurred in the test set might not have been detected. In fact, the infants retained considerable detail about the syllables during the delay. Even minimal changes of a single phonetic feature were detected. Nevertheless, there was little evidence that representations in long-term memory are structured in terms of phonetic segments at this stage of development. For example, performance was not affected by whether members of the familiarization set shared a common consonant ([bi], [ba], [bu]) or not ([si], [ba], [tu]).

More recently, Jusczyk, Jusczyk, et al. (in press) used a familiarization set of bisyllabic utterances that either shared a common CV syllable (the [ba] in the bisyllables [ba'lo], [ba'zi], [ba'dəs], [ba'mɪt]) or did not (i.e., [nɛ'lo], [pæ'zi], [ču'dəs], [ko'mɪt]). In this case, the presence of a common CV syllable in the familiarization set did lead to a significant improvement in detecting a new item in the test set. Only infants who were familiarized with the set containing the common syllable detected the addition of a new bisyllable ([pa'mʌl] or [na'bʌl]) during the test phase. It was concluded that the presence of the common CV syllable enhanced the encoding of these items during the delay and allowed them to be better remembered.

However, there is an alternative explanation for the results. The stimuli used in the study shared not only a common CV syllable but also two common phonetic segments, [b] and [a]. Thus, it may have been two common phonetic segments rather than a common syllable per se that led to better encoding and memory. To explore this possibility, an additional experiment was conducted in which the stimuli in the familiarization phase shared two common phonetic segments but in different syllables ([za'bi], [la'bo], [da'bəz], [ma'bɪt]). After the delay, a new bisyllabic item such as [ba'nʌl] or [na'bʌl] was added during the test phase. With these materials, the infants displayed no evidence of detecting the new item. The implication is that the common CV syllable, and not the individual phonetic segments, is critical for infants' encoding of speech.

More research is required to determine just what sort of information about speech infants encode into their long-term memories. To this point it appears that in the first few months of life, infants encode detailed information about speech in their perceptual representations and maintain it for at least a brief interval. Representations may become more detailed over the first couple of months of life. However, there is little evidence for representations structured in terms of phonetic segments at this period of development. Rather, any structuring of the input into representations in long-term memory may be in syllable-sized units.

Some studies with older infants address issues of the development of the lexicon. For example, Werker and Pegg (1992) report on several attempts to explore the nature of lexical representations in infants 12 to 20 months of age by testing them using a word-learning paradigm. They tried to teach infants to associate a nonsense label with an unfamiliar object and then tested for possible phonetic confusions between the learned nonsense label and a minimal-pair nonsense label. In the test phase, infants were shown two visual displays, one of the object that matched the original nonsense label and one that did not. Unfortunately, the results were inconclusive because for both the learned nonsense label and the minimal pair label the infants performed at chance levels (i.e., they looked at the correct and incorrect displays equally often). Pollock and Schwartz (1990) used a similar procedure but manipulated the amount of information in the foils by omitting the first phone, final phone, or a vowel. In one experiment, 18- to 20-month-olds showed some signs of treating the incomplete renditions of the test word as correct, but this pattern was not replicated in a second experiment.

Other investigations of word learning in older infants have focused on sensitivity to information about word boundaries in fluent speech, which is a likely prerequisite for correctly segmenting speech into words. Alternative solutions for achieving segmentation of fluent speech such as matching words in the lexicon that may have been learned in isolation against the input (Suomi, 1993) seem unlikely to get the infant very far. There are simply too many items that language learners are unlikely to hear in isolation (Jusczyk, 1993). Moreover, the acoustic structure of the same word heard in isolation and in casual speech is often very different. Finally, some words that might appear in isolation can also appear as syllables in larger words, leading to an incorrect segmentation of the input.

When mothers attempt to teach infants new words in sentential contexts, they may provide additional acoustic cues to word boundaries. Woodward and Aslin (1990) found that although mothers do not insert long pauses prior to the target word, they often enhance stress and frequently present the item in sentence final position. Of course, the effectiveness of these cues depends on the infant's ability to attend to them. Some recent work has examined infants' sensitivity to word boundaries in fluent speech. Kemler Nelson (1989) reported on a study by Myers et al. (submitted) in which infants' orientation times were recorded for passages that were interrupted either between two words or in the middle of words. Head-turn preference was used (Fernald, 1985; Hirsh-Pasek et al., 1987) to test infants at three ages: 4½, 9, and 11 months. Only the 11-month-olds displayed significantly longer orientation times for passages in which the interruptions occurred between two words. Thus there is some indication that 11-month-olds are sensitive to word boundaries in fluent speech. However, just what information they draw upon is unclear at present.

In conclusion, research on the way infant speech perception contributes to the development of the mental lexicon is still at an early stage. Research is only beginning on the way attentional factors influence what infants encode and remember about the speech signal. Nevertheless, there are indications that even the youngest infants do retain some information about the sound properties of words they hear and that the representations apparently have some internal structure.

Speech Perception and the Acquisition of Grammatical Units

When one travels to a foreign country for the first time, it is not uncommon to be overwhelmed by the speed at which the local language is spoken. Even visitors who have studied the language may have problems with the rate of speech. The situation is even worse for someone with no knowledge of the tongue. It is often difficult to determine where one sentence begins and another leaves off, let alone pick up boundaries between words.

In some respects, the situation may not be quite so bleak for the infant. Adults tend to modify their speech when speaking to young children by using fewer words per utterance, more repetitions of items, better articulation, and decreased structural complexity (Garnica, 1977; Newport, Gleitman, and Gleitman, 1977; Papousek, Papousek, and Bornstein, 1985; Cooper and Aslin, 1990). In addition, child-directed speech is often slower, contains more pauses, has higher overall pitch, and a wider pitch range (Broen, 1972; Snow, 1972; Garnica, 1977; Stern et al., 1982; Fernald and Simon, 1984; Fernald, 1985; Bernstein-Ratner, 1986; Morgan, 1986; Grieser and Kuhl, 1988; Fernald et al., 1989). There has been much debate in the literature about whether these and other properties of child-directed speech may facilitate the acquisition of language (Snow and Ferguson, 1977; Gleitman and Wanner, 1982; Gottfried and Gottfried, 1984; Gleitman et al., 1988; Rice and Schiefelbusch, 1989). Because the focus here is on speech perception capacities, our discussion will center on the acoustic properties of the input to the language learner.

As noted earlier, by now there is abundant evidence that infants are attracted to the acoustic properties of child-directed speech (Fernald, 1985; Fernald and Kuhl, 1987; Werker and McLeod, 1989; Cooper and Aslin, 1990). The possible functional values of using child-directed speech have been discussed by Fernald (1984), who suggested three possible functional roles: attentional (to elicit and maintain the infant's attention), social and affective (soothing, conveying approval or disapproval, etc.), and linguistic (directing attention to important information in the input). Fernald's (1989) research provides some interesting evidence about the way the prosody of child-directed speech may signal the intent of the talker. She examined the extent to which communicative intent could be derived from the prosody of child-directed and adult-directed speech in five different interactional contexts: attention bid, approval, prohibition, comfort, and game-telephone. Five different adult talkers produced examples of each type in interactions with infants and with adults. The resulting samples were low-pass filtered at 400 Hz so as to render the speech semantically unintelligible. A group of adult listeners was asked to use the prosody to categorize the filtered utterances according to their context. Judgments of communicative intent were significantly more accurate for infant-directed than for adult-directed speech. Fernald concluded that the infant-directed patterns are more distinctive and more meaningful than the adult patterns, hence

better at revealing the talker's intent. As she notes, because adults rather than infants were tested in the study, one cannot be absolutely certain that infants do derive such information from the input. However, given what has been demonstrated about their auditory capacities and interest in child-directed speech, it is not unlikely that the exaggerated melodies of infant-directed speech do function in this way.

A different role for speech perception capacities in language acquisition is suggested by what has come to be known as the **prosodic bootstrapping** hypothesis (Gleitman and Wanner, 1982; Morgan, 1986; Gleitman et al., 1988; Lederer and Kelly, 1991). The basic idea behind this hypothesis is that the language learner needs access to the correct phrase and clause bracketing of utterances and that prosody is one source of this information. Analyses of fluent speech suggest that boundaries between important grammatical units such as clauses and phrases often are marked by changes in prosodic structure such as drops in fundamental frequency, increases in syllable durations, pausing, and other changes (Martin, 1970; Klatt, 1975, 1976; Nakatani and Dukes, 1977; Nakatani and Shaffer, 1978; Cooper and Paccia-Cooper, 1980; Grosjean and Gee, 1987). Moreover, there is evidence that adult listeners are sensitive to such acoustic markers and that these may serve in locating syntactic boundaries (Collier and t'Hart, 1975; Lehiste, Olive, and Streeter, 1976; Streeter, 1978; Scott, 1982; Luce and Charles-Luce, 1983; Scott and Cutler, 1984; Price et al., 1991). Finally, there are indications that prosodic marking can facilitate adults' acquisition of artificial languages (Morgan, Meier, and Newport, 1987).

As noted earlier, child-directed speech tends to exaggerate prosodic marking in sentences (e.g., Broen, 1972; Fernald, 1984; Bernstein-Ratner, 1986). In this respect, it may be especially useful in providing infants with the necessary information for segmenting speech into the units required for grammatical analysis. Several recent investigations demonstrate that boundaries between important phrasal units are marked by changes in pitch and increases in duration of phrase-final syllables (Morgan, 1986; Fisher, 1991; Lederer and Kelly, 1991). Nevertheless, demonstrating the existence of such prosodic marking in the input is not sufficient to show that language learners make use of this marking to segment the speech stream. It is also

Coincident version

Cinderella lived in a great big house / but it was sort of dark / because she had this mean, mean, mean stepmother / And oh, she had two stepsisters / that were so ugly / they were mean. too /

Noncoincident version

. . . in a great big house but it was / sort of dark because she had / this mean, mean, mean stepmother And oh, she / had two stepsisters that were so / ugly they were mean. too. They were /

FIGURE 9-11 Coincident and noncoincident versions of one speech sample. Slashes indicate where 1-second silent pauses were inserted. (From Hirsh-Pasek, K., Kemler Nelson, D. G., Jusczyk, P. W., Wright Cassidy, K., Druss, B., & Kennedy, L. [1987]. Clauses are perceptual units for young infants. *Cognition, 26,* 269-286.)

necessary to demonstrate that infants actually do respond to the presence of these markers in fluent speech.

A number of recent studies have shown that infants are sensitive to **prosodic markers** of grammatical units. Hirsh-Pasek et al. (1987) tested 7- to 10-month-olds' sensitivity to the prosodic marking of clausal units in fluent speech. They first collected speech samples from a mother talking to her 18-month-old infant, and divided these into passages 15 to 20 seconds long. The passages were modified by inserting 1-second pauses in one of two ways (Fig. 9-11). It was reasoned that if the infants were sensitive to prosodic marking of clausal units, they might find the pauses less disruptive when they occurred between two successive clauses, as opposed to the middle of a clause. The infants tested with head-turn preference had significantly longer listening times for the coincident samples. A follow-up study by Kemler Nelson et al. (1989) investigated whether the exaggerated prosodic marking in child-directed speech is an important factor in how infants react to interruptions of clausal units. They tested 9-month-olds on passages of adult-directed and child-directed speech. The preference for the coincident over the noncoincident versions was significant for the child-directed samples but not for the adult-directed ones. Hence, there is some indication that child-directed speech is more effective in presenting cues to the marking of clausal units.

Subsequent research has focused on the basis for the marking of clausal units. Is experience with a particular language necessary to develop sensitivity to prosodic marking of clausal units, or is this a language universal? Prosodic marking of clausal units holds across a wide variety of the world's languages (Bolinger, 1978; Cruttenden, 1986). So there is reason to believe that infants respond to prosodic marking of clausal units in an unfamiliar language. Indeed, there is evidence that English-speaking adults are sensitive to the prosodic marking of clausal units in foreign languages (Wakefield, Doughtie, and Yom, 1974; Pilon, 1981). To determine whether infants are also sensitive to prosodic marking of clausal units in a foreign language, Jusczyk, et al. (in preparation; see also Jusczyk, 1989) presented American 6-month-olds with passages in Polish. In contrast to the earlier results for 6-month-olds listening to English samples, there was no evidence that listening times were significantly longer for the coincident versions of the Polish samples than for the noncoincident versions. It was speculated that the American infants were distracted by the unfamiliar phonetic structure of the Polish samples, an additional experiment was conducted using low-pass filtered versions of both the Polish and English materials. For the English materials, the infants did show a significant preference for the coincident samples. Since the phonetic content was unavailable in the filtered versions of the samples, this finding provides further evidence that they are responding to the prosody of the English input. By comparison, the infants still did not show a significant preference for the coincident versions of the Polish samples.

One possible interpretation of this result for the Polish samples is that some experience listening to a particular language is required to develop sensitivity to prosodic marking of clauses. However, there is an alternative explanation; namely, that after 6 months' experience with their native language, infants might not attend as closely to prosody in a foreign

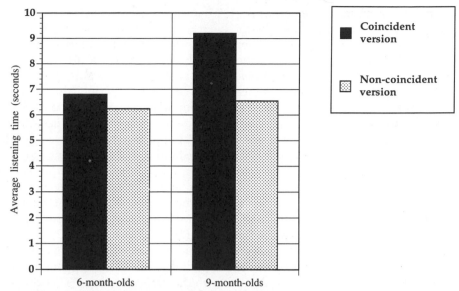

FIGURE 9-12 American infants' sensitivity to phrasal units in English sentences. The figure displays the average listening times of 6- and 9-month-olds to sentences with pauses inserted at boundaries between major phrasal units (coincident versions) or locations within major phrasal units (noncoincident versions).

language. To explore these possibilities, two groups of infants 4½-months-old were tested with the English and Polish materials. One group received the coincident and nonconcident versions of the English passages and the other received the comparable versions of the Polish passages. This time, both groups showed significant preferences for the coincident versions. Thus, at an earlier stage of development, American infants display sensitivity to prosodic marking of clausal units in a foreign language. One interpretation of these findings is that infants may be innately predisposed to respond to prosodic marking of clausal units in any language. However, as with the perception of nonnative phonetic contrasts, as they begin to focus more closely on the prosody characteristic of the native language that they are learning, sensitivity to these features in nonnative languages may decline.

Finally, some efforts have been made to examine sensitivity to phrasal units within clauses. Marking of phrasal units may vary considerably across different languages. For example, in languages that make heavy use of grammatical case-marking, words within the same phrasal unit may, but need not, be adjacent to one another. In contrast, in languages that use word order for syntactic marking, words from the same phrasal unit are much more apt to be adjacent. Thus, any marking of phrasal units in the acoustic signal may vary considerably by the structure of the language. Jusczyk et al. (1992) investigated American infants' sensitivity to prosodic marking of major phrasal units (i.e., subject and predicate phrases) in English. The materials for the study were analogous to the ones with the clausal units, only this time pauses were inserted either between two phrasal groups (coincident versions) or within a phrasal group (noncoincident versions). In contrast to the earlier results with clausal units, 6-month-olds displayed no significant preference for uninterrupted phrasal units over interrupted ones. Instead, sensitivity to prosodic marking of phrasal units was not evident until the infants reached 9 months of age (Figure 9-12). This finding suggests that in contrast to clausal units, sensitivity to prosodic marking of units within clauses may require greater experience with and attention to the sound structure of the native language.

In summary, infant speech perception may participate in more than just the acquisition of the sound structure of the native language. Specifically, attention to prosodic characteristics of the input can provide information about the communicative intent behind the acoustic signal as well as clues to the packaging of important grammatical units. One caveat pertains to the nature of the role of speech perception capacities in the acquisition of grammatical units. Their role is limited; they provide one means, but not the only one, of segmenting the input into the relevant grammatical units. As Morgan, Meier, and Newport (1987) observed, there are other kinds of markers that language learners may use in deriving grammatical units.

UNANSWERED QUESTIONS AND FUTURE DIRECTIONS FOR RESEARCH

Considerable information about the development of speech perception capacities can be gleaned from research over the past 20 years. Yet there are still many areas in which information is lacking. In some instances, the gaps in understanding are traceable to the lack of methodological tools for conducting the necessary investigations. In other cases, the progress in a particular area of research has made the holes in our understanding visible.

A number of unresolved issues in the field stem from the lack of an adequate measure for studying how infants categorize speech sounds. To this point, much of the information about infants' categorization comes from indirect measures, such as the head-turn conditioning procedure used by Kuhl (1979) and the modified HAS procedure (Bertoncini et al., 1988; Jusczyk et al., 1990). Investigators in the field would like some way of training infants to provide one kind of response to one speech sound category and a different response to another category so that generalization of new instances could be tested. This would provide an identification measure equivalent to the kinds of labeling tasks used in adult speech perception experiments (see Chapter 15). Unfortunately, despite efforts in many laboratories throughout the world, researchers have not been successful in devising this kind of measure. The report by Burnham, Earnshaw, and Clark (1991) is no better in this respect. Although they attempt to train responses to different speech sound categories and test for generalization, their infant subjects never achieved high levels of performance in responding distinctively to the best members of the categories. Thus, given that the infants showed considerable confusion in correctly identifying the training stimuli during testing, it is not possible to infer anything sensible about generalization.

A suitable procedure for testing categorization would have many applications. First, it produces labeling data concerning categorical perception. At present, all inferences about categorical perception during infancy are made strictly on the basis of discrimination data. By comparison, categorical perception in adults is inferred by comparing the way data from discrimination and categorization correspond (Liberman et al., 1967; Studdert-Kennedy et al., 1970; Repp, 1983) . Second, a procedure of this type would provide a more precise specification of the infant's speech sound categories in both native and nonnative languages. An identification measure would indicate whether phonetic categories are organized around prototypes, as Kuhl (1991; Kuhl et al., 1992) suggests. It would also aid the study of how the representations of speech develop as infants gain more familiarity with the native language. This kind of information is critical for understanding the organization and development of the mental lexicon. Third, the procedure would help clarify the nature of the mechanisms underlying infant speech perception capacities because it would allow for a more direct comparison of the way that speech and nonspeech stimuli are categorized. Finally, such a procedure is necessary to answer one of the important issues in phonological development, namely, when infants develop phonemic categories. The only way to answer this question is to find out when infants begin to treat different allophones of the same phonemic category as equivalent. One way to determine this would be to train them to respond to some **allophone** and see if they generalize to all and only allophones of the same phonemic category.

Some of the findings reported over the past few years have raised additional questions about the way speech perception develops. In most instances there are not enough data to draw firm conclusions. For example, consider the developments about the perception of nonnative language contrasts. It will be necessary to sample a much wider range of contrasts from more languages before we can reach firm conclusions about the conditions that lead to a decline in sensitivity to some contrasts but not others. Similarly, the research concerning prosodic markers of grammatical units is still in its early stages. Again, information from different languages is necessary to determine the role of such marking in language acquisition. Nor is it sufficient simply to show that infants are sensitive to these markers; one must also show that the units are actually extracted, processed, and remembered during fluent speech perception. More attention also should be directed to the way prosodic and phonetic information is extracted from the speech signal. Are the mechanisms responsible for processing suprasegmental information independent of those that deal with segmental cues?

Another interesting avenue of research is infant speech perception capacities in situations more like those of everyday life. Most procedures are intended to provide ideal conditions for infants to demonstrate some speech perception capacity. However, to understand how these capacities are used to acquire language, we have to gain some appreciation of how infants process and remember speech in a real world filled with many distractions. More careful study of the conditions that influence infants' attention to speech and a more precise description what they remember are critical for understanding the development of the mental lexicon.

Finally, an area not addressed in this chapter concerns the way developments in speech perception are related to speech production. Some intriguing developments in the production of speech occur as major changes are taking place in speech perception. For example, de Boysson-Bardies et al. (1989) note that vowel production in 10-month-olds from four different language backgrounds tends to parallel that of adult speakers of the native language. Hence there are some indications that speech production is taking on the character of the native language around the time sensitivity to nonnative contrasts begins to decline. Unfortunately, there is very little information about the way perception and production develop within the same child. Again, lack of appropriate methodological tools is a factor. The lack of an adequate perceptual categorization procedure is one factor. In addition, many perceptual measures are limited, either because they provide group data (like HAS), making it difficult to draw conclusions about the performance of individual infants, or because only one or two contrasts can be tested in a given session. A complete understanding of phonological development depends on relating developments in production and perception.

SUMMARY

Over the past 20 years sufficient progress has been made in delineating the speech perception capacities of infants that models of the development of speech perception capacities are being proposed (Jusczyk, 1985a; 1992; 1993; Mehler, Dupoux, and Segui, 1990; Werker, 1990; Suomi, 1992; Best, 1993; Kuhl, 1993). Early studies provided much information about the nature and range of capacities of infants for perceiving speech. These studies demonstrated that rather than requiring a long period of trial-and-error learning, the basic capacities for discriminating speech contrasts are more or less in place from birth (Bertoncini et al., 1987). In addition, findings suggest that infants discriminate contrasts that could appear in any language. Moreover, they show some signs of being able to compensate for differences in speaking rate (Eimas and Miller, 1980a) and changes in pitch contour and talker's voice (Kuhl, 1979, 1983; (Jusczyk et al., 1992). There are also indications that during the early stages, the mechanisms that underlie speech processing by infants may be a part of more general auditory processing capacities (Jusczyk et al., 1983; Krumhansl and Jusczyk, 1990).

Early findings provided a strong foundation for investigations into the way speech perception capacities develop. It is not surprising, then, that much recent research in the field has pursued developmental issues. One topic that has received a great deal of attention concerns the effects of acquiring a native language on the underlying speech perception capacities. Considerable evidence indicates that learning a native language affects speech perception capacities during the second half of the first year of life (Werker and Tees, 1984a; Best, 1991), if not sooner (e.g., Polka and Werker, 1991). There are indications that at the same time the formation of the mental lexicon is beginning. Infants show some capacity for retaining information about speech across short delay (Jusczyk, Kennedy, and Jusczyk, in press) and give some indication of being sensitive to word boundaries in continuous speech (Kemler Nelson, 1989). Several recent investigations have taken the first steps toward specifying the nature of infants' representations of speech sounds (Bertoncini et al., 1988; Greiser and Kuhl, 1989). Finally, one new direction of research has focused on the role of speech perception capacities in language acquisition. These studies have not been strictly limited to the way phonological categories develop. There also have been attempts to look at the role of these capacities in obtaining information about communicative intent (Fernald, 1989) and grammatical units (Hirsh-Pasek et al., 1987).

In conclusion, developmental speech research has entered an exciting new phase. Greater attention is being given to its role in language acquisition and to the interactions between experience and basic perceptual capacities. To pursue these new directions effectively, speech researchers will have to conduct more studies across different languages. New methods also will have to be developed to provide a more detailed picture of how infants represent speech sounds. In addition investigators will have to pay careful attention to the conditions in which infants attend to speech in the real world to understand the role of these capacities in language acquisition.

Review Questions

1. Years ago, the most popular view of how infants learn to discriminate speech sounds was that this was a learned ability gained through much practice in producing and listening to speech. With the findings from the first studies of infant speech perception, this view was replaced by one that held that speech discrimination capacities are part of the infant's innate endowment. Given what you have read in this chapter, what can you say about the roles of innate factors and experience in speech discrimination?

2. Some people have claimed that the capacities that underlie speech perception are highly specialized and separate from other auditory capacities. Others have taken the position that the capacities that underlie the infant's speech processing are general and apply to other domains of auditory processing. What sort of position would you take in this debate? What evidence would you use to support your stance?

3. What is perceptual normalization? Why is this an important ability in processing speech? What do we know about its development?

4. What kinds of changes occur in speech perception when the infant begins to acquire a native language? Why does the sound structure of the native language affect speech perception capacities? Would you expect that these changes are permanent or reversible?

5. What is the mental lexicon? Why might speech perception capacities be important to its development?

6. What is child-directed speech? How does it differ from adult-directed speech? How might the acoustic characteristics of child-directed speech assist in acquiring a native language?

7. What are some of the limitations of methodology used in studying infant speech perception? What kinds of features would you look at before deciding whether a given method was useful to a research question?

8. What is to be gained from studying the speech perception capacities of infants? Suppose you were interested in devising a model of how adults perceive continuous speech. Can you think of any reasons it might be valuable to know about infant speech perception capacities?

References

Aslin, R. N. (1987). Visual and auditory development in infancy. In Osofsky, J. D. (Ed.), *Handbook of infant development*. (2nd ed.) New York: Wiley (pp. 5-97).

Aslin, R.N., & Pisoni, D. B. (1980). Some developmental processes in speech perception. In Yeni-Komshian, G., Kavanagh, J. F., & Ferguson, C. A. (Eds.), *Child phonology: Perception and production*. New York: Academic Press (pp. 67-96).

Aslin, R. N., Pisoni, D. B., Hennessy, B. L., & Perey, A. J. (1981). Discrimination of voice onset time by human infants: New findings and implications for the effects of early experience. *Child Development, 52,* 1135-1145.

Aslin, R. N., Pisoni, D. B., & Jusczyk, P. W. (1983). Auditory development and speech perception in infancy. In Haith, M., & Campos, J. (Eds.), *Handbook of child psychology*, vol. 2. *Infancy and developmental psychobiology*. New York: Wiley. (pp. 573-687).

Bernstein-Ratner, N. (1986). Durational cues which mark clause boundaries in mother-child speech. *Phonetics, 14,* 303-309.

Bertoncini, J., Bijeljac-Babic, R., Blumstein, S. E., & Mehler, J. (1987). Discrimination in neonates of very short CV's. *Journal of the Acoustical Society of America, 82,* 31-37.

Bertoncini, J., Bijeljac-Babic, R., Jusczyk, P. W., Kennedy, L. J., & Mehler, J. (1988). An investigation of young infants' perceptual representations of speech sounds. *Journal of Experimental Psychology: General, 117,* 21-33.

Best, C. T. (1991). *Phonetic Influences on the perception of nonnative speech contrasts by 6-8 and 10-12 month olds.* Paper presented at the biennial meeting of the Society for Research in Child Development, Seattle, WA.

Best, C. T. (1993). The emergence of language specific constraints on the perception of native and non-native speech: A window on early phonological development. In de Boysson-Bardies, B., de Schoen, S., Jusczyk, P., MacNeilage, P., & Morton, J. (Eds.), *Developmental neurocognition: Speech and face processing in the first year of life.* Dordrecht: Kluwer (pp. 289-304).

Best, C. T., & McRoberts, G. W. (1989, April). *Phonological influences in infants' discrimination of two non-native speech contrasts.* Paper presented at the biennial meeting of the Society for Research in Child Development, Kansas City, MO.

Best, C. T., McRoberts, G. W., & Sithole, N. M. (1988). Examination of the perceptual reorganization for speech contrasts: Zulu click discrimination by English-speaking adults and infants. *Journal of Experimental Psychology: Human Perception and Performance, 14,* 345-360.

Best, C. T., McRoberts, G. W., Goodell, E., Womer, J., Insabella, G. Klatt, L., Luke, S., & Silver, J. (1990, April). *Infant and adult perception of nonnative speech contrasts differing in relation to the listeners' native phonology.* Paper presented at the International Conference on Infant Studies, Montreal.

Bladon, R. A., Henton, C. G., & Pickering, J. B. (1984). Towards an auditory theory of speaker normalization. *Language and Communication, 4,* 59-69.

Bolinger, D. L. (1978). Intonation across languages. In Greenberg, J. P., Ferguson, C. A., & Moravcsik, E. A. (Eds.), *Universals of human language,* vol. 2. Phonology. Stanford: Stanford University Press (pp. 471-524).

de Boysson-Bardies, B., Halle, P., Sagart, L., & Durand, C. (1989). A cross-linguistic investigation of vowel formants in babbling. *Journal of Child Language, 16,* 1-17.

Broen, P. (1972). The verbal environment of the language learning child. *ASHA Monograph, 17.*

Brown, R., & Fraser, C. (1964). The acquisition of syntax. *Monographs of the Society for Research in Child Development, 29,* 9-34.

Burnham, D. K., Earnshaw, L. J., & Clark, J. E. (1991). Development of categorical identification of native and non-native bilabial stops: Infants, children and adults. *Journal of Child Language, 18,* 231-260.

Carney, A. E., Widin, G. P., & Veimeister, N.F. (1977). Noncategorical perception of stop consonants differing in VOT. *Journal of the Acoustical Society of America, 62,* 961-970.

Carrell, T. D., Smith, L. B., & Pisoni, D. B. (1981). Some perceptual dependencies in speeded classification of vowel color and pitch. *Perception & Psychophysics, 29,* 1-10.

Collier, R., t'Hart, J. (1975). The role of intonation in speech perception. In Cohen, A. & Nooteboom, S. G. (eds.) Structure and process in speech perception. Heidelberg: Springer-Verlag, 107-121.

Cooper, R. P., & Aslin, R. N. (1990). Preference for infant-directed speech in the first month after birth. *Child Development, 61,* 1584-1595.

Cooper, W. E., & Paccia-Cooper, J. (1980). *Syntax and speech.* Cambridge, MA: Harvard University Press.

Cruttenden, A. (1986). *Intonation.* Cambridge, UK: Cambridge University Press.

DeCasper, A. J., & Fifer, W. P. (1980). Of human bonding: Newborns prefer their mothers' voices. *Science, 208,* 1174-1176.

Eilers, R. E. (1977). Context sensitive perception of naturally produced stops and fricative consonants by infants. *Journal of the Acoustical Society of America, 61,* 1321-1336.

Eilers, R. E., Gavin, W. J., & Wilson, W. R. (1979). Linguistic experience and phonemic perception in infancy: A cross-linguistic study. *Child Development, 50,* 14-18.

Eilers, R. E., & Minifie, F. (1975) Fricative discrimination in early infancy. *Journal of Speech and Hearing Research, 18,* 158-167.

Eilers, R. E., Wilson, W. R., & Moore, J. M. (1977). Developmental changes in speech discrimination in infants. *Journal of Speech and Hearing Research, 20,* 766-780.

Eilers, R. E., Wilson, W. R., & Moore, J. M. (1979). Speech discrimination in the language-innocent and language-wise: A study in the perception of voice onset time. *Journal of Child Language, 6,* 1-18.

Eimas, P. D. (1974). Auditory and linguistic units of processing of cues for place of articulation by infants. *Perception & Psychophysics, 16,* 513-521.

Eimas, P. D. (1975). Auditory and phonetic coding of the cues for speech: Discrimination of the [r-l] distinction by young infants. *Perception & Psychophysics, 18,* 341-347.

Eimas, P. D., & Miller, J. L. (1980a). Contextual

effects in infant speech perception. *Science, 209,* 1140-1141.

Eimas, P. D., & Miller, J. L. (1980b). Discrimination of the information for manner of articulation. *Infant Behavior and Development, 3,* 367-375.

Eimas, P. D., & Miller, J. L., & Jusczyk, P. W. (1987). On infant speech perception and the acquisition of language. In Harnad, S. (Ed.), *Categorical Perception.* New York: Cambridge University Press (pp. 161-195).

Eimas, P. D., Siqueland, E. R., Jusczyk, P., & Vigorito, J. (1971). Speech perception in infants. *Science, 171,* 303-306.

Fernald, A. (1984). The perceptual and affective salience of mothers' speech to infants. In Feagans, L., Garvey, C., & Golinkoff, R. (Eds.), *The origins and growth of communication.* Norwood, NJ: Ablex (pp. 5-29).

Fernald, A. (1985). Four-month-old infants prefer to listen to motherese. *Infant Behavior and Development, 8,* 181-195.

Fernald, A. (1989). Intonation and communicative intent in mothers' speech to infants: Is the melody the message? *Child Development, 60,* 1497-1510.

Fernald, A., & Kuhl, P. K. (1987). Acoustic determinants of infant preference for motherese speech. *Infant Behavior and Development, 10,* 279-293.

Fernald, A., & Simon, T. (1984). Expanded intonation contours in mothers' speech to newborns. *Developmental Psychology, 20,* 104-113.

Fernald, A., Taeschner, T., Dunn, J., Papousek, M., DeBoysson-Bardies, B., & Fukui, I. (1989). A cross-language study of prosodic modifications in mothers' and fathers' speech to preverbal infants. *Journal of Child Language, 16,* 477-501.

Fisher, C. (1991). Prosodic cues to phrase structure in infant directed speech. In *Papers and Reports on Child Language Development, 30,* Stanford, CA.

Fry, D. B., Abramson, A. S., Eimas, P. D., & Liberman, A. M. (1962). The identification and discrimination of synthetic vowels. *Language and Speech, 5,* 171-189.

Garnica, O. K. (1977). Some prosodic and paralinguistic features of speech to young children. In Snow, C. E., & Ferguson, C. A. (Eds.), *Talking to children.* Cambridge: Cambridge University Press (pp. 63-88).

Gerken, L. A. (1994). Sentential processes in early child language: Evidence from the perception and production of function morphemes. In Goodman, J. C., & Nusbaum, H. C. (Eds.), The transition from speech sounds to spoken words: The development of speech perception. Cambridge, MA: MIT Press (pp. 271-298).

Gerken, L. A., Landau, B., & Remez, R. E. (1989). Function morphemes in young children's speech perception and production. *Developmental Psychology, 25,* 204-216.

Gleitman, L.R., Gleitman, H., Landau, B., & Wanner, E. (1988). Where learning begins: Initial representations for language learning. In Newmeyer, F. (Ed.), *The Cambridge linguistic survey,* vol. 3. Cambridge, MA: Cambridge University Press (pp. 150-193).

Gleitman, L., & Wanner, E. (1982). The state of the state of the art. In Wanner, E. & Gleitman, L. (Eds.), *Language acquisition: The state of the art.* Cambridge, UK: Cambridge University Press (pp. 3-48).

Gottfried, H. W., & Gottfried, A. E. (1984). Home environment and cognitive development in young children of middle-socioeconomic-status families. In Gottfried, H. W. (Ed.), *Home environment and early cognitive development: Longitudinal research.* Orlando, FL: Academic Press (pp. 329-342).

Goodsitt, J. V., Morse, P. A., Ver Hoove, J. N., & Cowan, N. (1984). Infant Speech perception in multisyllabic contexts. *Child Development, 55,* 903-910.

Greiser, D., & Kuhl, P. K. (1988). Maternal speech to infants in a tonal language: Support for universal prosodic features in motherese. *Developmental Psychology, 24,* 14-20.

Greiser, D., & Kuhl, P. K. (1989). The categorization of speech by infants: Support for speech-sound prototypes. *Developmental Psychology, 25,* 577-588.

Grosjean, F., & Gee, J. P. (1987). Prosodic structure and spoken word recognition. *Cognition, 25,* 135-155.

Hillenbrand, J., Minifie, F. D., & Edwards, T. J. (1979). Tempo of spectrum change as a cue in speech sound discrimination by infants. *Journal of Speech and Hearing Research, 22,* 147-165.

Hirsh-Pasek, K., Kemler Nelson, D. G., Jusczyk, P. W., Wright Cassidy, K., Druss, B., & Kennedy, L. (1987). Clauses are perceptual units for young infants. *Cognition, 26,* 269-286.

Holmberg, T. L., Morgan, K. A., & Kuhl, P. K. (1977, December). *Speech perception in early infancy: Discrimination of fricative consonants.* Paper presented at the 94th meeting of the Acoustical Society of America, Miami Beach.

Jusczyk, P. W. (1985a). On characterizing the development of speech perception. In Mehler, J., & Fox, R. (Eds.), *Neonate cognition: Beyond the blooming, buzzing confusion.* Hillsdale, NJ: Erlbaum (pp. 199-229).

Jusczyk, P. W. (1985b). The high amplitude sucking procedure as a methodological tool in infant speech perception research. In Gottlieb, G., & Krasnegor, N. A. (Eds.), *Measurement of audition and vision in the first year of postnatal life: A methodological overview.* Norwood, NJ: Ablex (pp. 199-222.)

Jusczyk, P. W. (1986). Towards a model for the development of speech perception. In Perkell, J.,

& Klatt, D. H. (Eds.), *Invariance and variability in speech processes*. Hillsdale, NJ: Erlbaum (pp. 1-19).

Jusczyk, P. W. (1989, April). *Perception of cues to causal units in native and non-native languages*. Paper presented at the biennial meeting of the Society for Research in Child Development, Kansas City, MO.

Jusczyk, P. W. (1992). Developing phonological categories from the speech signal. In Ferguson, C. A., Stoel-Gammon, C., & Menn, L. (Eds.), *Phonological development: Models, research, implications*. Parkton, MD: York (pp. 17-64).

Jusczyk, P. W. (1993). From general to language-specific capacities: The WRAPSA model of how speech perception develops. *Journal of Phonetics, 21,* 3-28.

Jusczyk, P. W. (1994). Infant speech perception and the development of the mental lexicon. In Goodman, J. C., & Nusbaum, H. C. (Eds.), *The transition from speech sounds to spoken words: The development of speech perception*. Cambridge, MA: MIT Press (pp. 227-270).

Jusczyk, P. W., & Bertoncini, J. (1988). Viewing the development of speech perception as an innately guided learning process. *Language and Speech, 31,* 217-238.

Jusczyk, P. W., Bertoncini, J., Bijeljac-Babic, R., Kennedy, L. J., & Mehler, J. (1990). The role of attention in speech perception by young infants. *Cognitive Development, 5,* 265-286.

Jusczyk, P. W., Copan, H., & Thompson, E. (1978). Perception by 2-month-old infants of glide contrasts in multisyllabic utterances. *Perception & Psychophysics, 24,* 515-520.

Jusczyk, P. W., & Derrah, C. (1987). Representation of speech sounds by young infants. *Developmental Psychology, 23,* 648-654.

Jusczyk, P. W., Friederici, A. D., & Wessels, J. M. I., Svenkerud, V. Y., & Jusczyk, A. M. (1993). Infants' sensitivity to the sound patterns of native language words. *Journal of Memory and Language, 32,* 402-420.

Jusczyk, P. W., Hirsh-Pasek, K., Kemler Nelson, D. G., Kennedy, L. J., Woodward, A., & Piwoz, J. (1992). Perception of acoustic correlates of major phrasal units by young infants. *Cognitive Psychology, 24,* 252-293.

Jusczyk, P. W., Jusczyk, A. M., Kennedy, L. J., Schomberg, T., & Koenig, N. (in press). Young infants' retention of information about bisyllabic utterances. *Journal of Experimental Psychology: Human Perception and Performance.*

Jusczyk, P. W., Kemler Nelson, D. G., Hirsh-Pasek, K., & Schomberg, T. (in preparation). Perception of acoustic correlates to clausal units in a foreign language by American infants.

Jusczyk, P. W., Kennedy, L. J., & Jusczyk, A. M. (1995). Young infants' retention of information

about syllables. *Infant Behavior and Development 18,* 27-42.

Jusczyk, P. W., Pisoni, D. B., & Mullennix, J. (1992). Some consequences of stimulus variability on speech processing by 2-month-old infants. *Cognition, 43,* 253-291.

Jusczyk, P. W., Pisoni, D. B., Reed, M., Fernald, A., & Myers, M. (1983). Infants' discrimination of the duration of a rapid spectrum change in nonspeech signals. *Science, 222,* 175-177.

Jusczyk, P. W., Pisoni, D. B., Walley, A., & Murray, J. (1980). Discrimination of relative onset time of two-component tones by infants. *Journal of the Acoustical Society of America, 67,* 262-270.

Jusczyk, P. W., Rosner, B. S., Reed, M., & Kennedy, L. J. (1989). Could temporal order differences underlie 2-month-olds' discrimination of English voicing contrasts? *Journal of the Acoustical Society of America, 85,* 1741-1749.

Jusczyk, P. W., & Thompson, E. J. (1978). Perception of a phonetic contrast in multisyllabic utterances by two-month-old infants. *Perception & Psychophysics, 23,* 105-109.

Karzon, R. G. (1985). Discrimination of a polysyllabic sequence by 1- to 4-month-old infants. *Journal of Experimental Child Psychology, 39,* 326-342.

Kemler Nelson, D. G. (1989, April). *Developmental trends in infants' sensitivity to prosodic cues correlated with linguistic units*. Paper presented at the biennial meeting of the Society for Research in Child Development, Kansas City, MO.

Kemler Nelson, D. G., Hirsh-Pasek, K., Jusczyk, P. W., & Wright Cassidy, K. (1989). How the prosodic cues in motherese might assist language learning. *Journal of Child Language, 16,* 53-68.

Kemler Nelson, D. G., Jusczyk, P. W., Mandel, D. R., Myers, J., Turk, A., & Gerken, L. A. (1995). The head-turn preference procedure for testing auditory perception. Infant Behavior and Development *18,* 111-116.

Klatt, D. H. (1975). Voice onset time, friction and aspiration in word-initial consonant clusters. *Journal of Speech and Hearing Research, 18,* 686-706.

Klatt, D. H. (1976). Linguistic uses of segment duration in English: Acoustic and perceptual evidence. *Journal of the Acoustical Society of America, 59,* 1208-1221.

Krumhansl, C. L., & Jusczyk, P. W. (1990). Infants' perception of phrase structure in music. *Psychological Science, 1,* 70-73.

Kuhl, P. K. (1976). Speech perception in early infancy: the acquisition of speech-sound categories. In Hirsh, S. K., Eldridge, D. H., Hirsh, I. J., & Silverman, S. R. (Eds.), *Hearing and Davis: Essays honoring Hallowell Davis*. St. Louis: Washington University Press (pp. 265-280).

Kuhl, P. K. (1979). Speech perception in early infancy: Perceptual constancy for spectrally dissimilar vowel categories. *Journal of the Acoustical Society of America, 66,* 1668-1679.

Kuhl, P. K. (1983). Perception of auditory equivalence classes for speech in early infancy. *Infant Behavior and Development, 6,* 263-285.

Kuhl, P. K. (1985). Methods in the study of infant speech perception. In Gottlieb, G., & Krasnegor, N. A. (Eds.), *Measurement of audition and vision in the first year of postnatal life: A methodological overview.* Norwood, NJ: Ablex (pp. 223-251).

Kuhl, P. K. (1991). Human adults and human infants show a "perceptual magnet effect" for the prototypes of speech categories, monkeys do not. *Perception & Psychophysics, 50,* 93-107.

Kuhl, P. K. (1993). Innate predispositions and the effects of experience in speech perception: The native language magnet theory. In de Boysson-Bardies, B., de Schoen, S., Jusczyk, P., MacNeilage, P., & Morton, J. (Eds.), *Developmental neurocognition: Speech and face processing in the first year of life.* Dordrecht: Kluwer (pp. 259-274).

Kuhl, P. K., & Miller, J. D. (1975). Speech perception by the chinchilla: Voiced-voiceless distinction in alveolar-plosive consonants. *Science, 190,* 69-72.

Kuhl, P. K., & Miller, J. D. (1978). Speech perception by the chinchilla: Identification functions for synthetic VOT stimuli. *Journal of the Acoustical Society of America, 63,* 905-917.

Kuhl, P. K., & Miller, J. D. (1982). Discrimination of auditory target dimensions in the presence or absence of variation of a second dimension by infants. *Perception & Psychophysics, 31,* 279-292.

Kuhl, P. K., Williams, K. A., Lacerda, F., Stevens, K. N., & Lindblom, B. (1992). Linguistic experiences alter phonetic perception by 6 months of age. *Science, 255,* 606-608.

Lasky, R. E., Syrdal-Lasky, A., & Klein, R. E. (1975). VOT discrimination by 4 to 6½ month old infants from Spanish environments. *Journal of Experimental Child Psychology, 20,* 215-225.

Lederer, A., & Kelly, M. (1991). Prosodic correlates to the adjunct/complement distinction in motherese. In *Papers & Reports on Child Language Development, 30,* Stanford, CA.

Lehiste, I., Olive, J. P., & Streeter, L. A. (1976). The role of duration in disambiguating syntactically ambiguous sentences. *Journal of the Acoustical Society of America, 60,* 1199-1202.

Levitt, A., Jusczyk, P. W., Murray, J., & Carden, G. (1988). The perception of place of articulation in voiced and voiceless fricatives by 2-month-old infants. *Journal of Experimental Psychology: Human perception and performance, 14,* 361-368.

Liberman, A. M., Cooper, F. S., Shankweiler, D. P., & Studdert-Kennedy, M. (1967). Perception of the speech code. *Psychological Review, 74,* 431-461.

Lindblom, B. (1986). On the origin and purpose of discreteness and invariance in sound patterns. In

Perkell, J., & Klatt, D. H. (Eds.), *Invariance and variability in speech processes.* Hillsdale, NJ: Erlbaum (pp. 493-510).

Lisker, L., & Abramson, A. S. (1964). A cross-language study of voicing in initial stops: Acoustical measurements. *Word, 20,* 384-422.

Lisker, L., & Abramson, A. S. (1977). The voicing dimension: Some experiments in comparative phonetics. In *Proceedings of the Sixth International Congress of Phonetic Sciences.* Prague: Academia.

Luce, P. A., & Charles-Luce, J. (1983). *Contextual effects of the consonant/vowel ratio in speech production.* Paper presented at the 105th meeting of the Acoustical Society of America, Cincinnati.

Martin, J. G. (1970). On judging pauses in simultaneous speech. *Journal of Verbal Learning and Verbal Behavior, 9,* 75-78.

Mehler, J., Bertoncini, J., Barriere, M., & Jassik-Gerschenfeld, D. (1978). Infant recognition of mother's voice. *Perception, 7,* 491-497.

Mehler, J., Dupoux, E., & Segui, J. (1990). Constraining models of lexical access: The onset of word recognition. In Altmann, G. T. M. (Ed.), *Cognitive models of speech processing.* Hillsdale, NJ: Erlbaum (pp. 236-262).

Mehler, J., Jusczyk, P. W., Lambertz, G., Halsted, N., Bertoncini, J., & Amiel-Tison, C. (1988). A precursor of language acquisition in young infants. *Cognition, 29,* 143-178.

Miller, J. L., & Eimas, P. D. (1983). Studies on the categorization of speech by infants. *Cognition, 13,* 135-165.

Miller, J. D., Wier, L., Pastore, R., Kelly, W., & Dooling, R. (1976). Discrimination and labeling of noise-buzz sequences with varying noise-lead times: An example of categorical perception. *Journal of the Acoustical Society of America, 60,* 410-417.

Mills, M., & Meluish, E. (1974). Recognition of the mother's voice in early infancy. *Nature, 252,* 123-124.

Miyawaki, K., Strange, W., Verbrugge, R., Liberman, A., Jenkins, J. J., & Fujimura, O. (1975). An effect of linguistic experience: The discrimination of [r] and [l] by native speakers of Japanese and English. *Perception & Psychophysics, 18,* 331-340.

Moffit, A. R. (1971). Consonant cue perception by 20- to 24-week-old infants. *Child Development, 42,* 717-731.

Morgan, J. L. (1986). *From simple input to complex grammar.* Cambridge, MA: MIT Press.

Morgan, J. L., Meier, R. P., & Newport, E. L. (1987). Structural packaging in the input to language learning: Contributions of prosodic and morphological marking of phrases to the acquisition of language. *Cognitive Psychology, 19,* 498-550.

Morse, P. A. (1972). The discrimination of speech and nonspeech stimuli in early infancy. *Journal of Experimental Child Psychology, 13,* 477-492.

Myers, J., Jusczyk, P. W., Kemler Nelson, D. G., Charles-Luce, J., Woodward, A. L., & Hirsh-Pasek, K. (submitted).

Nakatani, L. H., & Dukes, K. D. (1977). Locus of segmental cues for word juncture. *Journal of the Acoustical Society of America, 62,* 714-719.

Nakatani, L. H., & Schaffer, J. A. (1978). Hearing "words" without words: Prosodic cues for word perception. *Journal of the Acoustical Society of America, 63,* 234-245.

Newport, E. L., Gleitman, H., & Gleitman, L. R. (1977). Mother, I'd rather do it myself: Some effects and noneffects of maternal speech-style. In Snow, C. E. & Ferguson, C. A. (Eds.), *Talking to children: Language input and acquisition.* Cambridge, UK: Cambridge University Press (pp. 109-150).

Nozza, R. J., Rossman, R. N. F., Bond, L. C., & Miller, S. L. (1990). Infant speech sound discrimination in noise. *Journal of the Acoustical Society of America, 87,* 339-350.

Papousek, M., Papousek, H., & Bornstein, M. H. (1985). The naturalistic vocal environment of young infants: On the significance of homogeneity in variability in parental speech. In Field, T., & Fox, N. (Eds.), *Social perception in infants.* Norwood, NJ: Ablex (pp. 269-297).

Pilon, R. (1981). Segmentation of speech in a foreign language. *Journal of Psycholinguistic Research, 10,* 113-122.

Pisoni, D. B. (1973). Auditory and phonetic memory codes in the discrimination of consonants and vowels. *Perception & Psychophysics, 13,* 253-260.

Pisoni, D. B. (1977). Identification and discrimination of the relative onset time of two-component tones: Implications for voicing perception in stops. *Journal of the Acoustical Society of America, 61,* 1352-1361.

Pisoni, D. B., & Tash, J. (1974). Reaction times to comparisons within and across phonetic categories. *Perception & Psychophysics, 15,* 285-290.

Polka, L., & Werker, J. F. Developmental changes in perception of non-native vowel contrasts. *Journal of Experimental Psychology: Human Perception and Performance, 20.*

Pollock, K., & Schwartz, R. G. (1990). Phonological perception of early words in 15- to 20-month-old children. Unpublished manuscript, Purdue University.

Price, P. J., Ostendorf, M., Shattuck-Hufnagel, S. & Fong, C. (1991). The use of prosody in syntactic disambiguation. *Journal of the Acoustical Society of America, 90,* 2956-2970.

Rand, T. C. (1971). Vocal tract size normalization in the perception of stop consonants. *Haskins Laboratories status report on speech research, SR-25/26,* 141-146.

Repp, B. H. (1983). Categorical perception: Issues, methods, findings. In Lass, N. (Ed.), *Speech and language: Advances in basic research and practice,* vol. 10. New York: Academic Press (pp. 243-335).

Rice, M. L. & Schiefelbusch, R. L. (1989). *The teachability of language.* Baltimore: Paul H. Brookes.

Samuel, A. G. (1977). The effect of discrimination training on speech perception: Noncategorical perception. *Perception & Psychophysics, 22,* 321-330.

Scott, D. R., (1982). Duration as a cue to the perception of a phrase boundary. *Journal of the Acoustical Society of America, 71,* 996-1007.

Scott, D. R., & Cutler, A. (1984). Segmental phonology and the perception of syntactic structure. *Journal of Verbal Learning and Verbal Behavior, 23,* 450-466.

Siqueland, E. R., & DeLucia, C. A. (1969). Visual reinforcement of non-nutritive sucking in human infants. *Science, 165,* 1144-1146.

Snow, C. E. (1972). Mothers' speech to children learning language. *Child Development, 43,* 539-565.

Stern, D. N., Spieker, S., Barnett, R. K., & MacKain, K. (1982). The prosody of maternal speech: infant age and context related changes. *Journal of Child Language, 10,* 1-15.

Stevens, K. N., Liberman, A. M., Studdert-Kennedy, M. G., & Öhman, S. E. G. (1969). Cross-language study of vowel perception. *Language and Speech, 12,* 1-23.

Strange, W., & Broen, P. A. (1971). The relationship between perception and production of /w/, /r/, and /l/ by 3-year-old children. *Journal of Experimental Child Psychology, 31,* 81-102.

Streeter, L. A. (1976). Language perception of 2-month-old infants shows effects of both innate mechanisms and experience. *Nature, 259,* 39-41.

Streeter, L. A. (1978). Acoustic determinants of phrase boundary perception. *Journal of the Acoustical Society of America, 64,* 1582-1592.

Studdert-Kennedy, M., Liberman, A. M., Harris, K. S., & Cooper, F. S. (1970). Motor theory of speech perception: A reply to Lane's critical review. *Psychological Review, 77,* 234-249.

Suomi, K. (1993). An outline of a developmental model of adult phonological organization and behavior. *Journal of Phonetics, 21,* 29-60.

Suzuki, T., & Ogiba, Y. (1961). Conditioned orientation reflex audiometry. *Archives of Otolaryngology, 74,* 192-198.

Swoboda, P., Morse, P. A., & Leavitt, L. A. (1976). Memory factors in infant vowel discrimination of normal and at-risk infants. *Child Development, 47,* 459-465.

Templin, M. (1957). Certain language skills in children. *Institute of Child Welfare Monographs, 26,* Minneapolis: University of Minnesota Press.

Trehub, S. E. (1973). Infants' sensitivity to vowel and tonal contrasts. *Developmental Psychology, 9,* 91-96.

Trehub, S. E. (1976). The discrimination of foreign speech contrasts by infants and adults. *Child Development, 47,* 466-472.

Trehub, S. E., Bull, D., & Schneider, B. A. (1981). Infants' speech and non-speech perception: A review and re-evaluation. In Schiefelbusch, R. L. & Bricker, D. B. (Eds.), *Early language: Acquisition and intervention.* Baltimore: University Park Press (pp. 11-50).

Trehub, S. E., & Rabinovitch, M. S. (1972). Auditory-linguistic sensitivity in early infancy. *Developmental Psychology, 6,* 74-77.

Verbrugge, R. R., Strange, W., Shankweiler, D. P., & Edman, T. R. (1976). What information enables a listener to map a talker's vowel space? *Journal of the Acoustical Society of America, 60,* 198-212.

Vince, M. A., Armitage, S. E., Baldwin, B. A., Toner, J., & Moore, B. C. J. (1981). The sound environment of fetal sheep. *Behaviour, 81,* 296-315.

Wakefield, J. R., Doughtie, E. B., & Yom, L. (1974). The identification of structural components of an unknown language. *Journal of Psycholinguistic Research, 3,* 261-269.

Werker, J. F., Gilbert, J. H. V., Humphrey, K., & Tees, R. C. (1981). Developmental aspects of cross-language speech perception. *Child Development, 52,* 349-355.

Werker, J. F., & Lalonde, C. E. (1988). Cross-language speech perception: Initial capabilities and developmental change. *Developmental Psychology, 24,* 672-683.

Werker, J. F., & McLeod, P. J. (1989). Infant preference for both male and female infant-directed talk: A developmental study of attentional and affective responsiveness. *Canadian Journal of Psychology, 43,* 230-246.

Werker, J. F.; & Pegg, J. E. (1992). Infant speech perception and phonological acquisition. In Ferguson, C., Menn, L., & Stoel-Gammon, C. (Eds.), *Phonological development: Models, research, implications.* Parkton, MD: York (pp. 285-311).

Werker, J. F., & Tees, R. C. (1984a). Cross language speech perception: Evidence for perceptual reorganization during the first year of life. *Infant Behavior and Development, 7,* 49-63.

Werker, J. F., & Tees, R. C. (1984b). Phonemic and phonetic factors in adult cross-language speech perception. *Journal of the Acoustical Society of America, 75,* 1866-1878.

Williams, L. (1977). The perception of stop consonants by Spanish-English bilinguals. *Perception & Psychophysics, 21,* 289-297.

Woodward, J. Z., & Aslin, R. N. (1990). *Segmentation Cues in Maternal Speech to Infants.* Poster presentation at the seventh biennial meeting of the International Conference on Infancy Studies, Montreal.

Suggested Readings

Overview of Developmental Speech Perception

Aslin, R. N. (1987). Visual and auditory development in infancy. In Osofsky, J. D. (Ed.), *Handbook of infancy* (2nd ed.). New York: Wiley (pp. 5-97).

Aslin, R. N., Pisoni, D. B., & Jusczyk, P. W. (1983). Auditory development and speech perception in infancy. In Haith, M., & Campos, J. (Eds.), *Handbook of child psychology,* vol. 2. *Infancy and developmental psychobiology.* New York: Wiley (pp. 573-687).

Kuhl, P. K. (1987). Perception of speech and sound in early infancy. In Salapatek, P., & Cohen, L. (Eds.), *Handbook of infant perception,* vol. 2. New York: Academic Press (pp. 275-381).

Categorical Perception

Harnad, S. (1987). *Categorical perception: The groundwork of cognition.* New York: Cambridge University Press.

Perception of Speech and Nonspeech Stimuli

Jusczyk, P. W., Rosner, B. S., Reed, M., & Kennedy, L. J. (1989). Could temporal order differences underlie 2-month-olds' discrimination of English voicing contrasts? *Journal of the Acoustical Society of America, 85,* 1741-1749.

Krumhansl, C. L., & Jusczyk, P. W. (1990). Infants' perception of phrase structure in music. *Psychological Science, 1,* 70-73.

Trehub, S. E. (1987). Infants' perception of musical patterns. *Perception & Psychophysics, 41,* 635-641.

Trehub, S. E., Thorpe, L. A., & Morrongiello, B. A. (1987). Organizational processes in infants' perceptions of auditory patterns. *Child Development, 58,* 741-749.

Cross-Linguistic Research and Developmental Change

Aslin, R. N., & Pisoni, D. B. (1980). Some developmental processes in speech perception. In Yeni-Komshian. G., Kavanagh, J. F., & Ferguson, C. A. (Eds.), *Child phonology: Perception and production.* New York: Academic Press (pp. 67-96).

Jusczyk, P. W., & Bertoncini, J. (1988). Viewing the development of speech perception as an innately guided learning process. *Language and Speech, 31,* 217-238.

Jusczyk, P. W. (1992). Developing phonological

categories. In Ferguson, C. A., Stoel-Gammon, C., & Menn, L. (Eds.), *Phonological development: Models, research, implications.* Parkton, MD: York (pp. 17-64).

Werker, J. F. (1991). The ontogeny of speech perception. In Mattingly, I. G., & Studdert-Kennedy, M. (Eds.), *Modularity and the motor theory of speech perception.* Hillsdale, NJ: Erlbaum (pp. 91-110).

Werker, J. F., & Tees, R. C. (1992). The organization and reorganization of human speech perception. *Annual Review of Neuroscience, 15,* 377-402.

Methods for Infant Perception Research

Gottlieb, G. & Krasnegor, N. A. (1985). *Measurement of audition and vision in the first year of postnatal life: A methodological overview.* Norwood, NJ: Ablex.

Biological Foundations of Speech Perception Capacities

Kuhl, P. K. (1988). Auditory perception and the evolution of speech. *Human Evolution, 3,* 19-43.

Miller, J. L., & Jusczyk, P. W. (1989). Seeking the neurobiological bases of speech perception. *Cognition, 33,* 111-137.

Models of the Development of Speech Perception Capacities

Jusczyk, P. W. (1986). Towards a model for the development of speech perception. In Perkell, J., & Klatt, D. H., (Eds.), *Invariance and variability in speech processes.* Hillsdale, NJ: Erlbaum (pp. 1-19).

Jusczyk, P. W. (1994). Infant speech perception and the development of the mental lexicon. In Nusbaum, H. C., & Goodman, J. C. (Eds.), *The transition from speech sounds to spoken words: The development of speech perception.* Cambridge, MA: MIT Press (pp. 227-270).

Mehler, J., Dupoux, E., & Segui, J. (1990). Constraining models of lexical access: The onset of word recognition. In Altmann, G. T. M. (Ed.), *Cognitive models of speech processing.* Hillsdale, NJ: Erlbaum (pp. 236-262).

Suomi, K. (1993). An outline of a developmental model of adult phonological organization and behavior. *Journal of Phonetics, 21,* 29-60.

Speech Perception Capacities and the Acquisition of Language

Fernald, A. (1989). Intonation and communicative intent in mothers' speech to infants: Is the melody the message? *Child Development, 60,* 1497-1510.

Gleitman, L.R., Gleitman, H., Landau, B., & Wanner, E. (1988). Where learning begins: Initial representations for language learning. In Newmeyer, F. (Ed.), *The Cambridge linguistic survey* (vol. 3). Cambridge, MA: Cambridge University Press (pp. 150-193).

Kemler Nelson, D. G., Hirsh-Pasek, K., Jusczyk, P. W., & Wright Cassidy, K. (1989). How the prosodic cues in motherese might assist language learning. *Journal of Child Language, 16,* 53-68.

Morgan, J. L. (1986). *From simple input to complex grammar.* Cambridge, MA: MIT Press.

Chapter 10

Auditory Processing
of Speech

Steven Greenberg

Key Terms

adaptation 394
autocorrelation (AC) 389
automatic gain control (AGC) 364
characteristic frequency (CF) 371
coincidence detection 386
efferent 393
Fourier theory 365
frequency-threshold curve (FTC) 382
inhibition 376
lateral inhibitory network (LIN) 379
linear, time-invariant (LTI) system 363
low pitch 392
neural delay lines 389
nonlinear system 380

INTRODUCTION

The auditory processing of speech is one of the most challenging and exciting domains of research in experimental phonetics and the speech sciences. For most of its history auditory research has focused on relatively simple signals with easy to characterize spectral (e.g., sinusoid) or temporal (e.g., click) features on the assumption that the representation of more complex signals (e.g., speech and music) could be extrapolated from the response to these more basic stimuli. In other words, the inner ear's response to sound was considered linear. A linear system's response to complex, time-varying signals such as speech is predictable from its response to mathematically more tractable stimuli as sinusoids, clicks and Gaussian (white) noise (see Oppenheim and Schafer [1975] or Lynn and Fuerst [1989] for a discussion of **linear, time-invariant (LTI)** systems). Because the ear was thought to function as an LTI system, there appeared to be no reason to use speech sounds in physiological or psychophysical studies. The linearity of the inner ear was first empirically challenged by Rhode's (1971) measurements of basilar membrane motion. While others (e.g., von Békésy, 1960; Johnstone and Boyle, 1967; Wilson and Johnstone, 1972) had found the membrane's motion to be completely linear, Rhode observed that over a certain portion of the membrane's response area, near its most sensitive region, the amplitude of motion was greater than expected. As other laboratories confirmed Rhode's observations and their implications became manifest, a shift to more sophisticated and realistic signals began.

It is within this historical context that Murray Sachs and Eric Young initiated a veritable revolution in our understanding of the auditory mechanisms underlying speech processing (Sachs and Young, 1979; Young and Sachs, 1979). Until that time little credence had been given to the idea that important features of the speech signal are based on the temporal properties of auditory neural response, as suggested by Wever (1949) and Licklider (1951). Most auditory researchers favored the **place theory** of frequency coding, in which the spectral characteristics of speech were thought to be encoded in terms of the spatial distribution of neural activity across a **tonotopically organized** population of cells (Whitfield, 1970). Over the past decade a substantial number of studies have confirmed Young and Sach's conclusions that temporal mechanisms play an important role in coding many features of the speech signal. At the same time, our understanding of the interplay between temporal and spatial dimensions has increased substantially, to the point where the traditional opposition between place models and temporal models for frequency representation no longer pertains. It is now generally recognized that speech is encoded through multiple representations, some primarily based on neural timing, others on place information. And there is increasing evidence that other cues, such as those pertaining to the spatial distribution of neural onset latency, are also involved (Shamma, 1985a,b; Holton, Love, and Gill, 1992).

Not only has our physiological knowledge of speech coding increased, but the approaches have also changed substantially. In the past, physiological studies were rarely undertaken with perceptual questions in mind, a notable exception being the work of Evans and Wilson (1974) and Evans (1978). Psychoacoustic experiments usually did not connect with the underlying physiology, Flanagan and Guttman (1960a,b) being an outstanding exception. Increasingly, auditory investigations are interdisciplinary, with physiologists, psychologists, linguists, electrical engineers, and computer scientists all working on the same questions from different perspectives. The advent of powerful, affordable computer technology is beginning to transform the field as it becomes possible to visualize the auditory representation of speech with a richness and clarity undreamed of only a decade ago (e.g., Cooke, Beet, and Crawford, 1993).

At first glance, auditory processing of speech appears to be straightforward and simple. The auditory periphery can spectrally analyze incoming sound, and it is natural to assume that the ear's primary responsibility, as far as speech is concerned, is to construct and transmit a running spectrum of the signal to higher cortical centers for conversion into linguistic units. In this rather commonly held view (e.g., Pisoni, 1982; Klatt, 1989), the auditory periphery functions merely as a biological frequency analyzer with little capability for intelligent processing or learning. Knowledge of complex auditory processing is largely confined to such peripheral structures as the auditory nerve and cochlear nucleus. However, it is apparent that even at these caudal stations of the auditory pathway, powerful and elegantly designed systems encode incoming speech and other biological sounds in a manner that provides a robust, reliable representation of the signal under an exceedingly wide range of acoustic conditions.

The importance of such adaptive processing is apparent to anyone who has ever had a serious hearing loss. Although such listeners generally understand speech well in quiet, nonreverberant environments, that ability is seriously compromised in noisy conditions. This suggests that the auditory periphery, locus of most hearing pathology, is far more than a mere spectrum analyzer. It is also an **automatic gain control**, adjusting the neural activity to the background level, and containing powerful, effective noise-reduction circuitry that allows the meaningful elements of speech to be successfully decoded, even in the presence of spectrally overlapping, competing sounds. Although the means by which the ear accomplishes these feats are not known in detail, a growing body of evidence suggests that much of this adaptive processing occurs in the inner ear and cochlear nuclei.

This chapter focuses on the physiological mechanisms underlying the ability to extract phonetically relevant information from the speech signal, particularly under realistically adverse acoustic conditions. The physiological basis of acoustic transduction in the auditory periphery will first be described, beginning with spectrally simpler signals than speech. This transduction pertains to the process of converting sound pressure into a pattern of mechanical vibrations in the middle ear and cochlea (basilar membrane) and thence to an electrochemical form in the cochlea (inner hair cells and auditory nerve).

Then how the speech spectrum is encoded in the auditory periphery as well as the transformations of these representations at the higher stations of the auditory pathway will be discussed. This chapter is concerned particularly with the mechanisms permitting robust encoding of speech in noisy environments and the utility of multiple representations for that end. Finally, auditory coding of speech will be addressed in relation to several other topics, including speech recognition, clinical assessment of hearing loss, and the structure of linguistic sound patterns.

RELEVANCE OF AUDITORY PHYSIOLOGY TO SPEECH PROCESSING

Inferences that can be made about speech coding in the auditory pathway are limited, because the overwhelming majority of physiological and anatomical studies by necessity have been performed on nonhumans, mainly cats and rodents. Because speech almost surely relies on neural circuitry unique to our species, it is necessary to be cautious in extending the insights garnered from animal studies to the processing of speech. Despite this limitation, several observations suggest that most of what we know about the mammalian auditory periphery in general applies to humans as well. The anatomy and physiology of this region (except the dorsal cochlear nucleus) is remarkably similar across most mammalian species, including primates, and much of the function of these structures is comparable across species. Differences among mammalian hearing organs generally involve parameters of relatively minor relevance to speech coding, such as sensitivity to ultrasonic signals and very low frequencies; however, the ability to make fine discriminations of frequency is an exception to this rule.

There are two additional caveats concerning the use of physiological data to infer the neural basis of human speech coding. Virtually all physiological studies are performed with the use of barbiturate anesthesia, which alters certain neural circuits, particularly inhibitory ones. Anesthesia probably has little or no effect on the response properties of cells in either the auditory nerve or ventral cochlear nucleus (Rhode and Kettner, 1987). However, the response properties of dorsal cochlear nucleus cells are known to change in the presence of barbiturates (Evans and Nelson, 1973a,b; Young and Brownell, 1976; Rhode and Kettner, 1987). In addition, one of the major circuits mediating the automatic gain control of the cochlea, the crossed olivocochlear bundle, is also affected by anesthesia.

The second concern involves linking physiology, particularly that of the auditory periphery, to the complex pattern of behavior underlying the perception of speech. Many auditory nuclei and millions of nerve cells lie between the auditory periphery and the destination of speech information in the cortical association areas of the parietal, temporal, and frontal lobes. For this reason the representation of the speech signal developed in the periphery is a crude one, far removed from such abstract linguistic entities as phoneme and distinctive feature. And because of the complex interactions among the auditory nuclei, it would be rash to link a specific behavioral capability to a single anatomical locus or population of cells. Nevertheless, certain inferences about the nature of the acoustic representation of speech, based on the physiological responses in the auditory periphery, are likely to have significant implications for general properties of the sound patterns of language.

AUDITORY FUNCTION

The role of the auditory periphery has traditionally been viewed as a frequency analyzer of limited precision represtating the spectrotemporal properties of the acoustic waveform for higher-level processing in the central auditory pathway (i.e., the auditory system above the level of the cochlear nuclei). According to **Fourier theory**, any waveform can be decomposed into a series of sinusoidal constituents that mathematically describe the acoustic waveform. By this analytical technique it is possible to describe all speech sounds in terms of an energy distribution across frequency and time. For example, the Fourier spectrum of a typical vowel is a series of sinusoidal components whose frequencies are integral multiples of a common fundamental frequency and whose amplitudes vary in accordance with the resonance (formant) pattern of the associated vocal tract configuration. The vocal tract transfer function modifies the glottal spectrum by selectively amplifying energy in certain regions of the spectrum. These regions of energy maxima are called *formants*. The spectra of nonvocalic sounds such as stop consonants, affricates, and fricatives differ from vowels in a number of ways possibly significant for the way they are encoded in the auditory periphery. In these sounds the energy peaks are generally considerably below those of vowels. In certain segments, such as the stop release and frication, the energy distribution is rather diffuse, with only a crude delineation of the underlying formant pattern. In addition, many of these segments are voiceless, their waveforms lacking a clear periodic quality that would reflect the vibration of the vocal folds. The amplitude of such consonantal segments is typically 30 to 50 dB sound pressure level (SPL), up to 40 dB less intense than adjacent vocalic segments. In addition, the rate of spectral change is generally greater for consonants, and they are usually brief compared with vocalic segments (see Chapter 5). These differences have significant consequences for the way consonants and vowels are encoded in the auditory periphery.

The traditional view of the ear as a frequency analyzer is probably inadequate to describe the auditory periphery's ability to process speech. Under many conditions the frequency-selective properties of the auditory periphery appear to be only tangential to its ability to convey the context of the speech signal, relying rather on integrative mechanisms to isolate the information-laden elements of the speech stream and provide a continuous event stream from which to extract the underlying message. Devotees of cocktail parties can attest to the fact that far more is involved in decoding speech than merely computing a running spectrum. In such conditions a faithful representation of the spectrum may even hinder the ability to understand because of its high noise content. The auditory system probably uses specific strategies to focus on the elements of speech most likely to extract the sense of the acoustic signal. Computing a running spectrum of the speech signal is singularly inefficient since much of the sound is extraneous to the message. Instead, the ear extracts the information-laden components of the speech signal and other biological communication sounds that may only slightly resemble the Fourier spectral representation. Such strategies are examined in later sections of this chapter.

ANATOMY AND PHYSIOLOGY OF THE AUDITORY PATHWAY

The auditory pathway has four primary zones. The first, encompassing the external and middle ears, the cochlea, and the auditory nerve, is the *auditory periphery*. The brain stem component of the system includes the cochlear nucleus, trapezoid body, superior olivary complex, lateral lemniscus, and inferior colliculus. The brain stem pathway projects into the auditory nuclei of the thalamus, incorporated in the medial

A

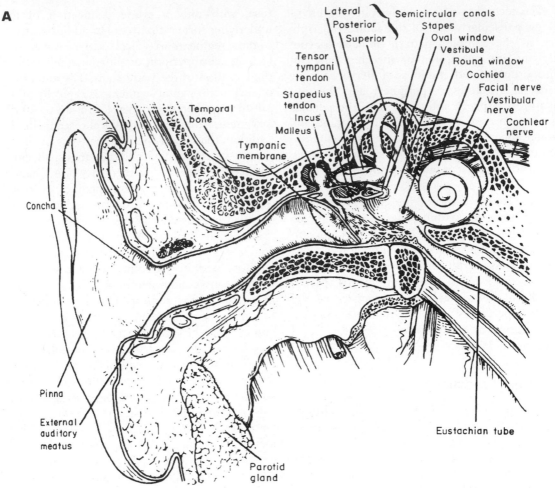

FIGURE 10-1   The principal anatomical structures of the auditory system. *A,* The auditory periphery, comprising the external, middle and inner ears. (From Kessel & Kardon, 1979.)

Continued.

geniculate body. From this third level fibers project into the primary auditory cortical areas, from which information is ultimately transmitted to the cortical association regions involved in speech recognition, such as Wernicke's area. The anatomy (Fig.10-1) and physiology of the auditory system will be considered only briefly in this chapter. For a more extended discussion, consult Pickles's (1988) excellent introduction to the anatomy and physiology of the auditory pathway. For more advanced treatment of anatomy see Webster, Popper, and Fay (1992), and for physiology, see Popper and Fay (1992).

The External Ear

The external ear, also known as the ear canal, funnels sound to the tympanic membrane, or eardrum. Directly outside the ear canal lies the

pinna, a cartilaginous appendage important for locating sound in space, particularly for frequencies above 4 kHz. In certain animals, such as cats, the pinnae can rotate to assist in tracking sound.

The contours of the human pinna, with the length of the ear canal, create a broad resonance resulting in an approximately 10 to 15 dB of amplification of the spectrum between 2.5 and 5 kHz, accounting for the enhanced sensitivity to signals in this region. This selective amplification is significant for speech, since many segments, such as stop consonants and fricatives, contain significant energy in this frequency region.

The Middle Ear

The tympanic membrane is a pressure transducer, responding to the pressure gradient in the external ear. Coupled to the other side of the tympanic membrane is the malleus, one of three

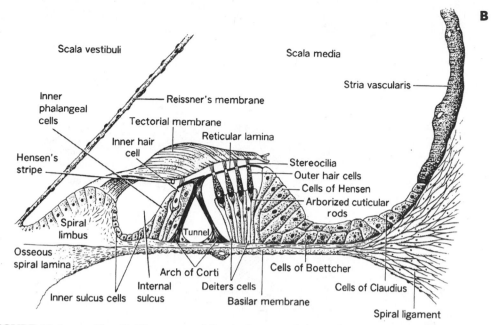

FIGURE 10-1, cont'd. *B,* The organ of Corti. (From Gulick, Will, Gelsand, S., Frisona, R., 1989.)

Continued.

exceedingly small bones (the other two being the incus and the stapes) that constitute the ossicles, or ossicular chain. The other end of the chain is the foot plate of the stapes, which articulates with a small membrane, the oval window. This membrane is about one-fifteenth the area of the tympanic membrane. Because of this area ratio and the tight linkage of the ossicular bones, the middle ear amplifies sound approximately 20 dB, effectively matching the impedance of air-borne sound with the fluid-filled vibrations of the cochlea. Because of their small mass the ossicles are less responsive to frequencies below 500 Hz, accounting for the falloff in sensitivity for very low frequencies. Without the middle ear the auditory system would be considerably less sensitive to sound and would lack the most peripheral of its automatic gain controls (AGCs). Two muscles, the tensor tympani and the stapedius, articulate with the ossicles. The stapedius attaches to the stapes and the tensor tympani to the malleus. The combined action of these muscles is to reduce the ossicular response to sound, particularly for frequencies below 2 kHz (Pang and Peake, 1986). These muscles contract in response to very intense sounds, reducing the risk of permanent trauma to the delicate sensory cells in the cochlea. They also enhance the processing of speech at high amplitudes.

Origins of Cochlear Frequency Selectivity

Much of the ear's frequency selective capability stems from physiological mechanisms of the inner ear, which contains three fluid-filled chambers. The middle chamber, the scala media, contains the principal anatomical structures of acoustic transduction. At the bottom of this partition is the basilar membrane (BM), underlying the organ of Corti, which contains the sensory hair cells, supporting cells, and tectorial membrane. The BM, relatively narrow and stiff at its base, becomes progressively wider and more massive toward the apex. Because of this taper the stiffness of the BM varies by a factor of a hundred over its 35-mm length. The basal (stiffest) portion responds most sensitively to very high frequencies and the apex is most sensitive to low frequencies (Fig. 10-2, *A*). The motion of the BM conforms to that of a traveling wave. For frequencies above 5 kHz this wave motion will quickly reach a maximum near the base of the membrane and damp out before traveling much further down the BM (Fig. 10-2, *B*). In response to frequencies below 1 kHz the pattern of motion is rather different. The BM vibrates along much of its length, particularly at SPLs typical of speech. At the place of resonance (i.e., peak response) the displacement amplitude will be maximum, but the motion does not

C

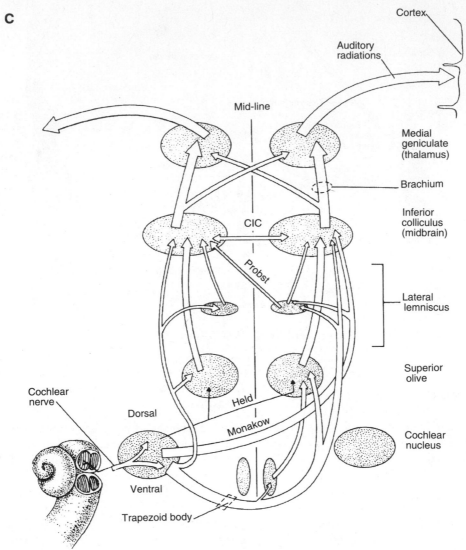

FIGURE 10-1, cont'd.   *C,* **The central pathway.** (From Gulick, Wil., Gelsand, S., & Frisina, R., 1989.)

diminish very rapidly as the wave proceeds toward the helicotrema, a gap in the cochlear partition through which endolymphatic fluid flows, at the apical end. Moreover, BM displacement in response to low-frequency signals can be of considerable magnitude across much of the cochlear partition at SPLs typical of speech. Because of this asymmetric characteristic of the traveling wave, the BM is sharply tuned to frequencies above 4 kHz and broadly tuned to most frequencies in the speech range. The tuning characteristics of neural elements all the way up the auditory pathway appear to stem from the mechanical tuning of the BM. This differential tuning has considerable significance for models of complex signal processing in the auditory periphery.

The motion of the BM filters the input waveform, distributing its local pattern of vibration in accordance with the traveling wave. Thus, the pattern of BM motion at the base may differ considerably from that at the apex. Consider the response of the BM to three different signals (Figure 10-2, *B*). An 8 kHz sinusoid produces a spatially discrete pattern of vibration confined to the basal portion of the membrane. The BM moves up and down at 8 kHz along a relatively small portion of its extent and otherwise is immobile. Increasing the amplitude of this signal to speech intensities (50 to 80 dB SPL) widens the area of response along the BM only slightly, consistent with the sharply tuned characteristic of the basal portion of the membrane. A 1 kHz signal will vibrate the BM at that frequency. At very low intensities the vibration will be largely confined to the apical portion, while

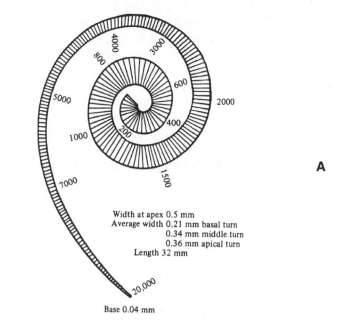

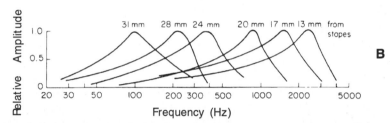

FIGURE 10-2   The mechanical basis for tonotopic organization. *A,* The spatial frequency mapping of the human cochlea. Because of the stiffness gradient of the basilar membrane, the basal portion is most sensitive to frequencies above 10 kHz, and the apical end is most responsive to frequencies below 200 Hz. In the human cochlea, approximately 60% of the 35 mm length of the basilar membrane is devoted to frequencies below 4 kHz, the core range of the speech spectrum. (From Stuhlman, O. [1943]. *An introduction to biophysics.* New York: Wiley.) *B,* Spatial segregation of the traveling wave associated with signals spanning a broad range of frequencies. High-frequency signals reach a maximum near the base of the basilar membrane and rapidly damp out. Low-frequency signals propagate to the apical end from the base and damp out much more slowly. Because of this traveling wave asymmetry, the cochlea appears to be considerably more highly tuned to high- frequency signals than to low. (Adapted from Békésy, G. von [1960]. *Experiments in Hearing.* New York: McGraw-Hill.)

higher SPLs much of the membrane, including the base, will move in synchrony to the 1 kHz tone. The pattern of BM motion resulting from concurrent presentation of these signals will depend on both relative and absolute amplitudes. If the intensity of the 1 kHz signal is relatively low, the membrane will vibrate in two spatially discrete modes, each synchronized to one of the frequencies. Under these conditions the mechanical response along the BM resolves the particular vibration associated with each spectral component. At higher SPLs BM motion is dominated by the response to the 1 kHz signal.

Traditional models of auditory frequency analysis assume that this place representation is the primary means by which spectral information is encoded in the cochlea and auditory nerve. The auditory nerve is the sole afferent path from the inner ear to the remainder of the auditory system and higher brain centers. In the human it consists of 30,000 fibers per ear whose most sensitive characteristic frequencies range from about 0.1 to 18 kHz.

The motion of the BM is transformed into nerve cell impulses, or spikes, through the membrane's coupling to the auditory nerve. The membrane's motion is converted into a modulation of the inner-hair-cell (IHC) **receptor potential** by the shearing action between the reticular membrane and the tectorial membrane overlying the IHC cilia. This modulation of the receptor potential, in turn, modulates the release of a chemical neurotransmitter, which depolarizes auditory nerve fibers (ANFs) innervating the cell. When the energy associated with a spectral component is high, the displacement of the BM at its maximum will be relatively large. In turn, the deflection of the ciliary bundle atop the IHC will also be large, producing large bursts of neurotransmitter release when the hair cell is depolarized. Up to a certain limit the displacement of the BM, the deflection of IHC cilia, the magnitude of the receptor potential, the amount of neurotransmitter released, and the rate of ANF discharge are all proportional to the amount of energy driving that portion of the cochlea. Under these conditions it is possible in principle to encode the spectrum of speech and other complex sounds in terms of the amount of ANF discharge at each location along the cochlear partition. This isomorphic coding can occur when the physiological elements of the system behave linearly, typically between threshold and 40 dB SPL. Thus, at low SPLs it is possible in principle to infer a sound's spectrum from the spatial pattern of neural activity in the auditory nerve if the filtering action of the basilar membrane is sufficiently sharp to resolve individual frequency components in the input signal. This is the basis of the rate-place coding of the spectrum.

Many auditory neurons, particularly in the periphery, discharge in the absence of sound. At the level of the auditory nerve this background activity is the result of neurotransmitter leakage from the inner hair cell, which is effective in depolarizing the innervating nerve fibers. There are three classes of AN fibers in terms of the level of background activity. Approximately 16% exhibit little or no spontaneous activity (low-SR group), another 25% fire between 0.5 and 18 times per second without acoustical stimulation (medium-SR group), while the third group (60%) has a relatively high level of spontaneous activity (18-120 spikes/s) (high-SR group).

Phase-Locking and Temporal Cues

The modulation of neurotransmitter release by the IHC receptor potential has an important consequence for the coding of speech in the auditory periphery. At frequencies below 4 or 5 kHz the receptor potential oscillation is large enough to modulate transmitter release so as to affect the temporal pattern of ANF discharge (Sellick and Russell, 1978). In response to sinusoidal stimulation, transmitter release occurs only during the rarefaction phase of the stimulus cycle. Because the probability of a fiber's discharge is highly correlated with transmitter release, the unit's firing pattern is itself modulated in a fashion analogous to but differing in important ways from the IHC receptor potential. The receptor potential modulation is large enough to produce a cadence of discharge activity in ANFs temporally synchronized to the driving waveform.

This phase-locked ANF response provides a second means by which frequency is encoded in the auditory periphery. In the absence of **phase-locking**, the probability of firing relative to the cochlear-filtered waveform is approximately uniform throughout. Under this condition the firing probability is uncorrelated with the fine temporal structure of the driving signal, hence provides no temporal information with which to infer the spectrotemporal characteristics of the stimulating waveform. This uniform firing distribution is characteristic of the ANF response to sinusoidal stimuli above 4 or 5 kHz. Contrast this pattern with that of lower-frequency stimuli. For such signals the probability of discharge is relatively high during a restricted time interval (or phase) of the stimulus cycle and relatively low otherwise (Fig. 10-3). Under such conditions potentially important information concerning the spectrotemporal characteristics of the driving waveform is carried in the cadence of auditory nerve discharge. A later section will discuss how such phase-locked patterns may be used by higher auditory centers to decode important features of the acoustic signal.

Lateral Suppression and Rate-Place Cues

Under certain acoustic conditions the discharge activity of single fibers diminishes in the presence of intense signals. In response to wideband noise the firing rate of certain fibers, usually of low spontaneous rate (SR), will first grow with increasing stimulus and then decrease with further increments of the noise level (Schalk and Sachs, 1980). A second instance of suppression

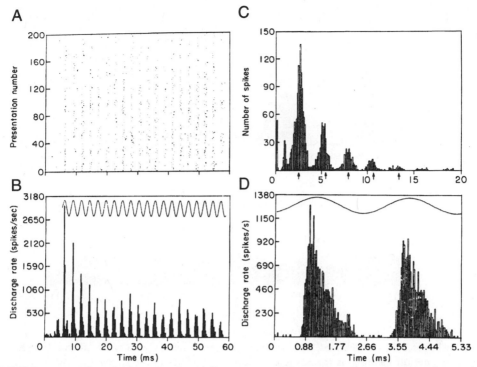

FIGURE 10-3   Phase-locking in the auditory nerve. The temporal distribution of neural discharge is highly synchronized to the stimulus waveform when the signal frequency is below 2 kHz. At higher frequencies, the correlation between waveform periodicity and neural discharge diminishes appreciably until it disappears around 5 kHz. Phase–locking of primary-like unit recorded from the anteroventral cochlear nucleus of the cat, in response to a 375-Hz sinusoid presented at 70 dB SPL. Stimulus duration was 50 ms. The unit's temporal response pattern is similar to that of an auditory-nerve fiber. A, Dot raster display, in which each dot represents the occurrence of a discharge, shows the stochastic nature of the phase-locked response. Binwidth = 250 μs. B, Post-stimulus-time (PST) histogram shows the probability of response as a function of time from stimulus onset. In this instance the probability is indicated in units of instantaneous discharge rate. The average rate was approximately 160 spikes/sec. Sinusoidal function whose period is equivalent to that of the input signal is shown for reference. Note the rapid adaptation of the response over the initial 5 to 10 ms. Binwidth = 250 μs. C, Interval histogram spanning a time window of 20 ms. Arrows mark the stimulus period and integral multiples thereof. Binwidth = 100 μs. D, Period histogram binned over a time window of 5.33 ms (equivalent to two periods of the input signal). Binwidth = 26.7 μs. The unit's discharge rate threshold was 25 dB SPL and its spontaneous rate was 36 spikes/sec. Histograms are based on 200 stimulus repetitions. (A–D, from Greenberg, S. (1988). Acoustic transduction in the auditory periphery. *Journal of Phonetics, 16*, 3-18.)   *Continued.*

is a response to the concurrent presentation of two sinusoidal signals. The response (average firing rate) to a sinusoid presented at the fiber's most sensitive tone, or **characteristic frequency (CF)**, will diminish upon presentation of a second tone, the suppressor (Sachs and Kiang, 1968). The effective frequency and intensity range of the suppressor tone is the suppression region (Fig. 10-4). This area generally lies outside the excitation region, the range of frequencies and intensities effective in driving the fiber to single-tone stimuli. Under most conditions the suppressor must be at least 20 dB more intense than the CF signal to drive down the fiber's discharge rate. It may be significant that the disparities in spectral magnitude required for suppression are common in many speech sounds. Sachs and Young (1980) have demonstrated that vowels can produce such suppression in the auditory nerve. The origins and consequences of this suppression remain controversial. Much of it appears to be mechanical, reflecting the nonlinear motion of the BM to complex signals.

E

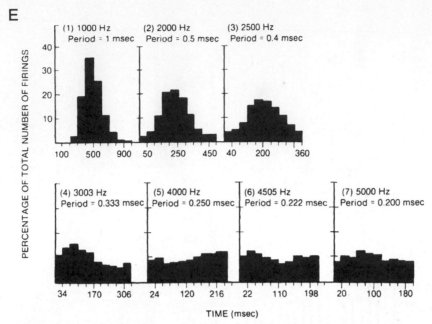

FIGURE 10-3, cont'd. *E,* The precision of synchronization to a sinusoidal signal is greatest for frequencies below 1 kHz and falls off sharply in response to frequencies above 2 kHz. Shown are period histograms for a single auditory nerve fiber in the squirrel monkey in response to sinusoidal signals ranging in frequency from 1 to 5 kHz. (From Hind, J. E., Anderson, D. J., Brugge, J. F., & Rose, S. E. (1967). Coding of information pertaining to paired low-frequency tones in single auditory nerve fibers of the squirrel monkey. *Journal of Neurophysiology, 30,* 794-816.)

ANATOMY AND PHYSIOLOGY OF THE COCHLEAR NUCLEUS

Information in the auditory nerve is integrated and processed in the cochlear nucleus (CN), which consists of the anteroventral (AVCN), posteroventral (PVCN), and dorsal (DCN) divisions (Fig. 10-5), each of which receives a strong, direct projection from the auditory nerve. Each division has a distinctive personality, both in cytoarchitecture and in the physiological response properties of its cells. Moreover, each division has a unique set of projections to the upper auditory brain stem nuclei and appears to behave as a separate system. Because of this anatomical and physiological diversity, as well as for reasons discussed below, the CN is probably the first locus in the auditory pathway where integrative operations concerned with extraction of biologically important acoustic features are performed (see Rhode and Greenberg [1992] for a detailed review).

Anteroventral Cochlear Nucleus

The anteroventral division is populated principally by primary-like (PL) and primary-like with notch (PLN) neurons, whose response properties closely resemble those of ANFs. These cells project via the trapezoid body to the superior olivary complex (SOC) and are thought to play an important role in binaural analysis for the localization of sound (Erulkar, 1972; Yin and Kuwada, 1984). A smaller population are stellate cells, which are physiologically identified as **chopper** units (Rhode, Oertel, and Smith, 1983). Choppers, the predominant physiological response pattern observed in the ventral cochlear nucleus, are also found in more centrally located nuclei such as the inferior colliculus. The name derives from the fact that the discharge level oscillates at a relatively regular interval, typically 1.5 to 10 ms. The function of these cells is not entirely clear, though they seem to be important for encoding spectral information. There are also a very few onset units, whose physiology and anatomy are discussed in the next section.

Posteroventral Cochlear Nucleus

The posteroventral division contains relatively few PL units but has a large concentration of chopper and onset units. These neurons project

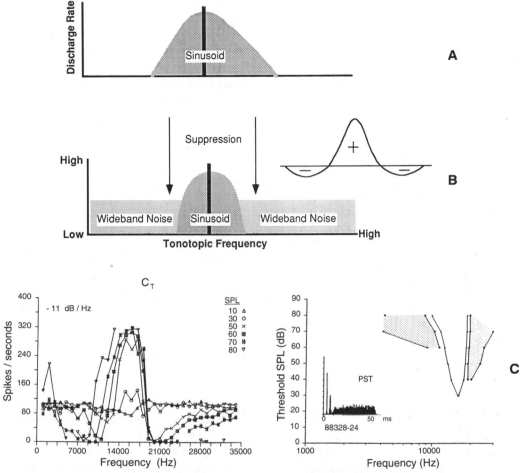

FIGURE 10-4   Lateral suppression and inhibition. Lateral suppression is the reduction in discharge rate evoked by a stimulus in the presence of an additional signal, such as a second tone or broadband noise. *A,* Without suppression. Lateral suppression/inhibition showing the excitation pattern (stippled area) evoked by a sinusoidal signal (black bar). *B,* With suppression. The excitation to the same sinusoidal signal in the presence of broadband noise. The noise effectively sharpens the rate-place representation of the sinusoidal component by suppressing the discharge on the skirts of the excitation pattern. *C,* Such discharge suppression is shown for a transient chopper unit from the posteroventral cochlear nucleus of the cat. Rather than record from many different cells spanning a broad tonotopic range, the discharge of a single cell is recorded in response to sinusoidal signals of variable frequency and sound pressure level. The degree of suppression is considerable, particularly on the high-frequency side of the excitatory component of the response area. The suppression contour is shown (stippled area) flanking the excitatory region, along with the poststimulus time histogram (PSTH) of the chopper unit. The response area delineated by sinusoidal signals is altered in the presence of broadband noise. The changes in the filtering principally affect the edges of the excitatory region, sharpening the contrast between the foreground excitatory signal and the background. This contrast enhance ment is clearly shown in the response areas of neurons obtained in the presence of broadband noise. The suppression results in clear delineation of the rate-place excitation pattern evoked by sinusoidal signals in the presence of the noise background. This contrast enhancement is augmented in the cochlear nucleus through inhibitory neural mechanisms. (From Rhode, W. S., & Greenberg, S. R. [1994]. Lateral suppression and inhibition in the cochlear nucleus of the cat. *Journal of Neurophysiology, 71,* 493-514.)

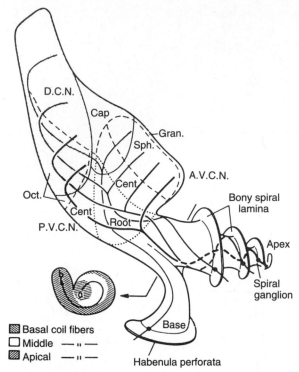

Basal coil fibers
☐ Middle — "" —
▨ Apical — "" —

FIGURE 10-5   A lateral view of the cochlear nuclei showing the projections of the auditory nerve into the three principal divisions of the complex (anteroventral [AVCN], posteroventral [PVCN] and dorsal [DCN]). The auditory nerve fibers from the base of the cochlea (high-frequency CF) are segregated from those coming from the apex (low-frequency CF). The spiral ganglion contains the cell bodies of auditory nerve fibers. The habenula perforata is the opening in the cochlear shell through which the AN fibers project to the cochlear nucleus. Certain cell populations such as granule (gran.) cells in the dorsal division, octopus (oct.) cells in the PVCN and spherical cells of the AVCN are shown. The auditory nerve projects to all three divisions of the cochlear nucleus in highly tonotopic fashion. (From Brodal, A. [1981]. *Neurological anatomy in relation to clinical, medicine* 3rd Ed. Oxford: Oxford University Press. Based on Arneson A. R., & Osen K.K., 1978. The cochlear nerve in the cat: Topography, cochleoptopy and fiber spectrum. *Journal of Comparative Neurology, 178,* 661-678.)

through the intermediate acoustic stria (IAS) to the lateral lemniscus and inferior colliculus, nuclei of the upper auditory brain stem pathway. Although the function of this IAS projection is less clearly defined than that of the AVCN-trapezoid body pathway, it appears to be involved in the coding of intensity and spectral information for complex sounds (Rhode and Smith, 1986a).

Choppers derive their name from their regularity of discharge. In response to high-frequency sinusoidal stimulation these units discharge at a regular interval independent of the stimulus frequency. This modal discharge interval typically ranges between 1.5 and 10 ms, with most choppers capable of discharging at rates up to 250 to 600 spikes per second. Choppers phase-lock to low-frequency sinusoidal and amplitude-modulated (AM) signals, but their ability to follow waveform modulations is generally limited to frequencies below 1 kHz (Rhode and Greenberg, 1991). Choppers appear to receive extensive inhibitory input, which enhances both the extent and magnitude of their lateral suppression relative to that observed in the auditory nerve. The way this enhanced suppression may encode gross spectral contours in terms of rate-place activity is discussed in a later section of this chapter.

The other major physiological response class of the PVCN comprises the onset units, so named because of their tendency to discharge at the onset of stimulation with a high degree of probability and temporal precision and thereafter to diminish their responsiveness. Although the instantaneous discharge rate declines appreciably after the initial onset spike, the sustained firing level of most onset units is relatively high. Their preferential response at stimulus onset pertains principally to signals whose frequencies are higher than 1.5 or 2 kHz. In response to low-frequency, sinusoidal, or AM signals, many of these units phase-lock to the modulation frequency with a remarkably high degree of temporal precision (Rhode and Smith, 1986a; Greenberg and Rhode, 1987; Rhode and Greenberg, 1991).

All onset units can phase-lock to frequency modulations below 0.5 kHz so that the cell fires virtually on every modulation cycle. This entrainment phenomenon may have significant implications for both temporal and rate coding of frequency. The entrainment drives the sustained discharge rate very high, between 500 and 1100 spikes per second, well beyond that observed in response to a high-CF tone (about 200 spikes per second) (Fig. 10-6). Consequently, the neuron is likely to be considerably more responsive to low-frequency signals than to stimuli to which it is most sensitive. This may be a very significant property of onset units, suggesting that they are optimized for processing of AM and low-frequency signals. It is thus

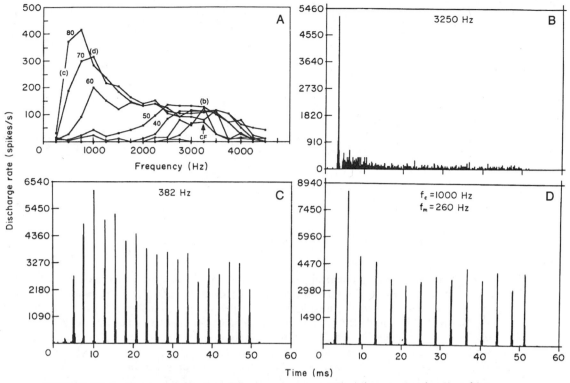

FIGURE 10-6 Temporal filtering. The response area *(A)* and post-stimulus-time histograms *(B,C,D)* of an onset-locker unit recorded from the posteroventral cochlear nucleus of the cat. The unit's characteristic frequency was 3250 Hz and its rate threshold was 20 dB SPL. The letters on the graph denote the frequency and amplitude of the signals used to evoke the responses shown in the PST histograms. *B,* The PST histogram of the unit's response to a CF signal of 3250 Hz, presented at 45 dB SPL. *C,* The PST histogram of the unit's response to a 382-Hz sinusoid, presented at 80 dB SPL. *D,* The response to an amplitude-modulated tone. Carrier frequency (fc) = 1 kHz; modulation frequency, (fm) = 260 Hz; modulation depth = 100%; sound pressure level of the carrier = 80 dB. (From Greenberg, 1988.)

not surprising that the **tonotopic organization** that so clearly characterizes the anteroventral division is not nearly so well defined in the PVCN (Adams, 1991).

The two basic types of onset units are the onset choppers (O_C) and onset lockers (O_L). Onset choppers differ physiologically from onset lockers in two principal respects. First, O_Cs are much more broadly tuned than O_Ls. The tuning properties of O_L units are roughly equivalent to that of ANFs of comparable CF. On average onset choppers are twice as broadly tuned as O_L units, meaning that the former are not very frequency selective, even at SPLs close to threshold (Rhode and Smith, 1986a). This property of O_C units is probably a result of the spatial orientation of their dendritic arborization, which lies at an angle relatively oblique to the isofrequency contour of ANF projections. Therefore, these cells sample the output of ANFs

spanning a relatively broad range of characteristic frequencies, suggesting that these cells are optimized to integrate AN activity over a large frequency range (Fig. 10-7).

One consequence of this broad tuning is that the discharge activity of a substantial proportion of the ANF projection will continue to grow with increasing SPL, implying that onset choppers have a much wider dynamic range than ANFs and other CN unit types. Indeed, this is the case. The dynamic range of most ANFs lies between 20 and 30 dB, a range typical of most CN units, including onset lockers. In contrast, the discharge rate of onset choppers grows with increasing intensity over 50 to 90 dB, suggesting that these cells are optimized to encode changes in intensity over the full range of hearing sensitivity (Fig. 10-7, *A,B*). At each intensity level the cell receives a significant proportion of ANF input whose rate is unsaturated. The CF

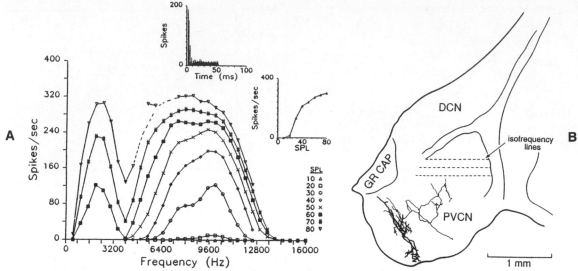

FIGURE 10-7 Physiological, anatomical, and morphological characterization of an onset-chopper (multipolar-stellate) cell of the posteroventral cochlear nucleus. *A*, The response area, rate-intensity curve and poststimulus time histogram of the multipolar-stellate (O_C) cell shown in *B*. CF = 10.4 kHz; threshold = 20 dB SPL. *B*, A labeled O_C multipolar cell in the PVCN illustrating the extent of its dendritic field and its orientation relative to the frequency plane of incoming ANFs. Horizontal lines indicate the approximate frequency isoclines for the ANF projection. Low frequencies are ventral and high frequencies are dorsal. Solid lines indicate dendrites and dashed lines axonal projection. (*A* and *B* from Rhode W. S., & Greenberg, S.R. [1992]. Physiology of the cochlear nuclei. In Popper A.N. & Fay, R. R. (Eds.), *The mammalian auditory pathway: Neurophysiology*. New York: Springer Verlag, pp. 94-152.)

range from which this unsaturated projection originates will change as a function of stimulus intensity. At low SPLs the input will come principally from ANFs most sensitive to the stimulus frequency. At higher intensities, when the rate of the on-CF fiber projection is saturated, other unsaturated ANFs with CFs above and especially below the signal frequency will dominate the afferent input activity to the onset choppers. The implications of onset-chopper and onset-locker response patterns for speech coding are discussed in a later section of this chapter.

Dorsal Cochlear Nucleus

The dorsal division is perhaps the most difficult region of the CN to describe and quantify in general terms. In contrast to the anteroventral and posteroventral divisions, which vary relatively little across mammalian species, there is appreciable diversity in the cytoarchitecture and morphology of the DCN, even among closely related species (Moore, 1991). Significantly, the morphology of the human DCN differs dramatically from that of cats and rodents, from which the bulk of physiological data derive. For this

reason we discuss the DCN's role in speech processing with the utmost caution, since much of the physiological data from animal studies may not pertain to the human. However, despite the morphological diversity, several properties of DCN physiology appear to apply across most, if not all, mammalian species.

Virtually all DCN cells have significant inhibitory input. This **inhibition** is reflected in two principal response properties. The input-output function (rate-intensity curve) of most cells is highly nonmonotonic. At low SPLs the unit discharge rate grows with increasing intensity. However, at moderate to high SPLs the rate neither grows nor saturates but actually declines with increasing intensity, often enough to shut down the cell at high SPLs. The basis of this decline in responsiveness is thought to lie in the complex interplay between excitatory and inhibitory inputs. At low SPLs the excitatory on-CF component of the ANF projection dominates the cell's discharge behavior. At increasing intensities the more diffusely organized inhibitory inputs overwhelm the excitatory component of the projection. One consequence of this interplay is that many DCN cells respond weakly if at all to broadband noise because of the prevalence of inhibitory inputs evoked by such signals (Young and Brownell, 1976). Such responses may be useful for extracting biologically significant signals in background noise (Rhode and Greenberg, 1991). This possibility is addressed in greater detail in later sections of this chapter.

A second manifestation of inhibition is observed in the magnitude and extent of lateral suppression observed in many DCN cells. The pauser-buildup (P/B) units of the dorsal division exhibit more suppression than any other CN unit type, including choppers. Moreover, the threshold of this suppression is very low, close to the cell's excitatory rate threshold, suggesting that these cells may be optimized to extract spectral contours of signals at relatively low and moderate intensities on the basis of rate-place information (Young, Spirou, Rice, and Voigt, 1992). The implications of this behavior for speech coding are discussed later on in this chapter.

Most neurons in the DCN of the cat, the species in which most physiological research has been conducted, are fusiform cells, which correspond to the P/B response type (Rhode & Smith, 1986b). They are the principal cell type in the dorsal cochlear nucleus. These cells have extensive inhibitory inputs, and their response patterns are exceedingly difficult to characterize. The temporal course of their discharge is highly sensitive to stimulus intensity. At low SPLs the unit is often unresponsive until 20 to 100 ms after stimulus onset, increasing the magnitude of its discharge gradually over the next 100 to 150 ms (buildup pattern). At higher intensities such a unit may exhibit either a chopper or pauser response pattern. The latter is similar to a buildup pattern except that the cell responds strongly at stimulus onset and then shuts down for an interval ranging between 20 and 100 ms. Both the pauser and buildup patterns possess certain properties consistent with the temporal integration capabilities of human and animal listeners.

The function of the dorsal division remains an enigma. In terms of its extensive inhibitory input and intricate, complex intrinsic neural circuitry, the DCN more closely resembles upper brain stem and cortical auditory nuclei than the ventral CN. The organization of its granule cell layer is reminiscent of the parallel and climbing fiber organization of the cerebellum (Mugnaini, 1991), suggesting that the DCN may dynami-

cally modify both its own and other regions' responses to sound. The DCN is also rich in zinc, which is associated with long-term synaptic changes in other regions of the brain thought to be involved in learning (e.g., the hippocampus).

The DCN also appears to have special noise-reduction circuitry that minimizes the effect of background sounds on the encoding of certain types of complex sounds, such as AM tones (Rhode and Greenberg, 1991). Environmental background noise varies from location to location and is highly dependent on the acoustic ecology of the species. For this reason it is possible that the variability observed in DCN morphology across mammalian species reflects the acoustic conditions under which different animals process sound. Short-term fluctuations in the sonic environment may make useful some means of dynamically modifying the noise-reduction circuitry of the DCN to optimize the signal-to-noise ratio of incoming acoustic information in real-time. If the DCN does filter out noise, its role in the processing of speech in humans should be particularly important.

SPECTRAL REPRESENTATIONS OF THE AUDITORY PERIPHERY AND PLACE CODING OF THE SPECTRUM IN THE AUDITORY NERVE AND COCHLEAR NUCLEUS

So far, the response properties of the auditory nerve have been discussed mostly in terms of single neural elements. However, the coding of speech and other complex sounds is based on the activity of thousands of nerve fibers whose tuning characteristics span a broad range of frequency sensitivity, threshold, and selectivity. It would be ideal to extrapolate from what is known about the response of single fibers to sinusoidal signals and noise to predict the response of the auditory nerve, as a whole, to various speech sounds.

Rate-Place Information

It is possible to infer the activity of the auditory nerve to speech by recording the response of hundreds of single fibers to the same stimulus. In the typical population study the characteristic frequency and spontaneous activity of the fibers recorded are distributed for accurate characterization of the underlying statistics of the auditory nerve. In this manner it is possible to infer how much information is contained in the distribution of activity across the tonotopic extent of the auditory nerve pertaining to the stimulus spectrum.

The representation of the spectrum for the steady-state vowel [ɛ], based on the distribution of average firing rate across the auditory nerve, is shown in Figure 10-8 for three stimulus intensities (Sachs and Young, 1979). At the lowest intensity, characteristic of very soft speech, the tonotopic distribution of firing rate approximates the gross spectral envelope of the vowel (Fig. 10-8, 38 dB). This correspondence is expected, since the cochlea is operating within the quasi-linear portion of its range. At this intensity most ANFs fire at a rate roughly proportional to the cochlear-filtered energy level. Increasing the SPL by 20 dB alters the distribution of discharge activity so that the spectral peaks are no longer so prominently resolved in the tonotopic place-rate profile (Fig. 10-8, 58 dB). This is a consequence of the fact that the discharge of fibers with CFs near the formant peaks has saturated relative to those with CFs corresponding to the spectral troughs. As the stimulus intensity rises to a level typical of conversational speech, the ability to resolve the spectral peaks on the basis of place-rate information is compromised even further (Fig. 10-8, 78 dB).

On the basis of such population profiles, it is difficult to envision how the spectral profile of vowels and other speech sounds can be accurately and reliably encoded on the basis of place-rate information at any but the lowest stimulus intensities. However, a small proportion of ANFs (15%) with spontaneous rates less than 0.5 spikes per second may encode the spectral envelope on the basis of rate-place information, even at the highest stimulus levels (Sachs, Winslow, and Blackburn, 1988; Blackburn and Sachs, 1990). These fibers exhibit extended dynamic ranges and are most sensitive to the mechanical suppression behavior of the BM (Schalk and Sachs, 1980; Sokolowski, Sachs, and Goldstein, 1989). Thus, the discharge rate of low-SR fibers with CFs close to the formant peaks will continue to grow at high SPLs, and the activity of low-SR fibers responsive to the spectral troughs should in principle be suppressed by energy associated with the formants. However, such rate suppression also reduces the response to the second and third formants (Sachs and Young, 1980), decreasing the resolution of the spectral peaks in the rate-place profile at

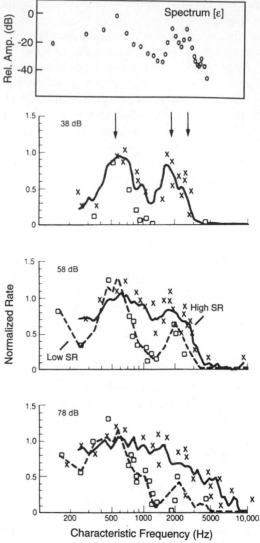

FIGURE 10-8 Place-rate representation of the vowel [ɛ] in the auditory nerve. The response of hundreds of auditory-nerve fibers to the vowel [ɛ] at three different sound pressure levels. The response to two separate populations of fibers is shown. The responses of the high-SR units are indicated with (x) and the solid line, while the low-SR responses are represented by squares and broken lines. At low SPLs (38 dB) the rate-place profile of the high-SR fibers (85% of the population) provides an adequate representation of the spectral envelope. At moderate and high SPLs representative of speech levels, the rate-place representation does not adequately resolve the spectral peaks. However, the activity of the low-SR fibers can provide such a representation at the same intensity levels. (From Handel, S. [1989]. *Listening.* Cambridge, MA: MIT Press. Adapted from Sachs, M.B. and Young, E. D. [1979].)

higher SPLs. For this reason it is not clear that lateral suppression by itself actually provides an adequate rate-place representation of speech and other spectrally complex signals in the auditory nerve.

The case for a rate-place code for vocalic stimuli is equivocal at the level of the auditory nerve. The discharge activity of a large majority of fibers is saturated at these levels in response to vocalic stimuli. Only a small number of ANFs resolve the spectral peaks across the entire dynamic range of speech, and the representation provided by these low-SR units is less than ideal, particularly at conversational intensity levels.

The rate-place representation of the spectrum may be enhanced in the cochlear nucleus and higher auditory stations relative to that observed in the auditory nerve. Such enhancement may be a result of preferential projection or through the operation of **lateral inhibitory networks (LIN)** that sharpen still further the contrast between excitatory and background neural activity.

Many chopper units in the AVCN respond to steady-state vocalic stimuli in a manner similar to that of low-SR ANFs (Blackburn and Sachs, 1990). The rate-place profile of these choppers exhibits clearly delineated peaks at CFs corresponding to the lower formant frequencies, even at 75 dB SPL (Blackburn and Sachs, 1990). In principle a spectral peak would act to suppress the activity of choppers with CFs corresponding to less intense energy, enhancing the neural contrast between spectral maxima and minima. Blackburn and Sachs have proposed that such lateral inhibitory mechanisms may underlie the ability of AVCN choppers to encode the spectral envelope of vocalic stimuli at SPLs well above those at which the average rate (defined as the number of times a cell fires per unit of time) of most ANFs saturate.

Winslow, Barta, and Sachs (1987) have suggested that the low-SR fibers have an influence out of proportion to their numbers, preferentially innervating certain chopper unit populations in the ventral CN. This idea is based on the anatomical studies of Fekete, Rouiller, Liberman, and Ryugo (1982) and Rouiller and Ryugo (1984). Blackburn and Sachs (1990) have amended this hypothesis in accordance with more recent anatomical evidence indicating that most chopper units receive significant projections from all SR fiber classes (Rouiller, Cronin-Schreiber, Fekete, and Ryugo, 1986). According to their selective listening model, the activity of

chopper units is dominated by the input of low-threshold, high-SR ANFs at low SPLs and by less sensitive low-SR fibers at higher intensities.

In their model this intensity-dependent domination of the chopper discharge behavior is a consequence of the differential projection pattern of ANFs. Low-SR fibers are presumed to innervate the portion of the cell closest to the soma (cell body) and the initial segment, while high-SR units contact the dendritic arborization distal from the stellate soma. At low SPLs only the high-SR fibers discharge. Their activity is integrated in the distal stellate dendritic complex, and this neural energy propagates down the dendrites to the cell body to drive the chopper's response pattern. At higher intensities both high- and low-SR units fire. The activity of the high-SR population is blocked from reaching the cell body by the discharge input of low-SR units, whose activity controls the chopper response.

Although this shunting inhibition model can account qualitatively for the ability of AVCN choppers to rate-place encode spectral peaks, there is as yet no anatomical or physiological evidence to support this conjecture. There is another means by which such selective listening could be accomplished without the operation of shunting inhibition. The ability of high-SR fibers to encode low-frequency amplitude modulation declines appreciably at moderate to high intensities (Rhode and Greenberg, 1991), while the low-SR units can still synchronize their discharge to the modulation frequency (Young and Sachs, 1979; Miller and Sachs, 1984). In the absence of phase-locked behavior, choppers typically fire between 250 and 600 spikes per second in response to signals 30 dB or more above threshold. In response to low-frequency AM stimuli, choppers can entrain their discharge to the modulation frequency. For vocalic stimuli with a fundamental frequency (F_o) as low as 100 Hz, the effect of such synchronization will often be to drop the cell's discharge rate well below that typical of sustained chopper firing rates. Therefore, the synchronization to F_o observed in the ANF population (Young and Sachs, 1979) may sharpen the rate-place representation of the vocalic spectrum as well.

The evidence is stronger for a rate-place representation of certain consonantal segments. The amplitude of most voiceless consonants is low enough (below 50 dB SPL) to evade the rate saturation in the coding of vocalic signals. The spectra of plosive bursts, for example, are generally broadband, with several local maxima. Such spectral information is not likely to be temporally encoded due to its brief duration and the lack of sharply defined peaks. Physiological studies have shown that such segments are adequately represented in the rate-place profile of all spontaneous rate groups across the tonotopic axis (e.g., Delgutte and Kiang, 1984).

The place-rate representation in the auditory nerve may also be enhanced in the DCN. Certain cells (with type II and IV receptive fields) in this region may be specialized to process spectral contours on the basis of rate-place information as a consequence of intrinsic neural circuitry (Young, Spirou, Rice, and Voigt, 1992). Although this system may have evolved originally for localization of sound based on monaural cues, it is likely that comparable inhibitory mechanisms operate at higher SPLs typical of interspecific communication and that such inhibitory processes may enhance the rate-place representation of spectral contour information.

Certain phonetic parameters, such as voice-onset time, are signaled through absolute and relative timing of specific acoustic cues. Such cues are observable in the tonotopic distribution of ANF responses to the initial portion of these segments (Sachs, Voigt, and Young, 1983; Delgutte and Kiang, 1984). For example, the articulatory release associated with stop consonants has a broadband spectrum and a rather abrupt onset, which evokes a marked flurry of activity across a wide CF range of fibers. Another burst of activity occurs at the onset of voicing. Because the dynamic range of ANF discharge is much larger during the initial rapid adaptation phase (up to 10 ms), there is relatively little or no saturation of discharge rate during this interval at high SPLs (Sachs, Voigt, and Young, 1983; Sinex and Geisler, 1983). Consequently, the onset spectra that distinguish the stop consonants (Blumstein and Stevens, 1980) are adequately represented in the distribution of rate-place activity across the auditory nerve (Delgutte and Kiang, 1984) over the short time of articulatory release.

This form of rate information differs from the more traditional average rate. The underlying parameter governing neural magnitude at onset is the probability of discharge over a very small interval. This probability is usually converted into effective discharge rate. If the analysis window (i.e., binwidth) is sufficiently small (e.g.,

100 μs), the apparent rate can be exceedingly high (up to 10,000 spikes per second). Such high onset rates reflect two properties of the neural discharge: the high probability of firing correlated with stimulus onset and the small degree of variance for this first spike latency. This measure of onset response magnitude is one form of instantaneous rate. *Instantaneous* in this context refers to the spike rate measured over an interval corresponding to the analysis binwidth, which generally ranges between 10 and 1000 μs. This is in contrast to average rate, which reflects the magnitude of activity over the entire stimulus duration. Average rate is essentially an integrative measure of activity that counts spikes over relatively long periods and weighs each point in time equally. Instantaneous rate emphasizes the clustering of spikes over small time windows and is a correlational measure of neural response. Upon repeated presentations, activity that is highly correlated in time will have very high instantaneous rates of discharge over certain intervals. Conversely, poorly correlated response patterns will show much lower peak instantaneous rates whose magnitudes are close to the average rate. The distinction between integrative and correlational measures of neural activity is critical for understanding how information in the auditory nerve is processed by neurons in the higher stations of the auditory pathway.

Phase-Place and Latency-Place Information

In a linear system the phase characteristics of a filter are highly correlated with its amplitude response. On the skirts of the filter, where the amplitude response diminishes quickly, the phase of the output signal also changes rapidly. The phase response by itself can thus be used in such a system to infer the properties of the filter (Huggins, 1952). For a **nonlinear system** such as pertains to signal transduction in the cochlea, phase and latency (group delay) information may more accurately estimate the underlying filter characteristics than average discharge rate because latency and phase are not necessarily so sensitive to such nonlinearities as compression of the input-output response (saturation). Although the average rate of a fiber may not continue to change with increasing intensity, the unit's phase response may continue to do so, providing information about the input spectrum beyond what is available in the rate-place population profile at high SPLs.

Several studies suggest that such phase and latency cues occur in the auditory nerve across a very broad range of intensities. A large phase transition is observed in the neural response distributed across ANFs whose CFs span the lower tonotopic boundary of a dominant frequency component (Anderson, Rose, and Brugge, 1971), indicating that the high-frequency skirt of the cochlear filters is sharply tuned across intensity. A latency shift of the neural response is observed over a small range of fiber CFs. The magnitude of the shift can be appreciable, as much as half a cycle of the driving frequency (Anderson, Rose, and Brugge, 1971; Kitzes, Gibson, Rose, and Hind, 1978). For a 500 Hz signal this latency change would be on the order of 1 ms. Because this phase transition may not be subject to the nonlinearities that saturate the discharge rate, fibers with CFs just apical to the place of maximal response have the potential to encode a spectral peak in terms of the onset phase across a wide range of intensities.

Interesting variants of this response-latency model have been proposed by Shamma (1985a, b, 1988) and Deng, Geisler, and Greenberg (1988). In principle, the phase transition for low-frequency signals should occur throughout the entire response, not just at the beginning, because of ANFs' phase-locking properties. They propose that such ongoing phase disparities are registered by some form of neural circuitry, presumably in the CN. The output of such networks would magnify activity in tonotopic regions over which the phase and/or latency changes rapidly through some form of cross-frequency-channel correlation. In the Shamma model the correlation is performed through a lateral inhibitory network, which subtracts the auditory nerve output of adjacent channels. The effect of this cross-channel subtraction is to null out activity for channels with similar phase and latency characteristics, leaving only the portion of the activity pattern where rapid phase transitions occur. The Deng model uses cross-channel correlation (i.e., multiplication) instead of subtraction to locate the response boundaries. Correlation magnifies the activity of channels with similar response patterns and reduces the output of dissimilar adjacent channels. Whether the cross-channel comparison is performed through subtraction, multiplication, or some other operation, the consequence of such neural computation is to provide pointers to tonotopic regions with a boundary that might be hidden if analyzed solely on the basis of average rate. In principle, these pointers may act in a manner analogous to peaks in the excitation pattern.

Synchrony-Place Information

Place and temporal models of frequency coding are generally discussed as if they are diametrically opposed perspectives. Traditionally, temporal models have deemphasized tonotopic organization in favor of the fine-temporal structure of the neural response. However, place and temporal coding need not exclude each other. The concept of the central spectrum (Goldstein and Srulovicz, 1977; Srulovicz and Goldstein, 1983) attempts to reconcile the two approaches into a single theory of frequency coding. In this model, both place and temporal information are used to construct the peripheral representation of the spectrum. Timing information, as reflected in the interval histogram of ANFs, is used to estimate the driving frequency. The model assumes that temporal activity is keyed to the tonotopic frequency representation. In some unspecified way the system knows what sort of temporal activity corresponds to each tonotopic location, analogous to matched filters in systems engineering.

The central spectrum model is the intellectual antecedent of the peripheral representational model of speech proposed by Young and Sachs (1979). Their model is based on the auditory nerve population response study discussed in a previous section of this chapter (Sachs and Young, 1979). As with place schemes in general, spectral frequency is mapped onto tonotopic place (i.e., ANF characteristic frequency), and the amplitude of each frequency is given by the magnitude of the neural response synchronized to that component by nerve fibers whose CFs lie within a quarter of an octave. The resulting average localized synchronized rate (ALSR) representation of the stimulus spectrum is illustrated in Figure 10-9. The ALSR is a computation for estimating the magnitude of neural response in a given frequency channel based on the product of firing rate and temporal correlation with a predefined frequency band. The spectral peaks associated with the three lower formants (F_1, F_2, F_3) are clearly delineated in the ALSR represen-

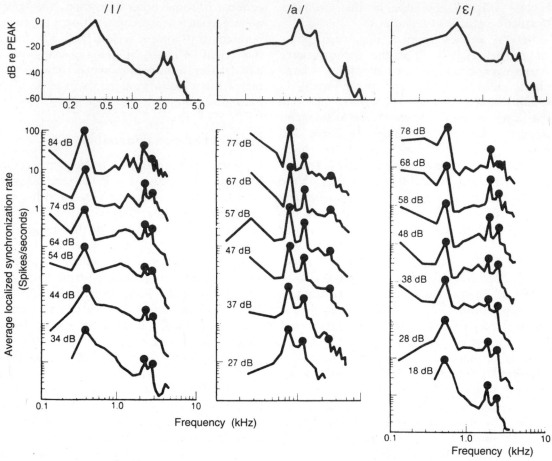

FIGURE 10-9   ALSR representation of vocalic spectra in the auditory nerve. Young and Sachs (1979) proposed the averaged localized synchronized rate (ALSR) metric for computing the temporal representation of auditory-nerve fibers to speech. The temporal activity of a nerve fiber goes through a matched filter corresponding to its characteristic frequency. Temporal activity in the range of the fiber CF is passed through without attenuation, while temporal activity to remote frequencies is suppressed. Thus the ALSR is a measure of the degree to which a fiber is synchronized to frequencies appropriate to its tonotopic affiliation. When computed thus, the temporal representation remains remarkably stable over a wide range of intensities. Shown are the ASLR representations across a 50 to 60 dB dynamic range for the vowels [I], [a] and [ɛ]. (From Handel, S. [1989]. *Listening*. Cambridge, MA: MIT Press. Adapted from Young, E.D. and Sachs, M. B. [1979].)

tation, in marked contrast to the rate-place representation.

The mechanism underlying the ALSR representation is suppression, or synchrony capture. At low SPLs, temporal activity synchronized to a single spectral component below 4 kHz is generally restricted to a circumscribed tonotopic region close to that frequency. Increasing the SPL spreads the synchronized activity, particularly toward the region of high-CF fibers. In this instance the spread of temporal activity occurs roughly in tandem with the activation of fibers in terms of average discharge rate. At high SPLs (about 70 to 80 dB) a large majority of ANFs with CFs below 10 kHz are phase-locked to low-frequency components of the spectrum. This upward spread of excitation into the high-frequency portion of the auditory nerve is a result of the unique filter characteristics of high-CF mammalian nerve fibers (see Greenwood [1986] and Shamma and Morrish [1987] for alternative views of synchrony suppression). Although the filter function for such units is sharply bandpass within 20 to 30 dB of rate threshold, it becomes broadly tuned and low-pass at high SPLs. This tail component of the high-CF fiber **frequency-threshold curve (FTC)** renders such fibers extremely responsive to low-frequency signals at SPLs typical of conversational speech (Figure 10-10). The conse-

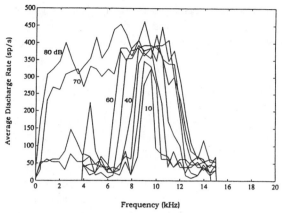

FIGURE 10-10   The intensity-level dependent nature of filtering in the auditory nerve. Response area for a cat auditory-nerve fiber with a CF of 9 kHz spanning an intensity range of 10 to 80 dB SPL. At low-to-moderate SPLs the filtering is bandpass in nature and relatively sharp. Above 60 dB the tuning becomes low-pass and broadens appreciably. (From Jenison, R., Greenberg, S., Kluender, K., & Rhode, W. S. [1991]. A composite model of the auditory periphery for the processing of speech based on the filter response functions of single auditory nerve fibers. *Journal of the Acoustical Society of America, 90,* 773-786.)

quence of this low-frequency sensitivity, in concert with the diminished selectivity of low-CF fibers, is the orderly basal recruitment toward the high-frequency end of the auditory nerve of ANFs as a function of increasing SPL.

Synchrony suppression is intricately related to the frequency selectivity of ANFs. At low SPLs most low-CF nerve fibers are phase-locked to components in the vicinity of their CF. At this amplitude the magnitude of a fiber's response, measured in either synchronized or average rate, is approximately proportional to the signal energy at the unit CF, resulting in rate-place and synchrony-place profiles relatively isomorphic to the input stimulus spectrum. At higher SPLs the average-rate response saturates across the tonotopic array of nerve fibers, significantly degrading the rate-place representation of the formant pattern, as mentioned above. The distribution of temporal activity also changes, but somewhat differently. The activity of fibers with CFs near the spectral peaks remains phase-locked to the formant frequencies. Fibers whose CFs lie in the spectral valleys, particularly between F_1 and F_2, become synchronized to a different frequency, most typically F_1.

The basis for this suppression of synchrony is

as follows. The amplitude of components in the formant region, particularly F_1, is typically 20 to 40 dB above that of harmonics in the valleys. When the amplitude of the formant becomes sufficiently intense, its energy spills over into neighboring frequency channels as a consequence of the broad tuning of low-frequency fibers. Because of the large amplitude disparity between spectral peak and valley, more formant-related energy passes through the fiber's filter than energy derived from components in the CF region of the spectrum. Suppression of the original timing pattern actually begins when the amount of formant-related energy equals that of the original signal. Virtually complete suppression of the less intense signal occurs when the amplitude disparity is greater than 15 dB (Greenberg, Geisler, and Deng, 1986). In this sense, encoding frequency as neural phase locking enhances the peaks of the spectrum at the expense of less intense components.

The result of this synchrony suppression is to reduce the amount of activity phase-locked to frequencies other than the formants. At higher SPLs the activity of fibers with CFs in the spectral valleys is indeed phase-locked, but to frequencies distant from their CFs. In the ALSR model the response of these units contributes to the auditory representation of the signal spectrum only indirectly, since the magnitude of temporal activity is measured only for frequencies near the fiber CF. In this model only a small subset of ANFs, those with CFs near the formant peaks, directly contribute to the auditory representation of the speech spectrum in the model.

Liabilities of Place Models

Place models of spectral coding do not function properly under intense background noise. Because the frequency parameter is coded through the spatial position of active neural elements, the representation of complex spectra is particularly vulnerable to extraneous interference (Greenberg, 1988). Intense noise and competing sounds with significant energy overlapping frequency regions containing primary information can damage the auditory representation of the spectrum. This vulnerability of place representations is particularly acute when the neural information is in the form of average rate. This is because there is no neural marker other than tonotopic affiliation to carry information about the frequency of the driving signal. When both foreground and background signals are sufficiently intense, it is exceedingly difficult to distinguish the portion of the place representation driven by the target signal from that driven by the interfering sounds. In other words, there is no systematic way of separating the neural activity associated with each source purely on the basis of rate place–encoded information.

The perceptual implications of a strictly rate-place model are counterintuitive, for it implies that the intelligibility of speech should decline as SPL increases above 40 dB. Above this level the rate-place representation of the vocalic spectrum for most ANFs becomes much less well defined, and only the low-SR fiber population continues to encode the spectral envelope with any degree of precision. In actuality speech intelligibility is somewhat better above 60 dB, where the rate-place representation is not nearly so well delineated.

At first glance the ALSR model offers an appealing alternative to rate-based models in that temporal information is more robust in the presence of noise. The ALSR model assumes the existence of a central mechanism that knows the synchrony pattern appropriate to the CFs of the projecting fibers and can filter out all other temporal activity. The ALSR model requires at some level of the auditory pathway a correlation between the temporal activity and a neuron's filter characteristics near threshold. However, physiological evidence for such a matched filter operation is entirely lacking, and it does not appear likely that any will be adduced in the near future. From a physiological perspective it is difficult to conceive of how such matched filtering would be implemented in the auditory pathway.

Another difficulty with place representations is their vulnerability to peripheral (i.e., cochlear) damage. Because in this representation the coding of frequency depends on the activity of discrete populations of nerve cells, significant damage to specific regions of the cochlea should result in the inability to encode whole regions of the spectrum. However, this does not occur except for frequency coding above 4 kHz (see a later section for further discussion of this topic).

Synchrony-Distributed Information In the Auditory Nerve

The mechanism that underlies synchrony suppression also ensures that under normal listening conditions temporal information pertaining to the formant peaks, particularly F_1, is distributed across ANFs spanning a broad tonotopic range. At low SPLs formant-related synchrony is confined to fibers with CFs close to the spectral peaks of the vowel [ɛ] (Fig. 10-11, 38 dB). As the signal amplitude rises, so does the number of fibers synchronized to F_1 (Fig. 10-11, 78 dB). At amplitudes typical of conversational speech, most fibers with CFs below 10 kHz are synchronized to the first formant (Young and Sachs, 1979). In Figure 10-11 there is a gap, centered at 1800 Hz, in the tonotopic distribution of F_1 synchrony, the frequency of the second formant. This circumscribed population of fibers maintains its synchrony to F_2 by virtue of the relatively large amplitude of the second formant peak.

The broadening of ANF frequency selectivity is the primary basis of this wide distribution of F_1 synchrony. At conversational levels the filtering of ANFs becomes almost low-pass, in contrast to the sharply bandpass characteristic observed in response to signals below 60 dB SPL (Fig. 10-10). In consequence, low-frequency signals can capture the activity of ANFs most sensitive to much higher frequencies. Jenison, Greenberg, Kluender, and Rhode (1991) have accurately simulated the tonotopic distribution of synchrony to the lower formants of vocalic stimuli using filter functions derived from the discharge-rate-based response areas (isointensity curves) of single ANFs. In that simulation the filter functions change with tonotopic frequency and SPL. Only at intensities 60 dB or greater is there observed a spreading of F_1 synchrony analogous to that reported by Young and Sachs (1979).

It is perhaps not coincidental that the broadening of auditory nerve filtering is always toward the low-frequency portion of the spectrum. Only low-frequency signals can label the neural response at any point along the tonotopic axis in terms of modulating (phase-locking) the fiber discharge pattern. Without phase locking, under many conditions it would be difficult to identify the signal frequency driving a unit's response. ANF discharge rate typically saturates 20 to 30 dB above threshold. Beyond this level there are few if any cues to distinguish excitation driven by frequencies close to the unit CF from those more distant. Under these conditions the auditory nerve population profile in response to an intense low-frequency tone would be virtually indistinguishable from the pattern evoked by a wideband noise. The rate-place patterns would be very similar. For this reason it is likely that the broadening of filter characteristics toward the low-frequency portion of the spectrum is associated with the capability of ANFs to synchronize to frequencies below 4 kHz.

In the mammalian auditory nerve there is a tendency for broad frequency selectivity to be associated with phase–locking and for very sharp tuning to be correlated with discharge-rate information. The tuning of ANF is relatively broad, as measured by the unit's Q_{10} dB (defined

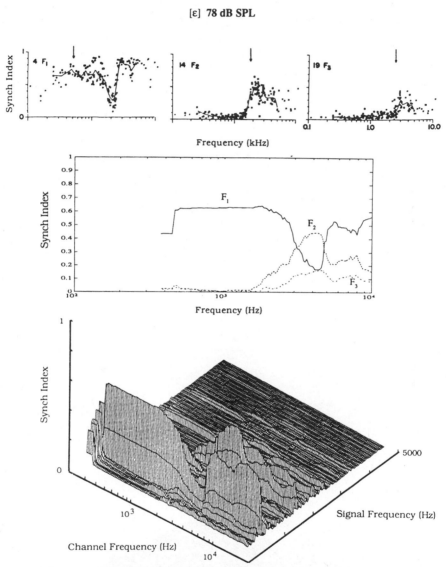

FIGURE 10-11 Distributed representation of vocalic spectra in the auditory nerve. The tonotopic distribution of neural synchronization to the first three formants of the vowel [ɛ] at two different sound pressure levels. The top row shows the distribution of activity phase-locked to F_1 (4th harmonic), F_2 (14th harmonic), and F_3 (19th harmonic) as recorded from the auditory nerve of the cat. Notice that distribution of activity to F_1 expands dramatically at 78 dB SPL, while islands of synchrony to F_2 and F_3 are preserved. The middle and lower rows show the output of a model based on physiological response areas such as that illustrated in Figure 10-10. The distribution of synchrony corresponds very closely to that of the cat. (From Jenison, R., Greenberg, S., Kluender, K., & Rhode, W. S. [1991]. A composite model of the auditory periphery for the processing of speech based on the filter response functions of single auditory nerve fibers. *Journal of the Acoustical Society of America, 90,* 773-786.)

as the fiber CF divided by BW_{10} minus the bandwidth of the response function 10 dB above threshold), for low-CF (below 2 kHz) units (Q_{10}s between 1 and 2) and rather sharp for fibers with CFs above 4 kHz (Q_{10}s between 4 and 20). Thus, at low intensities, where rate-place cues would be expected to dominate the coding of spectral information, the tuning of high-CF fibers is very sharp, and this high degree of selectivity is maintained up to approximately 50 or 60 dB SPL. Such sharp tuning may be the natural result of a reliance on rate-place cues for the encoding of spectral information beyond the range of phase locking (i.e., above 4 kHz).

There are at least two principal results of distributing temporal information pertaining to the lower formants over a large number of ANFs. First, such distributed coding emphasizes spectral peaks at the expense of other components of the acoustic waveform. Lower-amplitude components, particularly those in the spectral trough between widely separated formant peaks (e.g., F_1 and F_2 for high and midfront vowels, F_2 and F_3 for back vowels) will not be represented clearly, if at all, in such neural activity patterns. In this sense a distributed representation reduces the data encoded in the peripheral neural activity pattern. It is similar to the dominant frequency model proposed by Carlson, Fant, and Granström (1975) and elaborated by Sinex and Geisler (1983) and Ghitza (1988). These models assume that only a small

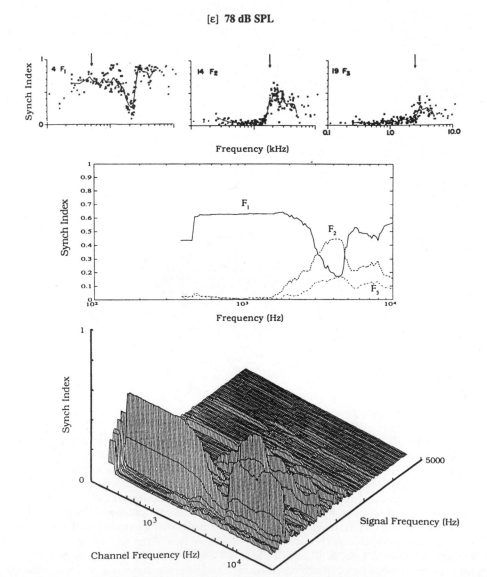

FIGURE 10-11, cont'd.   For legend, see opposite page.

portion of the spectrum is behaviorally significant and that the remainder is essentially "window dressing" with respect to biologically relevant information. A behavioral study by Kakusho, Hirato, Kato, and Kobayashi (1971) is consistent with this interpretation. In that experiment listeners were asked to discriminate between synthetic vocalic stimuli of variable spectral complexity. Reduced spectra were hardly distinguishable from full-spectrum vowels as long as the former contained the three lowest formants (each formant had to contain at least three harmonics). Remez, Rubin, Pisoni, and Carrell (1981) have demonstrated that intelligibility is preserved even when each formant is represented by only a single frequency component (speech sine wave).

A second consequence of distributed coding is the protection of the remaining information from background noise and acoustic interference. Distribution of key information-laden components (info-elements) of the acoustic signal across a broad tonotopic range reduces the probability that extraneous signals will severely compromise their representation. Since most interference is transient or narrowband, the neural activity evoked by the info-elements will be preserved across much of the tonotopic axis or will be interfered with only momentarily. However, it would be considerably more difficult to encode info-elements against sustained broadband interference. Under these conditions other strategies based on common modulation patterns and binaural correlation may be required (Bilsen, 1977; Bregman, 1990).

Synchrony-Distributed Information in the Posteroventral Cochlear Nucleus

Essential to the dominant frequency model is the means by which common **synchronous activity** distributed across the tonotopic axis is recognized and integrated at the level of the CN and beyond. Most cells in the CN receive direct excitatory input from a relatively narrow tonotopic range of ANFs (an isofrequency projection). For this reason their ability to monitor the spread of common synchronous activity over a broad tonotopic range is limited. Such cells, however, may serve to transmit synchronous neural activity to higher centers with the required integrative machinery.

One class of neuron in the CN does appear to have specific response properties required for the analysis of distributed temporal information. The onset choppers of the posteroventral division behave in a manner consistent with the dominant frequency model. In response to low-frequency sinusoidal or AM input the average rate of these cells grows with intensity over a broad dynamic range in tandem with the presumed tonotopic breadth of the active auditory nerve projections. Thus, discharge rate in these units appears to reflect both the tonotopic extent of coherent temporal activity and the intensity of the driving component.

The onset chopper's ability to integrate coherent synchronous activity in all probability relies on two different properties. One concerns the broad frequency selectivity that reflects the wide tonotopic extent of the ANF projection. The other involves some form of **coincidence detection**, in which a cell is sensitive to the relative arrival time of two or more nerve impulses from afferent inputs. Such neurons generally fire only if a certain minimum number of inputs discharge within a very small time (on the order of tens or hundreds of microseconds) (Fig. 10-12). Onset choppers behave like coincidence detectors in that the variance of their initial spike latency and the variance of their phase-locked response to low-frequency modulations are exceedingly small, far less variable than the analogous discharge measures for their ANF projections. In this sense onset units may correlate afferent temporal activity as in the cross-channel correlation model of Deng, Geisler, and Greenberg (1988).

Coincidence detection is potentially a very powerful means of protecting info-elements from the destructive effects of noise. Because noise by definition is without sustained correlation, neural elements particularly responsive to correlated inputs in principle can withstand appreciable levels of acoustic interference as long as the background is itself not highly correlated with the foreground signal. Under such circumstances the temporal pattern of neural activity will remain relatively unaffected at all but the lowest signal-to-noise ratios. Rhode and Greenberg (1994) have examined the ability of various cell types in the CN to encode amplitude modulation in noise. Although all response classes exhibit impressive AM coding in noise, onset-chopper units are among the least sensitive to background interference.

Another important aspect of coincidence detection pertains to learning and representational maps. Hebb (1949) suggested that coincidence detection formed the primary physiological mechanism underlying the creation of representational maps. Coincident input to neurons strengthens connections between nerve cells. As the connections between specific cells strengthen, connections with other cells will necessarily weaken. This Hebbian learning model has received substantial support in recent years from a wide variety of research (see Edelman [1987] and Brown, Kairiss, and Keenan [1990] for reviews). It is now thought that such physiological mechanisms underlie the modification of the brain through experience and may provide a basis for understanding how both the auditory system and higher cortical regions develop specializations for processing speech sounds (see Liberman and Mattingly [1989] for a discussion of the modularity of speech encoding).

In response to vocalic stimuli, synchrony to both F_1 and F_o will be dispersed across a broad tonotopic range of ANF inputs. At low SPLs the phase-locked response to F_o will be more broadly distributed than F_1-synchronized activity. Fibers with CFs below F_1, between F_1 and F_2, and above F_3 will exhibit appreciable phase-locking to the fundamental frequency. This common synchrony to a low-modulation frequency may encode important vocalic information in several ways. In the presence of compet-

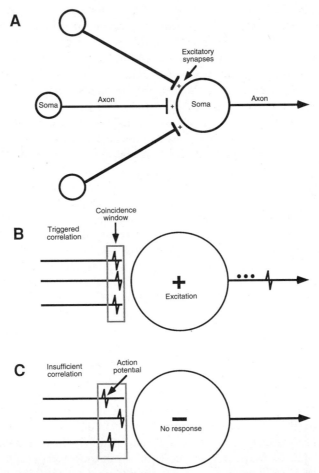

FIGURE 10-12 A coincidence detector cell receives neuronal input from two or more neurons. In the simplest form of coincidence detection, the projections are entirely excitatory. *A,* The hypothetical correlator is restricted to three inputs, though in practice the number is likely to be far higher. *B,* When the arrival times of nerve impulse inputs occur within a sufficiently narrow time range (coincidence), the nerve cell discharges because of the temporal summation of sufficient neurotransmitter to depolarize the cell. *C,* When the temporal dispersion of the impulses is greater than this coincidence range, sufficient summation does not occur and the cell remains silent.

ing speech or other background sounds, the common F_o-synchronized activity identifies tonotopically disjointed regions of the neural excitation pattern as originating from the same sound source. In noisy conditions the ability to track such common modulation patterns may be a powerful cue for segregation and grouping of acoustic information into coherent *event streams* (Bregman, 1990). Moreover, the phase-locked character of the common source coding would minimize the disruptive effects of background noise. Even in the absence of acoustic interference, F_o synchrony may bind disparate portions of the tonotopic activity pattern to form a single sound source.

At higher SPLs the dispersion of F_o synchrony decreases in the auditory nerve, and phase locking to F_1 expands appreciably. The tonotopic distribution of synchrony to F_o is generally complementary to that of F_1. Rarely are fibers in a CF region highly synchronized to both. Most fibers will be synchronized predominantly to either F_o or F_1, except the relatively small proportion phase-locked to F_2 and F_3. In consequence, the distribution of phase-locking to F_o can provide a negative image of the F_o dispersion of F_1 synchrony and vice versa. This complementary pattern may have significant consequences for coding vocalic stimuli in the upper reaches of the auditory pathway, as discussed in a later section of this chapter.

At the level of the CN virtually all cell types can synchronize to amplitude modulation within the frequency range of the speech fundamental (80 to 400 Hz). Onset-chopper units exhibit the greatest precision of phase locking to low-frequency amplitude modulation, followed by onset locker, chopper, P/B, and primary-like units. Thus, low-frequency modulation may be a powerful cue for informational encoding, source segregation, and signal extraction in noise.

Coherent low-frequency modulation of neural activity also may provide a form of pitch-synchronous analysis (PSA). A major drawback of conventional Fourier analysis is its reliance on a fixed time window of arbitrary length. In the analysis of acoustic signals of variable or unknown periodicity, such fixed-interval analyses may erroneously estimate the spectrum. Synchronizing the analysis to the pitch period circumvents this problem. Scott (1976) has suggested that F_1 is estimated by the auditory system completely in the time domain by a form of PSA. In Scott's model each glottal pulse

triggers the beginning of a new analysis frame, over which interval the number of major oscillations is counted. Category boundaries separating vowels are based not on the absolute frequencies of F_1, F_2 . . . F_n but rather on the number of modulations per pitch period. A related form of periodicity analysis has been proposed by Langner (1988, 1991), Patterson and Holdsworth (1991) and Holton, Love, and Gill (1992). In Langner's model onset units act as pitch-synchronous triggers, and choppers serve as **intrinsic oscillators** upon which the analysis of the signal's temporal fine structure is ultimately made. Activity from these two neural populations is presumably correlated in a more central auditory region such as the inferior colliculus.

CENTRAL AUDITORY MECHANISMS

At the higher reaches of the auditory pathway the ability of neurons to phase-lock diminishes appreciably. At the level of the inferior colliculus, in the upper brain stem, units rarely synchronize to frequencies above 1 kHz (Yin and Kuwada, 1984), and the upper limit of phase locking for units in the thalamic and cortical regions is only 200 to 300 Hz (de Ribaupierre, Goldstein, and Yeni-Komshian, 1972).

The question naturally arises as to how information encoded as synchrony in the auditory nerve and CN is converted into some form understood by the higher levels of the auditory pathway. What is the nature of this transformed temporal information, and what are the mechanisms responsible for the conversion?

Jeffress (1948) proposed a model for binaural analysis of signals from the two ears based on coincidence detection and **neural delay lines**. Jeffress's model was concerned exclusively with time-intensity trading for localization of sound sources. Licklider (1951) extended this model into the domain of pitch analysis for complex sounds, using the mathematical technique **autocorrelation**. Autocorrelation is used to estimate the periodicity of an arbitrary waveform. In Licklider's model an exact copy of the original waveform, as filtered and neurally transduced in the auditory periphery, is correlated (multiplied) with the reference signal after a variable time delay (Fig. 10-13). This delay is a result of neural circuitry that preserves the fine temporal details of the waveform but sends the signal down a longer path. This "high road" has at various

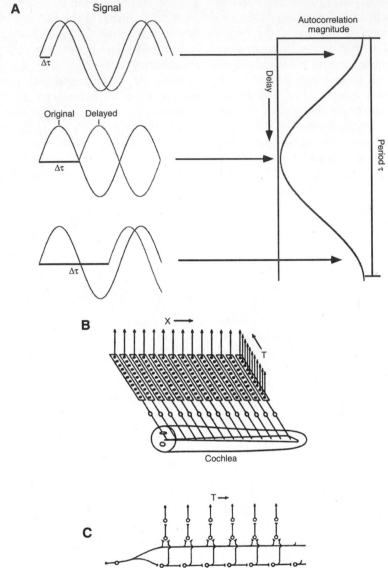

FIGURE 10-13 Autocorrelation in theory and in the nervous system. *A,* Autocorrelation with a sinusoidal signal. The signal is cloned and multiplied with a time-delayed version of itself. At each time step the two waveforms are multiplied and the product placed in a buffer (right). The process is a continuous function of time, but only three instances are shown here. Top, virtually no time delay, equal to a small fraction of the signal period. Middle, the product when the delay is half of the signal period, at which point the correlation shows a minimum. Bottom, the correlation when the delay is nearly a full period. For small time delays the correlation between the two signals is high. As the time delay of the clone increases, the correlation diminishes until it reaches a trough half a cycle away. As the delay increases still further, the correlation progressively increases until the function reaches another peak. The interval between this point and the starting frame is an estimate of the period (τ) of the signal. *B,* Autocorrelation is the basis of Licklider's (1951) duplex model of pitch. In his model the tonotopic frequency organization of the auditory nerve is supplemented by a second orthogonal topographic axis sensitive to neural periodicity (*dimension B*). Each frequency channel has a full complement of delays available to compute the periodicity of the activity encoded in that channel. *C,* The analysis is performed through the operation of neural delay lines using correlator circuits to estimate the waveform periodicity and segregate the output accordingly, so that a temporal property (periodicity) is converted into a place dimension. (B,C, from Licklider, J.C.R. [1951]. A duplex theory of pitch perception. *Experientia, 7,* 129-133.)

points along its route connections (taps) to the more direct "low road." Each successive tap represents an incremental delay. At each tap a correlational operation is performed. At most taps the original and delayed versions will not be highly correlated, since they are out of phase with one another. However, for periodic or quasi-periodic signals, such as voiced speech, there will be some delay over which the correlation between the two waveforms is high relative to that of other taps. This interval of maximum correlation provides an estimate of the signal periodicity. Because each tap has a well-defined location, the neural autocorrelation converts a temporal measure of periodicity into a spatial representation which in Licklider's model runs orthogonal to the primary isofrequency representation of afferent activity and encodes the waveform periodicity (fundamental frequency). Patterson's (1986, 1987) pulse-ribbon model of periodicity pitch follows Licklider's model closely, except that the tonotopic frequency axis is spatially organized as a spiral rather than as a linear array. The spiral organization has a built-in delay that functions similarly to an autocorrelation.

To date, anatomical and physiological support for a delay-line and autocorrelation analysis is equivocal. Carr and Konishi (1988) have published preliminary evidence for a delay line in the barn owl nucleus laminaris, the avian homologue of the medial superior olive, but without any direct support for neural correlation. Yin and Kuwada (1984) have adduced strong evidence in the cat inferior colliculus for some form of correlation operation pertaining to binaural analysis and have presented some preliminary evidence consistent with a delay line in the medial superior olive.

The most interesting results in this regard come from Langner and Schreiner (1988) and Schreiner and Langner (1988). They find in the inferior colliculus of the cat a topographic representation of waveform periodicity based on a rate measure of best modulation frequency (BMF), defined as the frequency of amplitude modulation to which a neuron is most responsive (i.e., discharges at the highest rate). This BMF spans a range between 50 and 500 Hz, and its spatial organization appears to cut across the tonotopic frequency axis. However, the anatomical and physiological basis of this BMF map remains obscure. Moreover, it is not entirely clear whether such a coarse topographic representation is adequate to account for the precision of pitch discrimination among human listeners (about 1 Hz at 1 kHz, or 0.1%).

A related issue is whether such a correlational analysis pertains to the processing of formant-related information. Lyon (1984) has used an autocorrelational model to provide front-end spectral information for a speech recognition system. The psychophysical constraints for spatial autocorrelation of speech are less stringent than for periodicity pitch because discrimination performance is one to two orders of magnitude less fine than for pitch (Flanagan, 1955; Mermelstein, 1978).

In the upper brain stem nuclei and especially in the auditory cortex the discharge rate of neurons is appreciably lower than observed among cells in the CN and auditory nerve. This decrease in excitability may reflect in part the behavioral state of the animal, which is usually anesthetized, and the prevalence of inhibitory inputs, which are particularly vulnerable to the effects of barbiturate anesthesia. However, there is reason to believe that even in the awake, behaving animal, cortical and thalamic neurons are less excitable than units in the periphery. Abeles (1982) has suggested that this lesser degree of responsiveness reflects the prevalence of encoding information through coincidence detection rather than energy integration. Most of the spectral analysis and preliminary acoustic feature extraction are performed, according to Abeles' logic, in the caudal stations of the auditory pathway. What remains to be done at higher levels is a synthesis of primitive elements into a unified, coherent picture of the acoustic stream. In essence, the role of the cortical regions of the auditory system may be to process auditory events, which consist of relatively concurrent neural elements and which form a distinctive pattern of excitation for encoding information. The features of these events change much more slowly than the acoustic spectrum, alleviating the need to update the neural stream more frequently than several times a second.

Steinschneider, Arezzo, and Vaughan (1982) have demonstrated that neurons in the thalamic radiations and auditory cortex of awake monkeys can synchronize highly to the F_0 of synthetic speech sounds, suggesting that the temporal capability of at least some central auditory neurons is sufficient to encode F_0. At this level of auditory processing such temporal information may encode other properties of the speech signal, including the lower formants, duration, and intensity.

AUDITORY SCENE ANALYSIS

The auditory system possesses a remarkable ability to distinguish and segregate sounds emanating from different sources, such as different musical instruments or speakers. This capacity underlies the so-called *cocktail party phenomenon*, in which a listener filters out background conversation and nonlinguistic sounds to focus on a single speaker's message. This feat is of particular importance in understanding the neural basis of speech coding. Auditory scene analysis is the process by which the brain reconstructs the external world through intelligent analysis of acoustic cues and information.

Today's computer programs for automatic recognition of speech (ASR) cannot reliably decode speech in the presence of most other sounds. This failure to process noisy speech can provide important insights into the functional organization of the auditory system, particularly in light of clinical data pertaining to conditions that impede speech comprehension among the hearing impaired.

A speech recognizer works in the following manner (Lee, 1989; Waibel and Lee, 1990). The recognizer attempts to build acoustic templates for each significant sound segment in the language. These segments usually are similar to phonemes, although for technical reasons they often deviate from the traditional units used by phoneticians and phonologists. These templates are constructed from the spectral analysis of speech from many speakers in the hope that the inherent variability in the acoustic structure of the phoneme-like units can be captured and sufficiently described through sophisticated mathematical techniques. The speech signal is digitized and a spectrum computed for each brief time frame (typically 20 to 30 ms). The recognizer then attempts to classify each frame as a phonological unit through pattern-matching algorithms. Information pertaining to preceding and following time frames is often used to facilitate the matching procedure and increase the likelihood of a correct guess. The techniques underlying these procedures are based on observed probabilities of co-occurrence of template sequences, and they work relatively well for isolated words and simple sentences when there is little audible background noise. Distor-

tion, noise of almost any variety, or competing speech dramatically reduces recognition under conditions that present no challenge to normal-hearing listeners (see Chapter 11, Lee [1989], Waibel and Lee [1990] for more details).

Careful analysis of how ASR fails yields some insight into the strategies used by the auditory system for coding speech-relevant information. Most recognition systems use templates based on Fourier analysis of the speech signal and do not explicitly differentiate between linguistically relevant information and noise. This strategy works well in a quiet, nonreverberant environment such as a sound-attenuated chamber but fails in conditions more typical of everyday life, such as a noisy office, computer room, or automobile. Several research groups have substantially improved the accuracy of their recognition systems in noisy conditions by incorporating certain properties of auditory function pertaining to neural phase locking (Ghitza, 1988, 1993; Holton, Love, and Gill, 1992), suggesting that temporal coding of information may suppress background noise, as suggested by Lewis (1987) and Greenberg (1988). This auditory representation consists of the pattern of neural excitation and inhibition across the tonotopic axis and time associated with specific events or features.

For these reasons it is difficult to imagine how the ensemble of frequencies associated with a complex acoustic event such as a string quartet could be encoded purely on the basis of place cues, as traditional auditory theory holds; there are just too many frequency components to track through time. In a manner yet poorly understood, the auditory system not only uses efficient parsing strategies to encode information pertaining to a sound's spectrum but also tracks that signal's acoustic trajectory through time and space, grouping neural activity into singular acoustic events attached to specific sound sources. An increasing body of evidence suggests that neural temporal mechanisms play an important role.

Neural discharge synchronized to specific properties of the acoustic signal, such as the modulation envelope of the waveform, (which is typically correlated with the signal's **low pitch**) and onsets, can mark activity as coming from the same source. The operative assumption is that the auditory system, like other sensory systems, has evolved to focus on acoustic events rather than merely performing a frequency analysis of the incoming sound stream. Signatures of biologically relevant events include common onsets and offsets, coherent modulation, and spectral trajectories (Bregman, 1990). In other words, the auditory system intelligently processes the incoming sound to recreate the physical scenario from which the sound emanates. With music such scene analysis might involve reconstituting the individual instruments of a string quartet or focusing on the piano solo in a concerto. This ecological acoustical approach to hearing stems from the pioneering work of Gibson (1950, 1966, 1979), who considered the senses to be intelligent computational resources designed to recreate as much of the external physical world as possible. Huggins (1952) proposed a similar framework for understanding auditory function.

According to classic auditory theory, proposed by Ohm (1843), sound is passively analyzed according to principles established by the mechanical properties of the middle and inner ears, coupled to the physiological properties of the auditory periphery and more central regions of the auditory pathway. The representation and interpretation of any sound were said to be determined by inherent properties of the sensory system, the product of constraints imposed by the anatomy and physiology of the auditory pathway. This theory emphasizes limits imposed by the system for providing a faithful rendition of the external world. Difference limens for frequency, intensity, localization, and other acoustic attributes are interpreted as the result of limitations in the construction and operation of the auditory pathway.

In contrast, Gibson emphasizes the deductive capabilities of the senses to infer the conditions behind the sound, using whatever cues are available. The limits of hearing are ascribed to functional properties of interacting with the environment. Sensory systems are no more sensitive or discriminating than they need to be in the natural world. Evolutionary processes have assured that the auditory system works well enough under most conditions.

Although there are merits to both approaches, neither really addresses the important evolutionary and developmental issues, particularly how the auditory system interacts with other sensory systems and with the cortical centers of the brain. Nor do they provide for a dynamic perspective in which the auditory system modifies representations and interpretations of incoming sounds through learning or neural feedback (under **efferent** control).

Within the past 10 years there has been considerable interest in how speech is processed and understood in the presence of acoustic interference, including noise and background speech. Bregman (1990) provides a thorough review, so this discussion will be brief and selective.

The perception of concurrently presented vowels has been explored by Assmann and Summerfield (1989, 1990), Chalikia and Bregman (1989), and Summerfield and Assmann (1989, 1991). They have shown that the identification of vocalic material is significantly better when F_0 and formant contours are rather different. F_0 by itself can substantially improve recognition performance. Stubbs and Summerfield (1990) have extended these insights to automatic procedures for separating voices.

INFORMATION CODING

Audition differs from vision in many ways, but perhaps the most significant is the importance of time. When using our eyes we usually can scan an object of interest several times, building a representation of the scene through multiple passes across the visual field. This is not to suggest that the visual system is incapable of handling movement; on the contrary, the eyes deal with motion continually. However, the eyes themselves are usually in motion, such as when we scan a page of text or a majestic outdoor scene or look for a friend in a crowd. When we listen, we are always dealing with a moving target. Sound by its very nature is characterized by change over time. Rarely are the ears afforded the luxury of a second look, and for this reason they must keep up with the incoming sound stream, processing the acoustic signal in real time. Thus, the temporal demands on the auditory system are considerable, and they imply the use of special-purpose strategies to reduce the amount of information with which it must cope.

One strategy for reducing the amount of data processing required is to focus attention on the portions of the signal likely to convey the most information and to ignore the remainder. Such data reduction mechanisms operate at even the most peripheral stations of the auditory pathway, the cochlea and auditory nerve, emphasizing spectral peaks and transitions associated with many speech sounds and temporal onsets, either singular (e.g., a burst associated with articulatory release of a stop consonant) or repetitive (e.g., voicing and fundamental frequency information).

The Importance of Onsets

Onsets usually indicate a motion-related event such as the beginning of speech, the slam of a door, or the backfire of an automobile. Such transient sounds rarely last more than a few milliseconds but are highly effective as alerting cues. Their neural correlate is the burst of discharge associated with the beginning of a stimulus of sufficient amplitude. In the auditory nerve the probability of firing is usually far higher during the first 5 ms after signal onset than afterward. In the CN are cells whose responses are heavily weighted toward stimulus onset, to the exclusion of the steady-state response. As one ascends the auditory pathway, emphasis on the initial component of the signal becomes even more pronounced; at the level of the auditory cortex it is unusual for a cell to respond beyond the initial few milliseconds of the sound (Clarey, Barone, and Imig, 1992). The signal representation has been transformed from a fine-grained analysis at the periphery to event detection and discrimination at the cortical level.

Perceptually the initial few tens of milliseconds of a sound are more important than what follows, even for relatively long signals. This has been most clearly demonstrated for music but pertains as well to speech (Darwin, 1981). Grey and Gordon (1978) have shown that the timbre of musical instruments (analogous to vowel quality in speech) stems principally from a signal's initial 50 ms. A violin's tone can be computationally transformed into a trumpet and vice versa by manipulating the rise-time properties of this initial interval while keeping the remainder of the signal constant.

The spectrum of musical tones changes very little over the course of a single note. However, the attack and decay of the tone are very different. The attack is the time versus amplitude characteristic of the beginning of a sound. For example, a plucked string tends to have a very rapid attack, but a bowed string has a more gradual, longer attack. It is possible to transform perception of a trumpet tone into that of a violin sound by manipulating only the initial 50 ms of the signal (Grey and Gordon, 1978). It is now thought that each instrument has its own attack signature in addition to its specific spectral characteristics. The classical theory of timbre, first espoused by von Helmholtz (1863), attributed differences among instruments and many speech sounds entirely to the envelope of the spectrum averaged over time. This classical theory is still in use for specifying vowels in terms of a formant series (e.g., Peterson and Barney, 1952; Pickett, 1980). However, it is easy to demonstrate just how important onset characteristics are by playing a musical tape backward. Although the melody is necessarily altered by this manipulation, the instrument should not, if the sense of timbre is based on the long-term spectral characteristics of a tone. In fact, a piano is heard as something akin to an organ when played backwards (Demonstration 22 of the Acoustical Society of America's *Auditory Demonstrations* compact disc), and comparable perceptual transformations occur for other musical instruments.

Thus, it appears that the auditory system is primed to focus on the beginning of a sound, performing a fine-grained analysis for the first 50 ms or so, and then relaxing on the assumption that what follows is part of the same acoustic event. Because of certain properties associated with neural **adaptation**, auditory nerve cells are usually far more responsive to a signal onset than to succeeding portions of the sound, particularly when the spectrum does not change over time, as with a sinusoidal signal. Under these conditions the cell's firing adapts over the course of the signal, decreasing its firing rate. At the higher levels of the auditory pathway the adaptation reaches a point where the cell discharges only at signal onset and shuts off thereafter. Thus, such higher-level cells appear to function as event detectors signaling some feature or combination thereof. In this sense neural adaptation may be regarded as a novelty detector, acting as a filter for changes in sensory input. Acoustic signals can reduce the effects of neural adaptation by two principal means. One is to tailor the signal so that it consists of a series of onsets analogous to the glottal pulsing in a voiced speech sound. The other is to change the spectrum over time.

Amplitude Modulation

The vibration of the vocal folds during speech, the rumble of a train engine, the beating wing of a moth all produce cyclic variations in the signal envelope that leave their neural imprint. Such signals may be analyzed as a series of onsets, each modulation cycle being treated as a separate event trigger. On the time scale of 3 to 12 ms is the vibration of the human vocal folds. Each glottal pulse produces in the auditory periphery and CN a burst of discharge activity correlated with the amplitude variation of the waveform, indicating the temporal locus of perceptually important information. Such discharge activity serves at least two purposes. First, it labels the acoustic source in terms of the temporal activity it produces, allowing the auditory system to group the responses of different cells driven by the same source. It also increases the likelihood that auditory neurons will remain active over the course of the signal, in effect stabilizing the response activity of the cell.

At the level of the auditory nerve, synchronization to the amplitude modulation characteristics of the waveform is pervasive (Brugge, Anderson, Hind, and Rose, 1969; Evans, 1978; Javel, 1980; Greenberg, 1986; Joris and Yin, 1992). It is also quite common in the CN (Møller, 1974; Frisina, Smith, and Chamberlin, 1990; Rhode and Greenberg, 1991). It is not uncommon for cells at this level to synchronize their discharge to frequencies between 100 and 1000 Hz, a range matching that of low pitch and the residue (de Boer, 1976). At more central stations of the auditory pathway the upper limit of phase locking to AM signals declines, so that at the level of the auditory cortex it is unusual to observe synchrony to modulation frequencies greater than 200 Hz (de Ribaupierre, Goldstein, and Yeni-Komshian, 1972; Schreiner and Urbas, 1986). One might consider that the auditory periphery performs a fine-grained analysis on a pitch-cycle-by-cycle basis and the higher auditory stations are more concerned with encoding events such as words and syllables with longer time courses (50 to 500 ms).

Frequency Modulation

Neural adaptation in the auditory pathway is frequency selective. The adaptation in any given neuron is greatest when the signal spectrum contains substantial amounts of energy in the frequency region close to the characteristic frequency of the cell. Because adaptation requires time to unfold, cells adapt most to signals

whose spectrum does not change substantially over time. If the spectrum changes rapidly enough, few neurons will be exposed to enough energy to reduce significantly the response activity as the signal traverses the frequency response area of the cell. Thus, signals with substantial frequency modulation, such as consonantal and vocalic transitions, are likely to produce a net increase in auditory activity, both in terms of the number of neurons activated and the magnitude of excitation.

Noise Reduction

Neural synchrony in the auditory periphery is an important means of improving the internal signal-to-noise ratio (Lewis, 1987; Greenberg, 1988). Normal-hearing listeners typically understand speech even with extremely low signal-to-noise ratios (about -5 dB) (Bronkhorst and Plomp, 1989) because ANFs and second-order neurons phase-lock to the spectral peaks (formants), which in effect suppress the background noise.

In the CN and higher auditory nuclei the noise filtering is even more effective because of coincidence detection and correlational mechanisms. Coincidence detector cells such as the onset-chopper units of the PVCN are most likely to discharge when innervating ANFs fire within a small time frame, usually less than 100 μs. Such coincident firing patterns typically are produced only for pulselike transients such as the release associated with stop consonants and phase-locked response to AM and formant-like signals. These cells are considerably less responsive to noise-like signals; they act as noise-rejection filters, cleaning up the primary signal.

Reliability of Coding

All sensory systems face coding reliability problems. Because organisms interact with a complex, multifaceted environment, it is difficult to anticipate all of the environmental contexts in which important signals will occur. Consequently, coding strategies optimized for automatic suppression of extraneous or interfering signals provide an advantage over more linear forms of processing. The auditory system has several such strategies, such as lateral suppression and inhibition, neural phase locking, and distributed representations of high-energy components of the signal.

Because of this reliability problem, far more is involved in decoding the speech signal than merely computing a running spectrum. In noisy conditions a faithful representation of the spectrum may even hinder the ability to decode or understand. Computing a running spectrum of the speech signal is singularly inefficient, since much of the sound is extraneous to the message. To compensate, the auditory system focuses on the elements of speech most likely to contain the sense of the signal.

CLINICAL IMPLICATIONS

The importance of adaptive processing is apparent to anyone who has ever experienced a serious hearing loss. Individuals with moderate to severe hearing loss often experience little, if any, difficulty understanding speech in quiet, nonreverberant environments but have major problems in noisy real-life conditions. For this reason the deleterious effects of a sensorineural hearing loss are often evident only under acoustically adverse circumstances. To date, the basis of this paradox remains unresolved. There are, however, certain indications that this situation reflects in part the distributed nature of the peripheral representation of the information-laden, low-frequency elements of the speech signal.

Severe hearing impairment is usually a result of damage to the sensory hair cells in the cochlea. The frequency range over which sensitivity (as measured by hearing threshold) suffers most lies above 3 or 4 kHz. Sensitivity to frequencies below 2 or 3 kHz is usually not much poorer than in normal listeners except in rare instances of profound, nearly total deafness.

In quiet, the low-frequency region of the cochlea appears to represent speech well enough to maintain nearly perfect intelligibility, probably because virtually all information in speech lies below 3.5 kHz (Miller, 1951). Why then should the integrity of the basal cochlea, most sensitive to high-frequency signals, have such a dramatic effect on speech intelligibility in noise?

It appears that for normal-hearing listeners the basal segment of the cochlea provides a set of redundant frequency channels with which to encode low-frequency, informationally important components of the signal. In the presence of intense low-frequency background noise, it seems, much of the apical low-frequency portion of the cochlea is responding to the noise as well

as to the speech signal, interfering with the neural representation of the lower formants. Under such circumstances it is possible that the high-frequency channels provide a more robust representation of the low-frequency spectrum, particularly F_1 and F_o, because the background sounds are not sufficiently intense to capture the synchrony behavior of high-CF neurons.

Consistent with this interpretation is the fact that audiometric predictors of speech intelligibility are not the same under quiet and noisy conditions. In quiet, performance is most highly correlated with the pure tone threshold at 0.5 and 1 kHz, while in noise the listener's sensitivity at 2 and 4 kHz most accurately predicts the magnitude of speech reception impairment (Smoorenburg, 1992). Interestingly, attempts to predict intelligibility by other measures of hearing function, such as frequency resolution, have failed to observe statistically significant correlations.

A distributed representation of speech also accounts for the failure of hearing aids to restore normal speech intelligibility. Hearing aid users often complain that these devices are of limited help, particularly in noisy conditions. Because these aids rely principally on amplification, they merely boost the gain of the portion of the spectrum over which the listener is least sensitive. In essence, hearing aid design is predicated on a place model of frequency coding. Unfortunately, amplification of the high-frequency portion of the spectrum provides little benefit to many hearing-impaired persons because most of the information in the speech signal lies in the region of normal sensitivity, below 3 kHz.

It is likely that many of the problems of hearing-impaired listeners with understanding speech are a consequence of damage to the redundant frequency channels in the auditory periphery. If this hypothesis is sustained, remediation of hearing deficits should focus on restoring representational redundancy through some form of frequency-compression hearing aid.

IMPLICATIONS FOR MODELS OF SPEECH RECOGNITION

Background noise is the principal demon of computer-based speech-recognition systems. Many systems achieve a high recognition score (95% to 98%) under ideal quiet conditions (see Klatt [1989] for a review), but few can withstand moderate to intense low-frequency noise.

This noise-induced impairment of automatic recognition may be a consequence of the front-end design, which operates very much along the lines of a bank of linear bandpass filters. Under such conditions background noise has the potential to mask the informationally significant portions of the input spectrum without the possibility of recovering the information from other unmasked frequency channels. In this sense, automatic recognition systems operate in an environment analogous to a sensorineural hearing loss.

Significant improvement in recognition in noise may require a redesign of the front-end component to withstand acoustic interference. One of the most successful recognition systems in noise focuses on the temporal aspects of peripheral coding and integrates the activity of such synchrony information across frequency channels (Ghitza, 1988, 1993). Such cross-channel summation emphasizes the output of those channels with the highest signal-to-noise ratio and minimizes the masking effect of noise, which is usually severe over a restricted range of frequency channels. This strategy may be analogous to the way in which onset-chopper units continue to encode signals in the presence of intense background noise.

Some researchers are exploring the ability of neural networks to perform automatic speech recognition (Bourlard and Morgan, 1993). These computational systems mimic certain gross properties of the auditory pathway, consisting of an initial input layer analogous to the auditory nerve, one or more hidden layers corresponding perhaps to the auditory brain stem nuclei, and an output layer. The interesting processes occur in the hidden layers, which adjust the strength (weights) of neuronal interconnections to optimize the accuracy of phoneme recognition. This adjustment of weights has been likened to neural learning. Waibel (1988) uses time delays, not unlike autocorrelation, to enhance the recognition performance, and Kohonen (1988, 1989) attempts to extract relevant acoustic features through constructing an appropriate topological space pattern. One of the principal advantages of using neural networks for speech recognition is that they generally encode the acoustic waveform redundantly, particularly in the hidden layers, and in so doing, make the information less vulnerable to interfering noise. It is likely that further improvements in speech recognition in noisy environments can be gained through a better understanding of the noise-reduction circuitry of the auditory periphery (Morgan, Bourlard, Greenberg, and Hermansky, 1994).

IMPLICATIONS FOR GENERAL MODELS OF SPEECH PERCEPTION

General models of speech perception are concerned with several principles of information coding relevant to issues discussed in this chapter. Of particular concern is the nature of the underlying representation of speech sounds: whether these perceptual units are continuous or discrete and whether they are based on auditory or articulatory templates or some other form.

One well-known model argues that speech is perceived as articulatory gestures rather than through the auditory analysis of the acoustic waveform (Liberman, Cooper, Shankweiler, and Studdert-Kennedy, 1967). The premise of this motor theory is that speech invokes a unique mode of analysis distinguished from general auditory processing in its specialization for speech-like features. At some very early stage this information is routed to linguistic-specific processors that convert the speech stream into its underlying articulatory form. The motor theory originated in response to the enormous amount of acoustic variability inherent in speech. A search for some level of invariance akin to perceptual experience suggested that the underlying representation is in the set of motor gestures producing the acoustic waveform. Unfortunately for the motor theory, there is also considerable variability at the articulatory level (Holmes, 1986). Nor is there firm evidence as yet for speech-specific acoustic analysis (Kluender and Greenberg, 1989).

An alternative approach is to seek the invariant cues in the acoustic waveform itself. For example, Blumstein and Stevens (1980) have observed that each of the three place-of-articulation categories of American English stop consonants is associated with a distinctive spectral template that varies little with phonetic context. In their view, other phonetic categories also have an acoustic essence that remains immutable across context, speaker, and production rate. Nonetheless, Kewley-Port, Pisoni, and Studdert-Kennedy (1983) suggest that the variable, spectrally dynamic properties of the speech signal convey the lion's share of acoustic information.

A principal motivation for the design of auditory front-ends in speech analysis and recognition is the expectation that some set of properties of the auditory periphery will provide an invariant representation of the speech waveform that is lacking in conventional spectral analyses. Is much of the acoustic variability in the speech signal filtered out during an auditory smoothing operation that discards most of the details? Or is the invariance of phonetic categories a function of higher-level, more cognitive operations that follow the auditory stage of analysis? Although the answers to such questions must await future research, some evidence suggests that much invariance arises from more central, probably cortical mechanisms that extract acoustic features and properties from peripheral analysis in accordance with semantic and syntactic expectation (Marslen-Wilson, 1989). In this view there is considerable advantage in postponing the final interpretation until the last possible moment, to avoid premature categorization inconsistent with the intention of the speaker. On the other hand, it is certainly desirable to reduce the amount of information transmitted through the auditory pathway to the barest essentials required for accurate decoding of the speech stream for reasons of reliability. It is likely that spectral features conveying little phonetic and prosodic information are discarded in the peripheral transduction of the speech signal.

At issue, then, is the nature of the representational code for phonetic features and categories in the auditory pathway. Miller and Sachs (1983), Sinex and Geisler (1983), and Delgutte and Kiang (1984) have shown that certain properties of the auditory nerve population response profile are generally associated with such phonetic features as voicing, frication, and plosives. And voice-onset time, an important cue for voiced-voiceless distinctions, may also have some correlates in the auditory nerve response (Sinex and MacDonald, 1989). However, it is still unclear whether phonetic categorization is based primarily on such peripheral representations (unlikely) or requires additional processing at higher levels of the auditory pathway.

IMPLICATIONS FOR THE SOUND PATTERNS OF LANGUAGE

The spectro-temporal properties of speech are thought to reflect constraints imposed principally by the vocal apparatus, with little significance attributed to the ear's role in shaping the acoustics of speech (Ladefoged, 1992). Current knowledge of the auditory processing of complex sounds calls this traditional view into question.

The auditory system is phylogenetically far older than the human vocal apparatus. Although the latter shares certain features with those of its primate and mammalian relatives, the human speech production system is highly specialized, reflecting the unique properties of spoken language. The human auditory periphery and brain stem, by contrast, do not differ much from those of most other mammals. For this reason it is likely that the auditory system has imposed far more constraints on the evolutionary design of the human vocal apparatus than vice versa.

It is likely that reliability and redundancy are major factors in shaping the evolution of both human and animal communication systems. For example, among certain species of monkeys in central Africa, the spectro-temporal characteristics of many vocalizations appear to be optimized for reliable transmission in their specific acoustic environment (Brown, 1986). Similar ecological factors may have shaped the evolutionary course of linguistic sound patterns. The similarity of sound features across the world's languages is likely to reflect constraints imposed as much by the acoustic ecology of reliable sound transmission as by articulatory and auditory factors (Lindblom, 1986). Indeed, many of the design features of both the articulatory and auditory systems may be principally motivated by reliable transmission and encoding in unpredictable, potentially noisy conditions. Several acoustic properties of speech appear to be especially well adapted for ensuring reliable transmission of information. We consider each in turn.

Energy Distribution

Although human speech uses high-frequency energy (e.g., the sibilants [f] and [s]), virtually all speech energy lies below 3.5 kHz. This low-frequency bias in the spectrum is usually attributed to a greater sensitivity for these frequencies among listeners. However, humans generally are more sensitive at 4 kHz than they are below 1 kHz, where most of the energy in speech lies. The upper limit of neural phase locking in the auditory nerve is approximately 4 kHz (Rose,

Brugge, Anderson, and Hind, 1967; Johnson, 1980), and this limit may well account for the predominance of low-frequency energy in the speech signal. There are obvious advantages for encoding information in terms of synchrony, the most important of which is reliability in the presence of noise. It is significant that, without exception, peripheral ANFs of vertebrate hearing systems can phase-lock their discharge to low-frequency signals and that the energy distribution of most vertebrate vocalizations lies below 4 kHz. Thus, a low-frequency bias in vocalizations is likely to be a phylogenetically ancient adaptation and may have originated to increase the reliability of information coding.

Prevalence of Spectral Maxima (Formants)

A good deal of the speech stream is marked by formant peaks in the spectrum, thought to encode much of the phonetic information in the signal. Why, for example, is the phonetic inventory of the world's languages dominated by vowels, semivowels, glides, liquids, and formant transitions rather than by bursts, frication, and sibilance? Which properties of these formant peaks make them better suited for information coding than other spectral features?

As discussed in an earlier section, the encoding of spectral maxima is most robust in the face of acoustic interference and noise. This robustness arises from two properties of the auditory periphery: neural phase locking and low-pass filtering, which at moderate to high SPLs distributes the formant-relevant information across a wide range of frequency channels. In this sense the auditory periphery can enhance the representation of spectral maxima relative to lower-intensity components or noise.

Prevalence of Voicing

All vowels in English and most other languages, semivowels, liquids, and many consonants are produced with the glottis in vibration. Although voicing is not necessary for continuous communication (as attested by whispered speech), we rarely speak voicelessly unless compelled by pathology or secretiveness. Voicing creates a common pattern of amplitude modulation across frequency, possibly useful for binding disparate portions of the spectrum during acoustic interference and competition (Scheffers,

1983; Assmann and Summerfield, 1989; Bregman, 1990). It also raises the resistance of high-frequency energy to noise by synchronizing the discharge of neural elements to the fundamental frequency. In addition, it takes advantage of the ability of higher auditory neurons to phase-lock to low modulation frequencies.

Alternation of Long and Short Elements

Much of the phonetic information in the signal resides in the consonants (Miller, 1951). Why, then, do we not speak in a stream of consonants rather than alternating them with vocalic segments? Consonants are generally briefer than vowels and would provide a much higher rate of information transfer if vowels were excluded from the phonetic inventory. And yet no language excludes vowels. Consonants may optimize the rate of information flow but spoken devoid of vocalic context may also be more vulnerable to the masking effects of extraneous noise.

Vocalic segments are more robustly encoded than consonants in the presence of noise, but their longer duration necessarily retards the rate of information flow, which in turn may preclude the integration of such phonetic information into higher-level syntactic and semantic units due to constraints imposed by short- and intermediate-term memory. Thus, the alternating pattern of consonants and vowels may reflect a compromise between speed of information transfer and robust encoding in the presence of noise.

High Intensity of Speech

The SPL of speech generally exceeds 70 dB at the receiver (Miller, 1951), yet most verbal communication occurs over relatively short distances. Although it is physiologically feasible to speak at a lower intensity, it is rarely done except for whispering. This may be because the spectral peaks in the signal are more robustly encoded at higher SPLs due to the low-pass-like filtering at those intensities which, in turn, distributes the information-laden elements of the speech waveform across many channels.

CONCLUSIONS AND FUTURE DIRECTIONS

The human auditory system has an evolutionary history reaching into the Cretaceous period more than 65 million years ago. Acoustic transduction, particularly in the auditory periphery, is remarkably similar across mammalian species, and certain basic properties of auditory function, such as phase-locking and tonotopic organization, extend back to the Paleozoic era 225 million years ago. The conservatism of the auditory system suggests that this uniformity of nature's design reflects effective solutions to common problems of acoustic transduction and encoding.

One of the most pervasive obstacles to communication is background interference. Because this interference is so variable and therefore largely unpredictable, elaborate mechanisms have evolved to filter out this background and enhance the encoding of the target signal. This makes it highly unlikely that the auditory mechanisms underlying the processing of speech are evolutionarily recent. Rather, it seems that much if not all of the acoustic properties of speech are the product of an evolutionary process in which the vocal apparatus, which is indisputably of recent origin, has developed to produce sounds readily detected and robustly encoded by the ear.

Future research will undoubtedly shed more light upon the evolutionary history of speech and will in all likelihood demonstrate that the vocal communication systems of other mammals and vertebrates share many acoustic traits with human speech. At present a detailed knowledge of nonhuman vocal communication systems is lacking for all but a few species, and so are the theoretical insights to reveal precisely why speech and other communication systems sound the way they do. For greater insight into the neural mechanisms underlying the processing of communication sounds it will be necessary to understand the acoustic ecology in which they evolved. This in turn will require intensive study of vocal communication systems, both in the laboratory and under natural field conditions.

Another promising approach is to use models of the human auditory system and higher cortical centers to simulate the ontogenetic and phylogenetic conditions shaping the evolution of specific linguistic sound patterns (Lindblom, 1986). It is to be hoped that insights from these models will assist physiologists and psychoacousticians in their search for the neural underpinnings of speech processing.

Review Questions

1. Describe the physiological mechanisms in the cochlea responsible for neural phase-locking in the auditory nerve. What factors account for the inability of ANFs to phase-lock to high-frequency signals? What are some functional consequences of this frequency limitation on neural synchrony?

2. How important is the tonotopic organization of the auditory pathway in the processing of spectrally complex signals, such as speech? What would be the consequence for speech coding of a hearing system that lacked such topographic structure?

3. Which physiological response classes in the cochlear nuclei would you anticipate being most effective in coding the following attributes of sound?

        Intensity
        Pitch
        Sound location

        Spectral envelopes
        Syllable boundaries

4. Compare the properties of rate-place and spatially distributed temporal representations of the speech spectrum. Which representation would you anticipate being more effective under noisy conditions? What factors account for the relative noise immunity of this representation? Which representation would you expect to be important at low SPLs?

5. How would you use your knowledge of auditory coding to improve the performance of automatic speech recognition systems?

6. How well matched are the spectro-temporal properties of speech to the physiology and anatomy of the auditory pathway? Are there ways to enhance intelligibility of speech by changing some of these properties?

References

Abeles, M. (1982). Role of the cortical neuron: integrator or coincidence detector? *Israel Journal of Medical Sciences 18*, 83-92.

Adams, J. C. (1991). Connections of the cochlear nucleus. In Ainsworth, W. A., Hackney, C., & Evans, E. F. (Eds.), *Cochlear nucleus: Structure and function in relation to modelling*. London: JAI Press.

Anderson, D. J., Rose, J. E., & Brugge, J. F. (1971). Temporal position of discharges in single auditory nerve fibers within the cycle of a sine-wave stimulus: Frequency and intensity effects. *Journal of the Acoustical Society of America, 49*,1131-1139.

Arneson, A. R., & Osen, K. K. (1978). The cochlear nerve in the cat: Topography, cochleoptopy and fiber spectrum. *Journal of Comparative Neurology, 178,* 661-678.

Assmann, P. F., & Summerfield, Q. (1989). Modelling the perception of concurrent vowels: Vowels with the same fundamental frequencies. *Journal of the Acoustical Society of America, 85,* 327-338.

Assmann, P. F., & Summerfield, Q. (1990). Modelling the perception of concurrent vowels: Vowels with different fundamental frequencies. *Journal of the Acoustical Society of America, 88,* 680-697.

Békésy, G. von (1960). *Experiments in Hearing.* New York: McGraw-Hill.

Bilsen, F. A. (1977). Pitch of noise signals: Evidence for a central spectrum. *Journal of the Acoustical Society of America, 61,* 150-161.

Blackburn, C. C., & Sachs, M. B. (1990). The representation of the steady-state vowel sound [ɛ] in the discharge patterns of cat anteroventral cochlear nucleus neurons. *Journal of Neurophysiology, 63,* 1191-1212.

Blumstein, S. E., & Stevens, K. N. (1980). Perceptual invariance and onset spectra for stop consonants in different vowel environments. *Journal of the Acoustical Society of America, 67,* 648-662.

Boer, E. de (1976). On the residue and auditory pitch perception. In Keidel, W. D., & Neff, W. D., (Eds.), *Handbook of Sensory Physiology,* Vol. 3. Berlin: Springer-Verlag (pp. 479-583).

Bourlard, H. A., & Morgan, N. (1993). *Connectionist speech recognition: A hybrid approach.* Boston: Kluwer.

Bregman, A. S. (1990). *Auditory scene analysis.* Cambridge, MA: MIT Press.

Brodal, A. (1981). *Neurological anatomy in relation to clinical medicine,* 3rd ed. Oxford, UK: Oxford University Press.

Bronkhorst, A. W., & Plomp, R. (1989). Binaural speech intelligibility in noise for hearing-impaired listeners. *Journal of the Acoustical Society of America, 86,* 1374-1383.

Brown, C. (1986). The perception of vocal signals by blue monkeys and grey-cheeked mangabeys. *Experimental Biology, 45,* 145-165.

Brown T. H, Kairiss, E. W., & Keenan C. L. (1990). Hebbian synapses: Biophysical mechanisms and algorithms. *Annual Review of Neuroscience, 13,* 475-511.

Brugge, J. F., Anderson, D. J., Hind, J. E., & Rose, J. E. (1969). Time structure of discharges in single auditory nerve fibers of the squirrel in response to complex periodic sounds. *Journal of Neurophysiology, 32,* 386-401.

Carlson, R., Fant, G., & Granström, B. (1975). Two formant models, pitch and vowel perception. In Fant, G., & Tatham, M. (Eds.), *Analysis and perception of speech.* London: Academic Press, (pp. 55-82).

Carr, C. E., & Konishi, M. (1988). Axonal delay lines create maps of interaural phase differences in the owl's brainstem. *Proceedings of the National Academy of Sciences of the United States of America, 85,* 8311-8315.

Chalikia, M. H., & Bregman, A. S. (1989). The perceptual segregation of simultaneous auditory signals: Pulse train segregation and vowel segregation. *Perception and Psychophysics, 46,* 487-496.

Clarey, J. C., Barone, P., & Imig, T. J. (1992). Physiology of thalamus and cortex. In Popper, A. N., & Fay, R. R. (Eds.), *The mammalian auditory pathway: Neurophysiology.* New York: Springer-Verlag (pp. 232-334).

Cooke, M., Beet, S., & Crawford, M. (1993). *Visual representations of speech signals.* New York: Wiley.

Darwin, C. J. (1981). Perceptual grouping of speech components differing in fundamental frequency and onset-time. *Quarterly Journal of Experimental Psychology. A. Human Experimental Psychology, 33A,* 185-207.

Delgutte, B., & Kiang, N. Y. S. (1984). Speech coding in the auditory nerve: IV. Sounds with consonant-like dynamic characteristics, *Journal of the Acoustical Society of America, 75,* 897-907.

Deng, L., Geisler, C. D., & Greenberg, S. (1988). A composite model of the auditory periphery for the processing of speech. *Journal of Phonetics, 16,* 93-108.

Edelman, G. M. (1987). *Neural Darwinism: The theory of neuronal group selection.* New York: Basic Books.

Erulkar, S. D. (1972). Comparative aspects of spatial localization of sound. *Physiological Reviews, 52,* 237-360.

Evans, E. F. (1978). Place and time coding of

frequency in the peripheral auditory system: Some physiological pros and cons. *Audiology, 17,* 369-420.

Evans, E. F., & Nelson, P. G. (1973a). The responses of single neurons in the cochlear nucleus of the cat as a function of their location and anesthetic state. *Experimental Brain Research, 17,* 402-427.

Evans, E. F., & Nelson, P. G. (1973b). On the functional relationship between the dorsal and ventral divisions of the cochlear nucleus of the cat. *Experimental Brain Research, 17,* 428-442.

Evans, E. F., & Wilson, J. P. (1974). Frequency selectivity of the cochlea. In Møller, A. R. (Ed.), *Basic mechanisms in hearing.* New York: Academic Press (pp. 519-551).

Fekete, D. M., Rouiller, E. M., Liberman, M. C., & Ryugo, D. K. (1982). The central projections of intracellularly labeled auditory nerve fibers in cats. *Journal of Comparative Neurology, 229,* 432-450.

Flanagan, J. L. (1955). A difference limen for vowel formant frequency. *Journal of the Acoustical Society of America, 27,* 613-617.

Flanagan, J. L., & Guttman, N. (1960a). On the pitch of periodic pulses. *Journal of the Acoustical Society of America, 32,* 1308-1319.

Flanagan, J. L., & Guttman, N. (1960b). Pitch of periodic pulses without fundamental component. *Journal of the Acoustical Society of America, 32,* 1319-1328.

Frisina, R. D., Smith, R. L., & Chamberlin, S. C. (1990). Encoding of amplitude modulation in the gerbil cochlear nucleus: A hierarchy of enhancement. *Hearing Research, 44,* 99-122.

Ghitza, O. (1988). Temporal non-place information in the auditory-nerve firing patterns as a front-end for speech recognition in a noisy environment. *Journal of Phonetics, 16,* 109-124.

Ghitza, O. (1993). Adequacy of auditory models to predict human internal representation of speech sounds. *Journal of the Acoustical Society of America, 93,* 2160-2171.

Gibson, J. J. (1950). *The perception of the visual world.* Boston: Houghton Mifflin.

Gibson, J. J. (1966). *The senses considered as perceptual systems.* Boston: Houghton Mifflin.

Gibson, J. J. (1979). *The ecological approach to visual perception.* Boston: Houghton Mifflin.

Goldstein, J. L., & Srulovicz, P. (1977). Auditory nerve spike intervals as an adequate basis for aural spectrum analysis. In Evans, E. F., & Wilson, J. P. (Eds.), *Psychophysics and Physiology of Hearing.* London: Academic Press (pp. 337-346).

Greenberg, S. (1986). Possible role of low and medium spontaneous rate cochlear nerve fibers in the encoding of waveform periodicity. In Moore, B. C. J., & Patterson, R. D. (Eds.), *Auditory frequency selectivity.* New York: Plenum (pp. 241-248).

Greenberg, S. (1988). The ear as a speech analyzer. *Journal of Phonetics, 16,* 139-150.

Greenberg, S., Geisler, C. D., & Deng, L. (1986). Frequency selectivity of single cochlear-nerve fibers based on the temporal response pattern to two-tone signals. *Journal of the Acoustical Society of America, 79,* 1010-1019.

Greenberg, S., & Rhode, W. S. (1987). Periodicity coding in cochlear nerve and ventral cochlear nucleus. In Yost, W. A., & Watson, C. S. (Eds.), *Auditory processing of complex sounds.* Hillsdale, NJ: Lawrence Erlbaum (pp. 225-236).

Greenwood, D. D. (1986). What is synchrony suppression? *Journal of the Acoustical Society of America, 79,* 1857-1872.

Grey, J., & Gordon, J. (1978). Perceptual effects of spectral modifications on musical timbres. *Journal of the Acoustical Society of America, 63,* 1493-1500.

Gulick, W. L., Gelsand, S., & Frisina, R. (1989) Hearing: Physiological acoustics, neural noding, and psychoacoustics. New York: Oxford University Press.

Handel, S. (1989). *Listening.* Cambridge, MA: MIT Press.

Hebb, D. O. (1949). *The organization of behavior: A neuropsychological theory.* New York: Wiley.

Helmholtz, H. L. F. von (1863). *Die Lehre von Tonemfindungen als Physiologie Grundlage für die Theorie der Musik* [On the sensations of tone as a physiological basis for the theory of music]. Braunschweige: F. Wieweg und Sohn. (Ellis, A. J., Trans.). New York: Dover (reprint of 1897 edition).

Holmes, J. (1986). Normalization in vowel perception. In Perkell, J. S., & Klatt, D. H. (Eds.), *Invariance and variability in speech processes.* Hillsdale, NJ: Erlbaum (pp. 346-359).

Holton, T., Love, S., & Gill, S. (1992). Formant and pitch pulse detection using models of auditory signal processing. In *Proceedings of the 1992 international conference on spoken language processing* (pp. 81-84).

Huggins, W. H. (1952). A phase principle for complex-frequency analysis and its implications in auditory theory. *Journal of the Acoustical Society of America, 24,* 582-589.

Javel, E. (1980). Coding of AM tones in the chinchilla auditory nerve: Implications for the pitch of complex tones. *Journal of the Acoustical Society of America, 68,* 133-146.

Jeffress, L. L. (1948). A place theory of sound localization. *Journal of Comparative Physiological Psychology, 41,* 35-39.

Jenison, R., Greenberg, S., Kluender, K., & Rhode, W. S. (1991). A composite model of the auditory periphery for the processing of speech based on the filter response functions of single auditory nerve fibers. *Journal of the Acoustical Society of America, 90,* 773-786.

Johnson, D. H. (1980). The relationship between spike rate and synchrony in responses of auditory-nerve fibers to single tones. *Journal of the Acoustical Society of America, 68,* 1115-1122.

Johnstone, B. M., & Boyle, A. J. F. (1967). Basilar membrane vibration examined with the Mössbauer technique. *Science, 158,* 389-390.

Joris, P. X., & Yin, T. C. T. (1992). Responses to amplitude-modulated tones in the auditory nerve of the cat. *Journal of the Acoustical Society of America, 91,* 215-232.

Kakusho, O., Hirato, H., Kato, K., & Kobayashi, T. (1971). Some experiments of vowel perception by harmonic synthesizer. *Acustica, 24,* 179-190.

Kessel, R. G., & Kardon, R. (1979). Tissues and organs: A text atlas of scanning electron microscopy. San Francisco. W. H. Freeman.

Kewley-Port D., Pisoni D. B., & Studdert-Kennedy M. (1983). Perception of static and dynamic acoustic cues to place of articulation in initial stop consonants. *Journal of the Acoustical Society of America, 73,* 1779-1793.

Kitzes, L. M., Gibson, M. M., Rose, J. E., & Hind, J. E. (1978). Initial discharge latency and threshold considerations for some neurons in cochlear nucleus complex of the cat. *Journal of Neurophysiology, 41,* 1165-1182.

Klatt, D. H. (1989). Review of selected models of speech perception. In Marslen-Wilson, W. (Ed.), *Lexical representation and process.* Cambridge, MA: MIT Press (pp. 169-226).

Kluender, K., & Greenberg, S. (1989). A specialization for speech perception? *Science, 244,* 1530.

Kohonen, T. (1988). The neural phonetic typewriter. *Computer, 21* (3), 11-22.

Kohonen, T. (1989). Speech recognition based on topology-preserving neural maps. In Aleksander, I. (Ed.), *Neural computing architectures.* Cambridge, MA: MIT Press (pp. 26-40).

Ladefoged, P. (1992). *A course in phonetics,* 3rd ed. New York: Harcourt, Brace and Jovanovich.

Langner, G. (1988). Physiological properties of units in the cochlear nucleus are adequate for a model of periodicity analysis in the auditory midbrain. In Syka, J., & Masterton, R. B. (Eds.), *Auditory pathway: Structure and function.* New York: Plenum (pp. 207-212).

Langner, G. (1991). A model for periodicity analysis in line with physiological properties and anatomical connections of neurons in cochlear nucleus and inferior colliculus. In Ainsworth, W. A., Hackney, C., & Evans, E. F. (Eds.), *Cochlear nucleus: Structure and function in relation to modelling.* London: JAI Press.

Langner, G., & Schreiner, C. (1988). Periodicity coding in the inferior colliculus of the cat: I. Neuronal mechanisms. *Journal of Neurophysiology, 60,* 1799-1822.

Lee, K. F. (1989). *Automatic speech recognition: The development of the sphinx system.* Boston: Kluwer.

Lewis, E. R. (1987). Speculations about noise and the evolution of vertebrate hearing. *Hearing Research, 25,* 83-90.

Liberman, A. M., Cooper, F. S., Shankweiler, D. P., & Studdert-Kennedy, M. (1967). Perception of the speech code. *Psychological Review, 74,* 431-461.

Liberman A. M., & Mattingly, I. G. (1989). A specialization for speech perception. *Science, 243,* 489-494.

Licklider, J. C. R. (1951). A duplex theory of pitch perception. *Experientia, 7,* 129-133.

Lindblom, B. E. F. (1986). Phonetic universals in vowel systems. In Yaeger, J. J. (Ed.), *Experimental phonology.* Orlando, FL: Academic Press (pp. 13-44).

Lynn, P. A., & Fuerst, W. (1989). *Introductory digital signal processing with computer applications.* New York: Wiley.

Lyon, R. F. (1984). Computational models of neural auditory processing. *Proceedings of the IEEE international conference on acoustics, speech and signal processing.* 3611-3614.

Marslen-Wilson, W. (1989). Access and integration: Projecting sound onto meaning. In Marslen-Wilson, W. (Ed.), *Lexical representation and process.* Cambridge, MA: MIT Press (pp. 3-24).

Mermelstein, P. (1978). Difference limens for formant frequencies of steady-state and consonant-bound vowels. *Journal of the Acoustical Society of America, 63,* 572-580.

Miller, G. A. (1951). *Language and communication.* New York: McGraw-Hill.

Miller, M. I., & Sachs, M. B. (1983). Representation of stop consonants in the discharge patterns of auditory-nerve fibers. *Journal of the Acoustical Society of America, 74,* 502-517.

Miller, M. I., & Sachs, M. B. (1984). Representation of voice pitch in discharge patterns of auditory-nerve fibers. *Hearing Research, 14,* 257-279.

Møller, A. R. (1974). Response of units in the cochlear nucleus to sinusoidally amplitude-modulated tones. *Experimental Neurology, 45,* 104-117.

Moore, J. K. (1991). Dorsal cochlear nucleus organization. In Ainsworth, W. A., Hackney, C., & Evans, E. F. (Eds.), *Cochlear nucleus: Structure and function in relation to modelling.* London: JAI Press.

Morgan, N., Bourlard, H., Greenberg, S., & Hermansky, H. (1994). Stochastic perceptual auditory-event-based models for speech recognition. In *Proceedings of the International Congress on Spoken Language Processing.* Yokohama, Japan.

Mugnaini, E. (1991). The granule cell-cartwheel neuron system in the cochlear nucleus complex. In Ainsworth, W. A., Hackney, C., & Evans, E. F. (Eds.), *Cochlear nucleus: Structure and function in relation to modelling.* London: JAI Press.

Ohm, G. S. (1843). Über die definition des Tones, nebst daran geknupfter Theorie der Sirene und ahnlicher Tonbildener Vorrichtungen. *Annalen der Physik 59*: 497-565.

Oppenheim, A. V., & Schafer, R. W. (1975). *Digital signal processing*. Englewood Cliffs, NJ: Prentice-Hall.

Pang, X. D., & Peake, W. T. (1986). How do contractions of the stapedius muscle alter the acoustic properties of the ear? In Allen, J., Hall, J. L., Hubbard, A., Neely, S. T., & Tubis, A. (Eds.), *Peripheral auditory mechanisms*. Berlin: Springer-Verlag (pp. 36-43).

Patterson, R. D. (1986). Spiral detection of periodicity and the spiral form of musical scales. *Psychology of Music, 14*, 44-61.

Patterson, R. D. (1987). A pulse ribbon model of peripheral auditory processing. In Yost, W. A., & Watson, C. S. (Eds.), *Auditory Processing of Complex Sounds*. Hillsdale, NJ: Lawrence Erlbaum (pp. 167-179).

Patterson, R. D., & Holdsworth, J. (1991). A computational model of auditory image construction. In Ainsworth, W. A., Hackney, C., & Evans, E. F. (Eds.), *Cochlear nucleus: Structure and Function in Relation to Modelling*. London: JAI Press.

Peterson, G., & Barney, P. (1952) Control methods used in a study of the vowels. *Journal of the Acoustical Society of America, 24*, 175-184.

Pickett, J. M. (1980). *The sounds of speech communication: A primer of acoustic phonetics and speech perception*. Baltimore: University Park Press.

Pickles, J. O. (1988). *An introduction to the physiology of hearing*, 2nd ed. London: Academic Press.

Pisoni, D. B. (1982). Speech perception: The human listener as cognitive interface. *Speech Technology, 1*(2), 10-23.

Popper, A. N., & Fay, R. R. (1992). *The mammalian auditory pathway: Neurophysiology*. New York: Springer-Verlag.

Remez, R. E., Rubin, P. E., Pisoni, D. B., & Carrell, T. D. (1981). Speech perception without traditional speech cues. *Science, 212*, 947-950.

Rhode, W. S. (1971). Observations of the vibration of the basilar membrane in squirrel monkeys using the Mössbauer technique. *Journal of the Acoustical Society of America, 49*, 1218-1231.

Rhode, W. S., & Greenberg, S. R. (1994). Encoding of amplitude modulation in the cochlear nucleus of the cat. *Journal of Neurophysiology, 71*, 1797-1825.

Rhode, W. S., & Greenberg, S. R. (1992). Physiology of the cochlear nuclei. In Popper, A. N., & Fay, R. R., (Eds). *The mammalian auditory pathway: Neurophysiology*. New York: Springer-Verlag (pp. 94-152).

Rhode, W. S., & Kettner, R. E. (1987). Physiological study of neurons in the dorsal and posteroventral cochlear nucleus of the unanesthesized cat. *Journal of Neurophysiology, 57*, 414-442.

Rhode, W. S., Oertel, D., & Smith, P. H. (1983). Physiological response properties of cells labelled intracellularly with horseradish peroxidase in cat ventral cochlear nucleus, *Journal of Comparative Neurology, 213*, 448-463.

Rhode, W. S., & Smith, P. H. (1986a). Encoding time and intensity in the ventral cochlear nucleus of the cat. *Journal of Neurophysiology, 56*, 262-286.

Rhode, W. S., & Smith, P. H. (1986b). Physiological studies on neurons in the dorsal cochlear nucleus of cat. *Journal of Neurophysiology, 56*, 287-307.

Ribaupierre, F. de, Goldstein, M. H. Jr. & Yeni-Komshian, G. (1972). Cortical coding of repetitive acoustic pulses. *Brain Research, 48*, 205-225.

Rose, J. E., Brugge, J. F., Anderson, D. J., & Hind, J. E. (1967). Phase-locked response to low-frequency tones in single auditory nerve fibers of the squirrel monkey. *Journal of Neurophysiology, 30*, 769-793.

Rouiller, E. M., Cronin-Schreiber, R., Fekete, D. M., & Ryugo, D. K. (1986). The central projections of intracellularly labeled auditory nerve fibers in cats: an analysis of terminal morphology. *Journal of Comparative Neurology, 249*, 261-278.

Rouiller, E. M., & Ryugo, D. K. (1984). Intracellular marking of physiologically characterized cells in the ventral cochlear nucleus of the cat. *Journal of Comparative Neurology, 225*, 167-186.

Sachs, M. B., Blackburn, C. C., & Young, E. D. (1988). Rate-place and temporal-place representations of vowels in the auditory nerve and anteroventral cochlear nucleus. *Journal of Phonetics, 16*, 37-53.

Sachs, M. B., & Kiang, N. Y. S. (1968). Two-tone inhibition in auditory nerve fibers. *Journal of the Acoustical Society of America, 43*, 1120-1128.

Sachs, M. B., Voigt, H. F., & Young, E. D. (1983) Auditory nerve representation of vowels in background noise, *Journal of Neurophysiology, 50*, 27-45.

Sachs, M. B., Winslow, R. L., & Blackburn, C. C. (1988). Representation of speech in the auditory periphery. In Edelman, G. M., Gall, W. E., & Cowan, W. M. (Eds.), *Auditory function: Neurobiological bases of hearing*. New York: Wiley (pp. 747-774).

Sachs, M. B., & Young, E. D. (1979). Encoding of steady-state vowels in the auditory nerve: Representation in terms of discharge rate, *Journal of the Acoustical Society of America, 66*, 470-479.

Sachs, M.B., & Young, E. D. (1980). Effects of nonlinearities on speech encoding in the auditory nerve. *Journal of the Acoustical Society of America, 68*, 858-875.

Schalk, T. B., & Sachs, M. B. (1980). Nonlinearities in auditory-nerve responses to bandlimited noise.

Journal of the Acoustical Society of America, 67, 903-913.

Scheffers, M. T. M. (1983). *Sifting vowels: Auditory pitch analysis and sound segregation.* Unpublished doctoral dissertation, University of Groningen, The Netherlands.

Schreiner, C., & Langner, G. (1988). Periodicity coding in the inferior colliculus of the cat: II. Topographical organization. *Journal of Neurophysiology, 60,* 1823-1840.

Schreiner, C. E., & Urbas, J. V. (1986). Representation of amplitude modulation in the auditory cortex of the cat: I. The anterior auditory field (AAF). *Hearing Research, 21,* 227-241.

Scott, B. (1976). Temporal factors in vowel perception. *Journal of the Acoustical Society of America, 60,* 1354-1360.

Sellick, P. M., & Russell, I. J. (1978). Intracellular studies of hair cells: Filling the gap between basilar membrane mechanics and neural excitation. In Naunton, R. F., & Fernandez, C. (Eds.), *Evoked electrical activity in the auditory nervous system.* New York: Academic Press (pp. 113-139).

Shamma, S. (1985a). Speech processing in the auditory system: I. Representation of speech sounds in the responses of the auditory nerve. *Journal of the Acoustical Society of America, 78,* 1612-1621.

Shamma, S. (1985b). Speech processing in the auditory system: II. Lateral inhibition and the processing of speech-evoked activity in the auditory nerve. *Journal of the Acoustical Society of America, 78,* 1612-1621.

Shamma, S. (1988) The acoustic features of speech sounds in a model of auditory processing: Vowels and voiceless fricatives. *Journal of Phonetics, 16,* 77-91.

Shamma, S., & Morrish, K. (1987). Synchrony suppression in complex stimulus responses of a biophysical model of the cochlea. *Journal of the Acoustical Society of America, 81,* 1486-1498.

Sidwell, A., & Summerfield, Q. (1986). The auditory representation of symmetrical CVC syllables. *Speech Communication, 5,* 283-297.

Siebert, W. M. (1970). Frequency discrimination in the auditory system: Place or periodicity mechanisms? *Proceedings of the IEEE, 58,* 723-730.

Sinex, D. G., & Geisler, C. D. (1983). Responses of auditory-nerve fibers to consonant-vowel syllables. *Journal of the Acoustical Society of America, 73,* 602-615.

Sinex, D. G., & Geisler, C. D. (1984). Comparisons of the responses of auditory-nerve fibers to consonant-vowel syllables with predictions from linear models. *Journal of the Acoustical Society of America, 76,* 116-121.

Sinex, D., & MacDonald, L. P. (1989). Synchronized discharge rate representation of voice onset time in the chinchilla auditory nerve. *Journal of the Acoustical Society of America, 85,* 1995-2004.

Smoorenburg, G. F. (1992). Speech reception in quiet and in noisy conditions by individuals with noise-induced hearing loss in relation to their tone audiogram. *Journal of the Acoustical Society of America, 91,* 421-437.

Sokolowski, B. H. A., Sachs, M. B., & Goldstein, J. L. (1989). Auditory nerve rate-level functions for two-tone stimuli: Possible relation to basilar membrane nonlinearity. *Hearing Research, 41,* 115-124.

Srulovicz, P., & Goldstein, J. L. (1983). A central spectrum model: A synthesis of auditory-nerve timing and place cues in monaural communication of frequency spectrum. *Journal of the Acoustical Society of America, 73,* 1266-1275.

Steinschneider, M., Arezzo, J., & Vaughan, H. Jr. (1982). Speech evoked activity in the auditory radiations and the cortex of the awake monkey. *Brain Research, 252,* 353-365.

Stubbs, R. J., & Summerfield, Q. (1990). Algorithms for separating the speech of interfering talkers: Evaluations with voiced sentences, and normal-hearing and hearing-impaired listeners. *Journal of the Acoustical Society of America, 87,* 359-372.

Summerfield, Q., & Assmann P. F. (1989). Auditory enhancement and the perception of concurrent vowels. *Perception and Psychophysics, 45,* 529-536.

Summerfield Q., & Assmann, P. F. (1991). Perception of concurrent vowels: Effects of harmonic misalignment and pitch-period asynchrony. *Journal of the Acoustical Society of America, 89,* 1364 1377.

Waibel, A. (1988). Consonant recognition by modular construction of large phonemic time delay neural networks. In *Neural information processing systems.* San Mateo, CA: Morgan Kaufman (pp. 215-223).

Waibel, A., & Lee, K.-F. (1990). *Readings in speech recognition.* San Mateo, CA: Morgan Kaufman.

Webster, D. B., Popper, A. N., & Fay, R. R. (1992). *The mammalian auditory pathway: Neuroanatomy.* New York: Springer-Verlag.

Wever, E. G. (1949). *Theory of hearing.* New York: Wiley.

Whitfield, I. C. (1970). Central nervous processing in relation to spatio-temporal discrimination of auditory patterns. In Plomp, R., & Smoorenburg, G. F. (Eds.), *Frequency analysis and periodicity detection in hearing.* Leiden: Sijthof (pp. 136-147).

Wilson, J. P., & Johnstone, J. (1972). Capacitive probe study of basilar membrane vibration. In *Symposium on Hearing Theory.* Eindhoven, Netherlands: IPO (pp. 172-181).

Winslow, R. L., Barta, P. E., & Sachs, M. B. (1987). Rate coding in the auditory nerve. In Yost, W. A., & Watson, C. S. (Eds.), *Auditory processing of complex sounds.* Hillsdale, NJ: Lawrence Erlbaum (pp. 212-224).

Yin, T. C. T., & Kuwada, S. (1984). Neuronal mechanisms of binaural interaction. In Edelman,

G. M., Gall, W. E., & Cowan, W. M. (Eds.), *Dynamic aspects of neocortical function.* New York: Wiley (pp 263-313).

Young, E. D., & Brownell, W. E. (1976). Responses to tones and noise of single cells in dorsal cochlear nucleus of unanesthetized cats. *Journal of Neurophysiology, 39,* 282-300.

Young, E. D., & Sachs, M. B. (1979). Representation of steady-state vowels in the temporal aspects of the discharge patterns of auditory-nerve fibers.

Journal of the Acoustical Society of America, 66, 1381-1403.

Young, E. D., Spirou, G. A., Rice, J. J., & Voigt H. F. (1992). Neural organization and responses to complex stimuli in the dorsal cochlear nucleus. *Philosophical Transactions of the Royal Society of London, Series B, 336,* 407-413.

Suggested Readings

Auditory Physiology

Altschuler, R. A. (1991). *Neurobiology of hearing: the central auditory system.* New York: Raven Press.

Altschuler, R. A., Bobbin, R. P., & Hoffman, D. W. (1986). *Neurobiology of hearing: The cochlea.* New York: Raven Press.

Dallos, P., Geisler, C. D., Mathews, J., Ruggero M., & Steele, C. (1990). *The mechanics and biophysics of hearing.* New York: Springer-Verlag.

Edelman, G. M., Gall, W. E., & Cowan, W. M. (1988). *Auditory function: Neurobiological bases of hearing.* New York: Wiley.

Greenberg, S. R., Rose, D., Brugge, J. F., Geisler, C. D., & Hind, J. E. (1991). *Acoustic transduction in the auditory periphery.* Department of Neurophysiology, University of Wisconsin, Madison, WI 53706. (This CD-ROM application for the Macintosh illustrates many basic concepts of acoustic transduction using two-dimensional color animations.)

Gulick, W. L., Gelfand, S., & Frisina, R. (1989). *Hearing: Physiological acoustics, neural coding, and psychoacoustics.* New York: Oxford University Press.

Irvine, D. R. F. (1986). *The auditory brainstem.* Berlin: Springer-Verlag.

Kiang, N. Y. S. (1984). Peripheral neural processing of auditory information. In Brookhart, J. M., & Mountcastle, V. (Eds.), *Handbook of physiology: The nervous system,* vol. 3, Sensory processes, part 2. Bethesda: American Physiological Society (pp. 639-674).

Pickles, J. O. (1988). *An introduction to the physiology of hearing,* (ed. 2.) London: Academic Press.

Popper, A. N., & Fay, R. R. (1992). *The mammalian auditory pathway: Neurophysiology.* New York: Springer-Verlag.

Webster, D. B., Popper, A. N., & Fay, R. R. (1992). *The mammalian auditory pathway: Neuroanatomy.* New York: Springer-Verlag.

Psychology of Hearing

Bregman, A. (1990). *Auditory scene analysis.* Cambridge, MA: MIT Press.

Handel, S. (1989). *Listening.* Cambridge, MA: MIT Press.

Houtsma, A. J. M, Rossing, T. D., & Wagenaars, W. M. (1987). *Auditory demonstrations.* Woodbury NY: Acoustical Society of America. (An audio CD containing several dozen simulations of important auditory experiments. A HyperCard stack to accompany and control the CD is available from Malcolm Slaney, Interval Research, Inc. [malcolm@interval.com].)

Marr, D. (1982). *Vision.* San Francisco: W. H. Freeman. (Why is a book on vision recommended reading for those interested in hearing and speech? Because the approach to seeing pioneered by Marr (heavy on neural modeling and computation) in the 1970s is as valid for hearing. An extremely influential work.)

Moore, B. C. J. (1989). *An introduction to the psychology of hearing,* ed 3. London: Academic Press.

Speech

Cooke, M., Beet, S., & Crawford, M. (1993). *Visual representations of speech signals.* New York: Wiley.

Greenberg, S. (1988). Representation of speech in the auditory periphery [Special issue] *Journal of Phonetics 16,* 1.

Schouten, M. E. H. (1992). *The auditory processing of speech.* Berlin: Mouton de Gruyter.

Periodicity Processing and Pitch Perception

Boer, E. de (1976). On the residue and auditory pitch perception. In Keidel, W. D., & Neff, W. D., (Eds.), *Handbook of Sensory Physiology,* vol. 3. Berlin: Springer-Verlag (pp. 479-583).

Langner G. (1992). Periodicity coding in the auditory system. *Hearing Research, 60,* 115-142.

Licklider, J. C. R. (1962). Periodicity pitch and related auditory process models. *International Audiology, 1,* 1-36.

Slaney, M., & Lyon, R. F. (1993). On the importance of time: A temporal representation of sound. In Cooke, M., Beet, S., & Crawford, M. (Eds.). *Visual representations of speech signals.* New York: Wiley (pp. 95-116).

General Auditory Processes

Brink, G. van den, & Bilsen, F. A. (1980). *Psychophysical, physiological and behavioral studies in hearing.* Delft: Delft University Press.

Cazals, Y. (1992). *Auditory physiology and perception.* New York: Pergamon Press.

Duifhuis, H., Horst, J. W., & Wit, H. P. (1988). *Basic issues in hearing.* London: Academic Press.

Evans, E. F., & Wilson, J. P. (1977). *Psychophysics and physiology of hearing.* London: Academic Press.

Klinke, R., & Hartmann, R. (1983). *Hearing: Physiological bases and psychophysics.* Berlin: Springer-Verlag.

Møller, A. R. (1974). *Basic mechanisms in hearing.* New York: Academic Press.

Moore, B. C. J., & Patterson, R. D. (1986). *Auditory frequency selectivity.* New York: Plenum.

Plomp, R., & Smoorenberg, G. F. (1970). *Periodicity Detection and Frequency Analysis in Hearing.* Leiden: Sijthoff.

Historical Background

Békésy, G. von (1960). *Experiments in hearing.* New York: McGraw-Hill.

Békésy, G. von (1967). *Sensory inhibition.* Princeton, NJ: Princeton University Press.

Helmholtz, H. L. F. von (1863). *Die Lehre von Tonemfindungen als Physiologie Grundlage für die Theorie der Musik.* Braunschweige: F. Vieweg und Sohn. (Translated as *On the sensations of tone as a physiological basis for the theory of music,* 4th ed., by A. J. Ellis. New York: Dover (reprint of 1897) edition).

Wever, E. G. (1949). *Theory of Hearing.* New York: Wiley.

Digital Signal Processing

Lynn, P. A., & Fuerst, W. (1989). *Introductory digital signal processing with computer applications.* New York: Wiley.

Chapter 11

Speech Recognition by Computer

Jared Bernstein, Horacio Franco

Chapter Outline

Key Terms

INTRODUCTION

When someone says a machine can recognize speech, it means the machine can take in a speech signal and produce a sequence of words that fairly represents what was said. In other words, a speech recognizer is a device that converts an acoustic signal into another form, like writing, to be stored or used in some way. This ability seems basic to a person who is highly literate, but you can get an appreciation for the difficulty of the task by attempting to transcribe or take dictation in a language that you do not know. Taking dictation in a new language requires that you learn the vocabulary and the pronunciation of the language. Getting good at this new skill requires a lot of practice hearing the language spoken. It helps to know what people are likely to talk about, how they express themselves, and what are the common constructions and idioms.

This same information must be learned by a machine if you expect it to recognize the words in a stream of spoken English. The machine must know some English words and how they are pronounced. Moreover, it will perform much more accurately if it has some information about common word sequences in English and how they are typically used in some domain of discourse. However, although computational methods for recognizing speech may now be sufficient to accomplish this task, the methods discussed in this chapter are probably not the best model for understanding speech perception or word recognition as performed by human listeners. Many human processes are demonstrably different; the human skills develop differently, they operate in a different context, they succeed in a different range of circumstances, and they fail in a different way.

The design and construction of systems that recognize speech are most often carried out by people trained in computer science or electrical engineering. Work is going on at many universities and at various commercial laboratories. In universities basic development is likely to take place in the department of computer science or electrical engineering, while new applications of speech recognition are developed in any department where someone sees a potential benefit. At

one university or another, linguists, psychologists, speech scientists, aerospace engineers, biologists, and medical specialists are all seeking new ways to apply speech recognition. The basic development efforts may involve the cooperative efforts of people trained in computers, mathematics, linguistics, speech science, and psychology.

The commercial efforts at speech recognition are generally found in small companies that specialize in speech technology and in the research and development laboratories of large companies involved with computers or telecommunication. For example, major efforts in speech recognition have been under way for more than 20 years at both IBM and AT&T. Until recently most of the work in these large laboratories has been focused on the core problem of getting a machine to identify the words in an acoustic stream. That capability improved significantly during the 1980s, and now these companies and others are building systems for the public that use speech recognition.

What are the current applications of speech recognition and what upcoming applications will justify the research investment by governments and industrial firms? We can briefly describe two current applications that suggest the limits and the promise of the technology: emergency medical reports and the handling of collect telephone calls. Future applications in education and in speech-language pathology and audiology will also be mentioned here and will be treated more fully at the end of the chapter.

CURRENT APPLICATIONS

An emergency room physician may see 36 patients in a 12-hour shift. Each patient's visit requires a report for the hospital and the insurer of the patient, and each report must include certain information. Many emergency room physicians dictate this information to a medical report system that uses speech recognition. The physician only speaks various phrases that fill in the blanks in a preset report template, and the process is faster and cheaper than conventional alternatives. Furthermore, the resulting reports

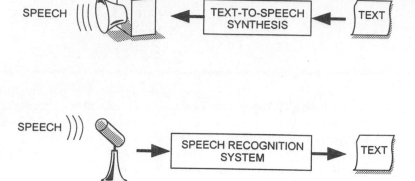

FIGURE 11-1   Text-to-speech synthesis and speech recognition shown as inverse processes.

are more satisfactory because they always include all the information that the various administrative channels need. The physician says the date and time of admission, date and time of injury, the nature of the injury and what treatment, if any, was administered or recommended. Of the many features of this scenario three are particularly significant: First, the speech to be recognized is not arbitrary. At certain points in the procedure the machine expects a date or an injury description or treatment, and these utterances will come in a fixed format. Second, the users of these machines are few, and they soon gain experience with it. They have been trained in medical school to describe injuries and treatments in a particular stylized format. Finally, the medical vocabulary itself is mostly polysyllabic and distinct and is therefore relatively easy to recognize. There are many well-formatted applications, like emergency room reports, whose vocabulary is known, and the user population is small and controlled. A more recent successful application accepts speech over the telephone.

Handling collect telephone calls has been a major activity for thousands of telephone operators. New systems at AT&T and other telephone companies handle the collect call transaction by computer. Callers are asked to say their names; the machine records the name as it is spoken and then puts the call through to the intended recipient. The person who answers the call at the receiving end hears the recording of the caller's name and is asked by the machine to say yes to accept the charges. A speech recognition system decides whether the recipient has said yes and then either puts the call through or rejects it.

FUTURE APPLICATIONS

There are many future applications of speech recognition in education, and speech-language pathology, and audiology. For example, imagine a machine that can teach spoken English to a recent immigrant who has only limited proficiency in English. Imagine a system that can automatically diagnose articulation disorders and measure progress during treatment. Imagine a system that can monitor and help a person who is learning to read or that engages students in a spoken dialogue in Spanish. Such a system is not like that found in a traditional language laboratory, where a student speaks onto tape; instead, the system hears whether the student's response is correct and judges how fluent the answer is and how well it was pronounced. All of these systems are now in operation in one laboratory or another.

Now, let us try to understand in more detail what speech recognition is and how it works. The potential and the limits of speech recognition for speech, hearing, and language research and treatment should be clearer if the nature of the technology is understood.

TECHNICAL OVERVIEW

Functional Description and Relation to Speech Synthesis

Take a closer look at the functional (external) behavior of a speech recognition device. It accepts acoustic signals as input and produces sequences of words as output. This is the inverse function of a text-to-speech synthesizer as described in Chapter 7. Figure 11-1 shows a text-to-speech synthesizer and a speech recog-

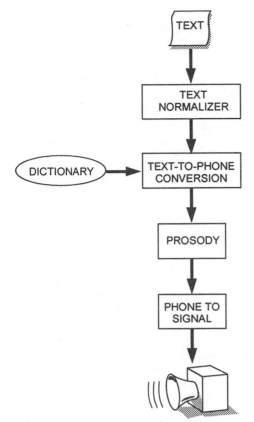

FIGURE 11-2   Component processes in text-to-speech synthesis.

forms such as abbreviations and monetary amounts. Then a phonological process takes the letter string that makes up each word and analyzes it into a sequence of phonemes. The phonological process of translating the spelled form of the word into a phoneme sequence is usually done by first looking for the whole word in a lexicon. If the whole word is not found, the process works by analyzing the word into morphological elements like a stem and affixes, which can be matched and transformed into phonemes and stress information.

This phonological process works with reference to a lexicon and a set of rules that look more or less like the kinds of rules and lexical forms proposed by linguists. After the prosody module constructs a rhythm and melody to impose on the phonemes in the sentence, the actual construction of the acoustic signal proceeds inside a speech synthesizer. The signal construction, however, is radically different from the coordinated muscular and aerodynamic processes in the vocal tract.

Internal Structure of Hidden Markov Model Speech Recognition

Figure 11-3 shows a schematic design of a speech recognition device. The acoustic signal is transduced by the microphone on the left and processed by the signal processor and search modules to the right until the best matching sequence of words is produced. Some stages of speech recognition may also be similar to simple models of human performance in similar tasks.

For example, the operation of a microphone and a frequency analyzer are somewhat similar to processes that occur in the auditory periphery. However, the methods used in speech recognizers to identify words and hypothesize sentences are probably fundamentally different from the corresponding processes in human listeners. The recognition system schematized in Figure 11-3 has two models, one of speech and the other of language. In the simple **hidden Markov model** (HMM) system that we will discuss below, the model of human speech acoustics is just the **spectrum** codebook— nothing more than a list of spectral shapes that are commonly found in speech signals. The language model in our example system is a small **finite state machine**—that is, a graph that describes exactly which words can start an utterance and which words can follow those words.

nizer in their simplest functional representation. The synthesis function is like a person reading aloud from a written text, and the recognition function is like a person taking dictation or transcribing a spoken message. If both systems worked perfectly, the operation of one could undo the operation of the other. That is, if a particular text were fed to a text-to-speech synthesis device and an ideal speech recognizer listened to the spoken output of the synthesizer, the recognizer would reproduce the original text.

The internal structures of the synthesis device and the recognition device may be very different. The typical text-to-speech synthesizer implements a series of processes that show some similarity to the processes discussed by linguists and psychologists when they are describing the structure and use of natural spoken languages. One simplified design for text-to-speech conversion is shown in Figure 11-2, with the text coming in at the top and a speech signal generated out the bottom. The first process normalizes the incoming text by expanding

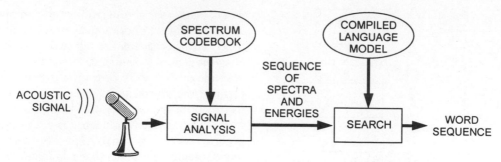

FIGURE 11-3   Component processes and static structures in speech recognition.

For each word the phones are given, and for each phone there is a list of spectral shapes that are likely to be realizations of it. The signal processor and search modules find the elements in these models that are the best match for the incoming acoustic signal. These operations are explained in the next section, which describes the design of a typical HMM-based speech recognition system.

Potential Intermediate Representations

In the schematic representation of speech synthesis shown in Figure 11-2 the text goes through many intermediate representations as it is converted to speech. As text is processed inside a text-to-speech converter, it takes several understandable forms that may be accessed for one use or another. For example, letters enter the text normalizer and words are produced. From these words morphemes and phonemes are produced by the text-to-phoneme conversion. The prosody module produces a specific intonation melody and an explicit rhythm to align with the words and phonemes.

The amount and kind of intermediate information normally calculated in the process of speech recognition is very different from the intermediate representations of a text-to-speech synthesis system. The only standard intermediate representation is the sequence of **spectra** produced by the signal processor, and then there is the final product, the best-matching word sequence. It takes significant engineering to allow most current recognition systems to produce a string of phonemes or a fundamental frequency pattern that is time-aligned with the words in a sentence. The search process, as explained below, is designed to find the optimum word sequence. Representations at other linguistic levels (e.g., the best matching sequence

of phones or morphemes) are not calculated as such. Thus, although recognition systems in principle can produce phonemic transcriptions, most systems are not designed so that this can be done easily or with optimum accuracy in isolation from the task of finding the best word sequence.

Task Types

Many types of tasks could be accomplished with a speech recognition device. From the acoustic signal, one could identify the speaker or the speaker's gender or the language being spoken or the speaker's physical condition or the speaker's skill in producing the language. In this chapter we focus on speech recognition, by which we mean the recognition of the words in the signal. Bear in mind that various systems may operate at different levels of complexity to accomplish tasks that could be identified as speech recognition. A system that accepts and answers spoken queries about commercial airline schedules and fares will have in it a *speech recognition system* as we have been using the term here, but it probably will also have many other component systems:

- A **syntactic parser** that assigns syntactic labels to words or phrases in the utterances.
- A semantic model of requests, times, flights, and destinations.
- A database of airlines, flights, times, aircraft, fares, and connections.
- A **user interface** that guides the user of the system and responds by graphic displays or by voice or both.

The focus in this chapter is on understanding just those processes involved in the extraction of word sequences from the acoustic signal. This single speech recognition function is essential in many larger system applications, and so far, speech recognition can be treated in isolation from the many other issues that affect its functioning in more complex systems. Furthermore, limiting the task domain should make the exposition of the technology simpler.

History from 1970 to 1990

You can better appreciate the strengths and limits of current speech recognition design if you know a bit of the history of speech recognition since 1970. There were some attempts at automatic speech recognition before 1970; the 12-page review of the field in Flanagan's comprehensive 1972 book, *Speech Analysis, Synthesis, and Perception* covers most of the significant work up to that time. Some systems used analog electronic circuits to recognize small vocabularies (like the English digits zero through nine in real time) and a few limited digital systems offered similar function (e.g., Reddy, 1967) but used digital computers.

Since 1970, speech recognition has advanced in two waves, both based on general pattern matching techniques and implemented in digital computers. First, there was the rise and decline of systems based on dynamic time warping (DTW); and second, there was the emergence and dominance of systems based on the HMM. A third major thread in the development of speech recognition during the 1970s and 1980s was the expert system based on speech and language insights. Although some systems based on expert knowledge of phonetics and linguistics could accurately recognize speech (Weinstein et al., 1975), most have not been as accurate, as fast, or as extensible as contemporaneous systems based on DTW or HMM algorithms. That is, systems based on more general approaches to optimizing the match between a signal and a preexisting pattern have consistently outperformed systems that seem more intuitive to the expert trained in linguistics or acoustic phonetics.

Typically, a DTW recognition system is designed to recognize isolated words spoken one at a time by a particular talker who has trained this DTW system by repeatedly speaking a fixed set of words to the system during a training session. DTW technology was developed and extended at AT&T Bell Labs during the 1970s (Itakura, 1975). DTW was the basis of most of the commercial speech recognition systems that were available during the late 1970s and early 1980s. A clear explanation of the internal operation of a DTW system can be found in Levinson and Liberman (1981).

Basically, a DTW system stores a separate template of each word in its vocabulary. The templates are based on example pronunciations that the system records during training sessions. The templates are sequences of acoustic spectra that represent the word. When a DTW system is recognizing, it captures each speechlike event in the incoming acoustic stream, reduces it to a sequence of spectra, and compares the sequence of incoming spectra with each word template by stretching and/or compressing the incoming spectral sequence to form a best match with each of the stored word templates. The incoming signal is identified with the word template that best matches the incoming signal. The dynamic programming technique used to map the incoming spectral sequence to the stored template is called *time warping*.

The limits of the classic DTW technique are that it is a **speaker dependent system** (each talker has to train the system), it is most suitable for recognizing isolated words or phrases, and it operates on each word as a unique template, so larger vocabularies have to be trained by having users say each word. Some of the limits of classic DTW recognition were overcome by the early 1980s. DTW techniques were extended to handle connected speech, and clustering methods were developed to allow accurate recognition in a **speaker independent system** for limited vocabularies. Furthermore, special-purpose computing elements supported DTW recognition of vocabularies of up to 1000 words by the mid-1980s.

However, the treatment of each word as a unique template makes the training of a DTW system extremely inefficient. Since the DTW technique recognizes no subword units like syllables or phonemes, word sets like {cable, table, fable, able, sable, label . . .} cannot share training material. Each word has to be trained separately by a population of speakers. Fortunately, an alternative method for representing words, HMM, has very efficient training methods and operates on words in terms of phoneme-sized units. Thus, with an HMM system, a fairly accurate speaker-independent model of a new word (for example, "chronic" [kranik]) can be constructed from material that was part of other words (like "crop", "crock", "Ronnie", "sonic", "nickel", and many others) that may be

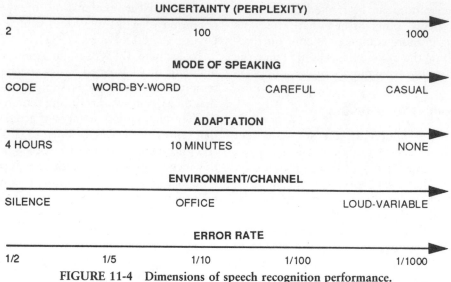

FIGURE 11-4 Dimensions of speech recognition performance.

part of a large speaker-independent training set covering the phonemes and common phoneme sequences of English.

Speech recognition systems based on hidden Markov models of words were first devised at IBM and Carnegie-Mellon University in the mid-1970s (Baker, 1975; Jelinek, 1976). By the early 1980s, it was shown that they could perform as well as DTW systems on those very tasks for which DTW had been optimized, and the long-term advantages of HMM techniques in large-vocabulary, speaker-independent systems were becoming clear. Thus, by the end of the 1980s, DTW systems had been generally supplanted by HMM systems, although DTW systems can operate very successfully in tasks for which a limited vocabulary like the digits is spoken by a limited number of speakers.

In a later section of this chapter, we describe an HMM-based speech recognition system without reference either to alternative techniques such as neural networks (Cohen et al., 1993) or to the possible integration of semantic and task-domain information into the recognition system design. As of 1995, almost all the high-performance experimental and commercial speech recognition systems share some of the major elements of the design that we describe in this chapter.

Performance Specification

Consider the concept of performance as it relates to speech recognizers. Just as with the

performance of a car, the performance of a speech recognizer has many aspects. Recognition systems are sometimes touted in terms of their accuracy. For example, many systems at various levels of complexity have been described as "99% accurate" in some task. This is vaguely similar to comparing automobiles in terms of top speed. The cars that have the highest top speed are often not the cars that most people want or need. A useful car typically offers some agreeable array of qualities including ease of operation, reliability, fuel economy, smooth ride, a quiet interior that seats five, and an affordable purchase price. The fastest racing cars are not suitable for general street use.

There are many dimensions along which speech recognizers vary. Five of these dimensions—perplexity, accuracy, adaptation, mode, and noise—are shown in Figure 11-4. **Perplexity** relates to the uncertainty of the task. If the possible distinct outcomes of the recognition are many, the perplexity is high, and if the recognition is only deciding between two possible options, the perplexity is low. The perplexity is like the effective or expected vocabulary size. **Error rate** in Figure 11-4 means raw accuracy, shown in the figure as average errors per number of words. **Adaptation** means how long the speaker has to use the system before it reaches its peak performance for that speaker—does it take 10 minutes or is it immediate? The *mode of speaking* is the manner in which the user is expected to speak. Is the form of input a code like {alpha, bravo, Charlie, delta . . .}, or is there a requirement to speak in an isolated word-by-word mode, or can the system recognize casual, continuous speech? The last dimension shown is *environment/channel*. Can the system operate in normal office noise, or does it require a very quiet acoustic environment? Is it immune to adverse noise conditions, and does it operate well in the loud and variable noise of a factory floor? Can it operate on speech signals over radio or telephone channels?

Notice that the right-hand ends of the arrows represent the desirable high-performance goal for speech recognition but that no recognition system, even a human listener, can operate at the right end of all the dimensions at once. People can simultaneously reach the right end of most of these dimensions, except for loud and variable noise. A current speech recognition system can achieve the right end of any one of the dimensions in Figure 11-4 by limiting the requirement on the other dimensions. Thus, for example, a system can achieve accuracies of just 1 error in 10,000 words if the active vocabulary is a set of three or four distinct words and if the system can adapt to (or train itself on) the speaker repeating those few words many times over several hours and the acoustic conditions are good. Similarly, we can design systems that will recognize any one of 20,000 or even 50,000 words if an error rate of 1 in 10 is acceptable and again if the speaker trains the system for several hours and the acoustic conditions are excellent.

We discussed two commercially viable applications of speech recognition: emergency room reports and collect call handling, at the beginning of the chapter. Where do these applications sit on the dimensions of Figure 11-4? The collect call handler requires the recognition of "yes" and "no" over the telephone from any person at any location. Phone company engineers say that a rejection rate of 1 in 10 is acceptable. Thus, the collect call handler is operating at the difficult end of the adaptation and mode dimensions; the machine has to deal with any unfamiliar person, and most people speak fairly casually in most circumstances. The noise and channel conditions are a challenge too, but the very low perplexity of the task—yes or no—and clever user interface design around the 1-in-10 rejection (the person just gets switched to a human operator) make the service a major commercial success.

The emergency room reporting system has quite a large overall vocabulary, but the speech recognition task is always constrained to be rather low perplexity in the way the system is used. Accuracies seem high (the emergency room physicians are satisfied with the accuracy), but only a small number of physicians use each system, and each is required to train the system for several hours before the system reaches its best performance. The physicians speak carefully and the noise environment is usually benign. In addition, the medical vocabulary is composed of fairly distinct polysyllabic words that also help the recognizer maintain adequate accuracy.

The Advanced Research Projects Agency (ARPA) has been the single largest U.S. government supporter of speech recognition development in the period between 1970 and 1990. Since about 1985 ARPA has been setting up a series of technology challenges that can be understood with reference to the dimensions of Figure 11-4. ARPA has focused mainly on speaker-independent recognition of sentence material read aloud in a normal fashion. This sets the adaptation to the right hand end of the arrow (no adaptation) and the speaking mode somewhere between careful and casual but certainly continuous. The sentence material has been taken from several sources (e.g., *The Wall Street Journal*), and the perplexity of the tasks has been held in the range between 50 and 100. For materials with an average sentence length of 10 words, a word perplexity of 50 implies that the recognition task is equivalent to a selection from among an equally probable set of 50^{10} different sentences; 50^{10} is about 100 quadrillion.

For readings recorded in a reasonable office environment, by 1993 the best laboratory systems had achieved speaker independent accuracies on *The Wall Street Journal* of about 1 error in 20 words. The ARPA challenge is to push upward on the error-rate and environment/channel dimensions, increasing accuracy in the presence of increasing levels of noise.

RECOGNITION SYSTEM DESIGN

This section discusses the operation of a complete but scaled-down version of an HMM speech recognition system, which we will call *Simple-HMM*. The system is missing several internal refinements that are needed for high accuracy; for example, it uses the technique *vector quantization* as an approximation of the spectrum estimation that is the first step in recognition. Furthermore, the system does not reject ill-formed input, nor does it "understand" the words that it recognizes, nor is there any provision for how the system may respond after it identifies what words have been said.

Assume that the Simple-HMM system has been trained, the spectrum codebook and language model as seen in Figure 11-4 are set, and the system is ready to process and recognize an incoming signal. The construction of the spectrum codebook and the language model from which the system works will be discussed in a later section.

This system can recognize which one of 81 possible sentences was spoken. More specifically, for each of the 81 possible word sequences specified in the grammar, the system will calculate how likely it is that the input signal is a realization of that word sequence. The word sequence that can account for the observed utterance with the greatest likelihood score is "recognized" to be the one spoken. Relevant parts of the system are illustrated and explained in turn as we progress through the example.

As shown in Figure 11-3, the Simple-HMM recognition system has two processes, the signal analysis and the search. The signal analysis takes an input signal and returns a sequence of spectra that more or less closely approximates the spectral shape of the input signal. The sequence of spectra is a greatly simplified representation of the original signal, yet if designed properly, this simplified representation is sufficient to identify words. The search process takes the sequence of spectra produced by the signal analysis and finds the path through the compiled language model that yields the word sequence with maximum probability for that spectrum sequence. The words traversed in that maximum-probability path are taken to be the recognized word sequence.

The next sections describe these processes and the related data structures in more detail. Much of the art of making an HMM system accurate, fast, and extensible is not included in the Simple-HMM, but the logic is essentially the same as in the best current recognition systems.

Signal Analysis

In the Simple-HMM system the first of the two recognition processes is signal analysis. In the first step of signal analysis an acoustic signal is converted to an electrical signal by a microphone. The microphone produces a voltage signal that varies as a function of time in a form that follows the acoustic pressure signal at the microphone. The next step is to convert this electrical signal into a **digital signal** so that it can be processed by a digital computer.

A digital signal is just a series of binary numbers. A small device called an analog-to-digital converter (ADC) replaces the electrical signal, which varies continuously over time, with a series of numbers that represent the amplitude of the original signal at fixed intervals. In a typical speech recognition system, the ADC samples the electrical signal 16,000 times per second, and the amplitude of the signal is represented by a 16-bit (or 16-place binary) number at each sample. Thus, the signal enters the computer in the form of numbers that require 256,000 (16 × 16,000) bits to represent each second of signal. These numbers are a very precise description of the speech, and if they are reconverted into an **analog signal,** amplified, and played back through a loudspeaker, they can sound nearly indistinguishable from the original acoustic signal.

Following the operation of the ADC, the signal is available for processing inside the computer. Inside the computer, the first process is *signal analysis.* The main purpose of the signal analysis is to reduce this flood of information (256,000 bits per second) into a more manageable form that still retains most of the important linguistic information. In the Simple-HMM system, the output of the signal analysis process is a much simpler stream of information: just two 3-bit numbers, 50 times per second. This is only 300 bits per second. A 3-bit number can have any of eight values, in this case zero through seven.

Figure 11-5 shows a waveform of the word [san] pronounced like the first three segments in the English word "sonic." The 1-second waveform displayed at the top of the figure is represented in the computer as 16,000 16-bit samples. A spectrogram of the same signal is displayed below it for reference, and the output of the coarse-grain signal analysis in the Simple-HMM is shown at the bottom.

The key operation in the Simple-HMM signal analysis is *vector quantization.* Vector quantization in this context is the process that approximates the continuously changing spectral shape of the signal by a sequence of spectral types (Gray, 1984; Furui, 1989). In the Simple-HMM

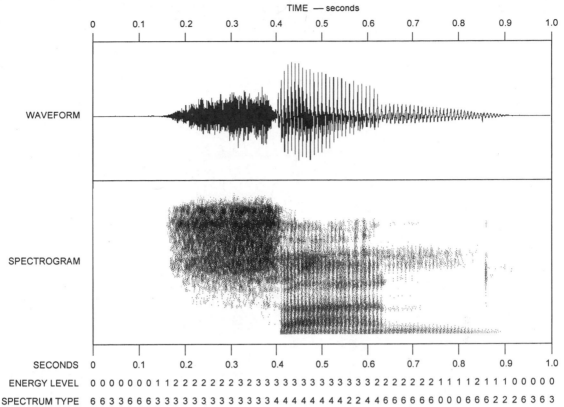

FIGURE 11-5   Waveform, spectrogram, and 20 msec frame parameters of a 1 sec signal of "san".

system, the signal is approximated by one of eight spectrum types every 20 ms, or 50 times per second.

In operation, the signal analysis process produces a spectral type for every 20 ms of incoming signal. First, the actual spectral envelope of the 20-ms speech signal is determined by calculating a **discrete Fourier transform** of the digital signal in that region. The signal analysis process then finds the spectrum type from among the set in the spectrum codebook that is most similar to the actual calculated spectrum. From this point forward everything in the Simple-HMM recognition process is done with reference to the energy level and spectrum type, as quantized by the signal analysis process. The signal analysis has reduced the intricate detail in the 1-second signal that entered the system to 50 pairs of 3-bit numbers per second.

Thus, the search process of the Simple-HMM ignores everything about the speech signal except this sequence of 50 pairs of derived 3-bit numbers. The energy level is a number that corresponds to a coarse linear quantization of the energy level in the digital signal. The spectrum type, however, is a vector quantization of the original spectrum. The Simple-HMM reduces all the infinitely subtle differences in sound quality and timbre into exactly eight different types. No matter what the spectrum of the incoming sound, the signal analysis classifies it as one of eight distinct types and sends that type identifier across to the search process. The subsequent search through the compiled language model operates with reference solely to this string of number-pairs (an energy level and a spectrum type), which encodes all the information about the original speech that the system will use. The spectrum types encode the actual spectra found in the incoming signal, and the set of available types is a *codebook*. The spectrum types are sometimes called *code words* (Figure 11-6).

Before running the system, we establish a set of spectra generally representative of the kinds of spectra observed in acoustic signals containing speech. (An algorithm for deriving a **vector codebook** is presented in a later section.) Although a typical speech recognition system might use a set of 256 spectra to approximate

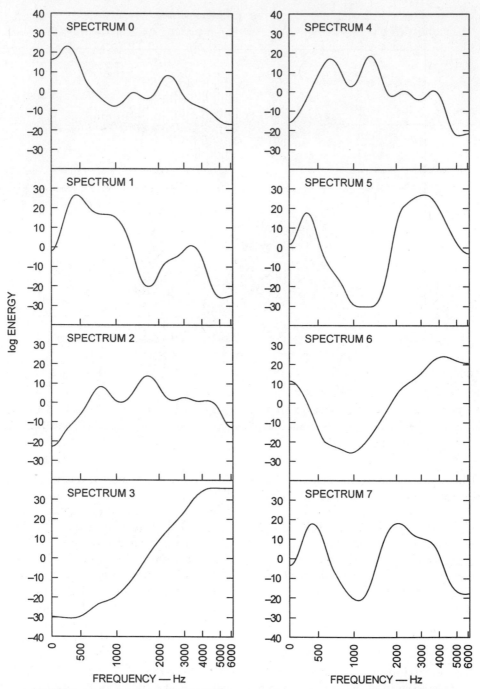

FIGURE 11-6   The set of eight different spectrum types used in Simple IIMM.

the speech signal, for the Simple-HMM system we derived a set of eight spectrum types, or vectors. These spectrum types are shown in Figure 11-6. Take time to verify that the spectrum types displayed in Figure 11-6 match the visible spectral properties of the speech signal displayed over time in Figure 11-5. In the middle of the [s] (the region around time 0.3 seconds), the best matching spectrum type is spectrum 3, which indeed has its predominant

energy in the high frequencies above 3000 Hz. The middle of the [a] (the region around time 0.55 seconds) yields spectrum types 2 and 4, which have energy concentrations (resonances) in the frequency range between 500 and 1500 Hz. The signal analysis matches the middle of the nasal (the region around time 0.75 seconds) to spectrum types 6 and 0, which have energy concentrated below 500 Hz and above 2000 Hz.

In high-performance HMM-based speech

recognition systems developed through 1990, the signal analysis process generally operated in the manner outlined above, except that the signal analysis produced four or six numbers 100 times per second (a 10-ms frame update), and the numbers represented a finer quantization of the incoming signal than those used in the Simple-HMM. The codebook of spectrum types typically had 256 members, and the energy levels were quantized to 32 levels. In recent high performance systems, the signal analysis modules also produce a delta energy and a **delta spectrum** for each frame of speech data. These delta parameters are derived by calculating the difference in energy or the difference in spectral shape between the current frame of the speech signal and a previous frame, usually two or three frames back. The delta parameters represent the rate and direction of change in the signal. For example, the delta parameters may indicate that the energy in the signal is increasing rapidly, although the spectral shape is changing only slightly toward a spectrum with more energy in the high frequencies. Lee (1989), Cohen et al. (1990), and Woodland et al. (1994) provide more details on the parameters of more recent high-performance systems.

Searching the Compiled Language Model

Signal analysis, the first major module of the recognition system, reduces the incoming signal to manageable dimensions, but the essential elements of HMM will become apparent only when the search through the compiled language model is understood.

To understand the search, it is necessary to understand the compiled language model and the way a sequence of number pairs produced by the signal analysis process yields a probability score for each path in the language model. The path with the best score is taken to be the system's best guess as to what words were in the signal. Some very efficient computational methods, like the Viterbi algorithm (Rabiner, 1989), find the best-scoring path.

The Compiled Language Model

A compiled language model, the central element in an HMM speech recognizer, contains the definition of the task that the recognizer is trying to solve. It specifies the grammar of the utterances that can be recognized as well as the words

and where they can fit in the grammar. It also specifies the pronunciation of the words and the acoustic events that are likely to be observed when these pronunciations are produced. That is, the language model is built as a series of structures embedded within larger structures. Figures 11-7 and 11-8 illustrate this concept. Figure 11-7 displays the outer four layers of the structure of the language model of the Simple-HMM recognizer, and Figure 11-8 shows the innermost three layers of a model for the syllable [sán] as in "sonic." The compiled language model *is* the hidden Markov model.

But what is *hidden* about a hidden Markov model? In concise form, the hidden Markov model is a multiply embedded probabilistic model of the language that is to be recognized by the device. The language model is a network of states and transitions between states in which each transition between states has a probability of occurring; thus, it is a **Markov model**. Simple-HMM has a sentence network that expands as the word-class models, word models, and phone models (as in Figure 11-7) are embedded. The innermost states of the Markov language model are subphone units (for example, the beginning of [a] or the middle state of [s]) that are not directly observable in the signal but have only a probabilistic relation to the observed signal parameters that are produced by the signal analysis. Thus, it is a *hidden* Markov model; the states are not directly observed but are inferred with more or less likelihood, depending on the sequence of signal analysis parameters that *are* directly observed.

At its heart, Simple-HMM assumes that words are composed of sequences of linguistic segments (like phonemes) and that each segment can be represented by a simple statistical model. Thus, the sentence "Sam went in" has three words, and the words have three, four, and two segments, respectively. Each segment, for example the /m/ in "Sam", is represented as a probability distribution reflecting the likelihood that various spectral shapes will be observed when the particular segment is pronounced.

The frequency spectra typical of various speech sounds are different: an [s] usually has much more energy higher in the frequency spectrum, and an /m/ usually has little high-frequency energy but more low-frequency energy. Thus, the HMM system represents the [m] as very likely to be observed with frequency spectra that have predominantly low-frequency energy, while the HMM system will expect to

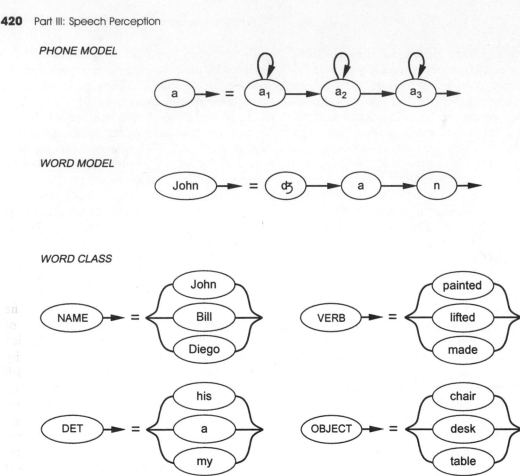

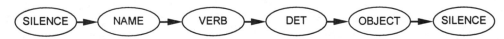

FIGURE 11-7 Embedded network elements for Simple HMM.

observe spectra with more high-frequency energy when an [s] is spoken.

The compiled language model of Figure 11-3 is disassembled in Figures 11-7 and 11-8. Consider it closely. The model has a grammar (shown at the bottom of Figure 11-7) that expects and accepts exactly one type of sentence: a name, followed by a verb, followed by a determiner, followed by an object. The whole sentence starts and ends in silence.

The name in the sentence can be any one of the three forms "John", "Bill", or "Diego". The verb must be one of the forms "painted", "lifted", or "made". Each word expands into a sequence of phones, as suggested by the word model for "John". "John" is exactly a directional network of three phones, and each phone

(e.g. [a]) is further represented as a sequence of subphone states in sequence. If we make some assumptions about how the words are pronounced and assign one phone per phoneme and three subphone states per phone, we can see that this simple grammar has about 126 states when fully expanded to its implicit subphone states.

What is a state? A state represents a phonetic subsegment like the beginning of [k] or the middle of [s]. In the computer the states are nothing more than tables that say how likely we are to observe a particular spectrum type or energy level when the **frame** in question is counted as being in that state. Figure 11-8 shows the probability distributions associated with the states in the phones [s], [a], and [n]. Only the probability distributions of the spectrum types

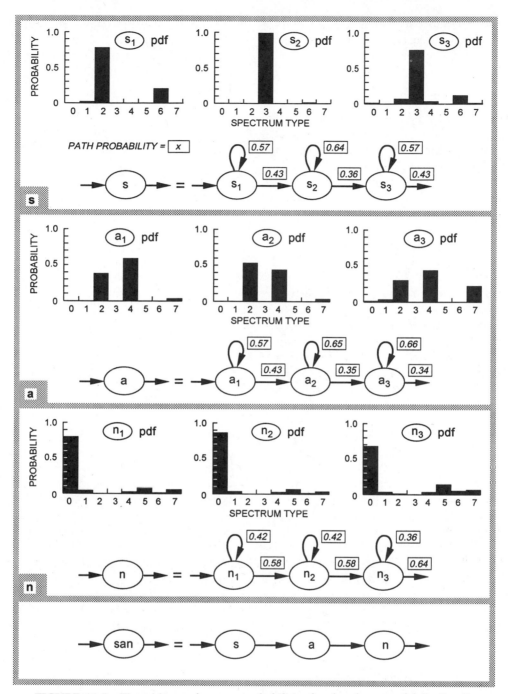

FIGURE 11-8 Transition and output probabilities for the phone models in "san".

are shown; those representing the relative likelihood of energy levels are not shown in Figure 11-8.

Note that the state structure is the same for all the phones: there is a sequence of three subphone states, each of which can loop back to itself or can pass to the next state. However, the probabilities associated with the various states like subphone s_1 or a_2 or n_3 are quite different.

So, for example, if the signal analysis identifies a frame as spectrum type 4, the probability density function (pdf) of a_1 suggests that the frame may well be part of an [a] but is not likely to be part of an [s] or an [n].

These pdfs (inside subphone states, inside phones, inside words, inside grammars) define how information about the speech signal is related to sound segments and therefore to words and therefore to sentences and therefore to the meanings that are conveyed, or at least intended, by the spoken utterance.

The Search

Figures 11-7 and 11-8 show what the language model is, but how does the machine decide which word sequence was said? We can take an example and work it through partially. Consider the signal shown in Figure 11-5. The sequence of 51 energy levels and spectrum types derived from it by the signal analysis are displayed at the bottom of the figure. To keep things simple and consistent with the simplification depicted in Figure 11-8, we will work only with the sequence of spectrum types, ignoring the information given in the sequence of energy levels.

Imagine that the signal that we are trying to recognize is the 1-second utterance shown in Figure 11-5 and that we are attempting to decide whether it is an example of the word "san" or "nap" or "and" or "snap". Each of these words has an utterance grammar consisting of (silence, <word>, silence), with the <word> part of the grammar expandable, much as the word "san" is expanded in Figure 11-8. Each utterance grammar starts with the same optional silence, but the words start with one of the four two-sound sequences [sa], [na], [an], [sn]. If the silence model common to all four utterance models has accounted for those first seven frames that have 0-level energy, we can start to decode the utterance at the eighth frame, where the energy level is 1 and the sequence of spectrum types begins a string of 13 consecutive 3s. If the final silence model takes care of the last five frames of the signal that have 0-level energy, we have 39 frames of speech signal for which we wish to find the best matching utterance model. Our task is to get the optimal state sequence for the observed sequence of frames. Figure 11-8 shows the state-to-state transition probabilities and the spectrum type probabilities for each of three phones: [s], [a], [n].

For the [s] model, the 13 consecutive 3s pass through the model with the highest probability by associating the first 3-type frame with the s_1 state, the next eleven 3s with the s_2 state, and the last of the 13 consecutive 3-type frames with the s_3 state. The probability of this sequence of 13 frames being from the the [s] model is then simply the product of probabilities of these

frames in these states, times the appropriate transition probabilities.

Assigning a minimum probability of 0.01 for spectral types that have no bar at all in a state's pdf, we could calculate probability for the best path through [s] for the 13 3s as

$$(.01 \times .43 \times (.98 \times .64)^{11}$$
$$\times .36 \times .78 \times .43) = 0.0000048$$

This 0.0000048 is a small number, but the probability of that sequence of 3s is much smaller for the other models or for the other possible paths through the [s] model. The pdf graphs in Figure 11-8 show that the probability of observing a spectrum type 3 appears to be zero for all three states of [a] and [n]. Thus, assigning 0.01 as the state probability of the 13 consecutive 3s being an [a] or an [n], we can calculate the probability for the 13 3s in the [a] model as

$$(.01 \times .43 \times .01 \times .35 \times$$
$$(.01 \times .66)^{10} \times .01 \times .34)$$
$$= 0.0000000000000000000000000000000080$$

which is really a very small number. It is important to understand that there are many different paths through these 3-state models, and these calculations are only the ones that generate the highest-probability paths for this data. Given the input sequence of spectrum types, every state sequence has a probability associated with it. From all the possible state sequences allowed by the model, the one with the highest probability is chosen. This may, in principle, be accomplished by exhaustive search. However, an exhaustive search is impractical, and the Viterbi algorithm (Rabiner, 1989) produces the optimal path without computing the probability associated with each particular path.

Methods and Materials for Training

When you build a speech recognition system, you have to select the structure of the compiled language model and then train the acoustic models that define the innermost states of the network that defines that model. In building a successful HMM-based recognition system, much of the subtle engineering art is involved in the construction and training of the language model. The language model and training method used for our Simple-HMM follow common practice from about 1990. Recently, several groups have described more subtle methods for extracting the most appropriate statistical models from a given body of **training data** for a specific task (see for example Young, Woodland, and Byrne, 1993; Woodland et al, 1994.) The following sections on vector codebook selection and acoustic model training describe methods that are relatively simple yet adequate to build useful recognition systems.

Vector Codebook Selection

Codebook training is the process by which we choose the set of spectral types used to characterize the speech signal. Large vocabulary, speaker-independent recognition systems are typically trained on databases of several thousand sentences, although a codebook of spectral types can be trained from a much smaller sample of utterances. The set of spectral types (or code words) is usually selected by the procedure *k-means,* which consists of the following steps:

1. Compute the mean or average of all the speech spectra in the training data set; this is the initial spectral type.
2. Perturb each spectral type by adding some small random values to its components and generate two spectral types from each.
3. Classify the speech training data into clusters by measuring the distance from each speech spectrum to each spectral type and then assigning the speech spectrum to the closest spectral type.
4. For each cluster compute the mean of all the spectra belonging to it and define this as the new spectral type.

Steps 3 and 4 are iterated until the spectral types do not change between successive iterations. The resulting set of spectral prototypes is a codebook of size 2. From the set of two spectral prototypes it is possible to obtain codebooks with more elements (4, 8, etc.) by repeating step 2, which gives us a new initial set of spectral types of twice the size of the previous set, and then iterating steps 3 and 4 for each new set of spectral types.

The underlying mathematical theory of this method shows that the spectral types incrementally move from their initial positions to an optimal position such that it minimizes the average distance between each member of the set of training speech spectra and the nearest member of the set of spectral types. That is, this procedure produces a set of spectra that in aggregate are the closest possible match to the speech in the training data set.

In this way, if we want a small set of spectral types for our Simple-HMM system, we find, for example, the set of eight spectra that as a group best matches the many spectra observed in speech. For a long sample of speech, this procedure yields the eight spectral types shown in Figure 11-6.

Acoustic Model Training

Training of the HMM models is the process that yields the values of the parameters of the phone models. That is, it yields the probability parameters for each state of each phone model and the values of the transition probabilities between the states of the model with reference to a criterion. The criterion is to choose the parameters of each phone model so that they represent the corresponding speech segments with the highest likelihood of match.

But how exactly do we train **continuous speech** models with continuous speech data? Consider the probability distributions associated with one state of a phone model (e.g., the middle state of an [a]). Each probability entry associated with a given spectral type (or code word) should be as close as possible to the actual rate of the occurrences of spectral type as observed over all the speech segments that should be associated with the state (e.g. $[a_2]$).

Imagine a large corpus of vector-quantized speech segmented into phones and subphone states (beginning, middle, final). We could count the occurrences of each code word in all the segments associated with a state and then simply divide them by the total number of collected code words in those states. If the corpus is very large, this procedure will yield a good estimate of the probabilities for each spectrum type (code word) for each state. This is the *estimation step.*

On the other hand, if we had trained models for each phone, we could segment each training sentence into states. To do so, we would only have to know the word sequence or orthographic transcription of each training sentence. This could be done in two steps: first, we build a *sentence HMM* that represents each sentence by concatenating the corresponding word models so that the final state of each word has a transition to the first state of the following word. Each word model is formed in turn by a concatenation (with possible alternative branches) of phone models, each of which is formed by a concatenation of subphone states. Second, we use the Viterbi algorithm to compute the best possible segmentation into states for each sentence, using as input both the quantized speech data and the sentence model just built from the transcription. This is the *segmentation step*.

Now we face a problem. If we had the speech segmented, we could obtain good models, but to get the segmentation, we need the models first. This problem can be solved by iteratively applying the segmentation and estimation steps outlined above. We start the procedure with some small database that has been segmented by hand. From this we obtain an initial set of *seed models*. We use these seed models to derive an approximate segmentation of the large unsegmented database, as described above in the segmentation step. After that we reestimate the model parameters from the new approximate segmentations. The theory shows that when these two steps are iterated, the models improve and provide a better match at each iteration. The iteration is stopped when no significant further improvement is found.

Characteristics of HMM Training for Continuous Speech

Consider some characteristics of HMM training:
- The training process imposes the linguistic structure on the speech data at a high level. By constructing a *sentence HMM* for each training sentence, we impose the word sequence, the allowed pronunciations for each word, and the sequence of subphonetic segments within each word.
- The fine details of the segmentation of the speech data into words and phone units are left to the training algorithm, which solves them iteratively so as to maximize the match of the models to the data across the set of training sentences.
- To start, or bootstrap, the training iteration we need a set of coarse models, called *seed models*. These seed models can readily be obtained from a small database of speech that has been hand-labeled and segmented.
- The full training database is just a set of recorded sentences with associated orthography. No information on where the different words start or end is needed, nor any phonetic transcription. This is a very important factor because the hand segmentation of a large database is an extremely expensive task that is difficult to accomplish accurately and consistently.
- To generate the sentence HMM mentioned above for each training sentence, it is necessary to have a dictionary, or lexicon, of pronunciations for the words in the relevant vocabulary. This dictionary tells us which sequence of phones (along with possible alternatives) corresponds to the pronunciation of each word. Compiling a good pronunciation dictionary can be easy or difficult, depending on the language. For example, it is very difficult to generate the pronunciations from the spelling of English words, while in Spanish it is a trivial task.

Evaluation

A speech recognizer should be evaluated with reference to a task. Depending on what is expected, what is valuable, and what is catastrophic in the task context, we can design a reasonable test to measure performance and propose a useful set of numerical measures to report from the test. In various task contexts a person might require the recognizer to align phone-length segments, return the best matching word string, find a particular database record, or present the best graphic or voice response. A good place to start understanding how speech recognition systems are evaluated is to review the evaluations conducted in the ARPA program and the databases developed for these evaluations (Price et al., 1988; Pallett et al., 1994).

APPLICATIONS

There are now many applications of speech recognition, and we expect that in the future the applications will be as widespread as they are for other types of actuators, controls, and data entry devices. Knobs, pushbuttons, switches, levers, keys, and pedals are found on innumerable devices around us. Because it is often used as a surrogate linguistic modality, the keyboard will be largely replaced through the application of speech recognition technology. In this section we will mention some commercial applications of speech technology and then discuss one particular educational application in some detail. Many aspects of other applications can be understood within the framework outlined below for the use of speech recognition in language education.

Commercial

The commercial uses of speech recognition started in the 1980s, when systems were installed on a trial basis in factories and other industrial settings where some operators have their hands and eyes busy. Hands-busy and eyes-busy preclude the convenient use of keyboards or even pen and paper as a way of recording information or routing items. More recently, the key area of activity has been in telecommunications. If speech input and output can be handled automatically, it should accomplish two things simultaneously: First, some proportion of the people who have been working the customer service phones will be freed to do other work. Second, every telephone will begin to work like a computer terminal. We will be able to record and retrieve many kinds of information, and we should soon be able to search files for information, skim and sort information, and generally interact with most local and remote services by voice directly to machines. Imagine ordering tickets and merchandise, asking for reference help at the library, getting bus and weather information by asking for it directly from a computer database over the phone. The next logical step is the replacement of the keyboards in the general entry of text. Automated voice dictation systems are now beginning to enter the general computer market, and they will see wide use when their accuracy is sufficient.

Educational

In education there has been a vision for some time that speech recognition, or at least speech processing, would open the talking world to hearing-impaired people. This dream has been pursued with great energy at several laboratories. Some work has focused on circumventing the hearing loss itself through the design of prosthetic receptors, and some research focused on speech training. A broad view of the history of technological aids for hearing-impaired people is provided in the book *Sensory Aids for the Hearing Impaired* (Levitt, Pickett, and

Houde, 1980; see also Bernstein, 1986a). More recently, there have been several very promising initiatives based on digital speech recognition equipment for use with people who have cerebral palsy (Carlson and Bernstein, 1988) and deaf people. Projects for teaching speech to deaf children and adults also have turned to speech recognition technology (Watson and Kewley-Port, 1989; Javkin et al., 1993; Uchanski et al., 1994). Stevens and Bernstein (1986) demonstrated that speech recognition systems could be used as telephone relay services are now used.

One long-term goal that is important for people with a hearing impairment is the real-time automatic captioner, a portable device that would display the text equivalent of any conversation. This hypothetical real-time, automatic captioner will come into reality at about the same time that large-vocabulary dictation systems reach significant commercial success (Bernstein, 1986b, 1989).

In the next subsection we outline some of the issues that suggest a large, near-term payoff in using speech recognition in language education. The subsequent discussion is based in part on the technical results presented in Bernstein et al. (1990) and Bernstein and Rtischev (1991); see also Watson et al. (1989).

Components of Foreign Language Competence

We will identify four components of language competence: reading, writing, listening, and speaking. Each of these competence components has aspects of skill that range from subtle and conceptual through conventionally linguistic to mechanical. For example, in reading, recognizing the political slant of a text is a subtle conceptual skill; recognizing the proper attachment of a clause is a linguistic skill; and recognizing the characters themselves (e.g., the Japanese kanji) is a mechanical skill. Similarly, in speaking, responding appropriately to a rude question is a subtle conceptual skill, using the right forms of address with their verbs is a linguistic skill, and pronouncing the words like a native is a mechanical skill.

In general, skills closest to the subtle and conceptual end of the continuum will require a native or near-native human teacher for some time to come, because many of the subtle aspects of language are still not understood or codified. Even some basic aspects of standard English syntax are not yet well described, certainly not understood well enough to be programmed into a computer. A computer can teach and test mechanical skills, but it also can present material that exemplifies some subtleties and check a student's recognition of them.

Live Instruction

TUTOR A skilled native tutor who has access to good multimedia materials and who can give individual attention to a student is the best method for teaching a language. If the tutor is energetic and encouraging and has a fine sense of the subtle aspects of the language, the situation should be ideal. Such teaching should be sensitive and flexible, with the only remaining issues the cost, availability, and patience of the tutor. The constraints of cost and availability, however, lead to the common practice of having classes with several students (or dozens) per teacher and having students taught by several different teachers during an instructional cycle.

CLASSROOM For listening to good examples of language spoken in a meaningful context, the classroom is nearly as good as the tutor. But for practice of productive skills like writing and speaking, the teacher can only spot-check student work as a task rotates around the room or check the work off-line when time allows. If the students speak in unison in class, the teacher can focus on one at a time or can have the students take turns with an exercise. For written work, it is more common that the students write one day and get feedback the next day. This feedback can be over the range of subtle, linguistic, and mechanical skills, but it will be delayed. With more than one student, the teacher is still limited to one-at-a-time serial processing. On the other hand, for the time being, only a teacher, like a tutor, can ask open-ended questions and deal appropriately with unpredictable answers. Machines are still generally limited to interactive formats that take a fixed response.

To use computers directly to provide instruction in spoken language skills, we need system functions that can recognize what has been said, when it was said, and how well it was said. These functions and their limits are explained and illustrated in the next section.

The uses of speech recognition in language education are determined in part by the charac-

teristics of the technology itself. We now understand how speech recognition works in general, and we need to see how it can be used specifically in language education. However, bear in mind that teachers and lesson designers do not need to be familiar with the internal details of a speech recognition system to use this technology. These functions can be used for instructional or testing purposes through a lesson editor or an authoring tool.

Language Education

In general, when a person interacts with another in a spoken language, several aspects of the person's speech provide information about the person's level of skill in the language. For example, when presented with a question, can the person give a correct answer? How long does it take to come up with an answer, and how fluently is the answer produced? How well is the answer pronounced? Consider both prosodic and segmental aspects of pronunciation. Do the rhythm and melody of the sentence sound native? Is each word formed correctly with each sound produced in the manner that natives produce it?

All of these questions can be answered by the speech recognition technology used in teaching systems and in systems for automatic scoring of pronunciation. When appropriately modified, speech recognition systems can handle speech from nonnative speakers and can determine the following:
- Which answer was spoken in response to a question
- How quickly it was produced
- How well it was pronounced

We will explain how a computer can do these things with particular reference to the scoring of segmental pronunciation. First, remember how an incoming utterance is recognized as one response selected from among a set of hypothesized possible responses in a compiled language model. Think about what it would mean to align an incoming signal with linguistic models and how pronunciation can be scored in a way that is similar to human scoring.

An implementation of an HMM speech recognition system for language education is shown schematically in Figure 11-9. Three primary processing modules, a spectrum analyzer, a search aligner, and a scorer, operate in series. The search aligner is the core process that

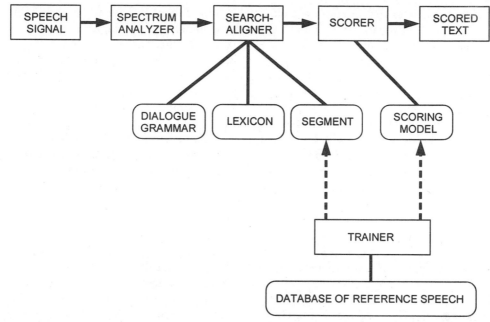

FIGURE 11-9 Schematic of a speech recognition system augmented for scoring speech quality.

decides at any given position in the dialogue grammar which of the permitted utterances was spoken and locates the words and segments in that utterance. To accomplish this, the search aligner makes reference to the dialogue grammar, the lexicon of the language, and the segment models.

In particular, the dialogue grammar specifies what sentences are expected or permitted at any particular point in the exchange between the student and the machine. It tells the search aligner what to look for. For example, check the next incoming utterance to find out which if any of a specified set of four sentences was spoken. The sentences in the dialogue grammar are listed in ordinary spellings, so the search aligner must check the lexicon to find the pronunciation of the words. The pronunciations of the words are listed in the lexicon as sequences of segments, and for each possible segment type there is a segment model that stores the likelihood of various spectral shapes, given that a particular segment type (e.g., /m/) was spoken.

When an utterance is spoken, the first step is to analyze the acoustic signal into a sequence of spectra. In this process a short sentence like "Sam went in" might be translated into a sequence of about 100 frequency spectra, or one spectrum for each hundredth of a second of incoming signal. The search aligner takes the spectra as input and selects the particular word-string hypothesis that best accounts for the spectra. If the system is asked to choose which one of two sentences (e.g., "In went Sam" and "Sam went in") was said, the system calculates how likely this particular sequence of spectra would be on the hypothesis of a segment sequence {samwentin} and on the alternative hypothesis of a segment sequence {inwentsam}.

The trainer is shown near the bottom of Figure 11-9. The trainer builds accurate segment models by processing a large database of spoken material. It uses actual pronunciations of the segments in the language to estimate the segment models and the scoring models referred to during the search aligner and scorer processes. The trainer is a development tool used by speech scientists and engineers in the design and preparation of the speech recognition system; it has already done its work before the first student ever speaks to the system. Some allowances must be made for the pronunciation of nonnatives, but the calculation of relative likelihood for the competing utterances that are possible according to the dialogue grammar is the basic method that answers the first question, "What answer did the person give?"

One more calculation has to be added to the method in order for the machine to interact with the student in a reasonable way: the system must reject spoken utterances that are not even close in form to any of the answers anticipated by the dialogue grammar. For example, if the system's dialogue grammar is designed to select material according to the student's last spoken response, simply calculating which sentence was closest to the incoming utterance is not enough. If the student says any random sentence like "Get me a soda while you're up," it will be closest acoustically to some one response sentence that is available at this point in the instructional dialogue. There has to be a rejection threshold such that if the incoming utterance from the student is a very unlikely match to all the available response sentences, the system can take it out of the discourse stream and still prompt and listen for the next contextually meaningful response.

Because, in general, computers can accurately track the time of various events, it is easy to calculate the promptness of the response to a particular spoken question or graphic display. Thus, the content accuracy and latency of a student's spoken responses can be measured by a computer with speech recognition capability.

Pronunciation Scoring

The challenge that remains is to score the pronunciation of the utterance. A particular utterance may be much more likely to be an instance of the word string "Uruguay está al sur de Brasil" than it is to be "Argentina está al este de Uruguay," yet the utterance may not be well pronounced at all. If it is too far off the mark, it will be rejected, but even if it is above the threshold of rejection, there may be quite a range of pronunciations observed in the speech of non-natives. The remainder of this section outlines the methods for determining how well an utterance was produced.

Alignment

Fundamentally, the method for scoring pronunciation is to align the speech and then score the various words and segments. As part of the speech recognition process, a search assigns each spectrum in the sequence of incoming speech spectra to a particular segment of a particular word. For each active sentence, the recognizer search produces two things: a likelihood score for that sentence and an alignment of the words and segments to the sequence of spectra. If a

likelihood score is above the rejection threshold, the sentence with the highest likelihood score is taken to be the sentence spoken, and its optimal alignment of the spectra and the linguistic units is taken to be the correct alignment of the sentence.

At this point the language education system has a good estimate of the location of every significant event in the speech signal. The system knows when the utterance starts and stops; it knows whether there are any internal pauses and how long they are; it knows the location and duration of every word and every segment of every word in the sentence about as well as an expert phonetician could know by ear and by examination of a speech spectrogram. This ability to align the speech—even the speech of beginning students—is a key to the operation of speech recognition in language education. Now that the system can find all the relevant events in the signal, it remains to score the prosodic and segmental aspects of the utterance.

Training Prosodic and Segmental Scorers

When expert human listeners hear a nonnative speaker of a language, they can judge the relative merit of several aspects of the pronunciation. Among the most salient aspects of pronunciation quality are the prosodics (rhythm and melody) and the segmentals (articulation of phones). Figure 11-10 presents a general procedure for the development and validation of automatic methods of pronunciation scoring. This procedure can be applied to scoring either prosodic or segmental aspects of pronunciation.

First, it must be understood that HMM-based speech recognition systems are developed with reference to large bodies of recorded speech used to train the segment models so that they accurately represent the distribution of spectral shapes observed in real speech. A similar process is needed to develop the scoring function. The first requirement is shown in the upper left panel of Figure 11-10: one has to collect a substantial sample of speech signals of nonnative speakers. The upper left panel of Figure 11-10 shows a portion of the time-amplitude waveform of a nonnative speaker's production of the English sentence "Mike's father owns that store."

In the development process that continues down the left side of Figure 11-10, the spectrum analyzer uses digital signal processing (DSP) techniques to derive a sequence of spectra

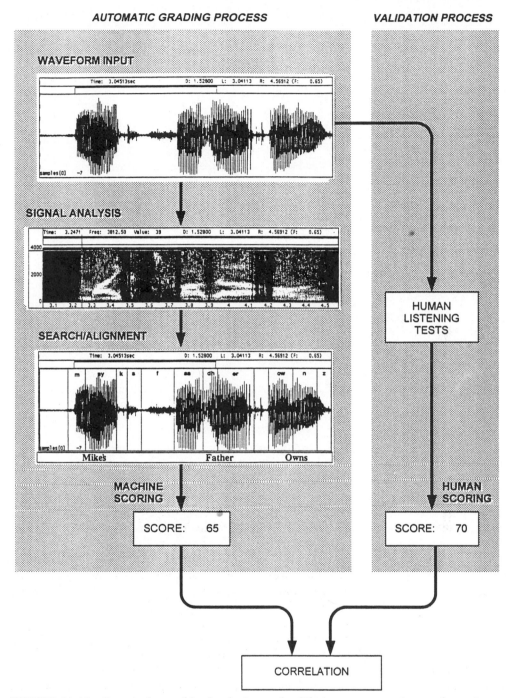

FIGURE 11-10   Data paths used in developing and validating an automatic speech scoring system.

shown as a speech spectrogram in the next panel down on the left side. The search-aligner then locates the words and their component segments in the sentence. A signal alignment for the first three words of the sentence is shown in the next lower panel on the left side of the figure. Finally, a set of algorithms calculates a set of scores for various aspects of the speech signals in the database of nonnative productions. Figure 11-10 shows a single aggregate score produced by both machine and human scoring.

General validation of this method and the further development of the component algorithms depend on the parallel process shown on the right side of Figure 11-10. The same database of nonnative utterances is played to

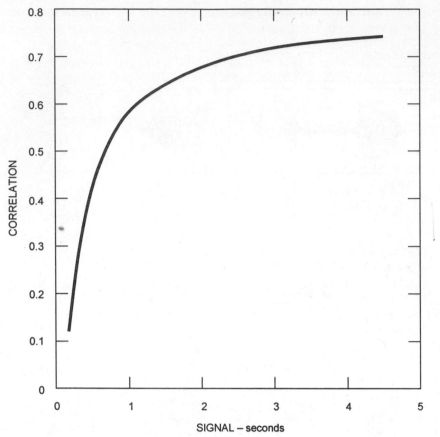

FIGURE 11-11   Correlation between ASR-based scores and human listener scores as a function of signal duration.

appropriate experts who score the pronunciation on one or more criteria. These human-generated scores can then be compared by correlation or by another method with the scores that were generated automatically. If the automatic scores are not in close agreement with the human-generated scores, the automatic scoring algorithms may have to be modified. Often the nature of the discrepancy between the two sets of scores provides useful information about how the automatic algorithms should be changed. When the automatic scoring is in close agreement with expert human scores for appropriate samples of spoken material that have not been part of the training set of the scoring algorithms, the scoring is deemed valid and the algorithm development is complete.

As seen in Figure 11-10, the correlation of the machine score with expert human scores determines the validity of the machine scoring method. The higher the correlation, the more reliable the machine score. Figure 11-11 displays an important characteristic of the automatic scoring procedures that have been developed in

prototype: the scores assigned to speech events increase in correlation (and therefore in reliability) as the length of the speech sample increases.

The graph in Figure 11-11 can be read thus: at the lower left end of the curve, it can be seen that the pronunciation scores calculated for a linguistic unit of short duration (approximately 0.2 seconds) will only correlate very roughly ($r \cong 0.12$) with human scores for the speech of this speaker. At the upper right end of the curve, it can be seen that automatically produced scores based on a 4- or 5-second sample of speech (about the length of a sentence) will correlate rather well ($r \cong 0.75$) with expert human scores. This means that with current techniques, recognition-based systems can provide more reliable scores for an utterance as a whole than for any particular short element in it. This is probably true of human judges as well; their judgments may also be more reliable when based on a longer sample of speech. If there is a need to judge a student's pronunciation of some particular speech sound like /s/ or /r/, a machine may be able to score it more reliably by a calculation over several occurrences of the sound that exhibit a total duration of a second or more. In this case, a lesson author might intentionally craft the student's part of the dialogue to contain many exemplars of the sounds of interest.

Authoring Lessons and Tests

Instructors who want to use a recognition-based system in teaching a language do not need to understand the details of speech recognition development that are presented above. However, an understanding of the general principles of the recognition and scoring process may be helpful in anticipating the strengths and limits of this technology in language education. After the speech system developer has set up the system and trained it on a well-designed database of spoken material, an instructor should be able to use the system to generate pedagogical materials by writing scripts in a lesson editor. The lesson editor can translate the teacher's flow plan into a lesson plan to be used as the dialogue grammar. This lesson plan controls the sequence of materials displayed by the system and defines what sentences are expected to be spoken by the student.

FUTURE RESEARCH

Missing Resources

Many resources that are simply not yet available would promote the application of speech recognition to a wider range of purposes. For example, you can imagine how the techniques outlined above for teaching a foreign language could be adapted for use in speech remediation or in remedial reading. But what about their application in the diagnosis of speech disorders? Or what about using speech recognition for automatic translation from Zulu to Dutch? To accomplish either of these goals—speech diagnosis or translation from spoken Zulu—we will need training data. Useful training data must be reliably categorized in a valid system. That is, we need a Zulu dictionary and a corpus of transcribed spoken materials. For speech disorder diagnosis, we need a large corpus of recordings of people with various kinds of speech disorders. For the vast majority of interesting applications of speech recognition, the first missing resource is training data.

Missing Science

Several areas of active research in the field of speech recognition may lead to systems with improved performance and bring speech recognition to more challenging environments and applications. These are some of the lines of research:

Fast Speaker Adaptation

The goal of **speaker adaptation** is to achieve recognition accuracy close to that of a speaker-dependent system with a speaker-independent system that adjusts its parameters using as input a small number of sentences (ideally one) spoken by the current speaker.

Source Separation

Often in real life there are other people talking close to the speaker of interest. Ideally we would like to keep track of each speech source to minimize the interference from the extraneous speech.

Noise Immunity

The speech signal is sometimes produced in a noisy environment or is transmitted on a noisy channel. For example, inside a car or a plane or from a public telephone in the street, different types of noise signals are superimposed on the speech signal, producing significant degradation in speech recognition performance. Some noise canceling methods have achieved some success when the noise has stable statistical properties (Neumeyer and Weintraub, 1994), but most noises in nature do not allow the application of these methods.

Language Modeling

Current methods for modeling the patterns of words in utterances during speech recognition use bigrams and trigrams (statistical estimates of the likely two- or three-word sequences) that only model local correlations among adjacent words. The modeling of more distant syntactic and semantic relations between words may offer other powerful constraints on the search process in the recognizer. Recent research is investigating the use of hybrid approaches that combine analytical and statistical language models in the HMM search.

Detail Acuity

Resolution of different minimal speech units (like features and phonemes) by machine is still not comparable with human performance. Current HMM-based systems are surprisingly good at finding a reasonable match to whole utterances, but they perform relatively poorly in identifying or discriminating single segments or syllables. Research is under way in the use of more sophisticated statistical or classification techniques like those based on neural networks and in the application of more powerful proces-

sors that will allow the use of these more complex models in real time.

SUMMARY

This chapter has introduced speech recognition as it is practiced in the 1980s and 1990s. We have explained what the devices do and how they operate inside. We hope that this presentation has spurred you to imagine new ways that speech recognizers can be used.

Review Questions

1. What are the characteristics of a successful automatic speech recognition (ASR) application?

2. Describe the internal structure of a word in an HMM system. Explain how data moves into, through, and out of a speech recognition system. Describe the various ways that speech is represented inside the system.

3. Make up an application for speech recognition technology that is not mentioned in this chapter. Describe what aspects of your task will be particularly easy and which aspects of the task will be particularly difficult for the recognizer.

4. How would you go about assessing the performance of an ASR system? How does this compare to the assessment of receptive language skills in a human subject?

5. What is the principal result of the process called *signal analysis?* How might you verify that a signal analysis produces a signal represen-

tation that should be adequate for speech recognition?

6. What advantages might an ASR-based system have over a clinician or tutor in working with a speech-impaired student?

7. Are there speech-related tasks that machines can perform better than human listeners or human speakers? and vice versa?

8. Describe the process of training an ASR.

9. Why have many speech recognition researchers switched from DTW to HMM systems? Explain how hidden Markov models provide a flexible, trainable model of human speech.

10. Which aspects of speech and language can be scored by an ASR device?

11. What happens when a person uses words that are not in the vocabulary of a speech recognizer when speaking to the recognizer?

References

Baker, J.K. (1975). The DRAGON system – an overview. *IEEE Trans. Acoust. Speech and Signal Processing,* ASSP-23(1), 24-29.

Bernstein, J. (1986a). Applications of speech recognition technology in rehabilitation. Paper presented at an Electronic Industries Foundation special session on speech recognition, 1986 RESNA meeting, Minneapolis, MN.

Bernstein, J. (1986b). New technologies and captioning. Paper presented at the National Conference on New Directions for Captioning, Gallaudet University. In *Framework for the future: The role of captioning in empowering hearing-impaired people*

Conference summary distributed by the U.S. Departpartment of Education, Washington, D.C. (pp. 123-133).

Bernstein, J. (1989). Technical and business issues in speech recognition technology for deaf and hard of hearing users. In Harkins, J., & Virvan, B. (Eds.), *Emerging Technologies Report Monograph from the Gallaudet Research Institute, Washington, D.C. (pp. 51-66).*

Bernstein, J., Cohen, M., Murveit, H., Rtischev, D. & Weintraub, M. (1990). Automatic evaluation and training in English pronunciation. In *1990 International conference on spoken language process-*

ing. Kobe, Japan: Acoustical Society of Japan (pp. 1185-1188).

Bernstein, J., & Rtischev, D. (1991). A voice-interactive language instruction system. Proceedings of Eurospeech-91, 2nd European Conference on Speech Communication and Technology, European Speech Communication Association (pp. 981-984).

Carlson, G., & Bernstein, J. (1988). Automatic speech recognition for speech impaired people. *Journal of the Acoustical Society of America* (Suppl. 1) 84, S46 (abstract).

Cohen, M., Franco, H., Morgan, N., Rumelhart, D., & Abrash, V. (1993). Context-dependent multiple distribution phonetic modeling with MLP's. In *Advances in neural information processing systems 5.* Morgan Kaufmann. San Mateo, CA (pp. 649-657).

Cohen, M., Murveit, H., Bernstein, J., Price, P., & Weintraub, M. (1990). The decipher speech recognition system. *Proceedings ICASSP-90,* S1, 77-80.

Flanagan, J. (1972). *Speech analysis, synthesis and perception.* New York: Springer-Verlag.

Furui, S. (1989). *Digital speech processing, synthesis, and recognition.* New York: Marcel Dekker.

Gray, R. (1984). Vector quantization. *IEEE ASSP Magazine,* 1,(2) 4-29.

Itakura, F. (1975). Minimum prediction residual principle applied to speech recognition. *IEEE Trans. Acoust. Speech and Signal Processing,* ASSP-23, (1) 68-72.

Javkin, H. N., Antonanzas-Barroso, A., Das, D., Zerkle, Y., Yamada, N., Murata, H., Levitt, & Youdelman, K. (1993). A motivation sustaining articulatory/acoustic speech training system for profoundly deaf children. *Proc. ICASSP-93,* Vol. 1., (pp. 145-148).

Jelinek, F. (1976). Continuous speech recognition by statistical methods. *Proceedings of the IEEE,* 64(4), 532-556.

Lee, K. F. (1989). *Automatic speech recognition: The development of the SPHINX system.* Norwell, MA: Kluwer Academic.

Levinson, S., & Liberman, M. (1981). Speech recognition by computer. *Scientific American,* April, 64-76.

Levitt, H., Pickett, J. M., & Houde, R. A. (Eds.) (1980). *Sensory aids for the hearing impaired.* New York IEEE Press, ASSP

Neumeyer, L. & Weintraub, M. (1994). Probabilistic optimum filtering for robust speech recognition. *Proc. ICASSP-94,* Vol. 1., (pp. 417-429).

Pallett, D., Fiscus, J., Fisher, W., Garofolo, J., Lund, B., & Pryzbocki M. (1994). 1993 Benchmark tests for the ARPA spoken language program. Proceedings of the ARPA Human Language Technology Workshop Notebook, (pp. 49-74). Morgan Kaufmann. San Francisco, CA.

Price, P., Fisher, W., Bernstein, J., & Pallett, D. (1988). The DARPA 1000-word resource management database for speech recognition. *IEEE Proc. ICASSP-88,* pp. 651-654.

Rabiner, L. (1989). A tutorial on hidden Markov models and selected applications in speech recognition. *Proceedings of the IEEE,* 77 (2), 257-286.

Reddy, D.R. (1967). Computer recognition of continuous speech. *Journal of the Acoustical Society of America,* 42, 329-347.

Stevens, G., & Bernstein, J. (1986). A system for telephone communication between hearing-impaired and normal-hearing people. *Volta Review,* 88 (7), 367-373.

Uchanski, R., Delhorne, L., Dix, A., Braida, L., Reed, C., & Durlach, N. (1994). Automatic speech recognition to aid the hearing impaired: Prospects for the automatic generation of cued speech. *Journal of Rehabilitation Research and Development, 31* (1), 20-41.

Watson, C., Reed, D., Kewley-Port, D., & Maki, D. (1989). The Indiana Speech Training Aid (ISTRA) 1: Comparisons between human and computer-based evaluation of speech quality. *Journal of Speech and Hearing Research,* 32, 245-251.

Watson, C., & Kewley-Port, D. (1989). Advances in computer based speech training: Aids for the profoundly hearing impaired. *The Volta Review,* 91, 29-45.

Weinstein, C., McCandless, S., Mondshein, L., & Zue, V. (1975). A system for acoustic-phonetic analysis of continuous speech. *IEEE Trans. Acoust. Speech and Signal Processing,* ASSP-23, (1) 54-67.

Woodland, P., Odell, J., Valtchev, V., & Young, S. (1994). Large vocabulary continuous speech recognition using HTK. *IEEE Proceedings ICASSP-94,* pp. II-125-128.

Young, S., Woodland, P., & Byrne, W. (1993). *HTK: Hidden Markov model toolkit,* V1.5, Washington, DC: Entropic Research Laboratory.

Suggested Readings

Speech Recognition Technology

Huang, X. D., Ariki, Y., & Jack, M. A. (1990). *Hidden Markov models for speech recognition.* Edinburgh University Press.

Levinson, S., & Liberman, M. (1981). Speech recognition by computer. *Scientific American,* April, pp. 64-76.

O'Shaughnessy, D. (1987). *Speech communication:*

Human and machine. Reading, MA: Addison-Wesley.

Rabiner, L. (1989). A tutorial on hidden Markov models and selected applications in speech recognition. *Proc. IEEE*, Vol. 77(2), (pp. 257-286).

Rabiner, L. R., & Juang, B. H. (1986), January. An introduction to hidden Markov models. *IEEE ASSP Magazine*, 4-16.

Rabiner, L. R., & Juang, B. H. (1994). *Fundamentals of speech recognition.* Englewood Cliffs, NJ: Prentice-Hall.

Waibel, A., & Lee, K. (Eds.). (1990). *Readings in speech recognition,* San Mateo: Morgan Kaufmann.

Speech Recognition Application

Carlson, G. S., & Bernstein, J. (1986). A system for telephone communication between hearing-impaired and normal-hearing people. *Volta Review, 88* (7), 367-373.

Carlson, G. S., & Bernstein, J. (1988). *A voice-input communication aid.* Final Report. National Institute for Neurological and Communicative Disorders and Stroke, Contract N01-NS-5-2394.

Harkins, J., & Virvan, B. (Eds.). (1989). *Speech-to-text: today and tomorrow: Proceedings of a conference at Gallaudet University,* December 1988 (Monograph Series B, No. 2). Washington, D.C.: Gallaudet Research Institute.

Uchanski, R., Delhorne, L., Dix, A., Braida, L., Reed, C., & Durlach, N. (1994). Automatic speech recognition to aid the hearing impaired: Prospects for the automatic generation of cued speech. *Journal of Rehabilitation Research and Development, 31,* 20-41.

Watson, C., Reed, D., Kewley-Port, D., & Maki, D. (1989). The Indian Speech Training Aid (ISTRA). 1: Comparisons between human and computer-based evaluation of speech quality. *Journal of Speech and Hearing Research, 32,* 245-251.

Chapter 12

Auditory Illusions and Perceptual Processing of Speech

Richard M. Warren

INTRODUCTION

Highly skilled perceptual processes, such as those employed for the comprehension of speech, seem immediate and direct, and so the underlying mechanisms remain hidden in everyday life. Illusions are breakdowns in perceptual accuracy, and when used as experimental tools, they can reveal these normally inaccessible processes. The idea of using illusions to study normal processing is not new. In the nineteenth century Helmholtz stated that illusions provide a "particularly instructive" method for discovering the laws governing perception (Warren and Warren, 1968). An analogous principle in medicine is the maxim that disorders in normal function lay bare the mechanisms used to maintain health.

This chapter describes research on several interrelated illusions and their implications for normal perceptual processing: (1) perceptual cancellation of masking leading to the illusory presence of obliterated sounds, (2) uncertainties and perceptual errors in the temporal ordering of sounds, (3) illusory verbal organization of vowel sequences, and (4) illusory changes in repeated words.

A basic assumption concerning speech has guided the content and organization of the following sections. It is that speech perception employs basic general mechanisms employed for nonspeech sounds. It follows that to understand how we perceive speech, we must understand the general rules governing auditory perception and how these rules have been modified for linguistic purposes.

ILLUSORY PRESENCE OF OBLITERATED SOUNDS: PHONEMIC RESTORATIONS AND AUDITORY INDUCTION

Phonemic Restorations

Our world is a noisy place, and when we are listening to a message, portions are often masked by louder sounds. However, we possess a mechanism capable of reversing the effects of masking and restoring obliterated segments. The process by which listeners restore portions of masked speech is **phonemic restoration** (Warren, 1970; Warren and Warren, 1970).

In the first study of phonemic restorations (Warren, 1970), listeners heard the sentence, "The state governors met with their respective legislatures convening in the capital city", in which the /s/ in "legislatures" (the first "s") was deleted and replaced with a variety of sounds (coughs, tones, and buzzes). To minimize transitional cues to the identity of the missing sound, adjacent parts of the preceding and following phonemes were also deleted. Removal of this portion of the sentence was not expected to affect intelligibility, since the /s/ is evident from the information before and after it. It might also be expected that listeners could readily identify the missing segment. However, they could not identify the missing sound even when told that one was absent: The /s/ was "heard" as clearly as the phonemes actually present and was perceptually indistinguishable from them. Attempts to identify the missing sound through the location of the simultaneous extraneous sound were unsuccessful because this cough, tone, or buzz could not be placed accurately; it seemed to coexist with the speech sounds in the sentence at some poorly defined position.

The inability to locate extraneous sounds in sentences was reported by Ladefoged (1959) and later described in more detail by Ladefoged and Broadbent (1960). They employed clicks and short hisses, and since they were careful not to obliterate any phoneme, phonemic restorations could not arise. Warren and Obusek (1971) compared mislocalizations of a short click within a phoneme with the mislocalizations of a spliced-in cough that completely replaced the same phoneme in an otherwise identical recording. It was found that the direction of localization errors was rather different. When the sentence was heard for the first time, the longer sounds producing phonemic restoration were judged to occur earlier in the sentence than the click. This finding suggested that a delay in perceptual organization occurring with phonemic restoration caused an earlier part of the sentence to be selected as simultaneous with the separate event corresponding to the extraneous sound. This delay in processing within a sentence heard for the first time should be reduced by familiarity with the sentence. In keeping with this reasoning, replaying the stimulus to the listener resulted in a pronounced shift toward a later localization of the long extraneous sound, with judgments of its location having a more nearly symmetrical distribution about the true position. Phonemic restoration itself was not reduced by replaying, and the listener's certainty that all speech sounds were physically present remained unchanged after four presentations. However, when the extraneous sound replacing the missing phoneme was eliminated and a silent gap was present, listeners could localize the gap accurately and identify which speech sound was missing.

A subsequent experiment showed that the context identifying the phoneme replaced by an extraneous sound need not precede the missing speech sound (Warren and Sherman, 1974). That study employed a variety of sentences, each having some of the information required for identification of the deleted segments following their occurrence. To avoid the possibility that cues to the missing sounds were furnished by **coarticulation** involving the neighboring phonemes, the deleted speech sounds were deliberately mispronounced in each of the stimulus sentences as they were recorded prior to deletion. Care was taken that the mispronounced phonemes to be deleted matched the durations of the contextually appropriate items. Under these conditions, the contextually appropriate phonemes were restored despite the misleading coarticulation cues and the requirement that subsequent context be used before restoration could be achieved.

It appears that phonemic restorations are a linguistic adaptation of a more general ability to restore portions of signals that have been masked or obliterated by other sounds. This illusory perception of one sound induced by the presence of another has been called **auditory induction.** Three basic types of induction have been suggested (Warren, 1984). *Homophonic induction* involves different amplitudes of the same sound; it was discovered when three levels of broadband noise, each lasting 300 ms, were presented sequentially (60, 70, 80, 60, 70, 80, 60, . . . 80 dB) (Warren, Obusek, and Ackroff, 1972). Paradoxically, the faintest level (60 dB) seemed to be on all of the time, coexisting with each of the two louder levels of the same sound. Homophonic induction did not require three levels; two levels would suffice, and the illusory continuity of the fainter sound was found to occur for tones as well as for noises when two levels of the same sound were alternated.

Heterophonic continuity consists of the illusory continuation of a sound interrupted by another sound of different spectral characteristics. It was discovered independently by Miller

and Licklider (1950), Thurlow (1957), Vicario (1960), Houtgast (1972), and Warren, Obusek, and Ackroff (1972). (For a review of these discoveries and related issues, see Warren [1984]). Houtgast as well as Warren, Obusek, and Ackroff suggested that the illusory continuity of the fainter of two alternating sounds requires that the neural units stimulated by the higher-amplitude sound include those stimulated by the fainter sound. This is a condition occurring normally when one sound masks another, so that auditory induction appears to be a rather sophisticated selective process capable of perceptually synthesizing a signal only if it could have been masked. If a signal could not have been masked by an interrupting sound, its absence is detected and continuity is not heard.

A third type of temporal induction was called *contextual catenation.* It does not involve continuation of a steady-state signal, but rather the perceptual synthesis of a time-varying signal for which the restored portion of sound differs from the portions of the signal preceding and following the interrupting noise. Phonemic restoration has been investigated much more thoroughly than other forms of contextual catenation, such as the restoration of segments of tonal glides replaced by noise (Dannenbring, 1976) and the restoration of notes of a familiar melody replaced by noise (Sasaki, 1980).

When listening to speech in everyday life, interference is not restricted to single interruptions, and a number of investigators have studied the effects of multiple interruptions of speech by noise. Multiple interruptions by silent gaps decrease intelligibility and impart a rough or harsh quality corresponding to the discontinuities. Miller and Licklider (1950) reported that when periodic gaps in word lists were filled with a louder noise, the rough quality disappeared. However, even though the speech sounded more natural, intelligibility was not improved. Quite different results were obtained by Cherry and Wiley (1967) when connected discourse rather than word lists were used: They deleted either the high-amplitude components (mainly vowels) or the low-amplitude components (mainly consonants) in a speech passage and found that a considerable restoration of the intelligibility of the interrupted speech occurred when the silent gaps were filled with noise. Cherry and Wiley suggested that the addition of noise prevented a disruptive effect of silence on the natural rhythm of speech (however, it is not evident why noise

Mean interruption thresholds for 20 subjects listening to narrowband speech (1500 Hz frequency) alternated with narrowband noises

Noise Band (Hz)	375	750	1500	3000	6000
Thresholds (ms)	136	221	304	129	128

Note: The interruption threshold with silence substituted for the interpolated noise bands was 79 ms.
(From Bashford, J. A., Jr., & Warren, R. M. [1987]. Multiple phonemic restorations follow the rules for auditory induction. *Perception and Psychophysics, 42*, 114-121.)

would not also disrupt this rhythm). In an unpublished portion of his doctoral dissertation, Wiley (1968) reported that intelligibility also increased when gaps placed at regular intervals in discourse were filled with noise. Powers and Wilcox (1977) obtained results similar to Wiley's and reasoned that the addition of noise might improve intelligibility by removing the abrupt transitions to silence, which could suggest stop consonants. But this explanation does not handle the observation of Miller and Licklider (1950) that the addition of noise to periodic gaps in word lists, although it did result in apparent continuity, did not improve intelligibility. A different explanation for the ability of noise to increase intelligibility was offered by Warren and Obusek (1971). They suggested that phonemic restorations occur when multiple gaps in connected speech are filled with noise, with the contextual cues associated with syntactic and sentential context furnishing the information required for appropriate restoration. Since word lists lack this context, intelligibility is not increased by the addition of noise.

The evidence presented thus far indicates that filling multiple gaps in speech with noise can restore both apparent continuity and intelligibility. However, the relation of speech restoration to the restoration of nonverbal sounds through temporal induction has not yet been discussed. In keeping with the spectral requirements for nonverbal induction, Layton (1975) found that phonemic restoration was enhanced when single phonemes were replaced by broadband sounds such as coughs and noises, but not when they were replaced by a sinusoidal tone. Bashford and Warren (1987a) examined the spectral correspondence of speech and noise needed for illusory continuity of speech. One experiment in this study employed a narrowband speech passage (a one-third octave band centered on 1500 Hz). This filtered speech was interrupted by one-third octave bands of noise having various center frequencies (375, 750,

1500, 3000, and 6000 Hz). The recorded speech and on-line noise were alternated regularly (equal durations for each), and the stimuli were presented at a peak speech amplitude and an average noise amplitude of 80 dB sound pressure level (SPL). The longest duration for which continuity was observed (304 ms) occurred when the noise and the speech had the same center frequency (box). However, the continuity limit for the 20 subjects was less than half that value when the noise bands with the lowest and the highest center frequencies were used. Thus, illusory continuity of speech is enhanced when the interrupting sound is a potential masker.

The second part of this study by Bashford and Warren examined the effect of contextual information on the continuity of broadband speech alternated with on-line broadband noise. The limit for illusory continuity was highest when the speech consisted of connected discourse: The same passage read with the word order reversed and lists of unrelated monosyllabic words each had continuity limits only half as long as that found for normal discourse (Table 12-1). The continuity limit (or discontinuity threshold) for discourse corresponded to the duration of the average word in the passage, while the discontinuity thresholds for backward reading and for the word lists were between the average duration for the syllables and for the individual phonemes of the stimuli.

The observation that the limit of restoration in connected speech corresponds to the average word duration suggests that normal contextual information permits the restoration of entire obliterated words. Lacking this information, restoration is diminished appreciably. If average word duration does indeed determine the limit for restoration of continuity in connected speech, changes in the duration of words should produce corresponding changes in restoration limits. Bashford et al. (1988) designed an experiment to test this prediction. A new passage of speech was recorded broadband and inter-

TABLE 12-1   Mean interruption thresholds in milliseconds for 20 subjects listening to each combination of interrupter and speech stimulus

Interrupting Stimulus	Speech Stimulus		
	Normal Discourse	Backward Discourse	Isolated Monosyllables
Noise	304	148	161
Silence	52	50	61
Tone	72		

Note: The tonal interrupter was paired only with normal discourse.
(From Bashford, J. A., & Warren, R. M. [1987]. Multiple phonemic restorations follow the rules for auditory induction. *Perception & Psychophysics, 42,* 114-121.)

rupted by broadband noise. In agreement with the results of Bashford and Warren (1987a), the discontinuity threshold once again approximated the average word duration. Separate groups of listeners then heard the speech played back at tape speeds 15% greater and 15% less than the original recording (the speech appeared normal when heard at each of the three rates). The faster playback reduced the interruption threshold by 17.7%, and the slower playback increased the interruption threshold by 12.2%. The average threshold change of these two values for a 15% rate change (ignoring the direction of change) is almost exactly 15%.

A subsequent study of multiple phonemic restorations examined the effects of contextual information on the restoration of intelligibility (Bashford, Riener, and Warren, 1992). Three basic types of stimuli were used: monosyllabic word lists, sentences having key words with low contextual probability (e.g., "Ruth hopes she called about the junk", where the key word scored for intelligibility was "junk"), and sentences with high contextual probability (e.g., "Throw out all this useless junk", where the key word scored for intelligibility again was "junk"). As anticipated, when the speech was interrupted regularly by silent gaps (on-off times of 200 ms), scores for intelligibility dropped for all stimuli, with the greatest decrement for the word lists and the lowest decrement for the sentences having high-probability key words. When the gaps were filled with noise, there was no improvement in the intelligibility of the word lists (in keeping with the report by Miller and Licklider, 1950), but intelligibility did increase for the low-probability key words in sentences with normal syntactic context but in low semantic contextual clues to the identity of the key words. A still greater increase in intelligibility of

sentences occurred when high-probability key words were used.

To recapitulate, filling gaps in speech with noise can increase both apparent continuity and intelligibility, and when these effects take place, each of these measures of restoration follows the rules governing nonlinguistic temporal induction. Although the increases in continuity and intelligibility are related, there are important differences. While noise does produce an increase in interruption thresholds for word lists (Miller and Licklider, 1950; Bashford and Warren, 1987), it does not produce an increase in intelligibility (Miller and Licklider, 1950; Bashford, Reiner, and Warren, 1992). However, the addition of noise to gaps in sentences not only produces illusory continuity but increases intelligibility as well (Cherry and Wiley, 1967; Holloway, 1970; Powers and Wilcox, 1977; Bashford and Warren, 1979; Verschuure and Brocaar, 1983; Bashford, Reiner, and Warren, 1992). The magnitude of this increase appears to depend on the extent of syntactic and semantic information concerning the identity of the missing fragments.

Samuel (1981, 1987, 1991) used a rather different task for studying phonemic restoration. Listeners in these experiments tried to distinguish between a replaced condition, in which noise was substituted for a phoneme in a word, and an added condition, in which the phoneme was present along with the noise. An inability to distinguish between these conditions was considered to be a measure of phonemic restoration. In the latest version of this procedure, the noise in both cases was not stochastic (random) as in other studies of phonemic restorations, but was speech-correlated and had the same amplitude envelope as the target phoneme (that is, the moment-by-moment amplitude matched that of the speech sound). Signal detection methodology was used to investigate a number of factors influencing the ability to discriminate between the two conditions, including attention, bottom-up and top-down influences, and the lexical uniqueness of a word. However, it was found by Bashford, Warren, and Brown (in press) that the speech-correlated noise used in Samuel's replaced condition provided strong cues to the identity of the missing phonemes. These cues are absent in other laboratory studies of phonemic restoration (and in restoration outside the laboratory) when unrelated sounds mask or replace speech segments. In the added condition, the amplitudes of speech and speech-shaped noise were mixed at equal levels and presented at an overall amplitude level matching that of the replacement condition. This added condition does not result in masking—sentences and word lists are quite intelligible when mixed with equal amplitude speech-correlated noise. Indeed, speech maintains much of its intelligibility when mixed with equal amplitude noncorrelased stochastic noise. Hence, the procedures used by Samuel, while of interest, do not measure the restoration.

As we have seen, both apparent continuity and intelligibility can be restored if the extraneous sounds filling gaps in sentences are capable of masking the missing segments. The restoration of nonverbal signals is also facilitated when the interrupting sound is a potential masker (Houtgast, 1972; Warren, Obusek, and Ackroff, 1972). However, there has been some controversy concerning whether some of the neural input corresponding to the louder extraneous sound is subtracted and used as the raw material for reconstructing the missing fragments of both verbal and nonverbal signals, as suggested by Warren (1984). Bregman (1990) has taken the position that phonemic restoration represents a schema-driven stream segregation for which the extraneous sound acts only as a trigger, contributing nothing of its own substance. Other types of temporal induction were stated by Bregman to be innate and primitive and to involve a parceling out of some of the energy of the interrupter, resulting in the reduction of its loudness, as described above. Since there was no direct experimental evidence testing these conflicting hypotheses concerning phonemic restoration, Repp (1992) undertook a study designed to determine which

was correct. His listeners compared the timbre, or brightness, of a target noise that replaced a fricative noise in a word (the speech sound /s/) with a probe noise that was the same as the target stimulus and either preceded or followed the speech. The target and probe had a different spectral profile than the /s/, and Repp reasoned that if phonemic restoration involved reallocation of a portion of the interpolated noise, then there should be detectable change in its timbre. In the initial two experiments, there was a significant change in timbre, but in the final three experiments no significant change in timbre was found. Warren et al. (1994) approached this problem in a different fashion. They reported a series of experiments using a procedure that measured directly any change in the apparent level of the sound producing restoration by having listeners match its loudness using a variable amplitude comparison sound. In addition to phonemic restoration, homophonic and heterophonic restoration of nonverbal sounds were examined, and a statistically significant reduction in the loudness of the inducer was found in each case. It was concluded that the general rules for auditory temporal induction apply to the restoration of both speech and nonspeech stimuli, and that an overlay of linguistic skills is employed for the reconstruction of appropriate missing segments of fragmented speech.

Contralateral Induction

Temporal induction fills in an obliterated signal across time, and contralateral induction fills in an obliterated signal across space. Contralateral induction occurs when a signal at one ear is masked or replaced at the other ear by a louder noise. Under appropriate conditions, the monaural signal becomes completely delateralized and is heard as centered on the medial plane. This illusion follows acoustic rules similar to those governing the restoration of masked signals described for temporal induction. Furthermore, in keeping with the principle that illusions in general reflect processes normally leading to veridical perception, contralateral induction appears to involve mechanisms employed in the normally hidden early stages of binaural processing.

A partial contralateral induction was reported by Egan (1948), who found that when speech was delivered to one ear and noise to the other,

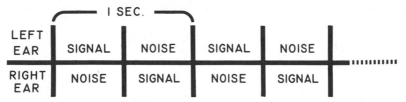

FIGURE 12-1   **Alternating pattern of stimulation at each ear used to produce delateralization of the signal through contralateral induction.** (From Warren, R. M., & Bashford, J. A., Jr. [1976]. Auditory contralateral induction: An early stage in binaural processing. *Perception & Psychophysics, 20,* 380-386.)

the position of the voice seemed to shift toward the side receiving the noise. Thurlow and Elfner (1959) found that a tone delivered to one ear moved toward the center when the contralateral ear received a tone of a different frequency. Related shifts in lateralization were observed by Butler and Naunton (1962, 1964) when their listeners were stimulated by both a monaural headphone and a loudspeaker that was moved to various positions. The qualitative nature of lateralization shifts are easy to observe but difficult to measure quantitatively for two reasons: (1) lateralized sounds seem to change position and drift slowly toward the medial plane with continued listening, and (2) at any given moment the exact extent of lateralization is difficult to measure because of the diffuse boundaries of the spatial image. However, there is a way of avoiding both of these problems.

Warren and Bashford (1976) described a technique permitting a precise threshold measurement for delateralization by a contralateral sound. A signal, either a tone or the recorded voice of someone reading an article, was delivered to one ear and a noise to the other, and the stimuli reversed sides each 500 ms (Fig. 12-1). This resulted in the signal appearing to be completely stationary at a diffuse location centered on the medial plane as long as the signal-to-noise ratio did not exceed a limiting value. Once this limit was exceeded, an abrupt change in the apparent location of the signal occurred, and it was heard to move from side to side. Contralateral induction requires appropriate intensity and spectral relations between the signal and noise. It was found that the rules governing contralateral induction parallel the rules governing temporal induction; that is, if the monaural noise could mask the contralateral signal if it were also present at the ear receiving the noise, the signal became delateralized, but if the noise could not mask

the signal, the signal was heard on the side of stimulation. These rules apply to both verbal and nonverbal sounds.

First, let us consider the experiment of Warren and Bashford dealing with tones. As shown in Fig. 12-2, sinusoidal tones of various frequencies were alternated (as in Fig. 12-1) with three types of noise. The upper limit of intensity for delateralization of the monaural signal occurred when noise components matching the frequency of the tone were present. The lower set of curves for contralateral masking were obtained using the same procedure, but instead of judging the position of the signal at supraliminal intensity levels, listeners were instructed to adjust the level of the monaural tone until it could just be heard in the presence of each of the three types of noise at 80 dB. These measurements of detection thresholds showed that the masking of the contralateral signal by the various monaural noises did not exhibit the same spectral effects as contralateral induction, and hence cross-ear masking artifacts could not be responsible for the spectral dependence of contralateral induction. Then monaural narrowband filtered speech was used with center frequencies of either 1000 Hz or 3000 Hz together with a contralateral narrowband noise at 80 dB with the various center frequencies shown in Figure 12-3. The upper limit for contralateral induction was highest when the center frequencies of the voice and the noise bands were the same.

An interesting change from one form of induction to the other was observed when a monaural broadband voice and a contralateral broadband noise switched sides at rates between 30 and 200 ms. A monaural temporal induction replaced contralateral induction at each ear, and listeners heard a highly unusual effect having some interesting neurophysiological implications: the same voice seemed to be saying the same thing at the same time at each

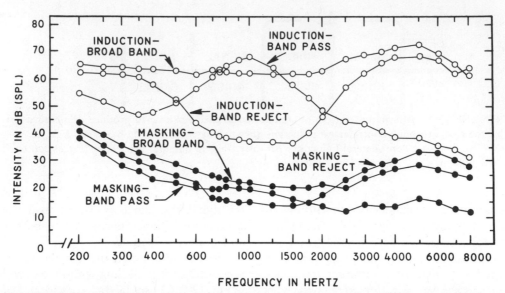

FIGURE 12-2   Upper limit of intensity for delateralization (contralateral induction) of pure tones (24 frequencies) delivered to one ear and presented along with three contralateral 80 dB SPL noises: broad-band (white) noise; narrow-band (⅓-octave) noise centered at 1000 Hz; and band-reject noise (spectral gap one octave wide) centered at 1000 Hz. The detection thresholds of the tones are shown as well, and the difference between the upper limit for delateralization and the masked detection thresholds represent the range over which contralateral induction occurred. (From Warren, R. M., & Bashford, J. A., [1976]. Auditory contralateral induction: An early stage in binaural processing. *Perception & Psychophysics, 20,* 380-386.)

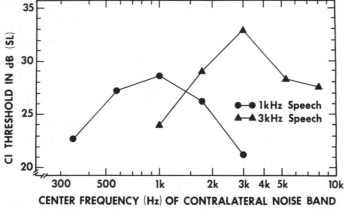

FIGURE 12-3   Upper intensity limit for delateralization (contralateral induction) of filtered speech bands (⅓-octave) centered at 1000 Hz and 3000 Hz delivered to one ear while contralateral 80 dB ⅓-octave noise bands of various center frequencies were presented to the opposite ear. Intensity of speech required for contralateral induction (CI) is given as sensation level (SL), or dB above threshold.   (From Warren, R. M., & Bashford, J. A., [1976]. Auditory contralateral induction: An early stage in binaural processing. *Perception & Psychophysics, 20,* 380-386.)

ear, and yet the identical simultaneous images did not fuse.

Delateralization through contralateral induction is a subtractive process, as is temporal induction; that is, the components corresponding to the signal are subtracted from the inducer when the signal moves to the medial plane. A condition involving uncorrelated noises demonstrates this clearly. When uncorrelated noises from separate generators having equivalent long-term spectra are delivered to opposite ears at the same level, both noises are delateralized and heard as a broad spatial blur centered on the medial plane. This effect has been described as the sound heard when standing under a waterfall or under a tin roof in the rain (Kock, 1950; David, Guttman, and van Bergeijk, 1958; Warren and Bashford, 1976). Thus, while the two inputs cannot be heard separately, neither do they fuse to form a single compact image as when noise from a single source is presented simultaneously to the two ears. When, for example, an 80-dB noise is delivered to one ear and an 82-dB uncorrelated noise to the other and the input to the two ears is switched every 500 ms, as shown in Figure 12-1, listeners perceive two images. One is a diffuse stationary sound centered on the medial plane, and the other is a lateralized faint noise corresponding to the residue remaining after subtraction of neural input corresponding to 80 dB from the ear receiving the 82 dB signal. This fainter residue is heard to switch from side to side while the louder noise remains centered. The residue can be made fainter or louder by decreasing or increasing the level of the noise having the greater amplitude. Of course, for the limiting case when the two levels of uncorrelated noises are matched, there is no residue, and switching sides of the two noises produces no perceptible effect on the centered diffuse image.

It was concluded that contralateral induction can be considered as a first stage in binaural processing. When appropriate information is available at each ear, further processing can lead to binaural fusion and accurate estimates of the location of a speaker or other sound source in space, as well as other types of binaural interaction.

Both temporal induction and contralateral induction are illusions, since these reconstructions of partially obliterated portions of signals do not represent the stimuli actually present at a listener's ears. However, considering that perception provides the basis for acting appropriately to events in the world outside the laboratory, auditory induction does not normally produce errors in judgment. Instead it can prevent false perception and erroneous judgments. Looked at from this vantage point, a fruitful direction for future research on speech perception under the noisy conditions of everyday life would be to examine in detail the cancellation of masking of speech by both temporal induction and contralateral induction, with special attention to limiting conditions and underlying mechanisms.

PERCEPTION AND CONFUSIONS OF TEMPORAL ORDER

Comprehension of speech, recognition of melodies, and many other aspects of hearing would be impossible without the ability to recognize and distinguish different temporal arrangements of the same sounds. Some years ago the literature on perception of sequential order seemed quite tidy. Auditory temporal acuity appeared analogous in some ways to visual spatial acuity: resolving power could be measured in milliseconds with one and in seconds of arc with the other. Hirsh (1959) and Hirsh and Sherrick (1961) reported that identification of order within a pair of sounds such as a tone and a hiss could be accomplished for onset disparities as brief as 15 or 20 ms. These studies were verified in other laboratories, although thresholds were generally a little higher (see Fay [1966] for a review). It was generally accepted that these experimental values were quite adequate to permit listeners to perceive the order of phonemes in speech. However, some subsequent observations concerning confusions and illusions in the identification of temporal order have led to new hypotheses concerning the nature of temporal resolution and its role in the perception of acoustic sequences.

A few curious reports in the 1950s did not seem to fit the concept of a general threshold for the perception of order. When Ladefoged (1959) and Ladefoged and Broadbent (1960) inserted brief extraneous sounds such as clicks in sentences, they found that listeners could not determine the position of the extraneous sound. (Ladefoged and Broadbent were careful not to remove or mask any phonemes, but of course errors in localization also occur for extraneous sounds completely replacing phonemes and producing phonemic restorations). Heise and Miller (1951) described a similar phenomenon with tones: if all but one of the tones in a series had frequencies close to one central value, then the odd tone seemed to pop out of the group, and listeners could not locate it in the sequence. However, these anomalous observations were considered to reflect special attentional and informational processing mechanisms associated with speech and music. Subsequently, another reported observation was quite difficult to reconcile with a general threshold for the perception of order, and it suggested a new look and reinterpretation of the literature on sequence perception.

At a conference on pattern recognition, some unusual observations involving iterating or recycling sequences were described (Warren, 1968a). A loop of tape was constructed by splicing together 200 ms statements of a tone, a hiss, a buzz, and a vowel. The four items were played in a fixed order that was repeated over and over, eliminating the special cues furnished by initial and terminal items of nonrepeated sequences. Subjects could listen for as long as they wished and could start naming the order with whichever sound they chose (there were factorial three, or six, possible arrangements of the four items presented in this fashion). Even when each of the sounds could be heard clearly and identified with accuracy, the order could not be reported correctly. It was not that a wrong arrangement was perceived by the listener but rather that no decision could be reached with confidence. Yet the duration of each sound was considerably longer than the previously accepted values for durations permitting the naming of order. However, it was possible to identify the order of four successive items in a repeated sequence when each item was a 200 ms word. As part of the initial study, a tape of four spoken numbers (eight, three, two, one) was repeated over and over, each complete statement of the four items taking 800 ms. To eliminate any transitional cues to order, each of the words was recorded separately, then cut and spliced into a loop. Despite the fact that each of the digits was itself complex (consisting of a sequence of phonemes), correct identification was accomplished easily by all of the listeners.

The last part of the initial study dealt with the identification of temporal order for vowels. Sequences of four vowels were constructed by cutting 200 ms segments from longer steady statements of each vowel and splicing the segments into a loop that repeated them without pauses. Although it was fairly difficult to judge the order, performance of a group of 30 subjects was significantly above chance. The task became easier when each steady-state vowel was reduced to 150 ms, with 50 ms of silence separating items, and it was easiest of all for single statements of each vowel with natural onset and decay characteristics for each statement, each vowel again

lasting about 150 ms, with 50-msec silences (Warren, 1968a; Warren and Warren, 1970). Subsequent work by Thomas, Cetti, and Chase (1971) with repeated sequences of synthetic vowels led them to conclude that differences in the ability to identify temporal order provide a possible method for measuring the speechlike quality of synthetic speech sounds. Under optimal conditions, listeners could identify order down to 100 ms/vowel. Dorman, Cutting, and Raphael (1975) also used recycled synthetic vowels, introducing formant transitions resembling normal coarticulation between adjacent vowels with some sequences, and formant transitions resembling stop consonants between the vowels with others. They concluded that the more their stimuli resembled sequences that could be produced by a speaker, the easier it became to identify the order of components. Nevertheless, as in the study by Thomas, Cetti, and Chase, the lower limit for identifying vowel order was about 100 ms/item.

The initial puzzling observations concerning the difficulty in identifying order for recycled sequences of three or four unrelated sounds (hisses, tones, buzzes) were examined further in a series of experiments dealing with the effects of experimental procedure on performance (Warren et al., 1969; Warren and Warren, 1970; Warren and Obusek, 1972). When thresholds for identification of order were measured, profound differences were found depending upon the method used for responding. When listeners called out the order of items (hiss, tone, buzz, and the vowel /i/), the threshold was found to be about 550 ms/item. But when different groups of subjects responded by arranging cards bearing the names of the sounds in the order of their occurrence, the threshold dropped to about 250 ms/item. Identification of order was made a little easier when the recycled sequences consisted of only three sounds (for which there are only two possible arrangements, compared with six possible arrangements with the four-item sequences). With three-item sequences, subjects can choose one sound as the anchor and make only a single decision concerning the following sound. The ordering is completed with this single decision, since the remaining sound must precede the anchor. When this process was used for card ordering with three-item sequences of nonverbal sounds, the threshold was about 200 ms/item (Warren and Ackroff, 1976).

Why is it not possible to identify the order of

nonverbal sequences below 200 ms/item? And why does the threshold for identification of vowel order have the considerably lower value of 100 ms/item? The answer seems to involve the time required for linguistic processing. Both Helmholtz (1870/1954) and Garner (1951) found that counting the number of identical acoustic events within extended sequences was not possible when the rate of occurrence exceeded five or six per second. Counting and the naming of items in the order of occurrence both require the fixing of distinctive verbal labels to successive events. The time required for verbal labeling may set the limit for both counting and the naming of order (Warren, 1974a). This suggestion also can explain why the threshold drops below 200 ms when recycled sequences consist of vowels or monosyllabic words. Verbal encoding of speech sounds may be facilitated not only because listeners are very familiar with these items but also because the sound itself is its own name. Teranishi (1977) independently arrived at the same explanation. Working with four-item recycled sequences consisting of either unrelated nonverbal sounds or Japanese vowels, he concluded that the rate-determining step in identification of order was the time required for naming, and that vowels can be ordered at high presentation rates because the sounds are equivalent to the verbal labels.

If verbal encoding time determines the threshold for identification of order, similar thresholds should be observed for visual and auditory sequences. Terence O'Brien and Anne Treisman (1970) recycled three visual items (successive geometric figures or successive colors) in a three-channel tachistoscope and found the threshold for identifying order to be about 200 ms/item (personal communication). Sperling and Reeves (1980) presented a rapid series of digits on an oscilloscope and reported that although the digits could be recognized, their order could not be named. They concluded that this difficulty was analogous to that for sequences of sounds.

The thresholds for identification of the order of sounds forming extended sequences are quite high, ranging from about 100 to 550 ms/item, depending on the nature of the sounds and the response procedure. Although the 100 ms threshold for order identification within vowel sequences is lower than for sequences of nonverbal sounds, this value is still higher than the average duration of phonemes in speech. These averages range from about 70 to 100 ms in normal discourse, and some intelligibility is possible down to average durations of 30 ms/phoneme (see Warren [1982]) for discussion). If we cannot identify the order of constituent phonemes, how can we understand speech? Before trying to answer this question, let us look further at some of the rules governing perception of acoustic sequences in general.

When recycled sequences consisting of different arrangements of the same sounds have item durations below the threshold for identification of order, they are not perceptually equivalent. Warren (1974a) found that the ability to recognize and discriminate permuted orders involves recognition of the overall patterns and does not require resolution of a pattern into an ordered series of items. Sequences consisted of four sounds (tone, noise, /i/, and buzz). The items in sequence A were always 200 ms (which was found to be below the threshold for identification of order). Sequence B had one of eight item durations (127, 160, 200, 215, 315, 415, 515, or 600 ms), and the order of items was either identical to that of sequence A for the same pairs or had the order of the noise and the buzz interchanged for different pairs (Fig. 12-4).

Accuracy declined as the item duration of sequence B decreased or increased from that of sequence A. Of especial interest is the low accuracy for the longest item durations in sequence B which would permit listeners to identify the order within that sequence. If the accurate same-different order judgments obtained when the two sequences had similar item durations involved a recognition of the actual order of components, then the accuracy of judgments should not decrease when the duration of items in sequence B was made longer. The results were interpreted in terms of a *temporal template* defining the extent of temporal mismatch permitting pattern recognition. This temporal specificity raises an interesting consideration that will become clearer if we turn a moment to vision. It is possible to recognize the same object at different distances, despite changes in the visual angle subtended, so that a pattern of stimulation corresponding to a retinal image need not match a stored template as a casting matches its mold. Thus, a smaller photograph may be placed alongside an enlargement of the same picture, and identity or difference can be recognized despite disparity in size. Since the temporal dimension in hearing is often

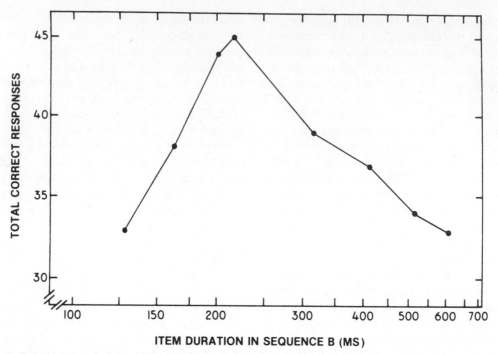

FIGURE 12-4 The extent of temporal mismatch permitting pattern recognition. Scores for correct same-or-different judgments are shown for pairs of recycled sequences consisting of the same four sounds arranged in either identical or permuted orders. Sequence A always had component sounds lasting 200 ms, and the duration of items in sequence B is given by the abscissa. The maximum score for correct responses is 60. Each data point is based on responses of separate groups of 30 subjects. (From Warren, R. M. [1974]. Auditory pattern discrimination by untrained listeners. *Perception & Psychophysics, 15,* 495-500.)

considered analogous to the spatial dimension in vision, we might expect that same-different judgments could be made over a wide range of temporal differences. However, the observed limits for temporal disparities permitting matching suggest that auditory pattern recognition uses temporal templates with rather strict durational limits for component items. Of course, with speech and music, some limited degree of durational flexibility is tolerated. Recently, both upper and lower durational limits of notes permitting the recognition of familiar melodic phrases were determined. When the phrases were played repetitively, the recognition limits corresponded to the range normally used for playing melodies (roughly 150 ms to 1 sec/note). The upper recognition limit was extended for those who could read and write musical notation (Warren et al., 1991).

Since same-different judgments are possible for pairs of recycled sequences of unrelated sounds having item durations of 200 ms, would listeners be able to distinguish identical from permuted orders at still briefer durations? To answer this question, Warren and Ackroff

(1976) used sequences of three items. In one experiment pairs of recycled sequences consisting of a tone, a square wave, and a noise were used. All the items within a pair had the same duration, but the order of components varied. The accuracy of judging whether the two sequences were the same or different was significantly above chance for a group of untrained listeners for all of the item durations, which ranged from 5 ms through 400 ms. At 200 ms and above, accurate same-different judgments could be made through direct identification of the components in their proper order for each of the arrangements. At durations below 200 ms, not only could order not be identified, but the component sounds themselves could not be recognized. It was suggested that the elements of brief sequences form *temporal compounds* with properties characteristic of their particular temporal arrangements, and which cannot be decomposed perceptually into their constituents (Warren, 1974b; Warren and Ackroff, 1976). However, it was quite easy for listeners to learn accurate analytical descriptions of temporal compounds through indirect means (Warren, 1974b). (For a more detailed description of the concept of temporal compounds and its implications for speech perception, see Warren, 1982, 1993).

Warren, Bashford, and Gardner (1990) demonstrated that the rules followed by sequences of brief nonverbal sounds were also followed by sequences of steady-state vowels, but with an interesting linguistic twist when the vowels had durations corresponding to phonemes in speech. Listeners could distinguish between different arrangements within recycled sequences of three vowels for the entire range of durations employed, extending from 10 ms/vowel (single glottal pulses) through 5 sec/vowel. At durations above 100 ms/vowel, the components could be named in their proper order with ease, and different arrangements were discriminated on that basis. From 30 to 10 ms/item the sequences of steady-state vowels did not resemble an assemblage of speech sounds, and discrimination was accomplished through differences in quality (such as one order described as "crisp" and the other as "dull"). However, for vowel durations of 30 through 100 ms (corresponding roughly to the range of phonemic durations occurring in conversational speech), different orders were distinguished through an especially interesting illusion. **Phonemic transformations** occurred, and the vowel sequences were heard as verbal forms—that is, as syllables and words—with different verbal organizations reported for different arrangements of the same vowels. These linguistic temporal compounds have a number of surprising characteristics now under investigation, as discussed in the next section. However, this initial study demonstrated that sequences consisting solely of vowels are heard as syllables consisting of consonants along with vowels other than those actually present. It was found that these verbal forms follow the phonotactic rules governing the permissible ordering of speech sounds in English (for example, syllables starting with /ts/ or /sr/ are not heard). Verbal organization was obligatory, and the listeners could not perceive the sequences as a succession of vowels even when they tried. Yet when the individual vowels (produced by the iteration of a single 10 ms glottal pulse excised from a recording of the vowel produced by a male speaker) were heard in isolation at the same durations (30 to 100 ms) that produced verbal organization, each could be identified by the listeners. Apparently the presence of the other

contiguous vowels results in formation of verbal temporal compounds, which as with nonverbal temporal compounds, cannot be resolved into the actual acoustic components.

Do phonemes in normal speech also form linguistic temporal compounds? If so, the ability to hear phonemic components and their orders within the syllables and words of normal speech may itself involve an illusion. That is, listeners may recognize temporal compounds corresponding to syllables and words and then infer the existence of the ordered series of phonetic components required to form these groupings. There is evidence along several lines that this may be the case. Savin and Bever (1970) found that the identification time for a nonsense syllable was always shorter than that for a phoneme within that syllable. These findings were confirmed in an independent study (Warren, 1971) completed shortly before their work was published. Besides employing stimuli consisting of nonsense syllables, as did Savin and Bever, the nature of both the syllables and their context was systematically varied. The four types of stimuli used were (1) a nonsense syllable list, (2) a word list, (3) sentences with the target word having a low contextual probability, and (4) sentences with the target word having a high contextual probability. For each type, the identification time for a phoneme was always greater than the identification time for the syllable containing that phoneme. The identification times for the words (and the longer identification times for phonemes within the words) were about the same for types 1, 2, and 3. When prior context made the target word's occurrence more probable with stimulus type 4, identification time for the word decreased, as might be expected. Furthermore, identification times for a phoneme within that word changed correspondingly, indicating that the phoneme identification was derived from a prior higher-level organization.

The second experiment in this study measured identification times for letter targets in the spelling of the same auditory stimuli by a separate group of subjects. (As in the first experiment, listeners were mostly staff, visiting scientists, and graduate students at an English university and so presumably were familiar with the vagaries of British orthography.) Some of the spoken words had irregular spelling, so auditory lexical recognition had to be achieved before the letters forming the word could be determined. Identification times matched those found for phonemic targets, suggesting that although grapheme and phoneme identification are functionally separate processes, each is derived from prior identification of the spoken word. Although there seem to have been no further studies dealing with the identification time for letters in spoken words, a considerable number of subsequent studies have confirmed the basic observation that identification of constituent phonemes takes more time than identification of the syllables or words in which they occur (see Massaro [1979] for a description of this work and a discussion of the implications for theory).

The evidence indicates that identification of the order of components in sequences of brief sounds (including those of speech) is a two-stage process: (1) identification of a global pattern, followed by (2) recitation of a learned analytical description of that pattern. The next section explores some of the processes in the perceptual organization of speech sounds using vowel sequences as an investigative tool.

TWEAKING THE SYLLABARY: IMPLICATIONS OF THE ILLUSORY ORGANIZATION OF LOUD AND CLEAR VOWEL SEQUENCES

As mentioned in the previous section, Warren, Bashford, and Gardner (1990) reported that sequences of steady-state vowels repeated loudly and clearly can become organized into either real words or nonsense words. From roughly 30 to 100 ms per vowel it is not possible to perceive the sequence as a series of vowels, and an obligatory verbal organization takes place. The characteristics of verbal organizations achieved with this unusual stimulus provide new insights into the processes employed for comprehending speech.

In the first of the experiments reported, recycled sequences of three vowels were used, and different words were heard for the two possible arrangements (/ʌæiʌ . . ./ and /ʌiæʌ. . ./), permitting easy discrimination between the two orders. A second experiment in this study employed much more complex vowel sequences consisting of recycled sequences of 10 40-ms steady-state vowels. There are factorial nine (362,880) possible arrangements of these vowels, and 48 were selected randomly for the experimental stimuli. In the initial portion of this experiment, the 48 sequences were divided

into 12 sets of 4 items. The sequences in each set were labeled A, B, C, and D, and listeners were told to write down the words heard next to the letters representing each sequence, so that the sequences could be identified subsequently. They were then presented with the same 4 sequences in scrambled order as unknowns. Matching of each of the 4 sequences with the corresponding verbal forms heard earlier was easy, and performance for all 12 sets was nearly perfect. Most of the verbal forms heard (65%) consisted of English words and phrases. The remaining verbal forms were nonlexical, but in this and subsequent studies, they not only followed the phonotactic rules of English but almost always were syllables actually occurring in English. The implications of this restriction will be discussed subsequently.

In the next part of the study, the same 48 sequences were used to construct 48 sequence pairs, members of each pair differing only in the transposition of 2 of the 10 40-ms contiguous vowels. Listeners made ABX judgments; that is, one member of the pair was designated as A and the other as B, and listeners were required to tell whether the vowel sequence X was the same as A or B. Listeners again used verbal mediation, and they reported different words characterizing each of the minimally different arrangements of the same components. Accuracy in identifying sequence X was near 100%. The task was repeated several days later with the same stimulus pairs, and performance was again nearly perfect. Listeners' verbal organizations of particular vowel sequences were stable over time: over half the forms reported by individual subjects on the second presentation of the 96 sequences were the same as the forms they heard earlier for the same sequence. A curious feature of vowel transformations is that only a limited portion of the acoustic signal is organized into a particular verbal form. A residue is perceived and occasionally is heard as a simultaneous nonverbal noise but more frequently as a second verbal organization. This second form has a different timbre or quality and appears to consist of different spectral components (the basis for this perceptual splitting is discussed later).

A subsequent study by Chalikia and Warren (1991) mapped the correspondence between the phonemes physically present and the illusory phonemes heard with recycled sequences of six 80-ms vowels. Three procedures that might seem appropriate for matching the stimulus

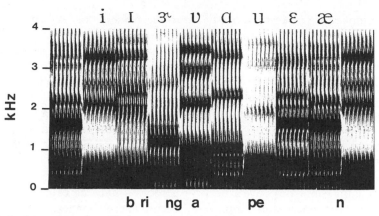

FIGURE 12-5 Mapping of an illusory phrase heard with a repeated sequence of eight 80-ms steady-state vowels. The vowels are shown above the spectrogram, and the onsets of the illusory speech sounds forming the phrase "bring a pen" are shown below.

phonemes and their transforms did not work. The reasons they failed provide additional information about the nature of verbal organization. (1) It might be thought that if one of the vowels was made louder, the listener could tell which portion of the illusory word increased in level. However, the listeners heard no change in the illusory words. Instead, the item having a louder level was heard as an isolated vowel that was identified accurately but could not be localized within the illusory word, which itself did not change. Thus, a type of duplex perception occurred in which a portion of the vowel was transformed into a different speech sound or sounds, while the remainder of the stimulus vowel was heard as a separate item and identified correctly. (2) Removing a vowel and then listening for the portion of the illusory word that seemed to become weaker or disappear failed to reveal that vowel's contribution to the verbal form, since the entire sequence was reorganized and a different verbal form was heard. (3) Superimposing a click as a marker for a particular vowel also failed, since nonspeech sounds cannot be localized accurately within a word (Ladefoged, 1959; Ladefoged and Broadbent, 1960).

Fortunately, there is a technique that can determine the stimulus vowels corresponding to illusory speech sounds. This mapping of illusory words employed a procedure used to locate the perceptual boundaries of phonemes within words (Warren and Sherman, 1974). This earlier study showed that when a sentence is terminated abruptly, the last speech sound can be identified with ease, and by adjusting the cutoff position, phonemic boundaries could be located with

considerable precision and accuracy (as measured by within-listener reproducibility and across-listener agreement as well as by inspection of sound spectrograms). Chalikia and Warren (1991) interrupted the vowel sequences at the middle and end of each steady-state vowel and asked listeners to report the last speech sound heard (Fig. 12-5). Before mapping the illusory verbal forms, each subject mapped a repeating real English word and a repeating nonsense word to ensure that they could match the perceptual phonemes with the corresponding physical phonemes of a repeated utterance. As anticipated, with these practice words, mapping agreed with estimates of the position of the interruptions based on inspection of the sound spectrograms. However, when a vowel sequence was interrupted, the terminal steady-state vowel invariably maintained its false identity as a portion of the illusory verbal form. Even when listeners, who knew that the stimulus consisted of a sequence of vowels, tried to identify the terminal vowel, they failed. Only the position of its illusory transform within the illusory syllable or word could be inferred. Considering this observation, why can listeners accurately identify the terminal phoneme when a real utterance is interrupted? Is it possible that the analysis of real utterances into an ordered succession of phonemes is also inferential, dependent on a prior higher-level organization?

Chalikia and Warren (1991) also reported results for mapping of the second, typically less salient form heard along with the first. Usually the primary form was of greater phonetic complexity than the secondary form. The two illusory organizations more often than not had no phonemes in common, and their onsets corresponded to different stimulus vowels. As in the Warren, Bashford, and Gardner (1990) study, the two illusory forms had different timbres and often seemed to be produced by speakers with different accents or enunciation characteristics.

The forms heard for the same sequence by individual listeners were not completely idiosyncratic but were often similar and sometimes identical, indicating that some objective acoustic features of the vowel sequences were employed the same way across listeners. This observation was confirmed in a subsequent study that used six different arrangements of four 60-ms vowels (Chalikia, Warren, and Bashford, 1992). A 300-ms silent gap separated two of the vowels, ensuring that the verbal organization of each subject started at the same position in the sequence. Listeners transcribed the forms heard for each of the arrangements. Then each subject was assigned randomly to a partner, and the pairs attempted to match the forms reported by the other person to the appropriate sequences. Most listeners achieved a perfect correspondence of sequences to the forms reported by their partner for each of the six stimuli, demonstrating common psychoacoustic bases for their phonemic transformations.

Warren, Bashford, and Gardner (1990) offered some speculations concerning the mechanisms responsible for the illusory transformation of vowels into syllables and words. They started with the assumption that a listener hearing a sequence of speech sounds tends to interpret the stimulus in terms of a verbal utterance. But how can this tendency cause a series of steady-state vowels to be heard as a word? It was suggested that listeners employ a set of criteria or auditory templates for identifying a syllable or word, and that repetition produces a shift in the criteria. According to the **criterion shift rule** for perceptual processing in general (Warren, 1985), the criteria for evaluation and classification of stimuli are displaced toward simultaneous or recent exemplars. These shifts can provide adaptive flexibility in everyday life, normally leading to a perceptual homeostasis under changing conditions. In psycholinguistic laboratory studies, application of this rule is reflected in shifts in the acoustic boundaries employed for categorizing speech sounds following exposure to repeated syllables. For example, after listening

to the syllable "ta" repeated over and over, the voice onset time corresponding to the perceptual boundary between /t/ and /d/ should shift in the direction of the /t/. Such shifts were reported by Eimas and Corbit in 1973, and since then have been studied extensively. There is considerable controversy concerning the underlying processes responsible for these changes in phonemic boundaries following repetition (see Diehl, Kluender, and Parker [1985] for discussion), but general acceptance of the evidence that repetition-induced category boundary shifts do occur. These changes in criteria are much more profound when observed while repetition is in progress (as with the repeated vowel sequences) than after repetition ceases (as in the typical studies measuring the extent of category boundary shifts). It appears that the effects produced during stimulation by a repeated sequence of steady-state vowels can change the acoustic requirements for perception of a particular syllable or word to the point where the vowel sequence is perceived as that verbal form. Similar conclusions emerged from a study of changes of one syllable to another heard while listening to a continuing repetition of the stimulus "to-do" (Warren and Meyers, 1987).

Warren, Bashford, and Gardner (1990) hypothesized that the verbal organization of vowel sequences is facilitated not only by criterion shifts but also by splitting the stimulus and using separate components for the simultaneous percepts. The different timbres of the concurrent verbal organizations suggested that different spectral components were used for the two forms. Chalikia and Warren (1994) used spectral filtering and found that one member of the paired verbal organizations corresponded to frequencies above roughly 1500 Hz and the other to frequencies below it. Many studies have shown that this frequency, about 1500 Hz, divides stimuli consisting of word lists or sentences into high and low ranges of equal intelligibility, and intelligibility scores of over 98% have been reported for standard test sentences that were either high-pass filtered at 1700 Hz or low-pass filtered at 1100 Hz (Bashford and Warren, 1987b). Warren, Bashford, and Gardner (1990) hypothesized that separate high-frequency and low-frequency templates are available for verbal organization when identification of utterances is difficult, and that broadband vowel sequences can undergo a spectral split and activate both types of templates following repetition-induced criterion shifts. If only one frequency-limited template is activated, the residual spectral components of a vowel sequence are heard not as speech but as a nonlinguistic noise. The existence of frequency-limited templates can be useful under noisy conditions when portions of the speech spectrum may escape masking.

We can now approach the nature of the organizational units of the initial processing of speech. The forms reported by listeners are frequently English words, but nonlexical forms are also heard. In addition to following the phonotactic rules governing the clustering of phonemes, the forms reported almost always correspond to syllables occurring in English. Although there are several thousand syllables that are English words or occur in English words, many more can be constructed that conform to the phonotactic rules governing the grouping of phonemes. The observation that the syllables heard with the repeated vowel sequences correspond to those occurring in English indicates that we possess a stored English syllabary in addition to a stored English lexicon, and that the syllabary can be tapped directly without prior access to the lexicon. It is not suggested, however, that speech perception normally proceeds stepwise from English syllable to English word and then on up to phrase and sentence. Speech perception appears to be variable and opportunistic, in keeping with the LAME (lateral access from multilevel engrams) model of speech perception (Warren, 1981), which considers that verbal organization can involve not only interactive bottom-up and top-down processing but also processing across comparable levels of linguistic complexity. Different listening tasks can limit organizational levels and restrict processing strategies. The organizations heard while listening to a sequence of brief vowels reveal a class of engrams or templates consisting of syllables that actually occur in English. Under these linguistically impoverished conditions, organization can be frozen at a syllabic level because of the lack of information normally leading to additional processing at lexical and sentential levels. The freezing of organization at the syllabic level can also be observed in jargon aphasia. Miller (1991, p. 83) said:

> "The rules for forming admissible syllables . . . seem to be learned at an extremely deep level. Even when injuries to the brain result in 'jargon aphasia,' a condition in which the victim can speak fluently but is largely unintelligible because the speech is dense with nonwords, nearly all the neologisms that are generated still conform to the conventional rules of syllable formation."

Perhaps the reason that nearly all of the neologisms of jargon aphasia conform to the rules of syllable formation is that while access to an inventory of lexical items is impaired, access to a prelexical inventory of English syllables is still available.

If one continues to listen to repeated vowel sequences after the initial organization into verbal forms takes place, illusory changes in what the voices seem to be saying can occur (Riener and Warren, 1990). A similar instability occurs when a recorded word is played over and over. This **verbal transformation** effect is discussed next.

ILLUSORY CHANGES IN REPEATED WORDS: THE VERBAL TRANSFORMATION EFFECT

It has been known for a long time that continued stimulation with an unchanging pattern can lead to illusory changes, or under some conditions, to perceptual fading and disappearance. In the seventeenth century John Locke noted, *"The mind cannot fix long on one invariable idea"* (Locke, 1690/1894, p. 244, italics his). He concluded (p. 245) that any attempt by an individual to restrict his thoughts to any one concept would fail, and new concepts or modifications of the old ". . .will constantly succeed one another in his thoughts, let him be as wary as he can."

Perceptually unstable figures have a long history as visual designs. A mosaic floor depicting stacked cubes that reverse in apparent perspective has been uncovered at the temple of Apollo at Pompeii. This design, as well as more intricate and ingenious reversible figures, can be seen in medieval and renaissance Italian churches (for photographs see Warren, 1981). Perhaps the richest collection is on the floor of St. Mark's in Venice, providing a dynamic counterpoint for the nonreversible devotional figures seen by raising the eyes heavenward to the ceiling mosaics. However, these reversible floor designs do not seem to have provoked any scientific curiosity. But Necker (1832) called attention to the illusory changes in apparent perspective of an outline drawing of a rhomboid and tried to explain the inversions in terms of perceptual processes. Many reversible figures have been constructed and studied since.

All of the visually reversible figures are actually ambiguous; that is, they have plausible alternative interpretations. These interpretations employ the same contours as parts of different perceptual organizations so that at any given time, one interpretation precludes the other. While three or more interpretations may be possible (especially with some classical mosaics), most figures have only two. A consideration of these facts led me to look for an auditory analog of the visual reversible figures using repeated words.

If a person repeats a word over and over, a lapse of meaning called semantic or **verbal satiation** usually occurs (Titchener, 1915; Amster, 1964). It is possible to create an ambiguous verbal stimulus by repeating aloud a word such as "ace" to oneself over and over without pauses; the stimulus should be acoustically equivalent to the repeated word "say." Would perceptual alternation occur between these two plausible interpretations of the stimulus and so prevent lapses of meaning? When I tried this for myself (as you can for yourself), such alternations did seem to occur. These observations suggested the desirability of further work in which articulation of the stimulus by the listener would be avoided. In a preliminary study, Richard Gregory and I prepared short loops of recorded tapes containing single words. When we played these tapes to ourselves and others in the laboratory, we found that changes of the sort anticipated seem to occur. But surprisingly, compelling illusory changes in phonetic structure were observed as well, even though the words were played clearly and listeners knew that each iteration was identical. Our bias was such that the note describing our observations was entitled "An auditory analog of the visual reversible figure" (Warren and Gregory, 1958). However, after subsequent work, I concluded that passive listening to repeated words produces both phonetic and semantic lability. This is in sharp contrast with the effects of restating a word to oneself, which produces only verbal satiation (or perceptual alternation for words that become ambiguous stimuli when repeated) without illusory changes in the phonetic structure. I came to believe that the auditory illusion that occurs while listening to recorded repetitions, which I named the **verbal transformation effect,** was not closely analogous to visual reversals.

To illustrate the sorts of changes reported for verbal transformations (VTs) in the first detailed study (Warren, 1961a), I will give a few examples obtained from subjects listening for 3 minutes to a loop of tape containing a clear statement of a single word repeated over and over. Subjects were instructed to call out what they heard initially and then to call out each change as it occurred, whether the change was to something new or to a form reported previously. The changes generally seemed quite real, and listeners believed that they were simply reporting what the voice was saying. The first example of illusory changes given below is based upon the stimulus "seashore" (since British naval ratings were used as subjects, a voice with standard English pronunciation was employed, and the terminal /r/ was not pronounced). The initial perceptual organization and all of the illusory changes reported by one subject during three minutes are listed in the order of occurrence: *seashore, sea-shove, seashore, she-saw, seesaw, sea-shove, seashore, she-saw-seesaw, seashore, she-saw-seesaw, seashore, she-sawve, seashore-seesaw, she-saw, seashore, seesaw-saw, seashell.* Another subject listening to "ripe" reported: *ripe, right, white, white-light, right, right-light, ripe, right, ripe, bright-light, right, ripe, bright-light, right, bright-light.* As a final example, a third subject listening to "fill-up" heard somewhat fewer changes and greater phonetic distortion than most: *fill-up, clock, fill-up, buildup, true love, build, broad, lunch, fill-up.* Note that changes that occur in going from one perceptual form to the next are frequently quite complex phonetically and sometimes suggest semantic linkages.

The main distinctions between VTs and visual reversible figures revealed by this study are these: (1) Visual reversible figures correspond to relatively few special configurations—VTs occur with all syllables, words, and phrases. (2) Reversible figures generally involve reinterpretation without appreciable distortion of the stimulus configuration—VTs usually involve considerable distortion of clear auditory stimuli. (3) Each of the reversible figures generally involves the same perceptual forms for different people—VTs vary greatly with individuals. (4) Reversible figures generally invoke changes between two and occasionally three or four forms—VTs usually involve more than four and sometimes more than a dozen different forms during 2 or 3 minutes. Yet there is some relation between these two types of illusions. In broad terms, both seem to reflect the principle stated by John

Locke (1690) that no particular thought or perceptual organization can be maintained without change for any length of time.

There is a visual effect that seems to resemble verbal transformations more closely than do reversible figures. If the small eye tremors (physiological nystagmus) that occur continuously during normal vision are canceled optically to produce a fixed or stabilized retinal image, perception becomes unstable. As Wheatstone (1835) concluded after considering the rapid perceptual fading of the shadows of retinal blood vessels when their images were fixed, the pattern of sensory input must change continually to maintain perceptual stability. Subsequent studies have shown that stabilized retinal images in general are seen to fade, fragment, disappear, and sometimes reappear in a dynamic display of illusory changes (Riggs et al., 1953; Pritchard, Heron, and Hebb, 1960). While the selective suppression of portions of a pattern is found for verbal transformations as well, the auditory illusion produces a greater distortion and synthesis of physically absent elements than do stabilized retinal images.

Subsequent studies have indicated that verbal transformations may be a valuable tool for studying speech perception. No attempt will be made to cover all aspects of VTs reported in the more than 50 papers published on this topic (for reviews, see Warren, 1968b, 1976, 1982). This discussion will deal briefly with acoustic and phonetic factors involved in VTs and, in somewhat more detail, implications concerning the mechanisms employed normally for perceptual processing of speech sounds. In addition, the relation of VTs to other phenomena in speech perception will be described. The measures traditionally used in experimental studies of the rate and variety of VTs are *transitions,* or numbers of changes, and *forms,* or different perceptual organizations, heard while listening to a particular repeated syllable, word, or sentence for periods ranging from 3 to 5 minutes.

The first detailed phonetic analysis of the verbal transformation effect was that of Barnett (1964). After using a variety of words as stimuli and examining the forms reported, she concluded that the articulatory positions of both vowels and consonants were relatively labile and subject to frequent illusory changes. Stability was noted for the voiced-voiceless property of consonants and the type of movement charac-

teristic of individual consonants and vowels. Intervowel glides were generally stable both in position and type of movement.

A study of the nature of phone-type substitutions by linguists and nonlinguists, each group consisting of native and nonnative speakers of English, listening to the repeated word "cogitate" was reported at a meeting of the Acoustical Society of America (Naeser and Lilly, 1970). In an unpublished manuscript based on this paper, they reported that people with linguistic training and those lacking such training gave similar responses. Consonants generally were substituted by the manner of articulation (not place) so that, for example, stops most often were substituted for other stops. On the other hand, vowels most often were substituted on the basis of similarity of place of articulation. A resemblance was noted to the articulatory feature-type substitution described by Wickelgren (1965, 1966) in his work on errors in short-term memory. Subsequently, Lass and Gasperini (1973) published a study comparing verbal transformations for a number of stimulus words presented to phonetically trained and phonetically untrained subjects. They noted some quantitative differences between the two groups, but emphasized that responses were qualitatively similar in agreement with the findings of Naeser and Lilly. The phonetically trained group reported more forms and transitions and required fewer repetitions of the stimuli to induce the first illusory change.

Clegg (1971) used 18 separate repeating syllables, each consisting of a different consonant followed by the vowel /i/. He ignored the illusory changes of the vowel, which he found minimal, and analyzed the transformations of the consonants. His analysis was in rough agreement with Naeser and Lilly's report but considerably more detailed. He concluded that a consonant and its transform tended to share the features of voicing, nasality, and affrication but not of duration and place of articulation.

Evans and Wilson (1968) also used a variety of consonants followed by the same vowel as stimuli for VTs. They analyzed responses only for changes in the initial consonant and reported a surprisingly high frequency of responses involving the aspirated phoneme /h/. Goldstein and Lackner (1974), in a more comprehensive study, used a variety of nonsense syllables as stimuli and found a large number of responses involving illusory /h/ and /j/. Not interested in these intrusions, they constructed matrices for illusory transformation of consonants and vowels for which /h/ and /j/ were excluded. Analysis of these matrices for distinctive features revealed a number of "very systematic" types of changes governing vowels and consonants, which they summarized. However, subsequent work by Lackner, Tuller, and Goldstein (1977) with repeated syllables suggested to them that feature detectors were not involved either in VTs or speech perception in general. This belief was not shared by Ohde and Sharf (1979), who attributed VTs to adaptation of feature detectors that respond selectively to particular acoustic aspects of the repeated stimulus. More recently, Debigaré (1984) has proposed that VTs are a consequence of changes in cortical "cell assemblies" described by Donald Hebb.

Lass and Golden (1971) employed repeating stimuli consisting of 200-ms statements of a single steady-state vowel separated by 500 ms of silence. Onset and decay characteristics of single utterances of the vowel were lacking, so the statements differed from normal speech productions. A high proportion of nonphonetic alternatives were reported (such as a telephone busy signal), perhaps reflecting the difference of the stimulus from normal speech productions. Changes usually involved illusory consonants, generally plosives, possibly due to the rapid onset and termination of the vowels. No analysis of distinctive features was offered.

The effects of noise on VTs are curious. When a voice can be heard but is not quite intelligible because of noise, the rate and variety of VTs are very different from those observed with words repeated clearly. While it seems reasonable to assume that a word that is heard less clearly should change more readily, such is not the case; partially masked speech has a considerably lower rate of VTs than clear speech (Warren, 1961a).

Sadler (1989) found that noise *per se* did not influence VTs. Rather it was the level above the threshold for intelligibility that determined the nature of verbal transformations, so the effects of noise could be duplicated by decreasing the amplitude of the voice in the absence of background noise. Once the voice was intelligible, further increase in level had little effect on either numbers of transitions or forms. However, when an intelligible voice was made louder, transitions from one form to the next involved fewer phonemes, and somewhat surprisingly, the ratio of nonsense forms to lexical forms increased.

Is it possible to observe any illusory changes while listening to repeated nonverbal stimuli? A number of experimenters have reported such illusory changes, but they seem different from VTs in important respects. Repetitions of white noise bursts were used by Lass, West, and Taft (1973); tone bursts by Fenelon and Blayden (1968), Perl (1970), and Lass, West, and Taft (1973); and melodic phrases by Guilford and Nelson (1936), Obusek (1971), and Lass, West, and Taft (1973). The changes reported in these studies generally were slight alterations in loudness, pitch, and tempo, with the rate of such changes sometimes similar to and sometimes slower than the rates corresponding to VTs. However, experimenters generally have ignored the fact that the analog tape recorders that they used produce slight variations in intensity (loudness) and speed (pitch and tempo). Even high-quality professional recorders can have moment-to-moment changes of about 1 dB in intensity and about 0.3% in both record and playback speed, which are at or just above the thresholds for detecting such differences. Anyone who has listened to an analog tape recording of an extended tone (e.g., 1000 Hz) rather than on-line output from an oscillator probably has encountered this instability. Of course, it may be that illusory variations are introduced with repetition of nonverbal stimuli that go beyond those corresponding to the instability of recordings. This hypothesis can be tested by using digital recording and playback that produce fluctuations well below threshold; I have found that verbal transformations still occur under these conditions of stimulus stability. Perhaps a general perceptual lability of unchanging patterns has been specially modified for speech. As we shall see, the verbal lability seems related to processes normally leading to improved intelligibility. Studies of age differences for VTs have suggested that this illusion employs mechanisms that normally aid in the comprehension of speech and that these mechanisms change systematically from childhood through old age.

A single tape recording of five repeated words was used in a cross-sectional age study of VTs in our laboratory. Experiments with children showed virtually no transitions at 5 years of age (Warren and Warren, 1966). At 6 years, almost half the subjects tested heard illusory changes, and those subjects heard them at the high rate found for older children. At age 8, all subjects heard illusory changes and during the 3-minute

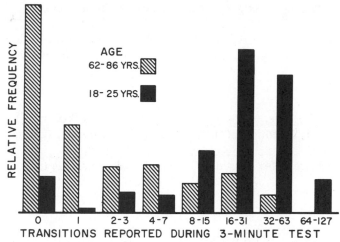

FIGURE 12-6 Distribution of scores for transitions heard by young and elderly adults. (From Warren, R. M. [1961]. Illusory changes in repeated words: Differences between young adults and the aged. *American Journal of Psychology, 74,* 506-516.)

stimulation time per word, the average number of transitions was 34. This rate remained about the same (32 changes in 3 minutes) at age 10 years. In a previous study using the same stimuli, the average rate of change (31 in 3 minutes) for young adults 18 to 25 years of age was equivalent to that of the 8- and 10-year-old children (Warren, 1961b). However, this study also revealed that the rate for adults aged 62 to 86 years was much lower (5.6 in 3 minutes), with many of the older listeners hearing no changes (Fig. 12-6).

Using subjects with a median age of 35 years and different stimulus words, Taylor and Henning (1963) reported a rate of illusory changes between that for young and aged adults, suggesting that the decrease in susceptibility during adulthood occurs gradually. The decrease in VTs with older adults does not seem to reflect a decrease in auditory acuity with age, since the aged not only maintain stability in what they hear but are more accurate as a group, generally reporting the correct word and staying with it. One might think that an increase in so-called *neural noise* associated with aging would reduce the effective signal-to-noise ratio for a given sound pressure level, and that this reduced ratio is responsible for the difference between young and old adults listening to a stimulus delivered at the same intensity. However, once a signal is intelligible, changes in the signal-to-noise ratio have only small effects upon the rate of VTs. A rather different suggestion will be offered after some additional factors have been addressed.

In addition to counting the numbers of illusory changes, the groupings of speech sounds were examined to determine the functional rules governing reorganization at different ages (Warren and Warren, 1966). Children responded in terms of the sounds of English, but they sometimes violated phonotactic rules and grouped these sounds in ways not permitted in the language. For example, with the repeated word "tress", a child reported "sreb", although the initial /sr/ sequence is not found in English words. Young adults also reported some nonsense syllables, but these always conformed to the phonotactic rules of English. An interesting question not addressed to date is whether nonlexical responses of young adults are restricted to syllables occurring in English, as Chalikia and Warren (1991) reported for forms heard with repeated vowel sequences. The group of adults over 62 years of age tended to report only meaningful words. Presented with "tress", they typically heard "tress" continuously, and when changes did occur, they usually were to such closely related forms as "dress" (Warren, 1961b). Even when presented with a nonsense syllable such as "flime", the older adults usually did not report the stimulus but distorted it into a meaningful word such as "flying", frequently hearing the distorted word throughout the 3-minute test. An interesting exception is the incorrect past participle "flyed", reported more frequently than the actual stimulus by the aged. The box compares the forms heard for the groups consisting of 20 younger

Forms reported while listening to single repeated words for three minutes

The total number of forms reported is given for each stimulus word followed by all forms reported by more than one listener, the number reporting each form given in the preceding parentheses.

TREES

Young: (72 forms). (19) tress; (11) press; (9) terez; (8) trez; (7) prez; (7) stress; (7) teress; (5) dress; (4) tressed; (3) tourist; (3) truss; (2) bread; (2) terass; (2) touress; (2) tred; (2) tresh; (2) trust.

Old: (39 forms). (18) tress; (4) tressed; (3) dress; (2) rest-tress; (2) trash; (2) tread; (2) truss; (2) trust.

SEE

Young: (73 forms). (20) see; (9) seeing; (8) pea; (6) thee [unvoiced 'th']; (5) bee; (5) tea; (4) fee; (3) dee; (2) bee-see; (2) being; (2) cease; (2) fee-see; (2) pink; (2) see-ink; (2) singing; (2) sink; (2) tea-see; (2) think.

Old: (26 forms). (20) see; (3) three; (2) fee; (2) pea; (2) see-seed; (2) tea; (2) tea-see.

FLIME

Young: (158 forms). (17) flime; (10) fly-'em; (8) fly; (7) slime; (6) climb; (6) fly-in; (6) flyed; (5) flying; (5) plime; (4) lime; (3) flibe; (3) flyer; (3) slide; (2) blime; (2) fline; (2) fly-in-flime; (2) flyumf; (2) fulime; (2) imply; (2) pline; (2) sly; (2) sulime; (2) wine.

Old: (65 forms). (8) flyed; (8) slide; (7) fly; (6) flime; (6) flying; (6) slime; (4) climb; (3) flime-slime; (2) flying-flyed; (2) fried; (2) plied.

POLICE

Young: (77 forms). (20) police; (15) please; (10) pleece; (10) peo-eece; (5) poe-eece; (4) police-please; (4) pulleys; (3) please-police; (2) oyce; (2) poyce; (2) boys; (2) pleece-police; (2) poe-iss; (2) poise; (2) pull-eece.

Old: (27 forms). (20) police; (7) please; (4) please-police; (2) peace-police; (2) police-please; (2) priest.

TRICE

Young: (101 forms). (20) trice; (9) tries; (7) price; (7) twice; (6) triced; (5) ter-ice; (5) try; (4) Christ; (4) right; (3) cry; (3) tries-trice; (3) try-ice; (2) krice; (2) estra; (2) her-eye; (2) prize; (2) ter-eyes; (2) thrice; (2) thrice-twice; (2) trice-tries; (2) try-ess; (2) try-est; (2) twiced; (2) twice-trice.

Old: (44 forms). (15) trice; (6) tries-trice; (5) twice; (4) triced; (4) tries; (3) trice-tries; (3) tripe; (3) trite; (2) Christ; (2) Christ-twice; (2) trice-Christ; (2) trice-triced; (2) trice-twice; (2) tries-twice; (2) twice-trice.

(From Warren, R. M. [1961b]. Illusory changes in repeated words: Differences between young adults and the aged. *American Journal of Psychology, 74,* 506-516.)

and 20 older adults by listing all forms heard by more than one listener in each group.

When the extent of phonemic differences between successive forms reported by individual subjects was analyzed, a regular change with age was found. For the five age groups (subjects 6 through 86 years of age), the number of phonemes changed in going from one form to the next decreased with increasing age. This decrease in the complexity of transformations seems to be associated with normal, healthy aging; the extent of phonemic changes observed with subjects diagnosed as having clear symptoms of senile deterioration approximated that of 10-year-old children (Obusek and Warren, 1973a).

These observations of the effect of aging on VTs, together with other considerations to be discussed shortly, suggest that (1) this illusion reflects reorganizational processes normally leading to the correction of errors in speech perception; and (2) the age differences observed for VTs mirror changes in processing strategies over our lifespan that can compensate for changes in functional capacity. Since performance as measured by the intelligibility of word lists and comprehension of sentences may be similar at different ages, it is all too easy to assume that the same perceptual processes are used. However, it may be necessary to change processing mechanisms to maintain performance accuracy over one's lifespan. In other words, adaptive changes in perceptual processing may be requisite for healthy maturation and aging.

Repetition of specially selected "reversible" words may produce changes more closely linked to perceptual reversals observed with such visual illusions as the Necker cube (Esposito, 1985; Roivainen, 1989; Radilova, Pöppel, and Ilmberger, 1990). Roivainen, working with repeated bisyllables, found that reversals in the order of syllables predominated, and the rate of these changes was only slightly slower for the aged subjects (64 to 86 years of age) than in that observed for young adults. This finding is in keeping with observations that changes in visual reversible figures decrease only slightly, if at all, with age (Miles, 1934). Roivainen considered that the great decrease in rate of VTs for nonreversible words in the aged resulted from the lack of some specific speech mechanism in this age group. The matter is at present unresolved, but perhaps changes in the ordering of syllables in bisyllabic reversible words should be considered as fundamentally different from verbal transformations.

Before dealing further with the changes occurring with repeated words, consider the evidence that reorganization is necessary to correct errors and resolve ambiguities while listening to speech. Bryan and Harter (1897, 1899) claimed that skilled telegraphers used a "telegraphic language" similar to other languages. Mastery required several years of continual application, perhaps 10 years, to achieve the speed and accuracy required for a press dispatcher. When this peak was obtained, the receiver could work effortlessly and automatically, often transcribing complex messages while thinking about something quite different. The expert usually delayed 6 to 12 words before transcribing the ongoing text. If redundancy and linkages between elements were reduced by transmitting in cipher or by sending stock market quotations, the task became much more difficult for expert receivers. Appreciating this difficulty, the sender slowed down the transmission rate, and the number of words held in storage by the receiver was reduced by decreasing the delay between receiving and transcribing. It seems that long storage was used only when context permitted useful interactions involving information received at different times, so that errors could be corrected and ambiguities resolved. Skilled storage similar to that observed for telegraphy has been reported for typing (Book, 1925), for reading aloud (Huey, 1968), and for tactile reading by the blind (Moore and Bliss, 1975). Storage with continuing processing and revision is probably important for comprehension of speech as well. The need for such mechanisms has been noted in the past, although the literature has been rather silent on how to study these covert processes. Brain (1962, p. 209) pointed out, "The meaning of a word which appears earlier in a sentence may depend upon the words which follow it. In such a case, the meaning of the earlier word is held in suspense, as it were, until the later words have made their appearance."

Lashley (1951, p. 120) gave a classic example of this process. He spoke of rapid writing to an audience and after creating a set for the word writing, several sentences later said, "Rapid *righting* with his uninjured hand saved from loss the contents of the capsized canoe." He pointed out that comprehension of the sentence was possible even though the context activating the proper meaning of the word did not occur until about 4 seconds after its occurrence.

It is not only meaning that depends on subsequent context. Chistovich (1962) has noted that subjects who repeated speech heard through headphones as quickly as possible made many phonemic errors. She suggested that these mistakes reflect the temporal course of speech identification, with an appreciable delay necessary to avoid such errors. Miller (1962) and Lieberman (1963) have emphasized that skilled speech perception cannot be a simple Markovian process, with perception occurring first on phonemic and then on higher levels. Such a process does not take advantage of the redundancy of the message and does not allow for the correction of mistakes. Without such correction, an error would continue to provide incorrect context, producing other errors until perception became completely disrupted.

Returning to VTs, I suggest that in addition to the perceptual instability associated with an unchanging pattern of stimulation, these illusory changes may involve reorganizational mechanisms that occur normally when the initial organization of a continuing message is inconsistent with subsequent context. With a repeated word there can be no stabilizing syntactic and semantic environment, so the stimulus is subject to successive reorganizations, none of which can receive contextual confirmation. It is important to note that these processes are considered to be quite automatic and under little cognitive control. They are not accessible through introspective search but only through their perceptual effects.

The age differences observed for VTs are consistent with this explanation. If VTs reflect skilled reorganizational processes, they should not appear in children until language skills have attained a certain level, normally by the age of 6 or 7. Certainly, the healthy over 60 years of age have mastery of language, so why do they exhibit a reduced susceptibility to VTs? The answer may be that they lack the requisite capacity for short-term storage of verbal information. It is well established that special difficulty is encountered by the aged for tasks involving complex storage that are interrupted by intervening activity (Welford, 1958). The concurrent coding, storing, and comparing required for appropriate verbal reorganization may not be possible for the elderly, so that their optimal strategy is to emphasize the previous context in organizing current input and to minimize reorganization contingent on subsequent context. The report that a higher proportion of meaningful words are reported by the aged than for young adults (Warren, 1961b) is consistent with the assumption that with a reduced capacity for reorganization, the elderly do not risk being locked to a meaningless speech fragment in their processing of discourse. VTs, when they do occur with the healthy aged, usually involve changes of a single phoneme to form another meaningful word, unlike the complex phonetic changes typical of younger listeners. The extensive phonetic changes in the infrequent VTs reported by Obusek and Warren (1973a) for senile elderly

listeners do not represent a strategy optimizing their capabilities; although this strategy may lead to meaningful organization when applied to discourse, the meaning may not match the speaker's intent. Thus, while children, young adults, and healthy elderly adults all can achieve accurate comprehension of speech, they may use different mechanisms. Equivalency in performance does not require equivalency of processing procedures.

The verbal transformation effect and the phonemic restoration effect may be linked, since each appears to be related to mechanisms employed normally for the prevention of errors and resolving ambiguities (Warren and Warren, 1970). Obusek and Warren (1973b), acting on this suggestion, combined these two illusions by presenting a repeated word ("magistrate") with a portion deleted and replaced by a louder noise. It was hypothesized that if illusory changes are indeed related to corrective mechanisms, they would be directed to the phonemically restored segment that lacked direct acoustic justification. This hypothesis was confirmed.

Figure 12-7 shows the baseline condition and the extent of illusory changes occurring at each speech sound and each syllable for the intact stimulus word. Figure 12-8 shows that when the /s/ of "magistrate" was removed and replaced by a louder noise, 42% of the illusory changes involved the position corresponding to the deleted /s/, compared with 5% when a different group of subjects heard the intact word as the repeated stimulus. Figure 12-9 shows the relative lability of phonemes for a third group of subjects when the /s/ was deleted and replaced by silence rather than noise (so that phonemic restorations were inhibited). Although the lability of phonemes heard in this position was greater than with the intact word, it was much less than that associated with noise: Only 18% of the changes involved the position of the silent gap.

When the noise replaced the /s/, listeners could not detect which phonemes were concurrent with the noise bursts, as reported earlier for restoration of a phoneme within a sentence (Warren, 1970). Yet it appears that at some level of processing, the distinction between speech-based and noise-based organization was maintained, and the perceptual reorganization was directed to the portion lacking acoustical confirmation.

As discussed earlier, phonemic restoration appears to be a special linguistic adaptation of

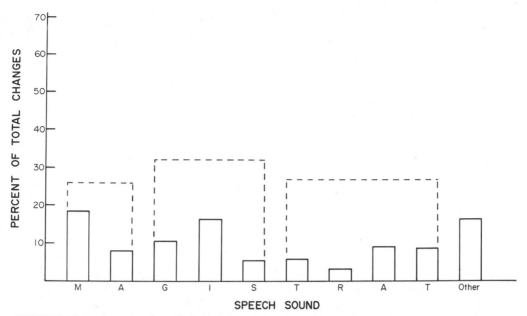

FIGURE 12-7   **Percent of total changes occurring at each speech sound and at each syllable for the intact repeated stimulus word "magistrate".** (From Obusek, C. J., & Warren, R. M. [1973]. Relation of the verbal transformation and the phonemic restoration effects. *Cognitive Psychology, 5,* 97-107.)

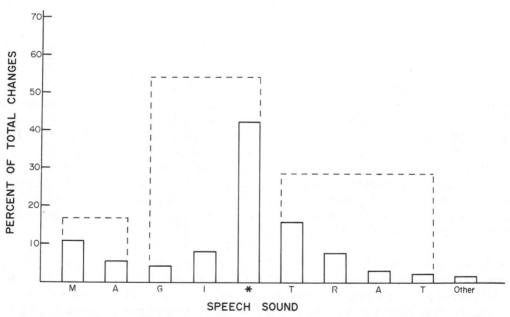

FIGURE 12-8   **Percent of total changes occurring at each speech sound and at each syllable for the repeated stimulus word "magi*trate" (the asterisk indicates the position of the speech sound deleted and replaced by noise).** (From Obusek, C. J., & Warren, R. M. [1973]. Relation of the verbal transformation and the phonemic restoration effects. *Cognitive Psychology, 5,* 97-107.)

the general phenomenon of temporal induction. It is also possible to consider verbal transformation as a special linguistic adaptation of broader perceptual rules. Two general principles appear to be involved in verbal transformations: the loss (or satiation) of a particular perceptual organization resulting from a continued exposure to a stimulus (see Amster [1964] for a discussion of verbal satiation), and the emergence of a new verbal form as a consequence of a shift in the

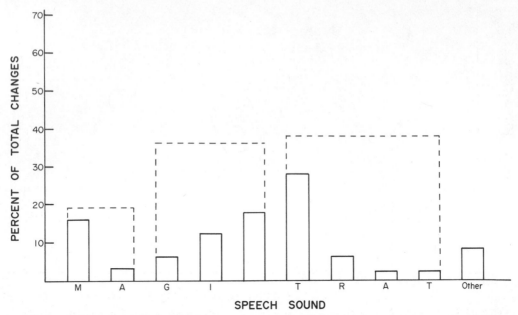

FIGURE 12-9   Percent of total changes occurring at each speech sound and at each syllable for the repeated word "magi trate" (the space indicates the position of the missing speech sound). (From Obusek, C. J., & Warren, R. M. [1973]. Relation of the verbal transformation and the phonemic restoration effects. *Cognitive Psychology, 5,* 97-107.)

auditory criteria corresponding to that form (see Warren [1984] for a discussion of criterion shifts). Changes in the criteria corresponding to a particular verbal organization also occur with repeated vowel sequences. These shifts bring the templates employed for syllabic or lexical recognition into a progressively closer correspondence to the repeated exemplar until the stimulus itself meets the changed criteria. To recapitulate the hypothesized sequence of events responsible for VTs: (1) With continued repetition any particular verbal form becomes satiated. (2) While satiation is taking place, concurrent shifts in perceptual criteria eventuate in the perceptual emergence of a different form. (3) This new form undergoes satiation and replacement. Of course, VTs are a linguistic phenomenon, and as such they tap into skills and strategies normally used to achieve a seemingly direct and effortless comprehension of speech. However, when applied to the unusual stimulus of a repeated word, they produce illusory effects that allow us to examine these otherwise inaccessible mechanisms.

It is possible to stimulate each ear with the same repeated word without hearing the word as a single fused image. When the stimulus word "tress" with a repetition period of 492 ms was passed through a digital delay line with two outputs, the delay between these outputs was adjusted so that the asynchrony was exactly half the repetition period (246 ms) (Warren and Ackroff, 1976). Listening was through a pair of headphones wired separately so that the temporally asynchronous but otherwise identical stimuli were heard in each ear. Neither ear could be considered as leading with the half-cycle delay, so there was lateral symmetry in the nature of simultaneous contralateral input. Since the interaural asynchrony was a few hundred milliseconds, there was no possibility of binaural fusion, and as would be expected, all listeners initially perceived the stimulus as two identical voices saying the same thing asynchronously on the right and left sides. The question was whether or not identical transformations would be heard on both sides. If the forms on the left and on the right remained linked, it would indicate that there was a sharing of a single set of neural linguistic processors. If independent changes were to occur at each ear, it would indicate that functionally separate processors were used for the acoustically identical verbal stimuli.

Verbal transformations occurred on both right and left sides, and these changes occurred at different times. Moreover, the forms heard at the two sides were independent, so that while the stimulus word "tress" might be perceived accurately at one ear, a word as far removed phonetically as "commence" might be heard at the other. Additional observations described by Warren (1976) demonstrated that independent changes of the same word were not limited to only two competing versions. Listeners were presented with three asynchronous versions of the same repeated word, each separated from the other two by exactly one-third of the word's duration. Two versions corresponded to monaural inputs (one on the right and one on the left), and one was diotic (synchronous stimulation at each ear). Listeners heard the three versions of the word (right, left, and center) change independently, a finding that Zuck (1992) replicated, employing the same procedure. It appears that three functionally independent sets of linguistic processors can be assembled for the same stimulus, so that there is a degree of equipotentiality for cortical units employed in speech processing. Thus, if one set of processors is occupied with a particular verbal stimulus, others can be employed for analyzing the stimulus, at least up to the level of the word.

The use of verbal transformations in psycholinguistic research permits experimenters to examine aspects of the perceptual organization of speech in ways not possible with other techniques. In a way, the inability to recognize a loud and clear stimulus word when repeated is a highly selective and reversible receptive aphasia. Verbal transformations show promise in providing information concerning both the architecture and functioning of the cortical processors responsible for the comprehension of speech.

SUMMARY

It appears that basic auditory mechanisms employed for nonverbal patterns have been modified in special ways for the comprehension of speech. Temporal auditory induction permits listeners to restore portions of verbal and nonverbal signals masked by extraneous sounds when the extraneous sounds meet appropriate criteria of amplitude and spectrum. The verbal form of temporal auditory induction (phonemic restoration) employs syntactic and semantic information in reconstructing obliterated fragments. Multiple phonemic restorations can restore intelligibility to speech that would otherwise be unintelligible, and can produce an illusion of continuous speech having no missing segments.

Another kind of auditory induction occurs when a signal is heard at one ear but obliterated by a louder sound at the other. Contralateral auditory induction permits restoration of the monaurally masked signal, so that mislocalization toward the side of the unmasked ear does not occur. The rules concerning spectral and intensity requirements for signal restoration are similar for temporal induction and for contralateral induction. It appears that contralateral induction corresponds to an early stage in binaural interaction. Additional detailed comparison of the input to the two ears can result in appropriate placing of a speaker or other sound source.

Experiments with speech and with sequences of nonspeech sounds such as hisses, tones, and buzzes have indicated that listeners employ two fundamentally separate processes for discriminating between different arrangements of the same items, whether the sequences are phonetic groupings, tonal groupings, or groupings of arbitrarily selected sounds: (1) a holistic recognition of overall patterns that does not require the resolution of individual components (this process can operate down to item durations of a few milliseconds) and (2) attaching verbal labels to items in order of occurrence, allowing direct identification of order within extended sequences—this process has a lower limit of resolution of about 100 to 500 ms/item depending upon the nature of components and the response procedure.

The individual phonemes in normal speech occur too fast to permit the direct identification of order. It is suggested that phonemic patterns are perceived globally rather than as a succession of individual speech sounds. This principle is illustrated by the perceptual transformation of sequences of steady-state vowels into illusory syllables and words when the duration of components is too brief to permit identification of the order of sounds. This organizational tendency is so strong that the individual concatenated vowels cannot be identified by phonetically trained listeners even if the individual vowels could each be named accurately when all of the others were deleted from the recycled sequence.

Rules governing the perceptual organization of speech sounds have been studied using the verbal transformation effect. Verbal transformations are a specialized linguistic form of the perceptual changes associated with unchanging patterns of stimulation. It appears that these verbal changes tap into mechanisms normally employed for correction of errors when listening to discourse and that this illusion permits us to examine these mechanisms. There is evidence that age differences in frequency and type of transformation reflect adaptive changes in the perceptual processing of speech, enabling listeners to compensate for changes in functional capacity accompanying normal maturation and aging.

Studies of auditory illusions and confusions have provided clues not only to the general mechanisms underlying auditory perception, but also to how these mechanisms have been modified for speech communication. Helmholtz's statement in the last century that illusions provide a "particularly instructive" way to study perception seems valid today. Research using verbal illusions will continue to be an exciting and rewarding method for studying normally hidden mechanisms employed for the perception of speech.

Acknowledgements

Preparation of this chapter and part of the research described were supported by the National Institutes of Health (Grant DC 00208).

Review Questions

1. Give three examples of how general rules of auditory induction have been specially modified for the perception of speech.

2. The susceptibility to verbal transformations changes markedly over an individual's life span. Explain why this occurs.

3. Why are repeated sequences of brief vowels perceived as syllables and words?

4. The perceptual boundaries of phonemes shift after listening to repeated syllables containing these phonemes. Give other examples of shifts in evaluative criteria following exposure to a stimulus.

5. Why can't the location of a cough in a sentence be identified?

References

Amster, H. (1964). Semantic satiation and generation: Learning? Adaptation? *Psychological Bulletin, 62,* 273-286.

Barnett, M. R. (1964). Perceived phonetic changes in the verbal transformation effect. Unpublished doctoral dissertation, Ohio University.

Bashford, J. A., Meyers, M. D., Brubaker, B. S., & Warren, R. M. (1988). Illusory continuity of interrupted speech: Speech rate determines durational limits. *Journal of the Acoustical Society of America, 84,* 1635-1638.

Bashford, J. A., Riener, K. R., & Warren, R. M. (1992). Increasing the intelligibility of speech through multiple phonemic restorations. *Perception & Psychophysics, 51,* 211-217.

Bashford, J. A., & Warren, R. M. (1987a). Multiple phonemic restorations follow the rules for auditory induction. *Perception & Psychophysics, 42,* 114-121.

Bashford, J. A., & Warren, R. M. (1987b). Effects of spectral alternation on the intelligibility of words and sentences. *Perception & Psychophysics, 42,* 431-438.

Bashford, J. A., & Warren, R. M. (1979). Perceptual synthesis of deleted phonemes. In Wolf, J. J. & Klatt, D. H., (Eds.), *Speech Communication Papers.* New York: Acoustical Society of America (pp. 423-426).

Bashford, J. A., Warren, R. M., and Brown, C. A. (1995). Use of speech-modulated noise adds strong "bottom-up" cues for phonemic restoration. *Perception & Psychophysics,* in press.

Book, W. F. (1925). *The psychology of skill with special reference to its acquisition in typewriting.* New York: Gregg.

Brain, W. R. (1962). Recent work on the physiological basis of speech. *Advancement of Science, 19,* 207-212.

Bregman, A. S. (1990). *Auditory scene analysis.* Cambridge, MA: MIT Press.

Bryan, W. L., & Harter, N. (1897). Studies in the physiology and psychology of the telegraphic language. *Psychological Review, 4,* 27-53.

Bryan, W. L., & Harter, N. (1899). Studies on the telegraphic language: The acquisition of a hierarchy of habits. *Psychological Review, 6,* 345-375.

Butler, R. A., & Naunton, R. F. (1962). Some effects of unilateral auditory masking upon the localization of sound in space. *Journal of the Acoustical Society of America, 34,* 1100-1107.

Butler, R. A., & Naunton, R. F. (1964). Role of stimulus frequency and duration in the phenomenon of localization shifts. *Journal of the Acoustical Society of America, 36,* 917-922.

Chalikia, M. H., & Warren, R. M. (1991). Phonemic transformations: Mapping the illusory organization of steady-state vowel sequences. *Language and Speech, 34,* 109-143.

Chalikia, M. H., Warren, R. M., & Bashford, J. A., Jr. (1992). The phonemic transformation effect: Intersubject agreement on verbal forms. *Journal of the Acoustical Society of America, 91,* 2422 (Abstract).

Chalikia, M. H., & Warren, R. M. (1994). Spectral fissioning in phonemic transformations. *Perception & Psychophysics 55,* 218-226.

Cherry, C., & Wiley, R. (1967). Speech communications in very noisy environments. *Nature, 214,* 1164.

Chistovich, L. A. (1962). Temporal course of speech sound perception. In *Proceedings of the Fourth International Commission on Acoustics* (Article H 18). Copenhagen.

Clegg, J. M. (1971). Verbal transformations on repeated listening to some English consonants. *British Journal of Psychology, 62,* 303-309.

Dannenbring, G. L. (1976). Perceived auditory continuity with alternately rising and falling frequency transitions. *Canadian Journal of Psychology, 30,* 99-114.

David, E. E., Guttman, N., & van Bergeijk, W. A. (1958). On the mechanism of binaural fusion. *Journal of the Acoustical Society of America, 30,* 801-802.

Debigaré, J. (1984). Le phénomène de la transformation verbale et la théorie de l'ensemble-cellules de D. O. Hebb: Un modèle de fonctionnement. *Revue Canadienne de Psychologie, 38,* 17-44.

Diehl, R. L., Kluender, K. R., & Parker, E. M. (1985). Are selective adaptation and contrast effects really distinct? *Journal of Experimental Psychology: Human Perception & Performance, 11,* 209-220.

Dorman, M. F., Cutting, J. E., & Raphael, L. J. (1975). Perception of temporal order in vowel sequences with and without formant transitions. *Journal of Experimental Psychology, 104,* 121-129.

Egan, J. P. (1948). The effect of noise in one ear upon the loudness of speech in the other. *Journal of the Acoustical Society of America, 20,* 58-62.

Eimas, P. D., & Corbit, J. D. (1973). Selective adaptation of linguistic feature detectors. *Cognitive Psychology, 4,* 99-109.

Esposito, N. J. (1985). Verbal transformation effect and auditory reversals. *Perceptual and Motor Skills, 61,* 1019-1022.

Evans, C. R., & Wilson, J. (1968). Subjective changes in the perception of consonants when presented as

"stabilized auditory images." *Division of Computer Science Publication No. 41,* National Physical Laboratory, England.

Fay, W. H. (1966). *Temporal sequence in the perception of speech.* The Hague: Mouton.

Fenelon, B., & Blayden, J. A. (1968). Stability of auditory perception of words and pure tones under repetitive stimulation in neural and suggestibility conditions. *Psychonomic Science, 13,* 285-286.

Garner, W. R. (1951). The accuracy of counting repeated short tones. *Journal of Experimental Psychology, 41,* 310-316.

Goldstein, L. M., & Lackner, J. R. (1974). Alterations in the phonetic coding of speech sounds during repetition. *Cognition, 2,* 279-297.

Guilford, J. P., & Nelson, H. M. (1936). Changes in the pitch of tones when melodies are repeated. *Journal of Experimental Psychology, 19,* 193-202.

Heise, G. A., & Miller, G. A. (1951). An experimental study of auditory patterns. *American Journal of Psychology, 64,* 68-77.

Helmholtz, H. L. F. (1954). *On the sensations of tone as a physiological basis for the theory of music.* (A. J. Ellis, Trans). New York: Dover. Original work published 1870.

Hirsh, I. J. (1959). Auditory perception of temporal order. *Journal of the Acoustical Society of America, 31,* 759-767.

Hirsh, I. J., & Sherrick, C. E. (1961). Perceived order in different sense modalities. *Journal of Experimental Psychology, 62,* 423-432.

Holloway, C. M. (1970). Passing the strongly voiced components of noisy speech. *Nature, 226,* 178-179.

Houtgast, T. (1972). Psychophysical evidence for lateral inhibition in hearing. *Journal of the Acoustical Society of America, 51,* 1885-1894.

Huey, E. B. (1968). *The psychology and pedagogy of reading.* Cambridge, MA: MIT Press.

Kock, W. E. (1950). Binaural localization and masking. *Journal of the Acoustical Society of America, 22,* 801-804.

Lackner, J. R., Tuller B., & Goldstein, L. M. (1977). Some aspects of the psychological representation of speech sounds. *Perceptual and Motor Skills, 45,* 459-471.

Ladefoged, P. (1959). The perception of speech. In *National Physical Laboratory Symposium No. 10, Mechanisation of Thought Processes.* Her Majesty's Stationery Office, London, 1, 398-418.

Ladefoged, P., & Broadbent, D. E. (1960). Perception of sequence in auditory events. *Quarterly Journal of Experimental Psychology, 12,* 162-170.

Lashley, K. S. (1951). The problem of serial order in behavior. In Jeffress, L. A. (Ed.), *Cerebral mechanisms in behavior: The Hixon Symposium.* New York: Wiley (pp. 112-136).

Lass, N. J., & Gasperini, R. M. (1973). The verbal transformation effect: A comparative study of the verbal transformations of phonetically trained and non-phonetically trained listeners. *British Journal of Psychology, 64,* 183-192.

Lass, N. J., & Golden, S. S. (1971). The use of isolated vowels as auditory stimuli in eliciting the verbal transformation effect. *Canadian Journal of Psychology, 25,* 349-359.

Lass, N. J., West, L. K., & Taft, D. D. (1973). A non-verbal analogue to the verbal transformation effect. *Canadian Journal of Psychology, 27,* 272-279.

Layton, B. (1975). Differential effects of two non-speech sounds on phonemic restoration. *Bulletin of the Psychonomic Society, 6,* 487-490.

Lieberman, P. (1963). Some effects of semantic and grammatical context on the production and perception of speech. *Language and Speech, 6,* 172-187.

Locke, J. (1690). *Concerning human understanding.* London: Holt, Book 2, Chapter 14, Section 13 (Reprinted Oxford: Clarendon, 1894).

Massaro, D. W. (1979). Reading and listening. In Kolers, P. A., Wrolstad, M. E., & Bouma H., (Eds.), *Processing of visible language.* New York: Plenum (pp. 331-354).

Miles, W. R. (1934). Age and the kinephantom. *Journal of General Psychology, 10,* 204-207.

Miller, G. A. (1962). Decision units in the perception of speech. *IRE Transactions on Information Theory, IT-8,* 81-83.

Miller, G. A. (1991). *The science of words.* Freeman: New York.

Miller, G. A., & Licklider, J. C. R. (1950). The intelligibility of interrupted speech. *Journal of the Acoustical Society of America, 22,* 167-173.

Moore, M. W., & Bliss, J. C. (1975). The Optacon reading system. *Education of the Visually Handicapped, 7,* 15-21.

Naeser, M. A., & Lilly, J. C. (1970). Preliminary evidence for a universal detector system: Perception of the repeating word. *Journal of the Acoustical Society of America, 48,* 85 (Abstract).

Necker, L. A. (1832). Observations on some remarkable optical phaenomena seen in Switzerland; and on an optical phaenomenon which occurs on viewing a figure of a crystal or geometrical solid. *London & Edinburgh Philosophical Magazine & Journal of Science, 1* (3rd Series), 329-337.

Obusek, C. J. (1971). An experimental investigation of some hypotheses concerning the verbal transformation effect. Unpublished doctoral dissertation, University of Wisconsin, Milwaukee.

Obusek, C. J., & Warren, R. M. (1973a). A comparison of speech perceptions in senile and well-preserved aged by means of the verbal transformation effect. *Journal of Gerontology, 28,* 184-188.

Obusek, C. J., & Warren, R. M. (1973b). Relation of the verbal transformation and the phonemic restoration effects. *Cognitive Psychology, 5,* 97-107.

Ohde, R. N., & Sharf, D. J. (1979). Relationship between adaptation and the percept and transformations of stop consonant voicing: Effects of the number of repetitions and intensity of adaptors. *Journal of the Acoustical Society of America, 66,* 30-45.

Perl, N. T. (1970). The application of the verbal transformation effect to the study of cerebral dominance. *Neuropsychologia, 8,* 259-261.

Powers, G. L., & Wilcox, J. C. (1977). Intelligibility of temporally interrupted speech with and without intervening noise. *Journal of the Acoustical Society of America, 61,* 195-199.

Pritchard, R. M., Heron, W., & Hebb, D. O. (1960). Visual perception approached by the method of stabilized images. *Canadian Journal of Psychology, 14,* 67-77.

Radilova, J., Pöppel, E., & Ilmberger, J. (1990). Auditory reversal timing. *Activas Nervosa Superior, 32,* 137-138.

Repp, B. H. (1992). Perceptual restoration of a "missing" speech sound: Auditory induction or illusion? *Perception & Psychophysics, 51,* 14-32.

Riener, K. R., & Warren, R. M. (1990). Verbal organization of vowel sequences: Effects of repetition rate and stimulus complexity. *Journal of the Acoustical Society of America, 88,* S55 (Abstract).

Riggs, L. A., Ratliff, F., Cornsweet, J. C., & Cornsweet, T. N. (1953). The disappearance of steadily fixated visual test objects. *Journal of the Optical Society of America, 43,* 495-501.

Roivainen, E. (1989). Verbal transformations in the aged. *Perception, 18,* 675-680.

Sadler, M. E. (1989). Effects of noise and amplitude upon the rate and nature of verbal transformations. Unpublished doctoral dissertation, University of Wisconsin, Milwaukee.

Samuel, A. G. (1981). Phonemic restoration: Insights from a new methodology. *Journal of Experimental Psychology: General, 110,* 474-494.

Samuel, A. G. (1987). Lexical uniqueness effects on phonemic restoration. *Journal of Memory and Language, 26,* 36-56.

Samuel, A. G. (1991). A further examination of attentional effects in the phonemic restoration illusion. *Quarterly Journal of Experimental Psychology, 43A,* 679-699.

Sasaki, T. (1980). Sound restoration and temporal localization of noise in speech and music sounds. *Tohoku Psychologica Folia, 39,* 79-88.

Savin, H. B., & Bever, T. G. (1970). The nonperceptual reality of the phoneme. *Journal of Verbal Learning and Verbal Behavior, 9,* 295-302.

Sperling, G., & Reeves, G. (1980). Measuring the reaction time of a shift of visual attention. In Nickerson, R. S., (Ed.), *Attention and Performance VIII.* Hillsdale, NJ: Erlbaum (pp. 347-360).

Taylor, M. M., & Henning, G. B. (1963). Verbal transformations and an effect of instructional bias on perception. *Canadian Journal of General Psychology, 17,* 210-223.

Teranishi, R. (1977). Critical rate for identification and information capacity in hearing system. *Journal of the Acoustical Society of Japan, 33,* 136-143.

Thomas, I. B., Cetti, R. P., & Chase, P. W. (1971). Effect of silent intervals on the perception of temporal order for vowels. *Journal of the Acoustical Society of America, 49,* 84 (Abstract).

Thurlow, W. R. (1957). An auditory figure-ground effect. *American Journal of Psychology, 70,* 653-654.

Thurlow, W. R., & Elfner, L. F. (1959). Continuity effects with alternately sounding tones. *Journal of the Acoustical Society of America, 31,* 1337-1339.

Titchener, E. B. (1915). *A beginner's psychology.* New York: Macmillan.

Verschuure, H., & Brocaar, M. (1983). Intelligibility of interrupted meaningful and nonsense speech with and without intervening noise. *Perception & Psychophysics, 33,* 232-240.

Vicario, G. (1960). L'effecto tunnel acoustico. *Rivista di Psicologia, 54,* 41-52.

Warren, R. M. (1961a). Illusory changes of distinct speech upon repetition: The verbal transformation effect. *British Journal of Psychology, 52,* 249-258.

Warren, R. M. (1961b). Illusory changes in repeated words: Differences between young adults and the aged. *American Journal of Psychology, 74,* 506-516.

Warren, R. M. (1968a). Relation of verbal transformations to other perceptual phenomena. *Conference Publication No. 12,* Institution of Electrical Engineers (London), Suppl. 1, 1-8.

Warren, R. M. (1968b). Verbal transformation effect and auditory perceptual mechanisms. *Psychological Bulletin, 70,* 261-270.

Warren, R. M. (1970). Perceptual restoration of missing speech sounds. *Science, 167,* 392-393.

Warren, R. M. (1971). Identification times for phonemic components of graded complexity and for spelling of speech. *Perception & Psychophysics, 9,* 345-349.

Warren, R. M. (1974a). Auditory pattern discrimination by untrained listeners. *Perception & Psychophysics, 15,* 495-500.

Warren, R. M. (1974b). Auditory temporal discrimination by trained listeners. *Cognitive Psychology, 6,* 237-256.

Warren, R. M. (1976). Auditory illusions and perceptual processes. In Lass, N. J., (Ed.), *Contemporary issues in experimental phonetics.* New York: Academic Press (pp. 389-417).

Warren, R. M. (1981). Perceptual transformations in vision and hearing. *International Journal of Man-Machine Studies, 14,* 123-132.

Warren, R. M. (1982). *Auditory perception: A new synthesis.* New York: Pergamon Press.

Warren, R. M. (1984). Perceptual restoration of obliterated sounds. *Psychological Bulletin, 96,* 371-383.

Warren, R. M. (1985). Criterion shift rule and perceptual homeostasis. *Psychological Review, 92,* 574-584.

Warren, R. M. (1993). Perception of acoustic sequences: Global integration versus temporal resolution. In McAdams, S., & Bigand, E., (Eds.), *Thinking in sound: The cognitive psychology of human audition.* Oxford: Oxford University Press (pp. 37-68).

Warren, R. M., & Ackroff, J. M. (1976). Two types of auditory sequence perception. *Perception & Psychophysics, 20,* 387-394.

Warren, R. M., & Bashford, J. A., (1976). Auditory contralateral induction: An early stage in binaural processing. *Perception & Psychophysics, 20,* 380-386.

Warren, R. M., Bashford, J. A., & Gardner, D. A. (1990). Tweaking the lexicon: Organization of vowel sequences into words. *Perception & Psychophysics, 47,* 423-432.

Warren, R. M., Bashford, J. A., Healy, E. W. & Brubaker, B. S. (1994). Auditory induction: Reciprocal changes in alternating sounds. *Perception & Psychophysics 55,* 313-322.

Warren, R. M., Gardner, D. A., Brubaker, B. S. & Bashford, J. A. (1991). Melodic and nonmelodic sequences of tones: Effects of duration on perception. *Music Perception, 8,* 277-289.

Warren, R. M., & Gregory, R. L. (1958). An auditory analogue of the visual reversible figure. *American Journal of Psychology, 71,* 612-613.

Warren, R. M., & Meyers, M. D. (1987). Effects of listening to repeated syllables: Category boundary shifts versus verbal transformation. *Journal of Phonetics, 15,* 169-181.

Warren, R. M., & Obusek, C. J. (1971). Speech perception and phonemic restorations. *Perception & Psychophysics, 9,* 358-362.

Warren, R. M., & Obusek, C. J. (1972). Identification of temporal order within auditory sequences. *Perception & Psychophysics, 12,* 86-90.

Warren, R. M., Obusek, C. J., & Ackroff, J. M. (1972). Auditory induction: Perceptual synthesis of absent sounds. *Science, 176,* 1149-1151.

Warren, R. M., Obusek, C. J., Farmer R. M., & Warren, R. P. (1969). Auditory sequence: Confusion of patterns other than speech or music. *Science, 164,* 586-587.

Warren, R. M., & Sherman, G. L. (1974). Phonemic restorations based on subsequent context. *Perception & Psychophysics, 16,* 150-156.

Warren, R. M., & Warren, R. P. (1966). A comparison of speech perception in childhood, maturity and old age by means of the verbal transformation effect. *Journal of Verbal Learning and Verbal Behavior, 5,* 142-146.

Warren, R. M., & Warren, R. P. (1968). *Helmholtz*

on perception: Its physiology and development. New York: Wiley.

Warren, R. M., & Warren, R. P. (1970). Auditory illusions and confusions. *Scientific American, 223* (December), 30-36.

Welford, A. T. (1958). *Ageing and human skill.* London: Oxford University Press.

Wheatstone, C. (1835). Remarks on Purkinje's experiments. *Report of the British Association, 551-553.*

Wickelgren, W. A. (1965). Distinctive features and errors in short-term memory for English vowels. *Journal of the Acoustical Society of America, 38,* 583-588.

Wickelgren, W. A. (1966). Distinctive features and errors in short-term memory for English consonants. *Journal of the Acoustical Society of America, 39,* 388-398.

Wiley, R. L. (1968). Speech communication using the strongly voiced components only. Unpublished doctoral dissertation, Imperial College, University of London.

Zuck, D. (1992). The verbal transformation effect: Auditory illusion as an index of lexical processing and homolog activation. *Brain and Language, 43,* 323-335.

Suggested Readings

General Articles on Auditory Illusions

Warren, R. M., & Warren, R. P. (1970 December). Auditory illusions and confusions. *Scientific American, 223,* 30-36.

Warren, R. M. (1983). Auditory illusions and their relation to mechanisms normally enhancing accuracy of perception. *Journal of the Audio Engineering Society, 31,* 623-629.

Phonemic Restorations and Auditory Induction

Warren, R. M. (1984). Perceptual restoration of obliterated sounds. *Psychological Bulletin, 96,* 371-383.

Samuel, A. G., & Ressler, W. H. (1986). Attention within auditory word perception: Insights from the phonemic restoration illusion. *Journal of Experimental Psychology: Human Perception and Performance, 12,* 70-79.

Confusions of Temporal Orders

Warren, R. M. (1982). *Auditory Perception: A New Synthesis.* Pergamon Press, New York (see Chapter 5, "Perception of Acoustic Sequences").

Bregman, A. S., & Campbell, J. (1971). Primary auditory stream segregation and perception of order in rapid sequences of tones. *Journal of Experimental Psychology, 89,* 244-249.

Dorman, M. F., Cutting, J. E., & Raphael, L. J. (1975). Perception of temporal order in vowel sequences with and without formant transitions. *Journal of Experimental Psychology: Human Perception and Performance, 104,* 121-129.

Illusory Organization of Vowel Sequences

Chalikia, M. H., & Warren, R. M. (1994). Spectral fissioning in phonemic transformations. *Perception & Psychophysics 55,* 218-226.

Warren, R. M., Bashford, J. A., & Gardner, D. A. (1990). Tweaking the lexicon: Organization of vowel sequences into words. *Perception & Psychophysics, 47,* 423-432.

Verbal Transformations

Warren, R. M. (1968). Verbal transformation effect and auditory perceptual mechanisms. *Psychological Bulletin, 70,* 261-270.

Obusek, C. J., & Warren, R. M. (1973). Relation of the verbal transformation and the phonemic restoration effects. *Cognitive Psychology, 5,* 97-107.

Part IV

RESEARCH TECHNIQUES

Chapter 13

Instrumentation for the Study of Speech Acoustics

Hisashi J. Wakita

INTRODUCTION

This chapter focuses on some digital speech analysis techniques for the study of acoustic phonetics. Although these techniques were developed exclusively as an efficient means of speech transmission and automatic speech recognition, not for the study of acoustic phonetics, they provide some powerful tools for the study of acoustic phonetics.

In the past two decades, digital techniques advanced greatly along with computer hardware. Particularly, faster microprocessors and large-capacity memory boosted the development of sophisticated software and made it easier to run experiments on large databases. The sound spectrograph, which used to be based on analog techniques, is now entirely digital, which allows more flexibility and more variety of operations. The advantages of digital techniques over analog ones are more precision, accuracy, and repeatability of a process.

The purpose of this chapter is to introduce digital techniques and methods used in speech analysis. The reader is assumed to be reasonably familiar with basic instrumentation such as microphones, amplifiers, and tape recorders and to have a fundamental knowledge of digital computers (see recommended readings).

SPEECH MODEL AND PARAMETERS

Speech Production Model for Analysis

Most natural phenomena are so complicated that we usually do not have adequate mathematical tools to describe them in general terms. Speech is no exception. There are not as yet sufficient mathematical tools to describe completely human speech, even if all the physiological processes of speech production and perception could be elucidated. In developing a method of speech analysis, we must simplify the actual event to the extent that existing mathematical tools can be applied to it but not to such an extent that its essential physical properties cannot be preserved satisfactorily. In some cases a greatly simplified model can be created by adopting very simple hypotheses and assumptions and by imposing strong constraints. Generally speaking, for acoustic analysis of speech, we consider production processes involving only the larynx, pharynx, and oral cavity. Obviously, this does not take into account the nasal cavity

or the subglottal activities that are important for speech production. However, it is necessary to ignore these in the analysis techniques, since they unduly complicate the model and associated mathematics.

In the simplification of speech production, three major factors are considered: excitation (glottal oscillation), transmission (pharyngeal and oral cavity configuration), and the radiation effect at the mouth. Although these factors are inseparable in actual speech, the strong assumption is that they are separable. Under this assumption it becomes possible to apply some of the concepts of mathematics and engineering to modeling of the speech production process. The system that satisfies this assumption is linear, and most models of speech analysis and synthesis are **linear systems.** It should be realized, therefore, that limitations exist from the starting point. Yet because of the assumption of separability of elements, we can describe characteristics of sounds in terms of simple parameters that can be extracted from the linear model of speech production. This assumption also allows specification of the acoustic characteristics attributable to the excitation source, the oral cavity, and the radiation effect. This basic model of speech production permits extraction of a specific set of parameters with a certain degree of accuracy.

Speech Parameters

Speech parameters that can be extracted include (1) spectral envelopes, (2) formant frequencies and bandwidths, (3) **fundamental frequency,** commonly called *pitch,* (4) amplitude of fundamental frequency, also called intensity, (5) average energy, and (6) vocal tract shapes. For the description of phonetic values of speech sounds, the formant frequencies are most important, although studies provide the possibility of computing from acoustic data vocal tract shapes from which some articulatory features can be estimated (Wakita, 1973).

SPEECH ANALYSIS

Background

Since the middle 1960s and early 1970s, digital computers have played an extremely important role in speech research. One major use of the digital computer is the simulation of a system, which is especially helpful in the development of sophisticated analysis techniques. The same development with only electronic hardware would take an exceedingly long time. The advantages of computer simulation are that processes can be repeated exactly and the control of parameters is easy. The only disadvantage is that in many cases the simulation cannot be accomplished in real time. After extensive study of a technique by computer simulation, it is relatively easy to replace it partly or entirely with special-purpose hardware. Particularly, the recent development of an LSI (large-scale integrated circuit) chip called DSP (digital signal processor) allows easy implementation of many digital techniques in real time. Since hardware implementation of a computer simulation or replacement of part of the simulation with hardware implementation (a hybrid system) is relatively easy, the following discussion will focus on the computer simulation of various techniques.

In the early 1960s there were no particular developments of new analysis techniques. Those quiet days ended with the development of the **cepstrum** techniques (Noll, 1964), a method of extracting the fundamental frequency of speech sounds. It interested many people because it provided a fresh concept for separating the periodic from the nonperiodic components of speech sounds. Although the term *cepstrum* became widely known among speech researchers, they seldom used the method itself, probably because of its sophistication. The cepstrum method continued to be investigated for application to automatic formant analysis (Schafer and Rabiner, 1970) as well as to fundamental frequency extraction (Noll, 1967).

Several years after the cepstrum method was developed, two new techniques for speech analysis and synthesis gained prominence: the maximum likelihood method (Itakura and Saito, 1968) and predictive coding of speech (Atal and Schroeder, 1968; Atal and Hanauer, 1971). The development of these techniques was truly epoch making, for they vastly improved efficiency, accuracy, and speed. However, their merits were not widely proved in the United States until 4 years later, when the **partial correlation (PARCOR)** method demonstrated its amazing fidelity in analysis-synthesis telephony (Itakura and Saito, 1972). Since then, PARCOR, maximum likelihood, and predictive

coding of speech have influenced the thinking of many speech researchers and now are known popularly as the **linear prediction method.** In the meantime, Markel (1971) pointed out the similarity between the maximum likelihood method and linear predictive coding and then developed the inverse digital filter method, which is more closely related to a physical model of speech production. I then showed that the inverse digital filter method is equivalent to PARCOR (Wakita, 1973), and Makhoul and Wolf (1972) investigated the equivalences and differences among various approaches in linear prediction. Through all those efforts the theoretical basis for linear prediction has become much better understood. This technique is now extensively used for formant frequency tracking and fundamental frequency extraction. It also plays an extremely important role in speech compression and automatic speech recognition. In fact, it has attracted so much attention that in a remarkably short time it has been further developed theoretically and practically in considerable detail. Details of linear prediction are discussed in a later section.

The fast **Fourier transform** (FFT) algorithm (Cooley and Tukey, 1965) greatly accelerated the improvement of computer simulation efficiency. The Fourier transform is an important mathematical tool used to obtain from time-domain acoustic speech waveforms their frequency-domain characteristics. After the development of digital computers, a faster algorithm for computing the Fourier transform was sought. FFT was revolutionary not only in numerical analysis but also in various areas of research using digital computers.

In developing speech analysis methods, efforts used to be exerted predominantly on formant tracking and fundamental frequency extraction. However, there were also a few attempts to obtain articulatory information from acoustic data. There was considerable interest in the relationships between the vocal tract configuration and its formant frequency characteristics because sometimes the physiological description of speech sounds is much easier and more definitive than a purely acoustic description. Despite considerable interest in this aspect of speech research (Dunn, 1950; Stevens, Kasowski, and Fant, 1953), there was little progress in this area until Mermelstein and Schroeder (1965) developed a method for computing the shape of the vocal tract from formant

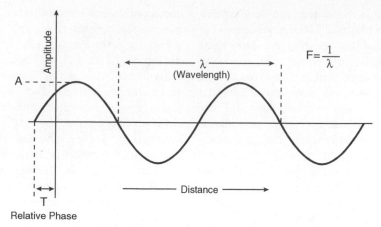

FIGURE 13-1   A sinusoidal wave.

frequencies. In this case shape of the vocal tract was represented in terms of the **vocal tract area function,** in which the cross-sectional areas along the tract are represented in a distance-area diagram. The vocal tract area function indicates gross features of configuration but not detailed structure. Nevertheless, this step was a breakthrough for obtaining a better understanding of speech sounds in the articulatory and frequency domains. Heinz (1967), Mermelstein (1967), and Schroeder (1967) further extended the method. The vocal tract area function was computed by measuring the input impedance (the ratio of air pressure to airflow) at the lips, which required the use of a cumbersome tube attached to the speaker's mouth. Sondhi and Gopinath (1971) avoided this difficulty by using the impulse response at the lips instead of the lip impedance. The impulse response is a system's output when an impulse is applied to it as an input. The system's frequency characteristics can be derived from the impulse response.

In the meantime, another possibility for computing the vocal tract area function from acoustic speech waveforms was investigated (Atal, 1970). A milestone in this technique was the development of a method for estimating the vocal tract area function directly from speech waveforms based on linear prediction (Wakita, 1973). Furthermore, it was demonstrated theoretically that linear prediction digital filtering is a discrete solution to the wave equations (from which Webster's horn equation can be derived) that describe the behavior of sound pressure and volume velocity in the models used by Schroeder (1967) and Mermelstein (1967), among others (Wakita and Gray, 1974). It is quite surprising

that a linear prediction digital filter is equivalent to an acoustic tube model or a transmission line analog of the vocal tract as proposed by Kelly and Lochbaum (1962). Yet the practical significance of linear prediction lies in its efficiency and accuracy in extracting speech parameters. In the following sections the details of some of this work will be discussed to clarify these analysis techniques. Although this research is conceptually and mathematically sophisticated, I will attempt to explain it in layman's terms with few equations.

Fourier Transform and Frequency Spectrum

Fourier transform constitutes a basis of spectral analysis and extraction of related speech parameters. Any speech signal can be decomposed into a set of sinusoidal waves. Mathematically, a sinusoidal wave is defined by its maximum amplitude (A), a frequency (F), and a phase (T) relative to the coordinate origin (Fig. 13-1). Thus, a sinusoidal wave can be represented by A, F, T, and a given speech signal can be decomposed into a number of sinusoidal waves, that is, into a set of A, F, T (Fig. 13-2, *A*). The set of A, F, T represents the distribution of the amplitude and phase of the components of a given speech signal and is called **frequency spectrum.** The set of A, F is the *amplitude spectrum* of a given speech signal, and the set of F, T is the *phase spectrum.* The *power spectrum,* a set of power (amplitude squared) and frequency, is also commonly used as well as the amplitude spectrum. A graphic plot of the amplitude spectrum is shown in Figure 13-2, *B.* This transformation from a

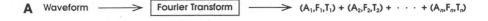

A Waveform ⟶ | Fourier Transform | ⟶ $(A_1, F_1, T_1) + (A_2, F_2, T_2) + \cdots + (A_n, F_n, T_n)$

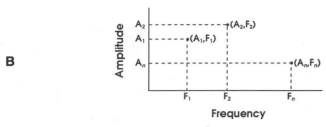

B

FIGURE 13-2 Fourier Transform. *A,* Input-output relationship. *B,* Graphic plot of an amplitude spectrum.

given speech signal to a set of A, F, T is called Fourier transform.

CEPSTRUM METHOD

Voice Pitch Extraction

Many fundamental frequency extraction techniques are based on the idea of detecting the recurrent peaks in the speech waveform. A difficulty with this approach was that peaks related to the periodicity of the laryngeal voice source could not always be distinguished from peaks resulting from the resonance behavior of the supraglottal spaces. However, the cepstrum method provides a means for separating the periodic components (the fundamental frequency and its harmonics) from the nonperiodic components (the vocal tract characteristics). To develop the cepstrum, assume a linear system in which the spectrum of a voiced sound can be expressed as a product of the source spectrum and the spectrum of the vocal tract resonance characteristics. Products are usually more difficult to handle than sums; therefore the description of the spectrum in terms of its components is simplified if we take the logarithm (log) of the speech spectrum. The product is thereby changed to a sum, and the resulting log spectrum can be expressed as the sum of the log source spectrum and the log spectrum of the vocal tract impulse response.

Figure 13-3, *A,* shows an example of the log spectrum of a voiced sound. Note that the log operation results in a vertical scale whose units are decibels. The slowly varying broken line denotes the log spectrum of the vocal tract impulse response on which the log spectrum of

the voice source is superimposed as the ripples. These ripples correspond to the harmonics of the fundamental frequency and are equally spaced along the frequency axis. The question is how to obtain information on the fundamental frequency from the log spectrum. That is, how can the regular spacing of the ripples be measured without interference from fluctuations attributable to resonance behavior? The approach that leads to the cepstrum is to look at the log spectrum in Figure 13-3, *A,* as if it were an ordinary time-domain waveform. If there are two sinusoidal waves of different frequencies and amplitudes superimposed in the time domain, how can they be separated? Can the frequency of each one be determined? In this case, the Fourier transform of the wave produces two line spectra in the frequency domain, and the frequency and amplitude of each sinusoidal wave are given by the positions and lengths of the two lines.

By applying the same concept to the present problem, we may take the Fourier transform of the log spectrum (formally, an inverse Fourier transform). Since the spectrum of a log spectrum is a new quantity, it is given a new name, the *cepstrum,* formed by inverting the first four letters in *spectrum.* The horizontal scale in the cepstrum is defined as the *quefrency* (Bogert, Healy, and Tukey, 1963) and has the unit of time. The cepstrum of Figure 13-3, *A,* is shown in Figure 13-3, *B.* Since the horizontal axis denotes the time scale, the periodicity of the source spectrum appears as a sharp spike in the higher range of the cepstrum, and the slowly varying components of the vocal tract spectrum appear in the very low range. The spike represents the period of the harmonic components

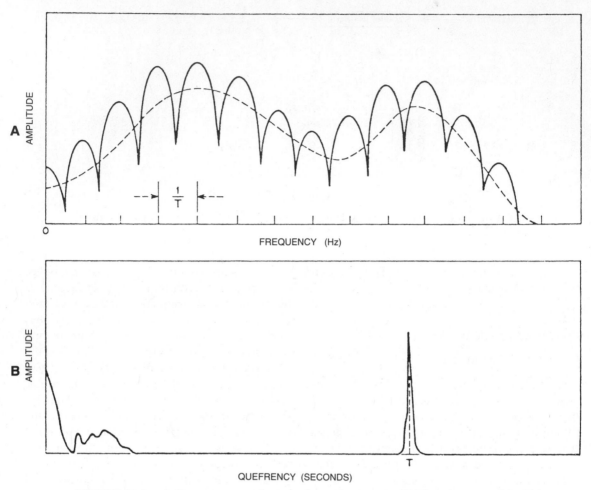

FIGURE 13-3   *A*, Log spectrum of a voiced speech segment. *B*, The spectrum of A. (From Noll, A. M. [1967]. Cepstrum pitch determination. *Journal of the Acoustical Society of America, 41,* 293-309.)

from which the fundamental frequency is computed as the reciprocal of the period. Since the period is determined from the periodicity of the harmonics in the cepstrum method, it is possible to determine pitch even for speech signals whose fundamental frequency is lost or filtered out, such as speech sent over a telephone line, the frequency band of which ranges between 300 Hz and 3400 Hz. In this case the periodicity is recovered from the regular spacing of the higher harmonics within the transmission band. Unvoiced sounds do not show any spike in the higher region of the cepstrum, and therefore no periodicity can be determined.

Formant Analysis

Since the characteristics of the excitation source and the vocal tract are separated in the cepstrum, it is also effective for obtaining formant frequen-

cies. To obtain the vocal tract characteristics from the cepstrum, the source characteristics in the higher region of the cepstrum are filtered out and the Fourier transform is applied to the vocal tract component in the lower range. This procedure yields the slowly varying log spectrum of the vocal tract resonance characteristics, the peaks of which correspond to formant frequencies. The ordinary spectrum of a speech segment also consists of the ripples corresponding to harmonics of the fundamental frequency. Thus, the vocal tract characteristics are not easily determined from it. What makes it easy to obtain vocal tract characteristics is the ability to find a smooth spectral envelope of the ordinary spectrum from which the peak frequencies can be determined. The cepstrum method makes this operation possible. A block diagram of the cepstrum method for pitch and formant frequency extraction is shown in Figure 13-4. In

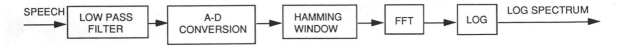

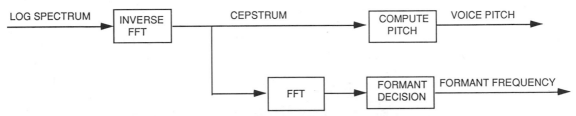

FIGURE 13-4   A block diagram of the cepstrum method.

practice, the speech signal to be analyzed is digitized after passing through the low-pass filter, the cutoff frequency of which is chosen as half the sampling frequency. One segment of the speech signal, normally 25 to 35 ms long, is passed through a *Hamming window* before the FFT is applied to it. The Hamming window is a special-purpose filter used for reducing distortion in the frequency domain. If the Fourier transform were applied to a short segment of unfiltered speech, discontinuities in the time domain of the two ends of the segment would distort the frequency domain. Figure 13-5 shows an example of the pitch period and formant data automatically processed from the utterance "we were away a year ago".

When the cepstrum method was first developed, its computer simulation was extremely time consuming because of frequent use of the Fourier transform. However, the development of the FFT algorithm improved the situation appreciably, although not to the point of satisfaction. With the recent development of DSP chips, real-time FFT analysis is easily implemented for speech signal processing.

LINEAR PREDICTION METHOD

Linear Regression

Linear prediction is analogous to the cepstrum method of computing formant frequencies in that both yield the smooth spectral envelopes

of speech sounds. The difference is in their approaches. Linear prediction manipulates sampled speech data mainly in the time domain, and the main processing of the cepstrum method is accomplished in the frequency domain and uses the Fourier transform three times, twice to get the cepstrum and once to get the smooth spectrum.

This may make it easier to understand the linear prediction of speech. Suppose there are two statistical quantities, the highest temperature (T_i) and the number of traffic accidents (N_i) in a day during the past several years. A question arises: Is it possible to estimate the number of traffic accidents by knowing the high temperature of the day, so that ambulances, physicians, hospital beds, and other important components, are available? The conditional distribution of the number of traffic accidents for a given temperature is known. The best possible estimate of N_i from a given T_i, according to the least-squares principle, is the mean (m_i) of the conditional distribution for T_i. Thus, in this example, the conditional mean, m_i, can be used as the best estimate for the number of traffic accidents when the high temperature, T_i, is recorded.

However, in many cases, especially when more than two statistical quantities are involved, it is more difficult to calculate the conditional mean. In such a case, past data can be used to determine a certain simple mathematical function that best approximates the least-squares conditional mean. In this example the aim is to

WE WERE AWAY A YEAR AGO

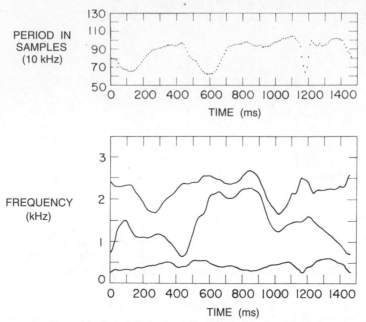

FIGURE 13-5 **Period and formant data obtained by the cepstrum method.** (From Schafer, R. W., & Rabiner, L. R. [1970]. System for the automatic analysis of voiced speech. *Journal of the Acoustical Society of America, 47,* 634-638.)

determine a straight line that will give the estimate of N_i, ($\hat{N}_i$), for a given T_i. Suppose the straight line is expressed as

$$N = \alpha T + \beta \qquad (1)$$

In Equation 1, α and β are constants, and α determines the slope of the straight line. The error e_i, the difference between the actual value N_i and the estimated value $\hat{N}_i$, is

$$e_i = N_i - \hat{N}_i. \qquad (2)$$

The straight line is determined from the statistical properties of the event by observing N_i and T_i for a sufficient range of i. It is computed by applying the least-squares principle so that the mean of the square errors between the actual values and the straight line is as small as possible. The straight line thus determined gives the best estimate of N_i for a given T_i. Of course, this best estimate is less accurate than the actual conditional mean but is as close to it as possible with a straight-line approximation. Once the formula in Equation 1 is determined, the number of traffic accidents can be predicted by ascertaining the highest temperature of a day. The smaller the standard deviation of a conditional distribution,

the greater the accuracy of prediction. This is *linear mean square regression,* and α in Equation 1 is the *regression coefficient,* which determines the slope of the straight line.

This example involves two different statistical quantities, but **linear regression** can be applied to a sequence of single statistical quantities. The question is whether it is possible to predict tomorrow's high temperature from today's. If tomorrow's temperature is N and today's is T, the same procedure yields the formula in Equation 1 for the linear mean square regression.

Imagine the expansion of this concept to an n-dimensional case. Suppose tomorrow's temperature is predicted from the temperatures in the past n days. Equation 1 expands to a straight line in the n-dimensional space, although it is difficult to visualize. As long as tomorrow's temperature correlates with the temperature of n days ago, the prediction accuracy will increase with n. Thus, the highest accuracy is attained by using all the past temperatures that correlate with tomorrow's temperature.

Linear Prediction of Speech

Consider an application of this concept to a time sequence of sampled speech instead of tempera-

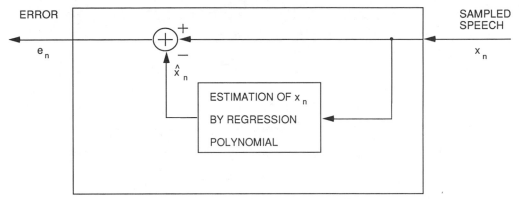

FIGURE 13-6 A linear regression filter.

tures. The problem is to obtain the best estimate of the next sample, x_n (corresponding to estimating tomorrow's temperature), by observing the past M samples. In this case, the error e_n, the difference between the actual sample x_n and the estimated sample $\hat{x}_n$, is given by

$$e_n = x_n - \hat{x}_n \qquad (3)$$

The estimated sample $\hat{x}_n$ is computed from a straight line in M-dimensional space as an expansion of the previous example and expressed as

$$\hat{x}_n = \alpha_1 x_{n-1} + \alpha_2 x_{n-2} \\ + ... + \alpha_M x_{n-M}. \qquad (4)$$

It is easily seen that this is the extension of Equation 1 into the Mth dimensional space. Here x_{n-1}, x_{n-2}, ..., x_{n-M} are M samples observed in the past, and α_1, α_2, ..., α_M are the regression coefficients to be determined. The regression coefficients are determined so that the mean square error is minimized. Speech events for a certain period are observed through a time window to determine the regression coefficients. It is assumed that the speech event during the observation is stationary. That is, the statistical distribution does not change; the mean and the standard deviation of the speech event are constant during the observation. This assumption is satisfied reasonably well for time windows of approximately 10 to 20 ms. The computation to determine the regression coefficients efficiently is the kernel of linear prediction. The procedure is so technical that it has to be omitted here except to say that autocorrelation coefficients have an important role in determining

the regression coefficients (Makhoul, 1975; Markel and Gray, 1976) (Fig. 13-6).

What significance do the regression coefficients α_i have in this speech production model? How are they related to formant frequencies? Assume the spectrum of a voiced nonnasalized sound is characterized only by the frequencies and bandwidths of the peaks in its smoothed spectrum. Strictly speaking, the speech spectra of voiced nonnasalized sounds sometimes have dips that arise from the glottal wave characteristics. They are usually not conspicuous, and the spectra, even in such cases, are well approximated by peaks only. By this assumption the spectral envelope of a voiced nonnasalized sound can be represented as the reciprocal of a polynomial of a certain kind:

Spectral envelope = 1/Polynomial A.   (5)

The roots of the polynomial in Equation 5 give the peak frequencies and bandwidths. Thus, determining the formant frequencies and bandwidths is reduced to determining this polynomial from speech waveforms.

Equation 5 can be interpreted as the relationship between input and output of a system. It is represented in the frequency domain as the product of an input and the transfer function of the system,

Speech(1/A) = Excitation(1) * System
transfer function(1/A)   (6)

The system as a production model (Fig. 13-7, *A*) illustrates this relationship. It is more convenient, however, to consider the system in terms of an analysis model (Fig. 13-7, *B*), to determine the polynomial A from a given speech input.

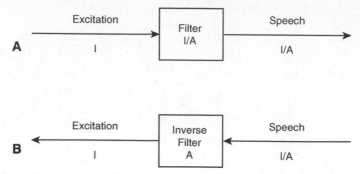

FIGURE 13-7   Models for the linear prediction method. *A*, The production model. *B*, The analysis model.

Since a constant in the frequency domain represents either an impulse or white noise in the time domain, the polynomial A is determined so that the excitation as output becomes either an impulse or white noise.

In the linear prediction technique in which speech sounds are handled in the form of sampled data, a special type of polynomial for A, in which z-transform notation is used, is expressed as

$$A = 1 + a_1 z^{-1} + a_2 z^{-2} + ... + a_M z^{-M} \quad (7)$$

Here a_1, a_2, ..., a_m are the *filter coefficients*. In Equation 7, z is a unit time delay in the time domain, and the filter coefficients are the impulse response of the inverse filter. Since the impulse response of a filter specifies the characteristics of that filter, to compute the filter coefficients is to obtain the characteristics of the filter. Thus, the expression A in Equation 7 is the transfer function of a filter. Expressing the polynomial A as in Equation 7 shows a very important fact: The filter coefficients a_i are identical to the regression coefficients α_i in Equation 4. That is, the coefficients of a polynomial that gives the best estimate of the next sample x_n equal the coefficients of the transfer function polynomial of an inverse filter. The prediction error is given as the output of the inverse filter. The formant frequencies and bandwidths are given by the roots of the polynomial A = 0. This is easily done by the use of a polynomial root-solving subroutine in the computer. However, a much easier way to obtain formant frequencies and bandwidths is to note the particular properties of the z-transform notation in Equation 7.

The z-transform notation of the inverse filter transfer function in Equation 7 represents both frequency domain and time domain. To obtain the spectral envelope, $\log |A|^2$ is computed for all frequencies of interest by substituting each frequency value into z, since z itself is a function of frequency. The result of this computation is precisely the smooth spectrum estimate; its local maxima therefore correspond to the formants. The formant frequencies and bandwidths can be measured directly from this smooth spectrum without solving for the roots of A = 0. One example of the inverse filter spectrum is shown in Figure 13-8, *A*. Figures 13-7 and 13-8, *A* and the reciprocal of the inverse filter spectrum, shown in Figure 13-8, *B*, define the resonance structure of the input speech spectrum. In the time domain the coefficients of A, {1, a_1, a_2, ..., a_M} denote the sampled values of the impulse response of the inverse filter. Since the inverse filter spectrum is obtained as the Fourier transform of the impulse response of the filter, the inverse filter spectrum shown in Figure 13-8, *A* is computed by taking the Fourier transform of a set of filter coefficients. Determination of formant frequencies and bandwidths from the spectrum is relatively easy.

Partial Correlation Coefficient

The filter coefficient is a new speech parameter, sometimes called the *a-parameter*, that is directly related to formant frequencies. This relation is not the only reason that linear prediction is interesting. Speech compression and automatic speech recognition have other parameters than formant frequencies, such as the filter coefficients themselves. These are preferred for their efficiency, especially when they are related to formant frequencies or have some other physical meaning in the speech production model of interest. One such speech parameter is the

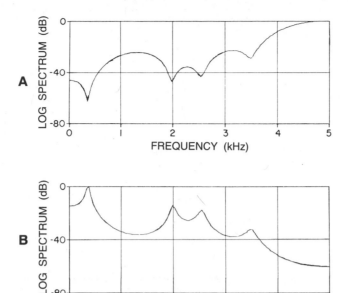

FIGURE 13-8   *A,* An inverse filter spectrum. *B,* Its reciprocal.

partial correlation coefficient (PARCOR coefficient), also called the *k-parameter* or the *reflection coefficient*. This parameter has a most important role in speech compression and automatic speech recognition because several of its properties are particularly suitable for these areas. This parameter is an intermediate result in the computation of the filter coefficients; thus it is indirectly related to the formant frequencies. When properly processed, it is equivalent to a set of acoustic reflection coefficients that determine the vocal tract area function. The partial correlation coefficient is so significant in linear prediction that an attempt will be made to explain some of its physical meanings even though it is very difficult to explain without the mathematical details.

Suppose there is a group of pairs of beautiful sisters; let A denote the beauty of the first sister of a pair and B, that of the second. The ordinary correlation between A and B for the whole group (called the *total correlation*) includes the effects of all the factors that contribute to their beauty: their parents are also beautiful, they exercise every morning, they use the most expensive cosmetics, and so forth. Sometimes it is desirable to consider the correlation between A and B so that one or two of the factors can be disregarded. For example, what correlation between A and B does not include the beauty of the parents? Let the beauty of the mothers be C and the handsomeness of the fathers be D. The best

estimates of the sisters' beauties ($\hat{A}$ and $\hat{B}$), based on C and D, can be computed with linear mean square regression. $\hat{A}$ and $\hat{B}$ can be interpreted as the best estimates of the contribution of C and D to A and B. Then the correlation between (A − $\hat{A}$) and (B − $\hat{B}$) is the correlation after the effects of the parents are subtracted. This is the *partial correlation;* essentially, it is the correlation between the errors of the estimates $\hat{A}$ and $\hat{B}$ for A and B. In this case, the partial correlation is the correlation between A and B of two beautiful sisters whose parents are equally beautiful. Thus, a statement such as "two sisters are beautiful because their parents are beautiful" is excluded.

Now consider partial correlation in the linear prediction of speech. Suppose there are m + 1 speech data $x_n, x_{n-1}, ..., x_{n-m}$ sampled 10,000 times per second. This means that speech is observed every 0.1 ms. If the length of the vocal tract is assumed to be 17.65 cm and the sound velocity is 35,300 cm/sec, it takes 0.5 ms for the acoustic wave at the glottis to travel to the lips. Two acoustic waves are considered to exist within the vocal tract; one is moving toward the lips, and the other is reflecting from the lips toward the glottis. Thus, it takes 1 ms for a wave to travel from the glottis to the lips and back to the glottis.

Now, consider wave A at the glottis, which is about to proceed toward the lips. At the glottis, wave A is affected by the waves coming toward

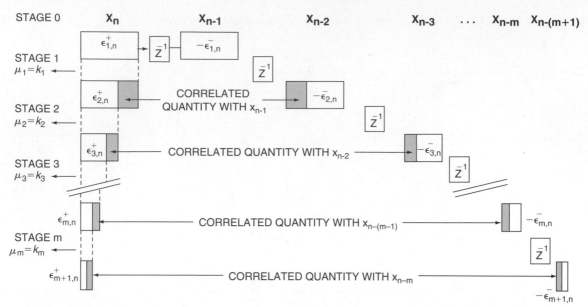

FIGURE 13-9   The inverse filtering process. (From Wakita, H. [1972]. *Estimation of vocal tract shape by optimal inverse filtering and acoustic to articulatory conversion methods.* Santa Barbara, CA: Speech Communication Research Laboratory. SCRL monograph no. 9.)

it from various positions along the vocal tract. The most distant position from which reflected waves arrive is the lips, and therefore wave A is affected by the behavior of A only as far back as 1 ms if the higher-order reflections are neglected. The way this effect on wave A affects the speech wave can be described in terms of the partial correlation between pairs of speech samples spaced 1 ms apart; that is, the partial correlation between x_n and x_{n-10}. Suppose wave A has proceeded for 0.45 ms and is 1.765 cm short of the lips. At that point it is further affected by the wave proceeding 0.1 ms ahead of wave A and is reflected at the lips. This effect is added to the speech wave via the partial correlation between pairs of samples spaced 0.1 ms apart; that is, between x_n and x_{n-1}. The intervening partial correlations have similar interpretations for the effects of the reflected waves at intermediate positions in the vocal tract.

In PARCOR analysis, one approach of linear prediction, the partial correlation between x_n and x_{n-1}, is computed first; it represents the effect added to the wave at a point 1.765 cm from the lips. In the next stage of analysis the partial correlation between x_n and x_{n-2} is computed by eliminating the effect from sample x_{n-1} by the use of the partial correlation between x_n and x_{n-2}. The partial correlation between x_n and x_{n-2} represents the effect

woven into the wave 3.53 cm from the lips. Thus successive stages unravel the effects accumulated into the wave at discrete points within the vocal tract (Fig. 13-9). At each stage the shaded portion represents the correlated quantity between pairs of samples; this quantity is subtracted from the original quantity at each stage of filtering. The residual signal is denoted as ϵ^+ and ϵ^-, and z^{-1} denotes a time delay corresponding to a sampling period. After subtraction of the correlated quantity at each stage, the partial correlation coefficient (k_i) to be used to determine the correlated quantity in the next stage is computed from the residual signal (Fig. 13-10). The triangles in the figure denote multipliers. From the partial correlation coefficients (k-parameters) thus computed, the filter coefficients (a-parameters) can be obtained easily with a *recursive relation,* in which successive members of a sequence are computed from a formula derived from the computed values of the preceding members of the sequence.

Some aspects of linear prediction are summarized here:

1. The coefficients of the transfer function polynomial of the inverse filter are identical to those of the regression polynomial that give the best estimate of the next speech sample in the least mean square principle.

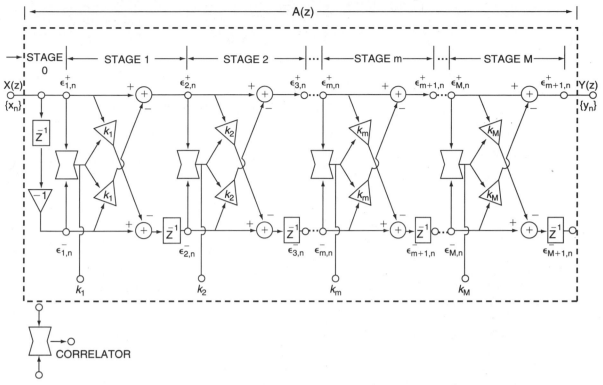

FIGURE 13-10   Detailed structure of the optimum inverse filter. (From Wakita, H. [1972]. *Estimation of vocal tract shape by optimal inverse filtering and acoustic to articulatory conversion methods.* Santa Barbara, CA: Speech Communication Research Laboratory. SCRL monograph no. 9.)

2. The peak frequencies in the speech spectrum are obtained either by solving for the roots of the transfer function polynomial of the inverse filter or by taking the Fourier transform of the filter coefficients.
3. The filter coefficients are obtained very efficiently through the partial correlation coefficients; these in turn give some physical insight into speech production.

Formant Analysis

It is easy to construct a block diagram for obtaining the peaks in the spectrum of a speech segment. Figure 13-11 shows a block diagram of inverse filtering. For a more accurate estimation of the higher formants, the higher-frequency components are emphasized by using the differencing network. The smooth spectral envelope is obtained by taking the FFT of the filter coefficients, which are computed by linear prediction analysis. An example of the smooth spectrum obtained by this analysis system and a comparison with the input spectrum are shown in Figure 13-12. The degree of the transfer func-

tion polynomial M, or the number of past data to be used for predicting the next sample, is 14. Various studies (e.g., Markel, 1972) show empirically that the optimum number for M depends on the sampling frequency used to digitize analog speech. If the sampling frequency is K kHz, the optimum number for M is between K and K + 4.

The next step is to track automatically the formant frequencies. However, a problem arises in choosing as precisely as possible the peaks attributable to vocal tract resonances, since the peaks do not always correspond to formants. Various schemes to choose the correct peaks have been attempted (e.g., Markel, 1973; McCandless, 1974). A simple peak-picking scheme applied to the smooth spectral envelope is fairly satisfactory for obtaining the formant trajectories for the first three formant frequencies. In it the three largest peaks of the speech spectrum in ascending order of frequency are defined as the formants. Although the input spectra will not produce correct results, peak picking of the inverse filter gives correct results approximately 90% of the time. This was tested on utterances

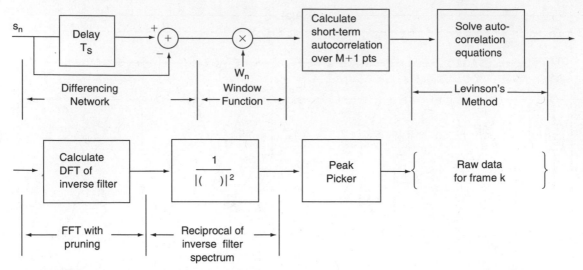

FIGURE 13-11 **A block diagram of inverse filtering for automatically extracting the raw data for formant trajectory estimation.** (From Markel, J. D. [1972]. Digital inverse filtering, a new tool for format trajectory estimation. *IEEE Transactions on Audio and Electroacoustics, AV-20,* 129-137.)

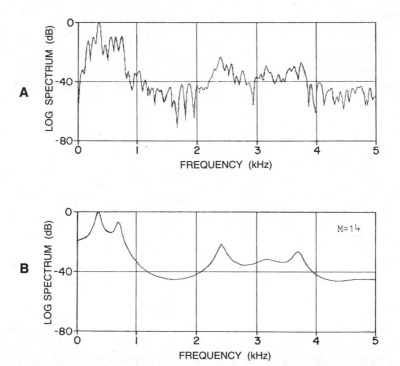

FIGURE 13-12 **A smooth spectral envelope produced by linear prediction. *A*, Input speech spectrum. *B*, Smooth spectrum.** (From Markel, J. D. [1972]. Digital inverse filtering, a new tool for formant trajectory estimation. *IEEE Transactions on Audio and Electroacoustics, AV-20,* 129-137.)

chosen as representative of a difficult form of voiced speech having close first and second formants, close second and third formants, and fast transition. One analysis for "we were away" is shown in Figure 13-13. Formant trajectories

are quite clear even from this raw data plotting. For this analysis, a sampling frequency of 10 kHz and a polynomial of order 14 were used. Each speech frame to be analyzed contained 256 samples spanning 25.6 ms, and analysis was

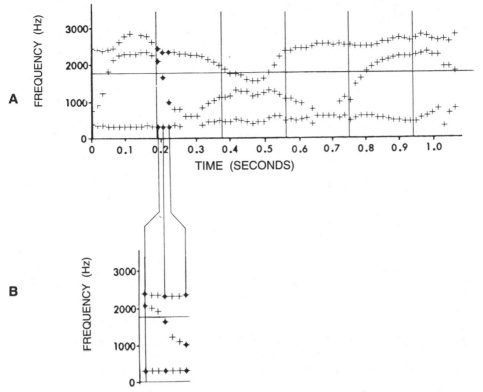

FIGURE 13-13 *A*, The raw data output for the utterance "we were away". *B*, An expanded resolution analysis for the interval indicated to illustrate the tracking of a rapid F_2 transition. (From Markel, J. D. [1972]. Digital inverse filtering, a new tool for formant trajectory estimation. *IEEE Transactions on Audio and Electroacoustics, AV-20*, 129-137.)

conducted every 16 ms. The portion where the formant frequencies are varying rapidly can also be analyzed more minutely by increasing the number of analyses.

Voice Pitch Extraction

Linear prediction processes speech so that an impulse or white noise is the residual signal. This ideal situation is actually realized as the degree of transfer function polynomial M approaches infinity. In practice, however, an optimum M was chosen to be at most the sampling frequency in kilohertz plus 4. Under this condition the residual signal is not an impulse or white noise. The linear prediction filter can extract the slowly varying frequency characteristics attributable to the glottal wave shape, the vocal tract, and the radiation, but it cannot extract the rapidly varying characteristics attributable to the fundamental frequency and its harmonics. The residual signal still contains this information; that is, the pitch information is well preserved in the residual signal (Fig. 13-14). The residual signal

contains clear peaks that are separated by a pitch period. The spikes correspond to the peaks of the original speech waveform. Thus, the largest prediction error occurs exactly at these peaks in the speech waveform.

There are various schemes to detect the periodicity of these spikes. The simplest is to compute the autocorrelation function of the residual signal. Two conspicuous spikes are found in the autocorrelation function, at the origin and at the point—that is, one pitch period from the origin. The pitch frequency is given by the reciprocal of the pitch period.

For signals that do not have a fundamental frequency component (such as telephone conversations, in which the fundamental may be too low in frequency to be transmitted), the harmonic relation is preserved in the residual signal even though the original signal does not have clear spikes in the time domain.

Although linear prediction was modeled for nonnasal voiced sounds, it has been demonstrated that it works for voiceless and nasal sounds as well, at least in analysis-synthesis

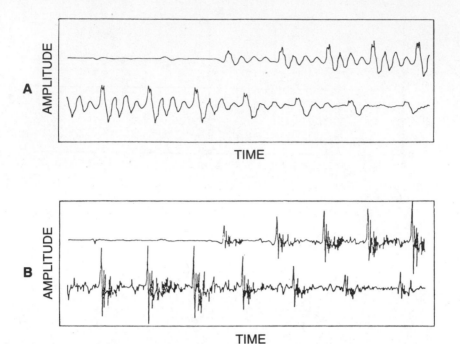

FIGURE 13-14 **Waveform from the segment "is".** *A,* Input speech. *B,* Residual signal. (From Markel, J. D., Gray, A. H., & Wakita, H. (1973). *Linear prediction of speech: Theory and practice.* Santa Barbara, CA: Speech Communication Research Laboratory. SCRL monograph no. 10.)

schemes. It is completely acceptable for voiceless and nasal sounds insofar as the peaks in their spectra are accurately extracted, although it becomes physically meaningless for these sounds, since it assumes the noise source always to be at the glottis for voiceless sounds and assumes no separate nasal tract for nasal sounds. A particular drawback of linear prediction is the inability to extract the spectral zeros (dips in the spectrum) attributable to the glottal waves and to the nasal tract. In addition to its computational convenience, a justification for using the linear prediction method to detect the spectral peaks is that the human ear is insensitive to the spectral zeros. Whether the detection of the spectral zeros is necessary and whether it is possible to determine them with reasonable accuracy remain unsolved.

Linear prediction is the most powerful analysis method in every respect. However, it is still essential to implement it in user-oriented analysis systems, either in software or in hardware. Otherwise, its merits as a research tool for phonetics may be lost. It is also important to be able to use other analysis methods, depending on the available instrumentation and the research problem at hand. For example, for the analysis of a small amount of speech data, the sound

spectrograph still may be the most useful instrument. On the other hand, if pitch is the only parameter to be extracted, easier and faster methods such as autocorrelation (Fujisaki, 1960) will suffice.

METHODS FOR COMPUTING VOCAL TRACT AREA FUNCTIONS

Background

Attempts to represent speech sounds as formant frequencies have been important in acoustic phonetics. There also has been considerable interest in the relationships between movements of articulators such as the tongue, jaw, and lips and formant frequency behavior (e.g., Chiba and Kajiyama, 1941; Dunn, 1950; Fant, 1960; Öhman, 1967; Lindblom and Sundberg, 1971). It is very difficult to determine formant frequencies directly from the positions of these articulators. Instead, the vocal tract configuration is first described as an area function determined by the position of the articulators. Although the actual vocal tract configuration is quite irregular and complicated, it is regarded for simplicity as a nonuniform acoustic tube having a cross-sectional area that varies along its length. To compute formant frequencies from a known vocal tract shape based on the acoustic tube model is relatively easy. However, it is open to question whether it is also possible to compute a unique vocal tract shape as an area function from acoustic data such as formant frequencies.

Until recently, the only way to obtain a vocal tract shape was to use x-ray film and palatograms, or plaster casts of the mouth, and so forth (Chiba and Kajiyama, 1941; Fant, 1960). Drawbacks of x-ray techniques are that processing the data is laborious and it requires guesswork and many assumptions. Yet even today the use of x-ray film is the most reliable method for observing the vocal tract area function, because it visualizes some details of the configuration. Probably x-ray film and direct measurement will continue for some time to be best for observing in detail the movements of articulators. On the other hand, it would certainly be convenient to have a simple, fast, efficient way to obtain information on the vocal tract shape, even if the information is less fine than that obtained through direct methods. There are two major recent developments in this area. The first is based on the mathematical formula *Webster's horn equation,* which describes the behavior of sound pressure and acoustic volume velocity of airflow within an acoustic tube. The other development is based on the linear prediction of speech.

Lip Impedance

The development of the lip impedance method was indeed an innovative attempt to estimate vocal tract shape from acoustic measurements (Mermelstein, 1967; Schroeder, 1967). To derive vocal tract shape from acoustic measurements or acoustic speech waveforms has been a dream of speech researchers for a long time. However, the lack of an appropriate analysis technique hindered development in this important area of speech research.

Lip impedance is based on Webster's horn equation. The vocal system is assumed to be lossless. That is, the input signal is assumed to transfer to output without any energy loss. This assumption allows the researcher to apply mathematical and engineering concepts to build a model. Introducing energy losses brings the model closer to reality, but it becomes very complicated to calculate the system's characteristics and responses. It is also assumed that the tract is closed at the glottis and open at the lips. For a given acoustic tube shape, Webster's horn equation gives an infinite number of resonance frequencies for a boundary condition not only with the glottis end closed and the lip end open but also with both ends closed. At the resonance frequencies for the first boundary condition, the input impedance looking into the tube from the lip end is *zero,* and it becomes infinite, or *pole,* at the resonance frequencies for the second boundary condition. Conversely, a theorem on the uniqueness of solutions demonstrates that a unique area function must exist, given a complete infinite set of zeros and poles of the input impedance. This means that to determine a unique vocal tract shape from a measured impedance, it is necessary to measure an infinite number of poles and zeros of the input impedance. In practice, however, we can observe only the first few zeros and poles of the lip impedance. Thus, the question is whether the use of the first few zeros and poles can produce a good representation of the original tube shape if the tube length is known.

A very significant finding was that the coefficients in the Fourier expansion of the logarithm of an area function are related to the zeros and poles of the lip impedance and their slight perturbations. Although the method was not straightforward, this finding permitted the computation of tube shape from given lip impedance zeros and poles and the condition of known tube length. The computation starts from a uniform tube for which the zeros and poles of the input impedance can be computed easily. Perturbing the first few zeros and poles yields a set of Fourier expansion coefficients and the first estimate of a perturbed tube shape. Exact zeros and poles of the input impedance are then recomputed for the perturbed tube shape, and further perturbations are introduced to bring them into coincidence with the measured values. This procedure is iterated until the computed zeros and poles draw as close to the given values as possible. A preliminary test on known area functions gave reasonably good results. However, difficulty lies in the measurement of the zeros and poles of the lip impedance. An impedance tube is connected to the subject's mouth, and a signal to measure the lip impedance is sent into the mouth via the tube; the

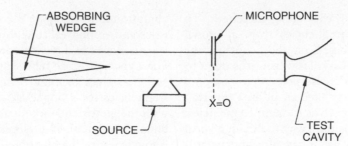

FIGURE 13-15 **Schematic of an experimental setup for estimating the vocal tract shape.** (From Sondhi, M. M., & Gopinath, B. [1971]. Determination of the vocal tract shape from impulse response at the lips. *Journal of the Acoustical Society of America, 49,* 1867-1873.)

subject is required to articulate without phonation (Fig. 13-15). This procedure imposes an unnatural condition on the subject, so it has not been pursued, even though it has been somewhat improved (Gopinath and Sondhi, 1970; Paige and Zue, 1970a; Wakita and Gray, 1975). However, the development of this method stimulated activities in this area, because it showed that a vocal tract shape actually could be deduced from acoustic data.

Lip Impulse Response

To avoid the drawbacks in the lip impedance method, Sondhi and Gopinath (1971) used an impulse to measure the acoustic impulse response at the lips. That eliminated the requirement of the boundary condition at the glottis, and the length did not have to be assumed (Fig. 13-15). An impulse generated by the source proceeds in both directions. The left-going signal is absorbed by the wedge so that no reflection of it takes place. The right-going signal is reflected at the lips according to the shape of the vocal tract. The microphone detects the right-going impulse and after some time delay, detects the reflected waves from the lips. Since the response dies down in a few milliseconds, rapidly recurring measurements allow study of the dynamics of a moving vocal tract. A subject again articulates without phonation. The procedure to construct the vocal tract shape from a measured impulse response is mathematically quite complicated, so its details will be omitted here. A test result obtained for a metal tube of known shape is reasonably good even though the tube has step discontinuities. Since this method assumes a lossless system, the losses should be considered for the impulse response measured from the actual lossy vocal tract (Sondhi, 1974).

Linear Prediction

In contrast to the previous two methods, linear prediction allows estimates of the vocal tract area function directly from acoustic speech waveforms. The mathematical procedure for computing the partial correlation coefficients is equivalent to a discrete solution for wave equations that describe the behavior of sound pressure and volume velocity inside an acoustic tube (Wakita and Gray, 1974). Thus, this theory applies to a model in which the vocal tract is regarded as a nonuniform acoustic tube represented by a concatenation of cylindrical tubes of equal length. The cross-sectional area denotes the average cross-sectional area of the corresponding portion of the vocal tract. For a discrete representation of an area function like this, the reflection coefficient μ_m can be defined at the boundary between two adjacent sections whose cross-sectional areas are S_m:

$$\mu_m = (S_m - S_{m+1})/(S_m + S_{m+1}) \qquad (8)$$

This relationship is actually a well-known result from elementary acoustics (Hunter, 1957). The sound pressure and the volume velocity within the acoustic tube can be represented in terms of the wave proceeding toward the lips (the forward-going wave) and the wave proceeding toward the glottis (the backward-going reflected wave). The two waves correspond to the error signals ϵ^+ and ϵ^-, respectively (Fig. 13-10). Interestingly enough, the partial correlation coefficients are equal to the respective reflection coefficients if the speech model is modified as follows. First, the transfer function we have considered so far includes all the contributions from the glottal and radiation characteristics as well as the vocal tract characteristics. This transfer function can be expressed as the reciprocal of a polynomial A for voiced

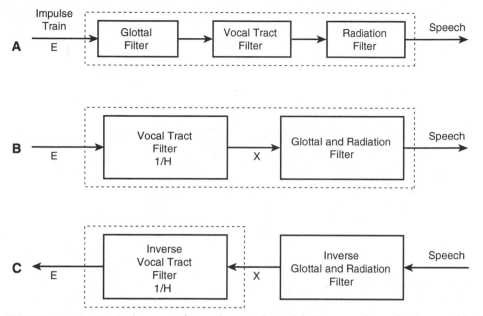

FIGURE 13-16 Equivalent transform of a speech model. *A*, a speech production model. *B*, an equivalent transform of A. *C*, a speech analysis model based on B.

and nonnasalized sounds. To obtain the true vocal tract transfer function, a speech production model (Fig. 13-16, *A*) is considered. Through the glottal filter an impulse train is shaped into a train of glottal waves that excites the vocal tract filter. Speech is generated after passing the output of the vocal tract filter through the radiation filter. Since the system is assumed to be linear, it can be modified into the system in Figure 13-16, *B* without changing the input-output relation. The vocal tract transfer function, 1/H, can then be computed from a knowledge of impulse train E and output X.

To determine the vocal tract transfer function from a given speech segment, consider the latter system in terms of an analysis model (Fig. 13-16, *C*). X is obtained through the inverse glottal radiation filter. Then the transfer function of the inverse vocal tract filter H can be determined by applying linear prediction, since it is formulated to produce the filter that with least squares will optimally transform X into an impulse train E. The partial correlation coefficients for this system are identical to the reflection coefficients of the vocal tract area function. Therefore, once the reflection coefficients are known, the area function is easily computed via Equation 8. In practice, the design of an optimum inverse glottal and radiation filter is one of the major problems in this method. However, since the

glottal and radiation characteristics in this case can be assumed to be slowly varying, they can be equalized approximately. For example, assuming a -12 dB/octave glottal characteristic and a +6 dB radiation characteristic, the glottal and radiation filter will have a -6 dB/octave characteristic. Thus, the inverse glottal and radiation filter are satisfied by a +6 dB/octave preemphasis of the input speech signal. In practice, even this crude equalization produces fairly reasonable results.

Another important factor is the length of the vocal tract (L). Since sampling period (T) is the time it takes for a sound wave to make a round trip between the ends of one of the cylindrical sections, the sampling frequency $F_s = 1/T$ must be adjusted to satisfy

$$L = cMT/2 = cM/(2F), \qquad (9)$$

where M is the number of sections in the model and c is a sound velocity approximately 353 m/sec under normal conditions. Figure 13-17 shows examples of area functions for five American vowels extracted from recordings of a male speaker. Gross features for each vowel are fairly well extracted, and smooth spectral characteristics of the vocal tract transfer function are shown alongside the area functions. One feature of linear prediction is its ability to perform simultaneous extraction of both area functions

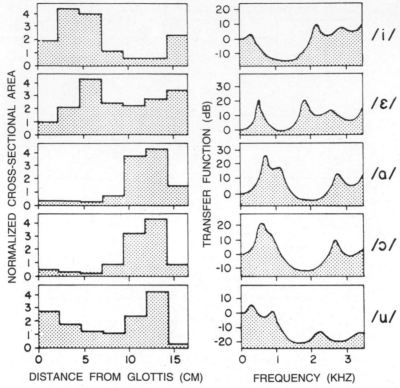

FIGURE 13-17   Vocal tract area functions and transfer functions obtained for five American vowels spoken by a male speaker. (From Wakita, H. [1972]. *Estimation of vocal tract shape by optimal inverse filtering and acoustic to articulatory conversion methods.* Santa Barbara, CA: Speech Communication Research Laboratory. SCRL monograph no. 9.)

and their corresponding smooth spectral envelopes. Dynamic changes in the area functions are also obtainable by analyzing successive frames of a recording.

The study of analysis techniques for observing vocal tract shapes is relatively new, and the capabilities and limitations of the linear prediction–acoustic tube method remain to be examined. For example, the method might be evaluated by comparing the results with those obtained from x-ray film. The accuracy of the x-ray film has not been established, since an accurate estimation of the lateral size of the vocal tract is rather difficult. Thus, the strict evaluation and comparison of these methods continues to be a problem. One study (Nakajima et al., 1973), using synthetic speech generated by a vocal tract analog synthesizer, reports that the original area functions are very well reconstructed by linear prediction.

Methods for estimating vocal tract length from given acoustic data also have been investigated (Paige and Zue, 1970b; Wakita, 1974). Continued studies in this area will be needed for

a better understanding of speech sounds. In addition, physiological studies of speech production will provide more information to interpret vocal tract area functions.

PERCEPTUALLY BASED ANALYSIS

Perceptually Based Linear Prediction

One interest in the study of acoustic phonetics is to extract parameters carrying the relevant phonetic information from a large amount of information obtainable from acoustic analysis of speech sounds. From the perceptual point of view, there are more consistent representations of vowels than formants, and a relatively small number of parameters is sufficient for complete phonetic specification of vowels. One is a two-peak representation of vowels based on perceptual experiments (Carlson, Fant, and Granstrom, 1975). In this study a vowel is specified by F_1 and F'_2, which is perceptually equivalent to higher formants.

Another proposal is that the vowel spectrum

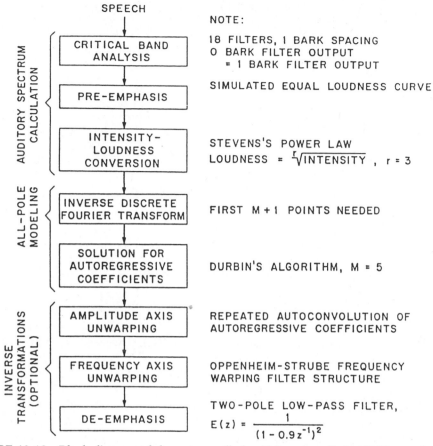

SPEECH

AUDITORY SPECTRUM CALCULATION

- CRITICAL BAND ANALYSIS
- PRE-EMPHASIS
- INTENSITY-LOUDNESS CONVERSION

ALL-POLE MODELING

- INVERSE DISCRETE FOURIER TRANSFORM
- SOLUTION FOR AUTOREGRESSIVE COEFFICIENTS

INVERSE TRANSFORMATIONS (OPTIONAL)

- AMPLITUDE AXIS UNWARPING
- FREQUENCY AXIS UNWARPING
- DE-EMPHASIS

NOTE:

18 FILTERS, 1 BARK SPACING
O BARK FILTER OUTPUT
= 1 BARK FILTER OUTPUT

SIMULATED EQUAL LOUDNESS CURVE

STEVENS'S POWER LAW
LOUDNESS = $\sqrt[r]{\text{INTENSITY}}$, $r = 3$

FIRST M + 1 POINTS NEEDED

DURBIN'S ALGORITHM, M = 5

REPEATED AUTOCONVOLUTION OF AUTOREGRESSIVE COEFFICIENTS

OPPENHEIM-STRUBE FREQUENCY WARPING FILTER STRUCTURE

TWO-POLE LOW-PASS FILTER,
$$E(z) = \frac{1}{(1 - 0.9z^{-1})^2}$$

FIGURE 13-18 **Block diagram of the perceptually based linear predictive (PLP) speech analysis method.** (From Hermansky, H., Hanson, B., & Wakita, H. [1985]. Low-dimensional representation of vowels based on all-pole modeling in the psychophysical domain. *Speech Communication, 4,* 181-187.)

is represented by major peaks obtained by two-stage peak extraction and auditory integration (Chistovich, Sheikin, and Lublinskaja, 1978). Stimuli with peaks closer than 3.5 Bark are found to be perceptually equivalent to one-peak stimuli with the peak position determined by the center of gravity of the two original peaks. When the distance between spectral peaks increases to more than 3.5 Bark, the one-peak representation is not possible.

A new approach introduced here models an auditory spectrum by an all-pole mathematical function, using autocorrelation linear prediction (Hermansky, Hanson, and Wakita, 1985; Hermansky, 1990). *Auditory spectrum* is the output of the critical-band filter bank followed by equal loudness curve preemphasis and intensity-loudness conversion. A fifth-order all-pole model is used to extract at most two major peaks from the auditory spectrum. All-pole modeling provides a compact representation of the audi-

tory spectrum shape in terms of its poles and corresponding bandwidths (Fig. 13-18).

The processing requires two steps: first, obtain the speech auditory spectrum, and second, approximate the auditory spectrum by an all-pole model. The auditory spectrum may be transformed back to the original amplitude frequency domain. The well-established psychophysical concepts of the critical band, equal loudness curves, and intensity-loudness power law are considered in this method.

In the **PLP method** (perceptually based linear prediction) the speech signal is first passed through critical-band bandpass filters. The 18 filters with a 1-Bark bandwidth are uniformly spaced on the Bark scale between 0 and 17 Barks. The roll-off characteristics of the filter are $+25$ dB/Bark toward lower frequency and -10 dB/Bark toward higher frequency. The filters can be simulated by weighted summation of a 20-ms short-time FFT power spectrum. The

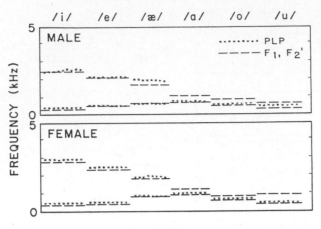

FIGURE 13-19   PLP-derived spectral peak frequencies (fifth-order analysis) and F_1, and F_2' frequencies. (From Hermansky, H., Hanson, B., & Wakita, H. [1985]. Low-dimensional representation of vowels based on all-pole modeling in the psychophysical domain. *Speech Communication, 4,* 181-187.)

value of the 0-Bark filter output is set equal to the value of the 1-Bark filter output, since the spectral slope of the subsequent all-pole model is always zero at 0 Bark. To approximate the auditory response over mid-range intensity levels, the critical-band output powers are weighted by an equal-loudness curve. The third root of the weighted critical-band power spectrum is used to approximate Stevens's power law to obtain the specific loudness representation.

Next, the 18-filter bank outputs are interpolated linearly in the power spectral domain to obtain a 256-point representation of the auditory spectrum. The interpolated auditory spectrum is then mapped into the autocorrelation domain by the inverse discrete Fourier transform and approximated by a fifth-order all-pole model using autocorrelation linear prediction. The dimensionality is reduced from the original 17 parameters (filter bank outputs) to 5 parameters of an all-pole model. The frequency resolution is effectively increased because positions of the peaks of the all-pole model are not restricted to the critical band center frequencies. Thus, the PLP method models the apparently conflicting auditory attributes of high resolution of spectral peaks and broad spectral integration.

Experimental Results

A set of vowels has been analyzed by the PLP method (Fig. 13-19). The peak trajectories for male and female speakers are similar. The front vowels /i/, /e/, and /æ/ are modeled by two peaks, and the back vowels /a/, /o/, and /u/ are modeled by one peak. This is in agreement with Delattre et al. (1952). The F_1, F_2' frequencies computed from LP-derived hand-edited vowel formant frequencies using the Carlson formula (Equation 1 in Carlson, Fant, and Granstrom, 1975) are also indicated in Figure 13-19 by the broken lines. Agreement of the PLP analysis results with this F_1, F_2' representation is good.

Figure 13-20 shows that while critical-band filtering yields a relatively smooth spectrum with at most two major peaks, the following low-order all-pole modeling removes the minor spectral peaks. The location of the local maxima of the all-pole model is consistent with the F_1, F_2' concept. The bandwidths of the poles indicate the spectral spread of the original formant cluster.

Analysis of Synthetic Speech

Chistovich, Sheikin, and Lublinskaja (1978) observed merging of the spectral peaks of the back vowels in experiments with two-formant synthetic speech stimuli. Their auditory integration theory simplifies the F_1, F_2' representation of the back vowels to a single peak. To examine this issue, a terminal analog serial synthesizer produced two-formant synthetic speech samples, and fifth-order PLP analysis was applied to them. The speech samples were generated like the ones Chistovich used in her perceptual experiments. The experiment was designed to de-

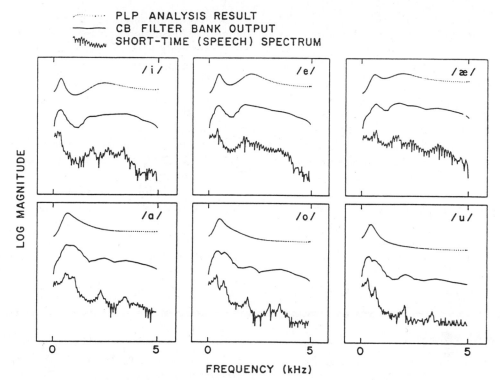

FIGURE 13-20   Spectra for vowels of a male speaker (short-time spectrum, interpolated critical band output, and PLP model). (From Hermansky, H., Hanson, B., & Wakita, H. [1985]. Low-dimensional representation of vowels based on all-pole modeling in the psychophysical domain. *Speech Communication, 4,* 181-187.)

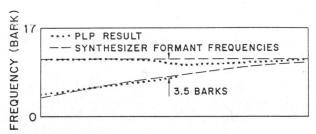

FIGURE 13-21   Comparison between PLP-derived spectral peak frequencies and formant frequencies for two-formant synthesized speech samples. (From Hermansky, H., Hanson, B., & Wakita, H. [1985]. Low-dimensional representation of vowels based on all-pole modeling in the psychophysical domain. *Speech Communication, 4,* 181-187.)

termine when the PLP method starts to integrate two spectral peaks into one peak. The first formant frequency varied from 350 Hz to 1600 Hz, and the second-formant frequency was fixed at 1800 Hz. The formant bandwidths were fixed at $B_1 = 150$ Hz and $B_2 = 200$ Hz. The synthesizer was pulse-excited with a fundamental frequency of 118 Hz. The combined effect of the glottal pulse and radiation characteristics was approximated by a real pole low-pass filter with a pole at $z = 0.5$ (Fig. 13-21). For comparison, the synthesizer formant frequencies are shown in the figure by broken lines, and arrows show where the 3.5-Bark separation between the synthesizer formant frequencies takes place. When the formants of the synthetic speech samples are far apart, PLP analysis estimates two distinct spectral peaks. As the formant frequencies become closer, the estimated peak frequencies start to deviate from the formant frequencies and finally merge into a single peak. The break point is in the vicinity of the 3.5-Bark separation. This finding agrees very well with Chistovich's results.

SUMMARY

This chapter discusses recent digital techniques for speech analysis. While there are techniques other than the ones discussed in this chapter, they have not been presented because of the limited space and their highly technical contents. One approach to be noted here is the time-frequency representation of speech signals based on generalized time-frequency analysis with higher-frequency resolution (Wakita and Zhao, 1993). This representation includes the conventional frequency spectrum by Fourier transform as well as spectrograms and further extends into an instantaneous spectral representation with higher frequency resolution.

Some of the remaining important and challenging issues in acoustic analysis are these:

1. An analysis method that is robust against noise and distortions
2. An articulatory model of speech production to generate clear, intelligible consonants
3. A method to relate acoustic parameters to articulatory parameters and vice versa
4. An analysis method for more accurately estimating formant frequencies for women's and children's speech.

It is hoped that future research and technological advancements will resolve these issues and thereby allow for more sophisticated analysis of the acoustic speech signal.

Review Questions

1. Draw the frequency spectrum of the following signals:

   A. A sinusoidal wave (frequency: 500 Hz, amplitude: 100)
   B. White noise.

2. Explain the principle of estimating the voice fundamental frequency.

3. Explain the basic concept used in linear prediction analysis.

4. What are the difficulties and problems in estimating the vocal tract shape from acoustic data?

5. What is the auditory spectrum?

References

Atal, B. S. (1970). Determination of the vocal tract shape directly from the speech wave. *Journal of the Acoustical Society of America, 47*, 65 (Abstract).

Atal, B. S., & Hanauer, S. L. (1971). Speech analysis and synthesis by linear prediction of the speech wave. *Journal of the Acoustical Society of America, 50*, 637-655.

Atal, B. S., & Schroeder, M. R. (1968). Predictive coding of speech signals. In Kohashi, Y. (Ed.), *Proceedings of the Sixth International Congress on Acoustics.* Tokyo: Acoustical Society of Japan (pp. C13-C16).

Bogert, B. P., Healy, M. J. R., & Tukey, J. W. (1963). The frequency analysis of time series for echoes: Cepstrum, pseudo-autocovariance, cross-cepstrum and shape. In Rosenblatt, M. (Ed.), *Proceedings of the Symposium on Series Analysis.* New York: Wiley (pp. 209-243).

Carlson, R., Fant, G., & Granstrom, B. (1975). Two formant models, pitch and vowel perception. In Fant, G., & Tatham, M. (Eds.), *Auditory Analysis and Perception of Speech.* New York: Academic Press (pp. 55-82).

Chiba, T., & Kajiyama, M. (1941). *The vowel, its nature and structure.* Tokyo: Kaiseikan.

Chistovich, L. A., Sheikin, R. L., & Lublinskaja, V. V. (1978). Centers of gravity and spectral peaks as the determinants of vowel quality. In Lindblom, B., & Öhman, S. (Eds.), *Frontiers of speech communication research.* New York: Academic Press (pp. 143-157).

Cooley, J. W., & Tukey, J. W. (1965). An algorithm for the machine calculation of complex Fourier series. *Mathematics of Computers, 19*, 297-301.

Delattre, P., Liberman, A. M., Cooper, F. S., & Gerstman, L. J. (1952). An experimental study of acoustic determinants of vowel color. *Word, 8*, 195-210.

Dunn, H. K. (1950). The calculation of vowel resonances and electrical vocal tract. *Journal of the Acoustical Society of America, 22*, 740-753.

Fant, C. G. M. (1960). *Acoustic theory of speech production.* The Hague: Mouton.

Fujisaki, H. (1960). Automatic extraction of fundamental period of speech by auto-correlation analysis and peak detection. *Journal of the Acoustical Society of America, 32*, 1518 (Abstract).

Gopinath, B., & Sondhi, M. M. (1970). Determination of the shape of the human vocal tract from acoustical measurements. *Bell System Technical Journal, 49*, 1195-1214.

Heinz, J. M. (1967, April). Perturbation functions for the determination of vocal tract area functions from vocal tract eigenvalues. *Speech Transmission Laboratory Quarterly Progress and Status Report.* Stockholm: Research Institute of Technology (pp. 1-14).

Hermansky, H. (1990). Perceptual linear predictive analysis of speech. *Journal of the Acoustical Society of America, 87*, 1738-1752.

Hermansky, H., Hanson, B., & Wakita, H. (1985). Low-dimensional representation of vowels based on all-pole modeling in the psychophysical domain. *Speech Communication, 4*, 181-187.

Hunter, J. L. (1957). *Acoustics.* Englewood Cliffs, NJ: Prentice-Hall.

Itakura, F., & Saito, S. (1968). Analysis synthesis telephony based on the maximum likelihood method. In Kohashi, Y. (Ed.), Proceedings of the Sixth International Congress on Acoustics. Tokyo: Acoustical Society of Japan (pp. C17-C20).

Itakura, F., & Saito, S. (1972). On the optimum quantization of feature parameters in the PARCOR speech synthesizer. In *Proceedings of the 1972 Conference on Speech Communication and Processing.* New York: IEEE (pp. 434-437).

Kelly, J. L., & Lochbaum, C. (1962). Speech synthesis. In *Preprints of the Stockholm Speech Communication Seminar.* Stockholm: Research Institute of Technology (pp. 30-37).

Lindblom, B. E. F., & Sundberg, J. E. F. (1971). Acoustical consequences of lip, tongue, jaw and larynx movement. *Journal of the Acoustical Society of America, 50*, 1166-1179.

Makhoul, J. (1975). Linear prediction: A tutorial review. *Proceedings of the Institute of Electrical and Electronic Engineers, 63*, 561-580.

Makhoul, J., & Wolf, J. (1972). *Linear prediction and the spectral analysis of speech* (Rep. 2304). Cambridge, MA: Bolt, Beranek, and Newman.

Markel, J. D. (1971). Formant trajectory estimation from a linear least-squares filter formulation. *SCRL Monographs, 7.* Santa Barbara: Speech Communications Research Laboratory.

Markel, J. D. (1972). Digital inverse filtering, a new tool for formant trajectory estimation. *IEEE Transactions on Audio and Electroacoustics, AU-20*, 129-137.

Markel, J. D. (1973). Application of a digital inverse filter for automatic formant and F_o analysis. *IEEE Transactions on Audio and Electroacoustics, AU-21*, 154-160.

Markel, J. D., & Gray, A. H. (1976). *Linear prediction of speech.* Berlin: Springer-Verlag.

Markel, J. D., Gray, A. H., & Wakita, H. (1973). *Linear prediction of speech: theory and practice.* Santa Barbara, CA: Speech Communication Research Laboratory. SCRL monograph no. 10.

McCandless, S. S. (1974). An algorithm for automatic formant extraction using linear prediction spectra. *IEEE Transactions on Acoustics, Speech, and Signal Processing, ASSP-22*, 135-141.

Mermelstein, P. (1967). Determination of vocal tract shape from measured formant frequencies. *Journal of the Acoustical Society of America, 41*, 1283-1294.

Mermelstein, P., & Schroeder, M. R. (1965). Determination of smoothed cross-sectional area functions of the vocal tract from formant frequencies. In Commins, D. E. (Ed.), *Proceedings of the Fifth International Congress on Acoustics.* Liege: (pp. 1a, A24).

Nakajima, T., Omura, H., Tanaka, K., & Ishizaki, S. (1973, February). *Estimation of vocal tract area function by adaptive inverse filtering.* Paper presented at the Speech Symposium of Acoustical Society of Japan, Sendai.

Noll, A. M. (1964). Short-time spectrum and cepstrum techniques for vocal pitch detection. *Journal of the Acoustical Society of America, 36*, 296-302.

Noll, A. M. (1967). Cepstrum pitch determination. *Journal of the Acoustical Society of America, 41*, 293-309.

Öhman, S. E. G. (1967). Numerical model of coarticulation. *Journal of the Acoustical Society of America, 41*, 310-320.

Paige, A., & Zue, V. W. (1970a). Computation of vocal tract area functions. *IEEE Transactions on Audio and Electroacoustics, AU-18*, 7-18.

Paige, A., & Zue, V. W. (1970b). Calculations of vocal tract length. *IEEE Transactions on Audio and Electroacoustics, AU-18*, 268-270.

Schafer, R. W., & Rabiner, L. R. (1970). System for the automatic analysis of voiced speech. *Journal of the Acoustical Society of America, 47*, 634-648.

Schroeder, M. R. (1967). Determination of the geometry of the human vocal tract by acoustic measurement. *Journal of the Acoustical Society of America, 41*, 1002-1010.

Sondhi, M. M. (1974). Model for wave propagation in a lossy vocal tract. *Journal of the Acoustical Society of America, 55*, 1070-1075.

Sondhi, M. M., & Gopinath, B. (1971). Determination of the vocal tract shape from impulse response at the lips. *Journal of the Acoustical Society of America, 49*, 1867-1873.

Stevens, K. N., Kasowski, S., & Fant, G. (1953). An

electrical analog of the vocal tract. *Journal of the Acoustical Society of America, 25,* 734-742.

Wakita, H. (1972). *Estimation of vocal tract shape by optimal inverse filtering and acoustic to articulatory conversion methods.* Santa Barbara, CA: Speech Communication Research Laboratory. SCRL monograph no. 9.

Wakita, H. (1973). Direct estimation of the vocal tract shape by inverse filtering of acoustic speech waveforms. *IEEE Transactions on Audio and Electroacoustics, AU-21,* 417-427.

Wakita, H., & Gray, A. H. (1974). *Some theoretical considerations for linear prediction of speech and applications.* Preprints of the Speech Communication Seminar. Stockholm: Speech Transmission Laboratory, KTH 1, (pp. 45-50).

Wakita, H., & Gray, A. H. (1975). Numerical determination of the lip impedance and vocal tract area functions. *IEEE Transactions on Acoustics, Speech, and Signal Processing, ASSP-23,* 574-580.

Wakita, H. (1977). Normalization of vowels by vocal-tract length and its application to vowel identification. *IEEE Transactions on Acoustics, Speech, and Signal Processing, ASSP-25,* 183-192.

Wakita, H., & Zhao, Y. (1993). On the time-frequency display of speech signals using a generalized time-frequency representation with a cone-shaped kernel. In Cooke, M., Beet, S., & Crawford, M. (Eds)., *Visual Representations of Speech Signals.* New York: Wiley (pp. 355-361).

Suggested Readings

Digital Computers

White, R. (1993). How Computer Works. Emeryville, CA: Ziff-Davis.

White, R. (1993). How Software Works. Emeryville, CA: Ziff-Davis.

General Acoustic Analysis

Borden G. J., Harris, K. S., & Raphael, L. J. (1994). *Speech science primer: Physiology, acoustics, and perception of speech,* (3rd ed.). Baltimore: Williams & Wilkins.

Flanagan, J. L. (1965). *Speech analysis, synthesis, and perception.* New York: Springer-Verlag.

Ladefoged, P. (1962). *Elements of Acoustic Phonetics.* Chicago: University of Chicago Press.

O'Shaughnessy, D. (1987). *Speech communication, human and machine.* New York: Addison-Wesley.

Cepstrum Method

Rabiner, L. R., & Schafer, R. W. (1978). *Digital processing of speech signals.* Englewood Cliffs, NJ: Prentice-Hall.

Linear Prediction

Wakita, H. (1980). New methods of analysis in speech acoustics. *Phonetica, 37,* 87-108.

Makhoul, J. (1975). Linear prediction: a tutorial review. *IEEE Proceedings, 63,* 561-580.

Markel, J. D., & Gray, A. H. (1976). *Linear prediction of speech.* Berlin: Springer-Verlag.

Vocal Tract Area Function

Wakita, H. (1980). New methods of analysis in speech acoustics. *Phonetica, 37,* 87-108.

Mermelstein, P. (1967). Determination of vocal tract shape from measured formant frequencies. *Journal of the Acoustical Society of America, 41,* 1283-1294.

Pitch Estimation

Hess, W. J. (1983). Pitch determination of speech signals: algorithms and devices. Berlin: Springer-Verlag.

Markel, J. D., & Gray, A. H. (1976). *Linear prediction of speech.* Berlin: Springer-Verlag.

Formant Estimation

Markel, J. D., & Gray, A. H. (1976). *Linear prediction of speech.* Berlin: Springer-Verlag.

McCandless, S. S. (1974). An algorithm for automatic formant extraction using linear prediction spectra. *IEEE Transactions on Acoustic, Speech and Signal Processing, ASSP-22,* 135-141.

Perceptually Based Analysis

Hermansky, H. (1990). Perceptual linear predictive analysis of speech. *Journal of the Acoustical Society of America, 87,* 1738-1752.

Chapter 14

Instrumentation for the Study of Speech Physiology

Maureen Stone

Chapter Outline

Key Terms

INTRODUCTION

The vocal tract is a complex system. It contains structures that are bony and therefore rigid as well as structures that are muscular and therefore flexible. The muscular soft tissue structures (tongue, lips, and velum) differ significantly in movement dimensionality from the hard tissue structures (jaw and palate). For example, the fluid deformation of the tongue needs quite different measurement strategies from the rigid body movements of the jaw. Jaw movement has three degrees of freedom: rotation about the temporomandibular joint (TMJ), anteroposterior translation, and superoinferior translation. Chewing uses lateral movements as well, but normal speech does not. The tongue, on the other hand, moves in a fluid manner. Local tongue regions will expand and compress to create displacement at a specific location on the tongue, forming a vocal tract constriction. For example, the tongue root pulls forward, helping to elevate the tongue tip. Local tongue displacement can occur in several places in the vocal tract, for example, alveolar displacement during [t] versus velar displacement during [k]. Not only are the constrictions in different parts of the vocal tract, but they are made using different parts of the tongue. Moreover, the shape of the tongue as it approximates the palate is a significant factor in distinguishing among sounds, such as [l] versus [s] versus [n]. Thus, whereas the rigid jaw has three degrees of freedom, the fluid tongue has many more.

A second feature of this complex system is the different speeds and movement patterns of the articulators. An instrument with a frequency response adequate for the slow-moving jaw will not necessarily be adequate for the fast-moving tongue tip. As for movement, the lips can spread, close, and round. The jaw is hinged at one end and swings open. An instrument with the range to measure jaw opening may have too great a range to measure the subtleties of lip rounding. Similarly, differences in articulator location significantly affect the type of transduction system needed. Structures that are visible to superficial inspection, such as the lips, are much easier to record than structures deep within the oral cavity, such as the velum.

The final and perhaps most important complication in measuring articulatory movement is the interaction among articulators. Some articulators are nested in others. Both the lower lip and the tongue nest on the jaw. Therefore, the movement of the jaw is highly correlated with the movements of the lower lip and tongue.

When measuring a nested structure, it is often useful to determine how much the support structure contributes and whether the measurement should include supporting behavior. The effect of the supporting structure is most dramatically observed in the tongue-jaw system. Although jaw height is a major factor in tongue height at the tip, the coupling of the two structures becomes progressively weaker as one moves posteriorly until in the pharynx tongue movement is only minimally coupled to jaw movement if at all. Thus, trying to measure the contribution of jaw movement to tongue movement is quite a difficult task. An equally important question is whether the research study must assess the tongue alone or as part of the tongue-jaw unit. In a complex system like the vocal tract, an instrument that accurately measures one articulator may be inadequate to measure another. For example, tracking one point on the jaw provides excellent jaw movement data. However, tracking one point on the tongue or lips fails to capture the complex, nonrigid nature of their movements. If a **transducer** is inserted into the mouth, it must not distort the speech event. This is very difficult to do, and virtually all intraoral transducers require at least a minimal adjustment on the part of the speaker.

Instruments that measure articulatory behavior must be unobtrusive. This can be achieved if the device rests flat against a surface (e.g., electropalatography [EPG]), is small and positioned on noncontact surfaces (e.g., pellet tracking systems), or does not enter the vocal tract at all (e.g., **imaging techniques**). Instruments that enter the oral cavity must also meet other criteria. They must be unaffected by temperature change, moisture, and air pressure. Adhesives must be unaffected by moisture, stick to expandable moist surfaces, and be removable without tearing the surface tissue. Devising instruments that are noninvasive and unobtrusive, meet the above criteria, and still measure one or more components of the speech event is quite difficult as evidenced by the larger number of acoustic than physiological studies on speech production in the literature. However, since those inferences are based on some initial physiological data, it is critical that new physiological data be added and refined, lest models of the vocal tract and our understanding of speech production stagnate. Physiological measurements are continually being developed and improved. Point-tracking systems are revealing interarticulator relationships that could be addressed only theoretically in the past. Imaging techniques have expanded our perception of the vocal tract as a three-dimensional system by providing recognizable images and cross-sectional surface information about structures deep within the pharynx. Finally, instruments with a relatively long history of use in speech science, such as electropalatography and electromyography, have been improved to provide better and more useful data. This chapter considers three types of nonacoustic instruments for measuring speech physiology: **point-tracking techniques**, imaging techniques, and measures of complex behaviors. It is not meant to be exhaustive but rather to provide an overview of most of the major instruments used to measure speech physiology.

POINT-TRACKING MEASUREMENTS OF THE VOCAL TRACT

Point-tracking systems measure individual **fleshpoints** by affixing pellets to the articulators and tracking their movement during speech. Typically, several articulators can be measured at the same time and tracking speed is fast, so that interarticulator timing measures are quite good. Three specific point tracking systems, the articulometer, the x-ray microbeam, and the Optotrak, are significantly improving the quality of vocal tract measurements.

Electromagnetic Midsagittal Articulometer

The electromagnetic midsagittal articulometer (EMMA) tracks fleshpoint movement by measuring the movement of small receiver coils through **alternating magnetic fields**. Several such instruments using roughly similar principles have been developed in Germany (Schonle et al., 1987, 1989), Sweden (Branderud, 1985), and the United States (Perkell, Cohen, and Garabi-

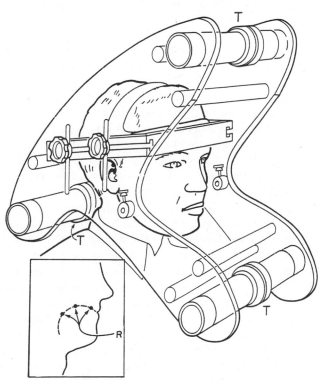

FIGURE 14-1   The electromagnetic midsagittal articulometer. T = transmitter coil; R = receiver coil. (After Perkell, J., Cohen, M., Svirsky, M., Matthies, M., Garabieta, I., & Jackson, M. [1992]. Electromagnetic midsagittal articulometer [EMMA] systems for transducing speech articulatory movements. *Journal of the Acoustical Society of America, 92,* 3078-3096.)

eta, 1988; Perkell et al., 1992). In the Perkell system a clear plastic assembly suspended from above fits around the subject's head (Fig. 14-1). Three transmitter coils (T) form an equilateral triangle, and each produces an alternating magnetic field. Each transmitter is driven at a different sinusoidal frequency to generate a different alternating magnetic field. The use of three transmitters, and therefore three overlapping fields, assures accuracy in locating the receiver coils (R). The best resolution in the field space is found in the center (i.e., in the oropharyngeal region), where measurement resolution is calculated at less than 1 mm. The receiver coils are small insulated coils attached with adhesive to articulatory structures at midline. As the alternating magnetic fields pass through the receiver coil, they induce an alternating signal in the receiver coils. The voltage of this signal is inversely related to the distance between the transmitter and the receiver coil. A computer algorithm calculates the actual location of the receiver coil as it moves in xy space over time.

One disadvantage of this system is that only points are measured, so the behavior of the entire articulator is largely inferred. This is most problematic for the soft tissue structures like the lips, tongue, and velum, whose movements are more fluid than rigid. A second disadvantage is that the data can be collected only at midline, and the receiver coils are subject to error when the articulators rotate left to right. The greatest advantages are the rapid tracking rate and the ability to track multiple articulators simultaneously. Because of these two advantages, interaction among the articulators can be measured and questions about interarticulator timing and programming can be asked. Although there has been some concern over possible health consequences from exposure to magnetic fields, the articulometer poses minimal biological hazards, since it uses short exposure times and low field strengths. Nonetheless, its use is not recommended with pregnant women.

X-ray Microbeam

The x-ray microbeam uses an extremely thin x-ray beam to track the motion of small gold pellets that are affixed to one or more articulators using dental adhesive (Westbury, 1991, 1994). The beam is 0.4 mm thick, and the pellets are 2 to 3 mm in diameter. Gold pellets are used because gold is inert and since the x-ray dosage is very small, only a very dense metal can be detected. The system was designed to reduce radiation dosage to well below that of a dental x-ray, to avoid radiosensitive areas (such as the eyes) and to reduce secondary photon scatter. The x-ray beam focuses primarily on the pellets so that the surrounding tissue receives only minimal radiation. The two-dimensional position of the beam is computer controlled. The x-ray beam originates at one side of the subject, passes through the subject's head, and is detected by a scintillation counter on the far side. Up to 1000 pellet positions are sampled per second. Thus, if 10 pellets are used, they can each be sampled 100 times per second. Differential sampling rates are also possible. Positioning accuracy of the beam is 62μ. Initially, the pellets are sampled in rest position to determine baseline xy displacement. A computer algorithm causes the beam to scan the area in which the pellet is predicted to move; the prediction is based on the pellet's previous displacement, velocity, and acceleration. Each pellet is scanned in order and the output is a tracking of pellet movement. Fig. 14-2 shows tongue surface shapes for the consonants [s] and [l] in three different vowel contexts with five pellets attached to the tongue surface.

There are several advantages to the x-ray microbeam. The rapid rate and accuracy of tracking make this an excellent system for examining timing-related coarticulatory effects, kinematic parameters such as velocity and acceleration, and the intercoordination of the articulators. In addition, the technique is unobtrusive and the low radiation dosage allows for reasonably large data sets to be collected on each subject. A disadvantage of the x-ray microbeam is that the large, costly facility and support staff needed will always be either unique or rare. Therefore, it requires considerable travel for most investigators and their subjects to reach the facility. The second disadvantage is that although the radiation dosage is low, the use of x-ray and its known biological hazards must still be considered a limitation of the system. A final disadvantage is that with a 450 kV beam, the x-ray will not pass through silver, and therefore subjects must have no fillings. However, a new or upgraded machine could produce a 600 kV beam level that will pass through silver fillings but not gold pellets, allowing the pellets to be better imaged.

Two other limitations are common to both

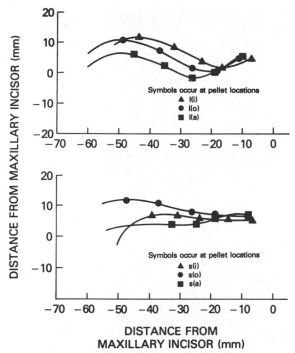

FIGURE 14-2 Tongue surfaces measured from ultrasound images for [s] (lower) and [l] (upper) in three vowel contexts. Five x-ray microbeam pellets are affixed to the tongue surface. (From Stone, M. [1990]. A three-dimensional model of tongue movement based on ultrasound and x-ray microbeam data. *Journal of the Acoustical Society of America, 87,* 2207-2217.)

the articulometer and the x-ray microbeam. First, only two-dimensional data are collected, and movements off-plane are lost or induce error. The second common problem is the difficulty of affixing pellets to the pharynx, velum, and posterior tongue due to the gag reflex, which limits their use with some subjects.

Strain Gauges

Strain gauges were developed for use in lip and jaw measurements in the early 1970s (Abbs and Gilbert, 1973; Muller et al., 1977; Barlow and Abbs, 1983). Strain gauge transducers are composed of two sequential, perpendicular, very thin cantilever beams (about 0.13 mm) on which are mounted miniature strain gauges. From the end of the outer beam a rigid wire extends and is affixed at midline to the articulator of interest; the wire moves with the articulator. The perpendicular arrangement of the beams causes one to bend in response to anteroposterior move-

ment and the other to bend in response to superoinferior movement. The bending of the beams is converted into a proportional voltage by the strain gauges mounted on them. The changes in voltage produce an analog waveform that can be recorded on an FM recorder, printed out on an oscillograph, or digitized and entered into a computer. In addition, the waveform can be differentiated to yield velocity and acceleration data (Fig. 14-3).

The method of attachment of the gauge to the jaw is of interest in both this instrument and the other jaw measurement instruments. Since the skin of the jaw moves with lower lip movement, an **artifact** in measures of jaw movement is created if the rigid wire is affixed to the skin below the chin rather than to a mandibular tooth. Kuehn, Reich, and Jordan (1980) used x-ray to calculate error in movement of a chin-mounted transducer relative to movement of the lower incisor. They found some error in both labial and nonlabial consonants with a chin mount. The tooth mount placement eliminated this problem. However, it may interfere with lip movement. Careful planning of speech materials and theoretical questions is needed to overcome these weaknesses. More recent modifications and applications of strain gauge technology have been used to measure lip and jaw closing force in nonspeech activities. Measurements of maximum voluntary closure force (Barlow and Rath, 1985) and controlled sustained closure force (Barlow and Burton, 1990) have provided normative data on lip and jaw forces. These data can be applied to dynamic models of lip and jaw movement as well as to comparisons of normal and disordered movements.

Optotrak

Another point tracking system, Optotrak, is a new and improved version of the older Watsmart. This device tracks the movement of points in three-dimensional (xyz) space. Thus, Optotrak can measure side-to-side movement as well as anteroposterior and superoinferior movement (Vatikiotis-Bateson and Ostry, in press). The system consists of markers placed on surface structures, sensors that track their position, and a system unit that controls the timing of the marker emissions and the sensor processing. The markers are lightweight disks that come in two diameters, 4.75 mm and 16 mm. Embedded in the center of each marker is a small

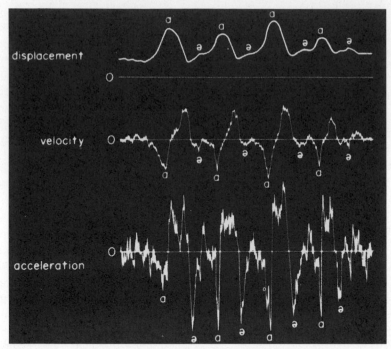

FIGURE 14-3 Strain gauge data showing displacement, velocity, and acceleration for jaw movement.

semiconductor chip that emits an infrared signal. Up to 256 markers can be used at one time. A strip of three sensors acts as a camera and tracks the movement of the markers. This is not a video system in which marker position is filmed. Rather, each sensor contains a lens and signal processing circuitry that records the infrared emissions of the marker. The sensors are prealigned so that they measure the position of each marker in three-dimensional space.

This instrument is particularly well suited to tracking lip and jaw motion in three dimensions and examining relationships between them and head position (Fig. 14-4). Its advantage over the other two point-tracking systems is that it provides three-dimensional motion data. The third dimension allows measurement of rotation and provides a better understanding of speech kinematics and motor control. The system's disadvantage is that unlike the x-ray microbeam and articulometer, it is limited to external use because its sensors track light-emitting diodes (LED) and must maintain visual contact with them. Therefore, it cannot be used inside the mouth and so does not reveal structures within the vocal tract. Two more disadvantages are common to all point-tracking systems. First, only fleshpoints are tracked, not the entire structure. For rigid structures such as the jaw,

the entire structure can be reconstructed. However, the flexibility of soft tissue structures, such as the tongue, lips, and velum, is incompletely measured and represented. Second, the markers or their attached wires may interfere, at least minimally, with truly natural speech.

IMAGING TECHNIQUES

The internal structures of the vocal tract are difficult to measure without impinging upon normal movement patterns. Imaging techniques overcome that difficulty because they register internal movement without directly contacting the structures. Four well-known imaging techniques have been applied to speech research: x-ray, computed tomography (CT), magnetic resonance imaging (MRI), and ultrasound. Imaging systems provide very different information from other physiological measures; they provide an image of the entire structure rather than a single point on the structure.

X-ray

X-ray is the best known of the imaging systems and is important because until recently most of our knowledge about the behavior of the pharyngeal portion of the vocal tract came from

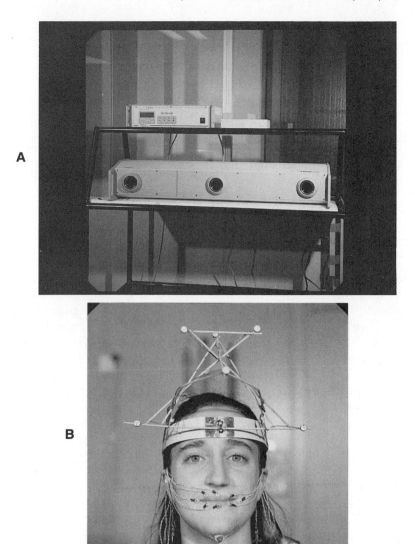

FIGURE 14-4   Optotrak. *A,* Three single-axis CCD position sensors compute the positions of multiple infrared LEDs in three dimensions. *B,* LEDs are attached to the subject's head, lips, and jaw and tracked during speech. (Courtesy of E. Vatikiotis-Bateson.)

x-ray data. To make a lateral x-ray image, an x-ray beam is projected from one side of the head through all the tissue and is recorded on a plate on the other side. The resulting image shows the head from front to back and provides a lengthwise view of the tongue. A frontal or anteroposterior x-ray is made by projecting the x-ray beam from the front of the head through to the back of the head and recording the image on a plate behind the head. The resulting image provides a cross-sectional, or side-to-side, view of the tongue, which appears as a dark shadow (Fig. 14-5). Usually soft tissue structures such as the tongue are difficult to measure with x-rays because the beam records everything in its path,

including teeth, jaw, and vertebrae. These strongly imaged bony structures obscure the fainter soft tissue.

A second problem with x-ray is that unless a contrast medium is used to mark the midline of the tongue, it is difficult to tell if the visible edge is the midline of the tongue or a lateral edge. This is particularly problematic during speech because the tongue commonly is grooved. Finally, the hazards of overexposure preclude the collection of large quantities of data with ordinary x-rays. The x-ray microbeam was devised to overcome this limitation by tracking points and vastly reducing the x-ray exposure. Considerable research has been conducted using

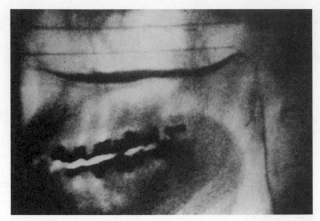

FIGURE 14-5   Lateral x-ray of the vocal tract. Anterior is on the left. The vertebrae can be seen on the lower right, the tongue and jaw on the left.

x-ray imaging. Most models of the vocal tract are based on x-ray data (Fant, 1965; Mermelstein, 1973; Harshman, Ladefoged, and Goldstein, 1977; Wood, 1979); Hashimoto and Sasaki, 1982; Maeda, 1989). X-rays have also been used to study normal speech production (Kent and Netsell, 1971; Kent, 1972; Kent and Moll, 1972) and speech disorders (Subtelney et al., 1989; Tye-Murray, 1991).

Xeroradiography

Xeroradiography, also a projection technique, uses a conventional x-ray tube to generate the x-rays. However, the image receptor is an aluminum plate coated with selenium, a photoconductive material, while the image receptor for a standard x-ray is x-ray film. The first stage in making a xeroradiograph is the formation of a latent image on the aluminum plate. The second stage is the development of that image into a xeroradiographic image. In stage 1, the selenium-coated aluminum plate is **electrostatically charged** before being exposed to the x-ray. The selenium coating acts as an insulator. When exposed to x-rays or light, selenium's insulating ability decreases in proportion to the amount of exposure, discharging a proportional amount of static electricity. This effect is extremely well localized. The x-ray exposure at one point does not cause discharge nearby, so that the edges of an object are very well defined. The plate at this point contains an invisible electrostatic representation of an x-ray image, called a *latent image*. The plate is taken to a light-tight chamber for stage 2, development. To develop the xeroradiograph, an aerosol of electrically charged pigmented powder is sprayed on the latent im-

age, trans ferred to paper, and fused by heating. Positive and negative xeroradiographs can be made. However, the plate must be cleaned (heated and cooled) before reuse to prevent shadow contours from previous images (Schertel et al., 1976; Zeman, 1976).

The advantage of xeroradiography is the extreme clarity at the edges of a structure, even a soft tissue structure (Fig. 14-6). However, the disadvantages are considerable. First, it is a very slow procedure, requiring two stages that can be used only for steady-state vocal tract measurements. Second, the technique uses considerably more radiation than conventional x-rays (Schertel et al., 1976). Third, the machines are difficult to maintain and are very sensitive to dust because of the static electricity. Last, these machines are quite old and difficult to find. Thus, this technique does not seem as well suited to speech research as the other imaging techniques available.

Tomography

Tomography creates images in a fundamentally different way from **projection x-ray.** **Tomographs,** or pictures of slices of tissue, are constructed by projecting a thin, flat beam through the tissue in a single plane. To interpret these data, four tomographic planes are used (Fig. 14-7). They are sagittal, coronal, oblique, and transverse. The midsagittal plane is a longitudinal slice from top to bottom down the median plane, or midline, of the body (broken line). The parasagittal plane is parallel to the midline of the body but off center. The coronal plane is a longitudinal slice perpendicular to the median plane of the body, and the oblique plane

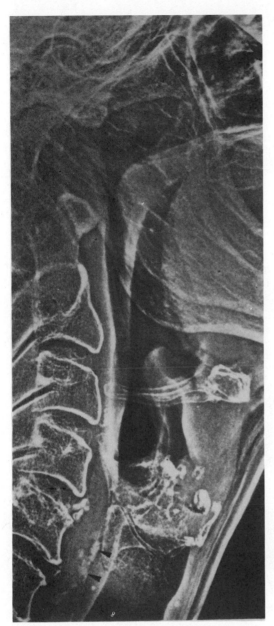

FIGURE 14-6 Xeroradiograph of the pharynx and posterior tongue. Anterior is on the right.

puter then creates a composite, including any structures that were visible in some scans but obscured in others. Fig. 14-9 shows a transverse section CT of the oropharynx at rest. Bone appears bright white in the image. The jaw can be seen at the top of the image and a vertebra at the bottom.

The hyoid bone is horseshoe shaped, in the middle of the image. The air in the vocal tract appears black, and the epiglottis can be seen within the vocal tract. The tongue and other soft tissue are gray. CT can image soft tissue more clearly than projection x-ray because it produces a composite section that has sharper edges and more distinct tissue definition. However, very few studies have used CT to image the vocal tract because of radiation exposure and because MRI provides much the same information. Studies that do depict the vocal tract using CT include those by Kiritani, Kakita, and Shibata (1977), Muraki et al. (1983), and Sundberg et al. (1987).

CT has three major limitations. The first is speed: most CT scans take 2.5 seconds per frame, too slow for real-time speech. The newer CTs can take several scans per second, so future technology may reduce this problem. The second limitation is the radiation exposure. CT is an x-ray; therefore, only limited data can be collected on a single subject. Finally, the scan images are limited to the transverse and oblique planes because the scanning table can only be tilted approximately 45 degrees. On the positive side, CT can image the entire tract, sectioning multiple planes for analysis. In addition, the images are extremely clear and the edges are easy to measure. The sections are quite thin (2 mm), allowing composite three-dimensional vocal tract shapes to be constructed by combining multiple sections.

Magnetic Resonance Imaging

Another tomographic technique is magnetic resonance imaging (MRI), sometimes called *nuclear magnetic resonance*. MRI uses a magnetic field and **radio waves** rather than x-rays to image a section of tissue. It is very effective at differentiating different types of tissue, and therefore a number of studies have used it to view vocal tract anatomy (Lufkin, 1983; Christianson, Lufkin, and Hanafee, 1987; McKenna et al., 1990). Several studies cross-validated or coupled MRI with other instruments, such as

is inclined between the horizontal and vertical planes. Finally, the transverse plane lies perpendicular to the long axis of the body and is often called the *transaxial* or *axial plane*.

Computed Tomography

Computed tomography (CT) uses x-rays to image slices of the body as thin as 2 mm. Fig. 14-8 depicts a CT scanner. The scanner rotates around the body, taking many images at different angles of a single section of tissue. A com-

IMAGING TECHNIQUES

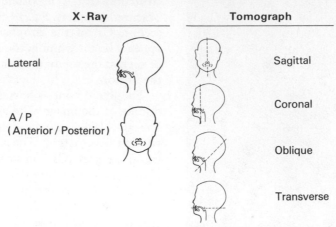

FIGURE 14-7 Scan types used in through-transmission (x-ray) and tomographic imaging. There are two x-ray angles contrasted with four tomographic scanning planes.

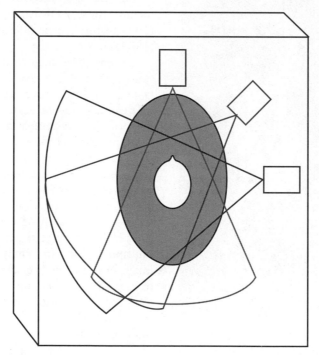

FIGURE 14-8 Schematic of patient lying in CT scanner with multiple scans being made and combined into an image.

ultrasound (Takashima et al., 1989; Wein et al., 1990), x-ray (Lakshminarayanan, Lee, and Mc-Cutcheon, 1990, 1991) and **glossometry** (Mc-Cutcheon et al., 1990). The last study cited validated both instruments by using tongue-palate spacers to generate known tongue positions.

MRI also has been used to calculate vocal tract volumes (Baer et al., 1987, 1991; Lakshminarayanan et al., 1990, 1991; Moore, 1992; Tiede, 1993). Lakshminarayanan et al. (1990) used a newer technique that allowed scan times as low as 4 seconds per image. This rapid rate was achieved through the use of a specially designed coil that highlighted the oral area and a gradient-echo technique. The **formant** patterns generated by the resultant model were generally comparable with real acoustic data, but individual formants varied by as much as 500 Hz. The authors hypothesized that the error might be due to their width-to-area conversion algo-

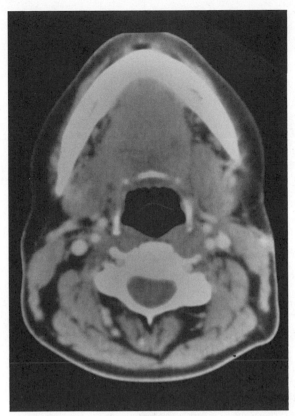

FIGURE 14-9 CT image of a transverse section of the oropharynx at rest.

rithm or to their assumptions of cross-sectional tube area. MRI is very useful for studying pathology that involves tissue changes, such as tumors, and highlights other speech-related pathologies as well. Takashima et al. (1989) used MRI and ultrasound in the staging of tongue cancers, while Cha and Patten (1989) described tongue postural abnormalities in amyotrophic lateral sclerosis (ALS) patients. In addition, Wein et al. (1991) employed sagittal images to demonstrate velopharyngeal insufficiency in five patients with varied pathologies.

An MRI scanner consists of electromagnets that surround the body and create a magnetic field. MRI scanning detects hydrogen atoms, which occur in abundance in water and therefore in tissue. In Fig. 14-10, *A* represents a hydrogen proton spinning about an axis which is oriented randomly. *B* shows what happens when a magnetic field is introduced. The proton's axis aligns along the direction of the field's poles. However, even when aligned the proton wobbles, or precesses. In *C*, a short-lived radio pulse, vibrating at the same frequency as the wobble, is introduced. This momentarily knocks

the proton out of alignment. *D* shows the proton realigning within milliseconds to the magnetic field. As it realigns, the proton emits a weak radio signal of its own. These radio signals are assembled as an image indicating hydrogen density, or water content, thus clearly differentiating between different types of tissue.

Fig. 14-11 shows a sagittal MRI image of [s] taken in the midsagittal plane. The subject held the [s] for 45 seconds to make this image. The vocal tract appears black, as do the teeth, since neither contain water. The marrow in the palate, which is high in water content, and the fat surrounding the head, which is high in hydrogen, are bright white. Although the edges are not as crisp as with CT, they are reasonably clear and easily measurable. A new application of MRI, the tagging snapshot technique, has been used by Kumada et al. (1992) and Niitsu et al. (1992) to examine tongue position at the beginning and end of a movement and to derive the direction of movement. In this technique tagging stripes are superimposed on a slice of tissue. As the tissue changes shape and position, the stripes move and deform, reflecting the changes in the tissue (Fig. 14-12). Thus, one can see compression and expansion within the body of the tongue.

As with CT, MRI has several drawbacks. The first is speed; the radio signal emitted by each proton is so weak that it must be summed over time. Image time for good resolution takes 3 seconds (Wein et al., 1991) to 6 minutes (Moore, 1992). Newer techniques, such as echo planar imaging, take as little as 50 ms per scan, but resolution is still poor (64 × 64 pixels), and the images can be very distorted by the air in the vocal tract. However, MRI speed is improving and progressing toward real time. The second drawback is the width of the section. Whereas CT sections are 2 mm wide, MRI scans are usually at least 5 mm wide. A tomographic scan compresses a three-dimensional space into two dimensions, like displaying a cylinder as a circle. Therefore, in a slice 5 mm wide, items that are actually 5 mm apart in the cross-sectional plane of the image will appear to be in the same plane. Thus the hyoid bone and epiglottis might appear in the same slice, even though one is several millimeters below the other. Narrower widths on MRI require longer exposure time. A third drawback is that many subjects, as many as 30%, suffer from claustrophobia and cannot tolerate the procedure. Fourth, metal clamps, tooth

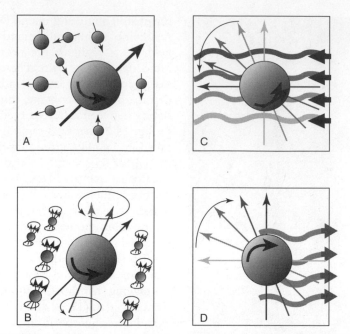

FIGURE 14-10   The effects of MRI scanning on hydrogen protons.

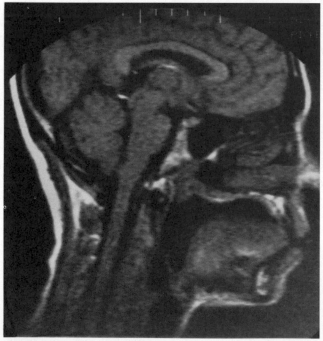

FIGURE 14-11   MRI image of a midsagittal section of the tongue during the production of [s].

crowns, and steel implants quench the signal, creating a diffuse dark spot surrounding the metal. A final drawback for both MRI and CT is that the subject must be lying supine or prone. This position changes the direction of gravity with respect to the oral structures and normal agonist-antagonist muscle relationships. It is not clear what effect this has on vocal tract shapes. However, one might speculate that the effects are greatest when at rest and minimal during

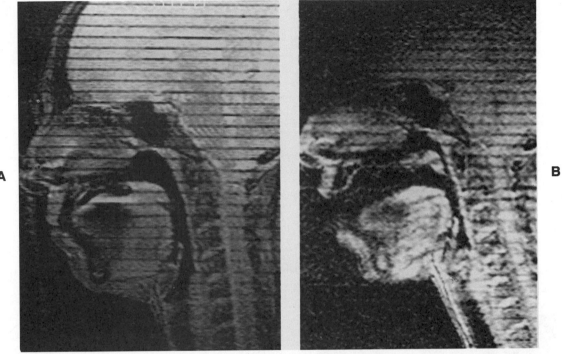

FIGURE 14-12   Tagging snapshot MRI. *A,* An MRI image of the vocal tract at rest. *B,* The tongue is deformed into an [ɑ]. The tags are no longer straight but reflect the compression and expansion occurring locally in the tongue.

speech, since acoustic constraints probably ensure relatively stable vocal tract behaviors. Nevertheless, despite these nontrivial drawbacks, MRI and CT provide unique and valuable information by imaging both the soft and hard tissue of the vocal tract with no obscuration. In addition, MRI is the only imaging technique that can image any plane of the body, providing outstanding cross-sectional vocal tract information.

Ultrasound

Ultrasound produces an image by using the reflective properties of sound waves. A **piezo-electric crystal** stimulated by electric current emits an ultrahigh-frequency sound wave. The crystal both emits a sound wave and receives the reflected echo. The sound wave travels through the soft tissue and bounces back when it reaches an **interface** with tissue of a different density, like bone, or when it reaches air. The best reflections are perpendicular to the beam (Fig. 14-13). To see a section of tissue rather than a single point, one needs a sector scanner or a linear array transducer. In a sector scanner transducer, multiple crystals rotate about a hub. The crystals are

on, or emit and receive waves, during a portion of the rotation cycle, and off during the remainder of the rotation. This creates a wedge-shaped image of up to 140 degrees (Fig. 14-14). In an array transducer, up to 128 crystals fire sequentially, imaging a rectangular section of tissue the size of the transducer. In both cases the returning echoes are processed by computer and displayed as a video image.

Fig. 14-15 shows a sagittal (lengthwise) image of the tongue during a bunched [r]. To create such an image, the transducer is placed below the chin and the beam passes upward through a 1.9 mm thick section of the tongue. When the sound reaches the air at the surface of the tongue, it is reflected, creating a bright white line. The black area immediately below is the tongue body, and the border between the white reflection and the black tissue is the surface of the tongue. Interfaces within the tongue are also visible. For example, the **genioglossus** muscle can be seen in the anterior tongue. Measurement error on such images is less than 0.7 mm. Fig. 14-16 depicts a three-dimensional tongue surface during the production of a bunched [r]. The front of the tongue is in the lower left, and its back is in the upper right portion of the figure. This illustra-

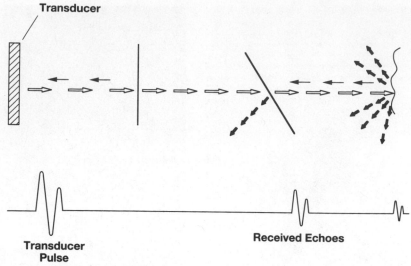

FIGURE 14-13 Schematic of ultrasound reflection patterns emanating from surfaces at different angles to the beam.

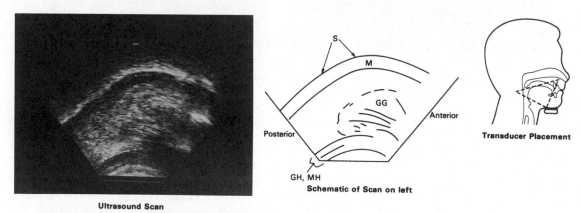

FIGURE 14-14 Schematic showing the submental position of the ultrasound transducer used during recording (*right*), the resulting midsagittal image (*left*) and the muscles of the tongue and floor of the mouth (*middle*). M = mucosa; S = tongue surface; GG = genioglossus muscle; GH = geniohyoid muscle; MH = mylohyoid muscle.

tion is reconstructed from 20 cross-sectional ultrasound slices of the tongue, each 3 degrees apart. A trading relationship can be seen between the upward displacement in the anterior portion of the tongue and the inward compression in its posterior portion (Stone and Lundberg, 1994). In addition, the vocal folds may also be imaged by placing the ultrasound transducer at the Adam's apple and pointing it directly back in the transverse plane.

A number of studies have used real-time ultrasound to explore tongue movements during speech (Stone et al., 1987, 1988; Watkin and Rubin, 1989; Stone, 1990; Wein et al., 1990) and swallowing (Sonies, 1991).

There are several disadvantages of ultra-sound. The first is that about 1 cm of the tongue tip may not be imaged because the ultrasound beam is reflected by the interface between the floor of the mouth and the air above it, hence never reaching the tongue tip. However, the tip may be imaged if there is a great deal of saliva in the mouth or if the tongue is resting against the floor. The second disadvantage is the inability to see beyond a tissue-air or tissue-bone interface. Since the air at the tongue's surface reflects the sound wave, the structures on the far side of the vocal tract, beyond the air gap (like the palate and pharyngeal wall) cannot be imaged. Similarly, when ultrasound reaches a bone, the curved shape refracts the sound wave, creating an acoustic shadow or dark area. Thus,

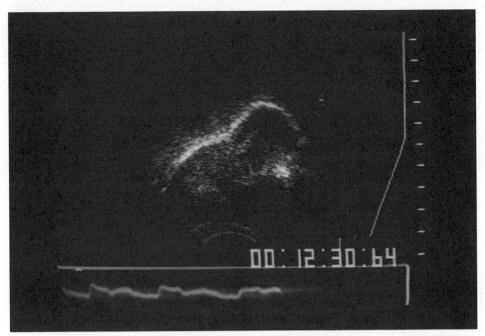

FIGURE 14-15   Midsagittal ultrasound of [r]. Anterior is on the right.

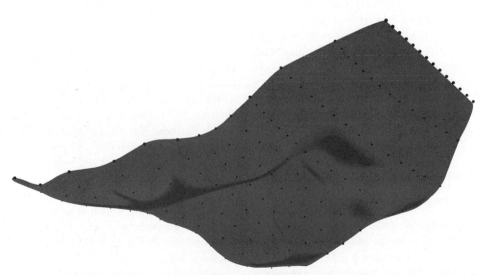

FIGURE 14-16   Three-dimensional tongue surface for the sound [r]. Anterior is on the left. A step midline groove is visible in the posterior tongue.

the jaw and hyoid bone appear as shadows, and their exact position cannot be reliably measured. However, ultrasound is relatively fast. The scan rate is as fast as 60 per second and is recorded on 60 video fields per second. It can image tongue movement for vowels and most consonants, although it is not fast enough to measure vocal fold vibration. A second advantage is that it involves no known biological hazards, since the transduction process uses only sound waves. In addition, the real-time multiple-plane capabilities capture tongue movements, not just positions, allowing reconstruction of complex three-dimensional movements of the tongue surface.

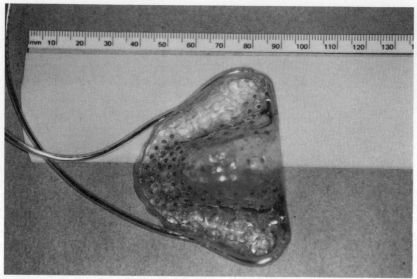

FIGURE 14-17 Electropalate with 96 electrodes embedded along the palatal surface and inner edges of the teeth.

This is more complete movement data on the tongue than can be obtained from any other instrument.

Imaging techniques provide more complete information about vocal tract behavior than is available from direct measures like point-tracking techniques or electropalatography (EPG), because imaging techniques measure the inaccessible parts of the tract (e.g., the pharynx), and they measure planes rather than points. In the future, as scan rates increase, imaging systems will become more accessible and more widely used, providing expanded data sets and multiple perspectives.

MEASUREMENT OF COMPLEX BEHAVIORS

Electropalatography

EPG measures tongue-palate contact in real time during speech. EPG is the only instrument that reveals the shape of tongue-palate contact patterns and their changes over time. Therefore, data from EPG provide a unique perspective on the interaction of the tongue and palate, as well as information on the cross-sectional vocal tract shape in the palatal area. A very thin (0.5 mm) acrylic pseudopalate is molded to fit a palatal cast of the speaker. A series of very small electrodes (up to 96) are embedded in the palate and along the inner surface of the teeth (Fig. 14-17). Thin wires (42 gauge) attached to each electrode leave the palate by winding behind the back molars on each side and out through the corners of the mouth. A ground electrode, usually placed on the wrist, completes the circuit. The pseudopalate is electrically isolated from the computer, and the wires that connect to it are driven by an undetectable direct current. When the tongue contacts an electrode, the circuit is completed and the contact registered. The electrodes are sampled 100 or more times per second in most systems. EPG has been in use for three decades (Kuzmin, 1962; Kydd and Belt, 1964; Shibata, 1968; Hardcastle, 1972, 1974; Palmer, 1973; Fletcher, McCutcheon, and Wolf, 1975; Kiritani, Kakita, and Shibata, 1977). It has been used to study both normal and speech-disordered subjects and has been an instrument of choice when available because it is only minimally invasive yet provides unique information. Data analysis is also relatively straightforward using a personal computer (see Hardcastle, Gibbon, and Nicolaides [1991] for a complete review).

Normative studies using EPG include demographic studies of palatal growth (Hiki and Itoh, 1986) as well as normative data on children (Fletcher, 1989) and adults (Fletcher and Newman, 1991). EPG also has been used in conjunction with other instruments to add to its power. Such instruments include acoustical measures (Hoole et al., 1989), articulography (Hoole, Nguyen-Trong, and Hardcastle 1993), ultrasound (Stone, Faber, and Cordaro, 1991; Stone et al., 1992), aerodynamics, (Hardcastle and Clark, 1981), fiber optics, air pressure, and transillumination (Manuel and Vatikiotis-Bateson, 1988).

There have been three major applications of EPG to linguistics. The first is the documentation of physiology for palatal sounds during speech production across languages. Alveolar sounds, such as [t,d,l,n,s,z] flap and trill, have been studied extensively in Japanese (Fujimura, Tatsumi, and Kagaya, 1972; Miyawaki et al., 1974; Mizutani et al., 1988); Italian (Farnetani, Vagges, and Magno-Caldognetto, 1985; Farnetani and Faber, 1992); Spanish (Recasens, 1991); German (Kohler, 1976); and English (Palmer, 1973; Hardcastle and Clark, 1981; Manuel and Vatikiotis-Bateson, 1988; Hardcastle and Barry, 1989). Velar sounds are less studied, since the traditional pseudopalate usually ends before the soft palate (Hardcastle, 1985). However, some velopalatography has been conducted (Suzuki and Michi, 1986).

The second area of interest has been fricatives. For intraoral fricatives, the size and shape of the constrictions are difficult to ascertain, yet they are very important to the spectrum and energy of the noise produced. EPG provides the width, length, and curvature of the palatal portion of the constriction, as well as the upper surface of the vocal tract tube throughout the palatal region (Hardcastle and Clark, 1981; Flege, Fletcher, and Homiedan, 1988; Hoole et al., 1989; Fletcher and Newman, 1991; Hoole, Nguyen-Trong, and Hardcastle, 1993). A third area of interest is **coarticulation**. The effects of neighboring vowels on tongue-palate contact during consonants reveal the nature of how we sequence sounds and strategies of motor control (Hardcastle and Roach, 1977; Marchal, 1983, 1988; Recasens, 1984a, 1984b, 1984c; Farnetani, Vagges, and Magno-Caldognetto, 1985; Farnetani and Faber, submitted; Farnetani, 1990; Gibbon, Hardcastle, and Nicolaidis, 1993).

Another contribution of EPG is to the study of disorders (Gibbon, 1990). EPG has been used to study cleft palate (Fletcher, 1985, Michi et al., 1986; Hardcastle et al., 1989), open bite (Suzuki et al., 1981), deaf speech (Fletcher et al., 1979), apraxic speech (Hardcastle and Edwards, 1992), and as a biofeedback tool to allow deaf speakers, who have an essentially normal speech production system, to receive biofeedback about the state of their vocal tract during speech (Fletcher and Hasegawa, 1983; Fletcher et al., 1991;

1979; Dagenais and Critz-Crosby, 1992). A review of literature on clinical aspects of EPG may be found in Hardcastle, Gibbon, and Jones (1991) and Nicolaides, Hardcastle, and Gibbon (1992). Two other applications of EPG are in the study of speech compensation to changes in oral morphology (Hamlet and Stone, 1978) and the study of word recognition from EPG patterns (Fletcher, 1990).

EPG has two principal drawbacks. The first is that it provides information on only one component of the vocal tract event. This can, of course, be said of most of the instruments discussed here. The second and more important drawback is that EPG provides information only when the tongue touches the palate. Thus it is less useful when the jaw lowers the tongue away from the domain of the palate. This occurs during mid and low vowels, and as a result the interpretation of EPG during continuous speech requires much inference (Stone, Faber, and Cordaro, 1991).

Electromyography

Electromyography (EMG) is the study of the electrical activity of a muscle. When a muscle contracts, a chemical change produces electrical activity. The amount of electrical activity depends on the size and function of the muscle. A muscle is composed of a number of motor units; a motor unit is a bundle of muscle fibers, the smallest unit of activity for that muscle. As more motor units are activated, the muscle's contraction increases, and the EMG signal increases as well.

Instrumentation includes three types of electrodes: needle, surface, and hooked wire electrodes. Needle electrodes are used only in small muscles because the large-scale movements of large muscles may dislodge the needle and cause discomfort. Surface electrodes are affixed to the skin above the muscle and are the most comfortable of the three. If the muscle is bundled and superficial, as with **orbicularis oris**, this technique yields considerable success. Hooked wire electrodes are used in muscles that move substantially when they contract because hooked wires maintain their position in the muscle quite well. A computer is employed to average the output voltage of the electrodes. Fig. 14-18 shows an EMG signal for a single motor unit and the contraction of an entire muscle (interference pattern).

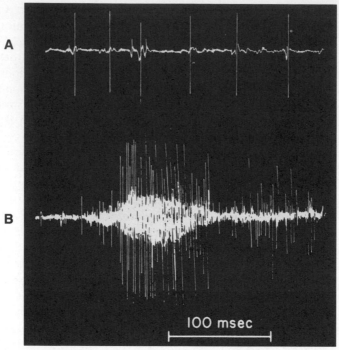

FIGURE 14-18 *A,* EMG signal from a single motor unit and *B,* the interference pattern from an entire muscle. (Adapted From Abbs & Watkin, 1976).

Considerable research has focused on developing this technique and interpreting its data (Hirose, 1971; Port, 1971; Kewley-Port, 1973; Doble et al., 1985; Palmer, 1989). Applications to oral musculature research have involved studies of nonspeech, normal speech, and speech disorders. Nonspeech behaviors include correlating specific lip, tongue, and jaw movements with EMG activity of corresponding muscles (Miyawaki et al., 1975; Sauerland and Mitchell, 1975; Abbs, Gracco, and Blair, 1984; Moore, Smith, and Ringel, 1988), and the study of reflexive vocal tract behaviors like swallowing (Palmer, 1989; Perlman, Luschei, and DuMond, 1989). EMG of normal and disordered speakers has been used to expose underlying motor control strategies for sequencing phonemes used in speech production (Harris, 1971, Gay, 1977). The tongue has been studied extensively because it is composed entirely of muscles and deforms in complex ways when it moves (Smith, 1971). Vowels have been of great interest not only because the tongue is the primary articulator for vowels but also because the entire tongue is integral to their production (MacNeilage and Sholes, 1964; Miyawaki et al., 1975; Raphael and Bell-Berti, 1975; Baer, Alfonso, and Honda,

1988). Other studies have examined velar muscles with respect to velopharyngeal function (Bell-Berti, 1976) and nasal sounds (Dixit, Bell-Berti, and Harris, 1987), lip muscles (Abbs, Gracco, and Blair, 1984), and jaw muscles (Tuller, Harris, and Gross, 1981; Moore, Smith, and Ringel, 1988). In addition, Hirose (1986) examined temporal patterns of muscle activity during speech in a dysarthric population.

There are several drawbacks to EMG. The first is that the signal is noisy and therefore difficult to interpret. Often the signal is averaged over multiple repetitions of a speech token to provide a more recognizable peak (Hirose, 1971; Kewley-Port, 1973). However, averaging masks token-to-token differences (Cooper and Folkins, 1982). A second drawback is the insertion problem. In muscles that are not neatly bundled, such as the tongue, it is almost impossible to be certain that the signal comes from the muscle of interest. Even where muscles are bundled, different insertion locations will affect signal strength (Cooper and Folkins, 1981; Perlman, Luschei, and DuMond, 1989). The third problem is that the procedure is physically uncomfortable. In a long session the electrodes can cause tissue swelling and speech distortion.

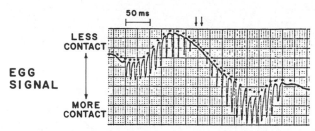

FIGURE 14-19 Electroglottograph of vocal fold vibration during [ʌh] portion of "the hut." Voicing stops—is impeded by air—when the vocal folds are open during the [h]. (From Rothenberg, M., & Mahshie, J. [1988]. Monitoring vocal fold contact through vocal fold contact area. *Journal of Speech and Hearing Research, 31,* 338-351.)

INDUCTANCE AND IMPEDANCE MEASURES OF RESPIRATION AND PHONATION

Inductance is the momentum of a current through a wire. The flow of current through a wire creates a magnetic field whose strength is proportional to the current that surrounds the wire. Therefore, changes in the current cause changes in the magnetic field. Conversely, a magnetic field will produce a current in a wire placed within the field. These two effects occur simultaneously so that a wire that is conducting a current (a conductor) produces a magnetic field, which induces a new current in the original conductor. The induced current will be in the opposite direction of the original current and 90 degrees out of phase. The interference of this out-of-phase opposing current is called *reactance;* it slows down and speeds up the flow of the original current. An inductive transducer takes advantage of this effect. An increase in current enlarges the magnetic field and slows down the rate of flow. The slower flow reduces the magnetic field, which increases the flow. The effect works with only alternating current, since a constant magnetic field would slow the current to a constant degree. Only during alternating current does the current flow change in systematic ways (Baken, 1987). The inductance properties of a coil of wire (i.e., the specific changes in the current) depend on the diameter-to-length ratio of the wire. Thus, stretching or compressing a wire will alter its inductance properties. An application of this technique is the inductance plethysmograph, used to measure respiration.

Impedance transduction measures the degree to which an electric current is impeded, or disrupted, by a physiological event. Impedance is a combination of resistance and reactance; thus, it is closely related to inductance. In this case, an electric current is passed through part of the body. Changes in the conduction of the current reflect changes in body activity because the diameter-to-length ratio of the wire is constant. An alternating current source is placed at one electrode and an impedance detector at the other. The physiological event is placed between two electrodes so that the event will alter the flow of current, causing a change in impedance. An example of this technique is the electroglottograph, which measures the impedance of vocal fold vibration. When the vocal folds are closed the current passes through; when they are open the current is impeded. Electric current can be passed through the body without sensation or harm if the current is of a sufficiently high frequency and low amplitude. Frequencies that are too low, below the kilohertz range, will cause stimulation of sensory receptors, and amplitudes that are too high will heat the tissue.

Electroglottography

The electroglottograph (EGG) measures the conductance of the vocal folds as they vibrate during phonation. From that the device estimates changes in vocal fold contact area (Rothenberg and Mahshie, 1988; Rothenberg, 1992). As vocal fold contact area increases and decreases during phonation, so does the conductance. Thus, the EGG indirectly measures the vibratory pattern of the vocal folds during speech. When the vocal folds are completely closed, the conductance is high; when they are open, it is zero. Fig. 14-19 shows the "uhu" portion of "the hut". The cessation of vibration during the [h] is clearly visible. This is an analog system having an infinite sampling rate. The high

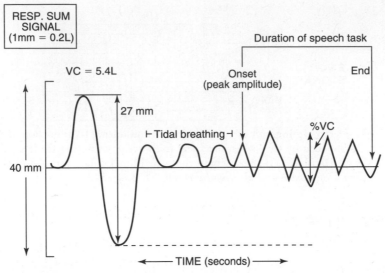

FIGURE 14-20   Schematized trace of a Respitrace sum signal. Baseline is the end expiratory lung volume at rest. First peak and trough indicate vital capacity (VC), or maximal inhalation and exhalation volume. Three tidal (quiet) breaths follow. The speech task is last and involves five breaths. (From Russell, N. K., & Stathopoulos, E. T. [1988]. Lung volume changes in children and adults during speech production. *Journal of Speech and Hearing Research, 31*, 146-155.)

temporal resolution afforded is a major advantage of the system. EGG provides key information on vibratory pattern, such as open quotient, speed quotient, duty cycle, aperiodicity, and irregularities. Another advantage is that the instrument is comfortable, with no sensation resulting from the current passing through the tissue. Furthermore, the EGG overcomes the vocal folds' inaccessibility to measurement. The current used in the EGG is of low amplitude and several MHz in frequency. This ensures that the current will neither produce heat nor be felt. The disadvantage is that it is sensitive to extraneous movement, so the subject must be still.

Respiration Measures

The inductance plethysmograph, marketed as Respitrace, measures changing lung volume during respiration as well as the relative contribution of the rib cage and abdomen (Baken, 1987). A wire band is fitted around the chest and/or abdomen, and as the body expands and contracts during respiration, the wire stretches and compresses. The change in inductance is caused by the change in diameter-to-length ratio of the wire, which varies with the cross-sectional area of the body part that it surrounds. The contributions of the rib cage and abdomen to

breathing are assessed independently and can be combined to calculate lung volume (Fig. 14-20).

The disadvantages of both EGG and Respitrace systems are that the events, lung volume, and vocal fold vibration are derived from other measures, reducing resolution. In addition, extraneous movements cause variation in inductance and produce unwanted signals. Therefore, the subject must be still. However, these are not insurmountable problems; impedance transduction has much potential for measuring biological events. The advantages of these measures are several. They are practical and simple to use. The electrodes are simple to apply, do not penetrate the skin, and are comfortable for the subject. Finally, the electrodes are affected very little by temperature and barometric pressure.

APPLICATIONS

Speech Disorders

Evaluation and treatment of speech disorders are usually performed using a clinician's listening skills. However, often a more thorough examination is needed, or detailed information would be useful in developing treatment strategies. While some of these instruments have been used clinically for diagnosis and treatment, the greater application has been in research

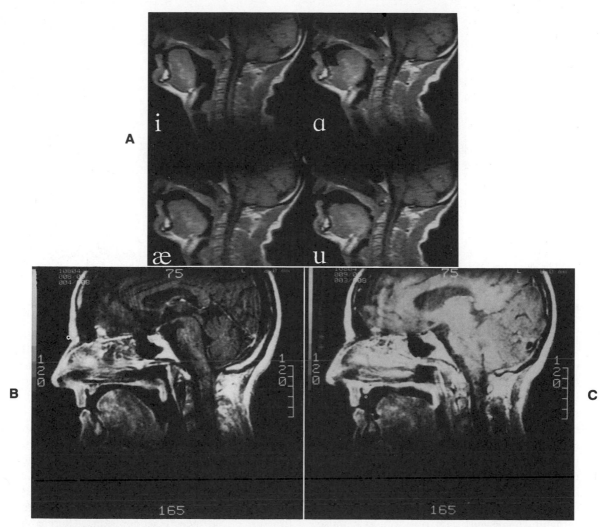

FIGURE 14-21   MRI images of *A*, normal vowels ([i], [u], [æ], and [a]), *B*, and dysarthric production of the vowel, [i] and *C*, dysarthric production of the vowel [a]. (Courtesy of C. Gracco.)

studying disordered populations. Fig. 14-21 shows MRI images of the vocal tract of a normal speaker and one with Parkinson's disease. Fig. 14-22 displays ultrasound measures of the tongue surface of a normal and a cerebellar ataxic speaker. In both cases the difference in tongue shape is apparent. Real-time measures, such as ultrasound images, EMMA, and EPG, allow the clinician to see disordered movement as well as disordered position.

Vocal Tract Models

Since only bits and pieces of the vocal tract system are available to instrumentation, it is often convenient to develop a model of the vocal tract or part of it. A model provides a theoretical explanation of how the system works, taking into account known information and hypothesizing about the missing pieces. Thus, one can simulate a system without complete knowledge of how it works. It is useful to simulate or model the vocal tract because the model can be used in experiments that help explain natural phenomena. For example, if a certain disorder resulted in abnormally slow tongue movement, a model of tongue movement control could explain the observed abnormality on the basis of the underlying control deficits that might have caused it. This would provide insight into both the disorder and normal speech production. However, the model might not be correct. There might be too many missing pieces, or the hypotheses might be in error. Vocal tract models must be tested against real data and modified as new, more complete data become available.

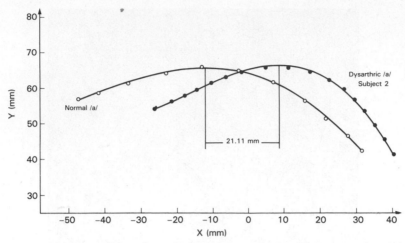

FIGURE 14-22   Tongue surfaces, fit with quadratic curves showing a normal and dysarthric production of [ɑ]. Anterior is on the left. The dysarthric patient's tongue is more arched.

Motor Control

Of great interest to physicians, cognitive scientists, speech-language pathologists, linguists, and many others is how the articulators of the vocal tract are controlled. Researchers who study speech motor control develop models of how the human system moves from linguistic concepts (e.g., words) to articulatory behaviors (e.g., lip rounding). They need models because measuring the human system becomes more difficult as we move away from the peripheral body structures and toward the central ones. In other words, it becomes progressively more difficult to measure jaw position, jaw muscle activity, jaw innervation, upper motor neuron activity, cerebellar control of jaw behavior, and cerebral programming of jaw movement. The instruments discussed in this chapter measure the two most peripheral levels of articulatory behavior: articulator state (e.g., jaw position) and muscle activity. It is almost impossible to measure the higher-level functions involved in speech motor control. Models fill in the enormous gaps in our knowledge of the motor control system; as much data as possible are needed to develop these models and to test the results of their predictions.

Speech Synthesis and Speech Recognition

Speech synthesis and speech recognition are fields in which computers are developed to produce and recognize human speech. These are exceedingly difficult tasks, because although the computer is often used as a model for the human brain, it has nowhere near the actual capabilities of a human brain. Data on vocal tract shapes and movements allow researchers to incorporate into the programs speech production rules, coarticulatory effects, rhythmic effects, and interarticulator coordination.

For the past decade or so most strides in speech processing were made using statistical measurements applied to analyzing the acoustic wave. However, recently, it has become clear that those advances have reached a plateau, and just interpreting acoustic features is inadequate for successful speech recognition. Therefore, new approaches are being sought, including the use of linguistic knowledge, vocal tract physiology, and human perception strategies. Vocal tract physiological data are now being incorporated into speech synthesis and recognition systems (Schroeter and Sondhi, 1992).

FUTURE RESEARCH AND UNRESOLVED ISSUES

Clinical Use of Instrumentation

As mentioned above, the instruments described in this chapter are typically used for research. However, many of them have clinical potential. The greatest possible application is biofeedback. Information on the movement, coordination, and shape of articulators deep within the oral cavity and pharynx can be obtained using many of the instruments discussed previously. Some are too expensive to be used clinically on a

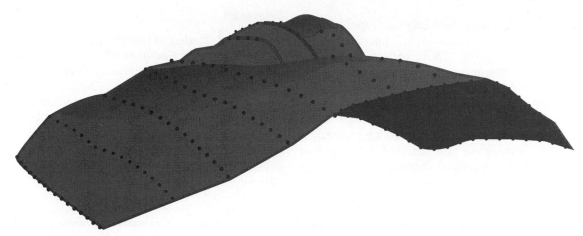

FIGURE 14-23   Three-dimensional tongue surface for the vowel [i] reconstructed from 20 ultrasound slices. The image has been rotated so that anterior is lower left and posterior is upper right.

routine basis, and others provide information that is too limited. However, some are quite well suited to provide biofeedback to patients whose disorders involve coordination of the articulators, particularly if cognition is intact. For example, deaf and hearing-impaired speakers, patients with functional articulatory disorders, partial glossectomies, those with excised pharyngeal, nasal, or oral tumors, people who stutter, and those with dysarthrias all may respond well to biofeedback. An instrument like ultrasound provides images of overall tongue shape. Such information can be invaluable to patients not only in the initial training of tongue positions and movements, but also in maintaining correct behaviors by means of regular biofeedback sessions. In a similar vein, EPG can be used to feed back tongue-palate contact patterns during speech. Positioning of linguapalatal consonants is immediately apparent, and patients' productions can easily be compared with correct productions (Fletcher, Dagenais, and Critz-Crosby, 1991). Of all the instruments described in this chapter, EPG is the one most frequently used clinically.

Modeling the Vocal Tract in Three Dimensions

Our understanding of the vocal tract is two-dimensional. Most instruments track the structures of interest at midline. Alternatively, as in x-ray, they collapse the three-dimensional tract to a two-dimensional picture from which the parallel planes cannot be easily separated. The use of tomographic images (ultrasound, MRI,

CT) and other nonmidline measures like EPG, EMG, and tracking points off midline (Optotrak) provide data that are not midline. For this reason, among others, the use of these techniques is growing rapidly. Three-dimensional models involve a great deal more detail than two-dimensional ones. Such complete detail is often cumbersome, particularly when the goal of the model is to provide the simplest reasonable representation of the system. However, three-dimensional data can be useful even in the simplest models. For example, the tongue is usually modeled for vowels as a flat surface. A better representation of cross-sectional shape would be a continuum from a grooved to an arched surface. The lower the tongue for vowels, the deeper the groove, the higher the tongue, the greater the arch (Stone et al., 1988). Thus, the more displaced portion of the tongue would be more arched (i.e., the front for [i] and the back for [a]), and the most compressed portion of the tongue would be more grooved (i.e., the back for [i] and the front for [a]) (Fig. 14-23). Since tongue shape correlates with height, it would add no computational complexity to tongue models and yet would be much more accurate to include shape information.

Understanding Articulator Motion and Cross-Dependencies

Most models of the vocal tract start with steady-state end points for each phoneme and interpolate between them to simulate movement. The simulated movement can now be achieved much more accurately because many instruments have a sampling rate rapid enough to look at real movement trajectories and model their paths. Thus, path nonlinearities and the influences of coarticulation, syllabic stress, and rate can be determined easily and described simply for multiple articulators. In the future, we hope to see more work on the patterns of interaction among articulators, how these are affected by linguistic constraints, and how they are disturbed in speech pathologies.

SUMMARY

Instrumental studies of physiology are challenging in that the instruments may be difficult to use or the data difficult to interpret. They are also limited in that no one technique provides complete information. However, our understanding of speech physiology, motor control, coarticulation, phonetics, and speech disorders has been greatly enhanced by such data. The benefits of physiological data collection far outweigh the difficulties.

Review Questions

1. Name three types of nonacoustic instruments used for measuring speech physiology.

2. How do point-tracking systems differ from imaging techniques in measuring speech physiology?

3. What components of speech production do the following instruments measure: electromagnetic midsagittal articulometer (EMMA), X-ray microbeam, strain gauges, Optotrak, x-ray, xeroradiography, imaging, ultrasound, electropalatography, electromyography, electroglottography, and inductance plethysmography.

4. What are some advantages and disadvantages of each instrument listed in #3 above?

5. What are the clinical applications, if any, of each of the instruments listed in #3 above?

References

Abbs, J., & Gilbert, B. (1973). A strain gauge transduction system for lip and jaw motion in two dimensions: Design criteria and calibration data. *Journal of Speech and Hearing Research, 16,* 248-256.

Abbs, J., Gracco, V., & Blair, C. (1984). Functional muscle partitioning during voluntary movement: Facial muscle activity for speech. *Experimental Neurology, 85,* 469-479.

Baer, T., Alfonso, P., & Honda, K. (1988). Electromyography of the tongue muscles during vowels in /pVp/ environment. *Annual Bulletin of the Research Institute of Logopedics and Phoniatics Tokyo, 22,* 7-19.

Baer, T., Gore, J., Boyce, S., & Nye, P. (1987). Application of MRI to the analysis of speech production. *Magnetic Resonance Imaging, 5,* 1-7.

Baer, T. Gore, J., Gracco, C., & Nye, P. (1991). Analysis of vocal tract shape and dimensions using magnetic resonance imaging: Vowels. *Journal of the Acoustical Society of America, 90,* 799-828.

Baken, R. (1987). *Clinical measurement of speech and voice.* Boston: Little, Brown and Company.

Barlow, S., & Abbs, J. (1983). Force transducers for the evaluation of labial, lingual, and mandibular motor impairments. *Journal of Speech and Hearing Research, 26,* 616-621.

Barlow, S., & Burton, M. (1990). Ramp-and-hold force control in the upper and lower lips: Developing new neuromotor assessment applications in traumatically brain injured adults. *Journal of Speech and Hearing Research, 33,* 660-675.

Barlow, S., & Rath, E. (1985). Maximum voluntary closing forces in the upper and lower lips of humans. *Journal of Speech and Hearing Research, 28,* 373-376.

Bell-Berti, F. (1976). An electromyographic study of velopharyngeal function in speech. *Journal of Speech and Hearing Research, 19,* 225-240.

Benguerel, A., Hirose, H., Sawashima, M., & Ushijima, T. (1977). Velar coarticulation in French: An electromyographic study. *Journal of Phonetics, 5,* 159-167.

Branderud, P. (1985). Movetrak: A movement tracking system. In *Proceedings of the French-Swedish Symposium on Speech* (pp. 113-122.) GALF, Grenoble, France, 1985.

Cha, C., & Patten, B. (1989). Amyotrophic lateral sclerosis: Abnormalities of the tongue on magnetic resonance imaging. *Annals of Neurology, 25,* 468-472.

Christianson, R., Lufkin, R., & Hanafee, W. (1987). Normal magnetic resonance imaging anatomy of the tongue, oropharynx, hypopharynx and larynx. *Dysphagia, 1,* 119-127.

Cooper, D., & Folkins, J. (1981, December). *The*

spatial sampling problem in electromyographic studies of speech musculature. Paper presented at the meeting of Acoustical Society of America, Miami Beach.

Cooper, D., & Folkins, J. (1982, April). *The temporal sampling problem in electromyographic studies of speech musculature.* Paper presented at the meeting of Acoustical Society of America, Chicago.

Dagenais, P., & Critz-Crosby, P. (1992). Comparing tongue positioning by normal-hearing and hearing-impaired children during vowel production. *Journal of Speech and Hearing Research, 35,* 35-44.

Dixit, R. P., Bell-Berti, F., & Harris, K. (1987). Palatoglussus activity during nasal/nonnasal vowels of Hindi. *Phonetica, 44,* 210-226.

Doble, E., Leiter, J., Knuth, S., Daubenspeck, J., & Bartlett, D. (1985). A noninvasive intraoral electromyographic electrode for genioglossus muscle. *Journal of Applied Physiology, 58,* 1378-1382.

Fant, G. (1965). Formants and cavities. In *Proceedings of the Fifth International Congress of the Phonetic Sciences,* Basel, Karger (pp. 120-141).

Farnetani, E. (1990). V-C-V lingual coarticulation and its spatiotemporal domain. In Hardcastle, W. J. and Marchal, A., (Eds). *Speech Production and speech modelling.* Kluwer (pp. 93-130).

Farnetani, E., & Faber, A. (1992). Tongue-jaw coordination in vowel production: Isolated words vs. connected speech. *Speech Communication, 11,* 411-419.

Farnetani, E., Vagges, K., & Magno-Caldognetto, E. (1985). Coarticulation in Italian /VtV/ sequences: A palatographic study. *Phonetica, 42,* 78-99.

Flege, J., Fletcher, S., & Homiedan, A. (1988). Compensating for a bite block in /s/ and /t/ production: Palatographic, acoustic, and perceptual data. *Journal of the Acoustical Society of America, 83,* 212-228.

Fletcher, S. (1985). Speech production and oral motor skill in an adult with an unrepaired palatal cleft. *Journal of Speech and Hearing Disorders, 50,* 254-261.

Fletcher, S. (1989). Palatometric specification of stop, affricate and sibilant sounds. *Journal of Speech and Hearing Research, 32,* 736-748.

Fletcher, S. (1990). Recognition of words from palatometric displays. *Clinical Linguistics and Phonetics, 4,* 9-24.

Fletcher, S., Dagenais, P., & Critz-Crosby, P. (1991). Teaching consonants to profoundly hearing-impaired speakers using palatometry. *Journal of Speech and Hearing Research, 34,* 929-942.

Fletcher, S., & Hasegawa, A. (1983). Speech modification by a deaf child through dynamic orometric modeling and feedback. *Journal of Speech and Hearing Disorders, 48,* 178-185.

Fletcher, S., Hasegawa, A., McCutcheon, M., & Gilliom, J. (1979). Use of linguapalatal contact patterns to modify articulation in a deaf adult. In McPherson, D., & Schwab, M. (Eds.), *Advances in Prosthetic Devices for the deaf: A technical workshop,* Rochester: NTID Press (pp. 127-133).

Fletcher, S., McCutcheon, M., & Wolf, M. (1975). Dynamic palatometry. *Journal of Speech and Hearing Research, 18,* 812-819.

Fletcher, S., & Newman, D. (1991). [s] and [ʃ] as a function of linguapalatal contact place and sibilant groove width. *Journal of the Acoustical Society of America, 89,* 850-858.

Fujimura, O., Tatsumi, I., & Kagaya, R. (1972). Computational processing of palatographic patterns. *Journal of Phonetics, 1,* 47-54.

Gay, T. (1977). Cinefluorographic and EMG studies of articulatory organization. *Haskins Labs Status Reports, SR-50,* 77-93.

Gibbon, F. (1990). Lingual activity in two speech disordered children's attempts to produce velar/alveolar stop contrasts: evidence from electropalatographic (EPG) data. *Reading University Speech Research laboratory Work in Progress, 6,* 1-4.

Gibbon, F., Hardcastle, W., & Nicolaidis, K. (1993). Temporal and spatial aspects of lingual coarticulation in /kl/ sequences: a cross-linguistic investigation. *Language and Speech, 36,* 261-277.

Hamlet, S., & Stone, M. (1978). Compensatory alveolar consonant production induced by wearing a dental prosthesis. *Journal of Phonetics, 6,* 227-248.

Hardcastle, W. (1972). The use of electropalatography in phonetic research. *Phonetica, 25,* 197-215.

Hardcastle, W. (1974). Instrumental investigations of lingual activity during speech: A survey. *Phonetica, 29,* 129-157.

Hardcastle, W. (1985). Some phonetic and syntactic constraints on lingual coarticulation during /kl/ sequences. *Speech Communication, 4,* 247-263.

Hardcastle, W., & Barry, W. (1989). Articulatory and perceptual factors in /l/ vocalisation in English. *Journal of the International Phonetic Association, 15,* 3-17.

Hardcastle, W., & Clark, J. (1981). Articulatory, aerodynamic and acoustic properties of lingual fricatives in English. *Phonetics Laboratory University of Reading Work in Progress, 1,* 27-44.

Hardcastle, W., & Edwards, S. (1992). EPG-based description of apraxic speech errors. In Kent, R. (Ed.), *Intelligibility in speech disorders,* Amsterdam: Benjamins (pp. 287-328).

Hardcastle, W., Gibbon, R., & Jones, W. (1991). Visual display of tongue palate contact: Electropalatography in the assessment and remediation of speech disorders. *British Journal of Disorders of Communication, 26,* 41-74.

Hardcastle, W., Gibbon, F., & Nicolaides, K. (1991). EPG data reduction methods and their implications for studies of lingual coarticulation. *Journal of Phonetics, 19,* 251-266.

Hardcastle, W., Morgan-Barry, R., & Nunn, M. (1989). Instrumental articulatory phonetics in assessment and remediation: Case studies with the electropalatograph. In Stengelhofen, J. (Ed.), *Cleft palate: The nature and remediation of communication problems.* Edinburgh: Churchill Livingstone (pp. 136-64).

Hardcastle, W., & Roach, P. (1977). An instrumental investigation of coarticulation in stop consonant sequences. *Phonetics Laboratory University of Reading Work in Progress, 1,* 27-44.

Harris, K. (1971). Action of the extrinsic tongue musculature in the control of tongue position. *Haskins Lab Status Reports, SR 25/26,* 87-96.

Harshman, R., Ladefoged, P., & Goldstein, L. (1977). Factor analysis of tongue shapes. *Journal of the Acoustical Society of America, 62,* 693-707.

Hashimoto, K., & Sasaki, K. (1982). On the relationship between the shape and position of the tongue for vowels. *Journal of Phonetics, 10,* 291-299.

Hiki, S., & Itoh, H. (1986). Influence of palate shape on lingual articulation. *Speech Communication, 5,* 141-158.

Hirose, H. (1971). Electromyography of articulatory muscles: Current instrumentation and technique. *Haskins Labs Status Reports, SR 25/26,* 73-86.

Hirose, H. (1986). Pathophysiology of motor speech disorders (dysarthria). *Folia Phoniatrica, 38,* 61-88.

Hoole, P., Ziegler, W., Hartmann, E., & Hardcastle, W. (1989). Parallel electropalatographic and acoustic measures of fricatives. *Clinical Linguistics and Phonetics, 3,* 59-69.

Hoole, J. P., Nguyen-Trong, N., & Hardcastle, W. (1993). A comparative investigation of coarticulation in fricatives: Electropalatographic, electromagnetic and acoustic data. *Language and Speech, 36,* 235-260.

Kent, R. (1972). Some considerations in the cinefluorographic analysis of tongue movements during speech. *Phonetica, 26,* 16-32.

Kent., R., & Moll, K. (1972). Cinefluorographic analyses of lingual consonants. *Journal of Speech and Hearing Research, 15,* 453-473.

Kent, R., & Netsell, R. (1971). Effects of stress contrasts on certain articulatory parameters. *Phonetica, 24,* 23-44.

Kewley-Port, D. (1973). Computer processing of EMG signals at Haskins Laboratories. *Haskins Labs Status Reports; SR-33,* 173-184.

Kiritani, S., Kakita, K., & Shibata, S. (1977). Dynamic palatography. In Sawashima, M., & Cooper, F., (Eds.), *Dynamic aspects of speech production.* Tokyo: Tokyo University Press (pp. 159-170).

Kohler, K. (1976). The instability of word-final alveolar plosives in German: An electropalatographic investigation. *Phonetica, 33,* 1-30.

Kuehn, D., Reich, A., & Jordan, J. (1980). A cineradiographic study of chin marker positioning: Implications for the strain gauge transduction of jaw movement. *Journal of the Acoustical Society of America, 67,* 1825-1827.

Kumada, M., Niitsu, B., Niimi, S., & Hirose, H. (1992). A study on the inner structure of the tongue in the production of the 5 Japanese vowels by Tagging Snapshop MRI. In *Research Institute of Logopedics and Phoniatrics Annual Bulletin,* No. 26, University of Tokyo (pp. 1-12).

Kuzmin, Y. (1962). Mobile palatography as a tool for acoustic study of speech sounds. In *Proceedings of the 4th International Congress in Acoustics,* Copenhagen.

Kydd, W., & Belt, D. (1964). Continuous palatography. *Journal of Speech Hearing Disorders, 29,* 489-494.

Lakshminarayanan, A, Lee, S., & McCutcheon, M. (1990). *Vocal tract shape during vowel production as determined by magnetic resonance imaging.* Paper presented at the thirteenth annual meeting of Society of Computed Body Tomography, Palm Springs, CA.

Lakshminarayanan, A, Lee, S., & McCutcheon, M. (1991). MR imaging of the vocal tract during vowel production. *Journal of Magnetic Resonance Imaging, 1,* 71-76.

Lubker, J., Fritzell, B., & Lindqvist, J. (1970). Velopharyngeal function in speech: An electromyographic study. *Speech Transmission Laboratory Quarterly Progress and Status Report,* Royal Institute of Technology, Stockholm, 4, 9-20.

Lufkin, R., Larsson, S., & Hanafee, W. (1983). Work in progress: NMR anatomy of the larynx and tongue base. *Radiology, 148,* 173-175.

MacNeilage, P, & Sholes, G. (1964). An electromyographic study of the tongue during vowel production. *Journal of Speech and Hearing Research, 7,* 211-232.

Maeda, S. (1989). Compensatory articulation during speech: Evidence from the analysis and sythesis of vocal tract shape using an articulatory model. In Hardcastle, W., & Marchal, A. (Eds.), *Speech production and speech modeling.* Boston: Kluwer (pp. 131-150).

Manuel, S., & Vatikiotis-Bateson, E. (1988). Oral and glottal gestures and acoustics of underlying [t] in English. *Journal of the Acoustical Society of America, 84,* S84A.

Marchal, A. (1983). Coarticulatory patterns in stop sequences: EPG evidence. In *Proceedings of the Tenth International Congress of Phonetic Sciences.* Foris, Utrecht, Dordrecht (p. 473).

Marchal, A. (1988). Coproduction: EPG evidence. *Speech Communication, 7,* 287-295.

McCutcheon, M., Lee, S., Lakshminarayanan, A., & Fletcher, S. (1990). A comparison of glossometric measurements of tongue position with magnetic resonance images of the vocal tract. *Journal of the Acoustical Society of America, 87,* S122A.

McKenna, K., Jabour, B., Lufkin, R., & Hanafee, W. (1990). Magnetic resonance imaging of the tongue and oropharynx. *Topics in Magnetic Resonance Imaging, 2,* 49-59.

Mermelstein, P. (1973). Articulatory model for the study of speech production. *Journal of the Acoustical Society of America, 53,* 1070-1082.

Michi, K., Suzuki, N., Yamashita, Y., & Imai, S. (1986). Visual training and correction of articulation disorders by use of dynamic palatography: Serial observation in a case of cleft palate. *Journal of Speech and Hearing Disorders, 51,* 226-238.

Miyawaki, K., Hirose, H., Ushijima, T., & Sawashima, M. (1975). A preliminary report on the electromyographic study of the activity of lingual muscles. *Ann Bull. Research Institute of Logopedics and Phoniatrics, University of Tokyo, 9,* 91-106.

Miyawaki, K., Kiritani, S., Tatsumi, I., & Fujimura, O. (1974). Palatographic observations of VCV articulations in Japanese. *Annual Bulletin of the Research Institute of Logopedics and Phoniatrics, University of Tokyo, 8,* 51-57.

Mizutani, T., Hashimoto, K, Wakumoto, M., Hamada, H., & Miura, T. (1988). *Analysis of tongue motion for the dental consonants based on high-speed palatographic data.* Second Joint Meeting of the Acoustical Society of America and Acoustical Society of Japan, Honolulu, HI.

Moore, C. (1992). The correspondence of vocal tract resonance with volumes obtained from magnetic resonance images. *Journal of Speech and Hearing Research, 35,* 1009-1023.

Moore, C. Smith, A., & Ringel, R. (1988). Task-specific organization of activity in human jaw muscles. *Journal of Speech and Hearing Research, 31,* 670-680.

Muller, W., Abbs, J., Kennedy, J., & Larson, C. (1977). *Significance of biomechanical variables in lip movements for speech.* Paper presented at the Annual Convention of the American Speech and Hearing Association, Chicago, IL.

Muraki, A, Mancuso, A., Harnsberger, H., Johnson, L., & Meads, G. (1983). CT of the oropharynx, tongue base and floor of the mouth: Normal anatomy and range of variations, and applications in staging carcinoma. *Radiology, 148,* 725-731.

Nicolaides, K., Hardcastle, W., & Gibbon, F. (1992). Bibliography of electropalatographic studies in English (1951-1992), Parts I, II and III. *Speech Research Laboratory, University of Reading Work in Progress, 7,* 26-147.

Niitsu, M., Kumada, M., Niimi, S., & Itai, Y. (1992). Tongue movement during phonation: A rapid quantitative visualization using Tagging Snapshot MR imaging. In *Research Institute of Logopedics and Phoniatrics Annual Bulletin, University of Tokyo, No 26.*

Palmer, J. (1973). Dynamic palatography. *Phonetica, 28,* 76-85.

Palmer, J. B. (1989). Electromyography of the muscles of oropharyngeal swallowing: Basic concepts. *Dysphagia, 6,* 1-6.

Perkell, J., Cohen, M., & Garabieta, I. (1988). Techniques for transducing movements of points on articulatory structures. *Journal of the Acoustical Society of America, 84,* Suppl. 1, S145A.

Perkell, J., Cohen, M., Svirsky, M., Matthies, M., Garabieta, I., & Jackson, M. (1992). Electromagnetic midsagittal articulometer (EMMA) systems for transducing speech articulatory movements. *Journal of the Acoustical Society of America, 92,* 3078-3096.

Perlman, A., Luschei, E., & DuMond, C. (1989). Electrical activity from the superior pharyngeal constrictor during reflexive and non-reflexive tasks. *Journal of Speech and Hearing Research, 32,* 749-754.

Port, D. K. (1971). The EMG data system. *Haskins Lab Status Report, SR 25/26,* 67-72.

Raphael, L., & Bell-Berti, F. (1975). Tongue musculature and the feature of tension in English vowels. *Phonetica, 32,* 661-673.

Recasens, D. (1984a). Vowel-to-vowel coarticulation in Catalan VCV sequences. *Journal of the Acoustical Society of America, 76,* 1624-1635.

Recasens, D. (1984b). Timing constraints and coarticulation: Alveolo-palatals and sequences of alveolar + [j] in Catalan. *Phonetica, 41,* 125-139.

Recasens, D. (1984c). V-to-C coarticulation in Catalan VCV sequences: an articulatory and acoustical study. *Journal of Phonetics, 12,* 61-73.

Recasens, D. (1991). On the production characteristics of apicoalveolar taps and trills. *Journal of Phonetics, 19,* 267-280.

Rothenberg, M. (1992). A multichannel electroglottograph. *Journal of Voice, 6,* 36-43.

Rothenberg, M., & Mahshie, J. (1988). Monitoring vocal fold contact through vocal fold contact area. *Journal of Speech and Hearing Research, 31,* 338-351.

Russell, N. K., & Stathopoulos, E. T. (1988). Lung volume changes in children and adults during speech production. *Journal of Speech and Hearing Research, 31,* 146-155.

Sauerland, E., & Mitchell, S. (1975). Electromyographic activity of intrinsic and extrinsic muscles of the human tongue. *Texas Reports on Biology and Medicine, 33,* 445-455.

Schertel, L., Puppe, D., Schnepper, E., Witt, H., & Winkel, K. (1976). *Atlas of Xeroradiography.* Philadelphia: Saunders.

Schonle, P., Grabe, K., Wenig, P., Hohne, J., Schrader, J., & Conrad, B. (1987). Electromagnetic articulography: Use of alternating magnetic fields for tracking movements of multiple points inside and outside the vocal tract. *Brain and Language, 31,* 26-35.

Schonle, P., Muller, C., & Wenig, P. (1989). Echtzeitanalyse von orofacialen Bewegungen mit Hilfe der elektromagnetischen Artikulographie. *Biomedizinische Technik, 34,* 126-130.

Schroeter, J., & Sondhi, M. (1992). Speech coding based on physiological models of speech production. In Furui, S., & Sondhi, M. (Eds.), *Advances in Speech Signal Processing,* New York: Marcel Dekker (pp. 231-268).

Shibata, S. (1968). A study of dynamic palatography. *Ann Bull. Research Institute of Logopedics and Phoniatrics, Univ. of Tokyo, 2,* 28-36.

Smith, T. (1971). A phonetic study of the function of the extrinsic tongue muscles. *UCLA Working Papers in Phonetics 18,* 1-131.

Sonies, B. (1991). Ultrasound imaging and swallowing. In Donner, M., & Jones, B. (Eds.), *Normal and abnormal swallowing: imaging in diagnosis and therapy.* New York: Springer (pp. 237-260).

Stone, M. (1990). A three-dimensional model of tongue movement based on ultrasound and x-ray microbeam data. *Journal of the Acoustical Society of America, 87,* 2207-2217.

Stone, M., Faber, A., & Cordaro, M. (1991). Cross-sectional tongue movement and tongue-palate movement patterns in [s] and [ʃ] syllables. Paper presented at Twelfth International Congress of Phonetic Science, Aix-en-Provence, France.

Stone, M., Faber, A., Raphael, L., & Shawker, T. (1992). Cross-sectional tongue shape and linguopalatal contact patterns in [s], [ʃ], and [l]. *Journal of Phonetics, 20,* 253-270.

Stone, M., & Lundberg, A. (1994). Tongue-palate interactions in consonants and vowels. In *Proceedings of the Third International Conference on Spoken Language Processing,* Yokohama, Japan, V. 1, pp. 49-52.

Stone, M., Morrish, K., Sonies, B, & Shawker, T. (1987). Tongue curvature: A model of shape during vowels. *Folia Phoniatrica, 39,* 302-315.

Stone, M., & Shawker, T. (1986). An ultrasound examination of tongue movement during swallowing. *Dysphagia, 1,* 78-83.

Stone, M., Shawker, T., Talbot, T., & Rich, A. (1988). Cross-sectional tongue shape during vowels. *Journal of the Acoustical Society of America, 83,* 1586-1596.

Subtelny, J., Li, W., Whitehead, R., & Subtelny, J. D. (1989). Cephalometric and cineradiographic study of deviant resonance in hearing impaired speakers. *Journal of Speech and Hearing Disorders, 54,* 249-265.

Sundberg, J., Johansson, C., Wilbrand, H., & Ytterbergh, C. (1987). From sagittal distance to area: A study of transverse vocal tract cross-sectional area. *Phonetica 44,* 76-90.

Suzuki, N., & Michi, K. (1986). Dynamic velography. In *Proceedings of the Twentieth Congress of the International Association of Logopedics and Phoniatrics,* Tokyo (p. 172-173).

Suzuki, N., Sakuma, T., Michi, K., & Ueno, T. (1981). The articulatory characteristics of the tongue in anterior openbite: Observation by use of dynamic palatography. *International Journal of Oral Surgery, 10,* 299-303.

Takashima, S., Ikezoe, J., Harada, K., Akai, Y., Hamada, S., Arisawa, J., Morimoto, S., Masaki, N., Kozuka, T., & Maeda, H. (1989). Tongue cancer: Correlation of MR imaging and sonography with pathology. *American Journal of Neuroradiology, 10,* 419-424.

Tiede, M. (1993). An MRI-based study of pharyngeal volume contrasts in Akan. *Haskins Laboratories Status Report on Speech Research,* SR-113, 107-130.

Tuller, B., Harris, K., & Gross, B. (1981). Electromyographic study of the jaw muscles during speech. *Haskins Laboratories Status Report on Speech Research, SR-59/60,* 83-102.

Tye-Murray, N. (1991). The establishment of open articulatory postures by deaf and hearing talkers. *Journal of Speech and Hearing Research, 34,* 453-459.

Vatikiotis-Bateson, E., & Ostry, D. J. (1992). Rigid body reconstruction of jaw motion in speech. *Journal of the Acoustical Society of Japan, 4(10),* 281-283.

Watkin, K., & Rubin, J. (1989). Pseudo-three-dimensional reconstruction of ultrasonic images of the tongue. *Journal of the Acoustical Society of America, 85,* 496-499.

Wein, B., Bockler, R., Huber, W., Klajman, S., & Willmes, K. (1990). Computer sonographic presentation of tongue shapes during formation of long German vowels (in German). *Ultrasound in Medicine, 11,* 100-103.

Wein, B., Drobnitzky, M., Klajman, S., & Angerstein, W. (1991). Evaluation of functional positions of tongue and soft palate with MR imaging: Initial clinical results. *Journal of Magnetic Resonance Imaging, 1,* 381-383.

Westbury, J. (1991). The significance and measurement of head position during speech production experiments using the x-ray microbeam system. *Journal of the Acoustical Society of America, 89,* 1782-1791.

Westbury, J. (1994). On coordinate systems and the representation of articulatory movements. *Journal of the Acoustical Society of America, 95,* 2271-2273.

Wood, S. (1979). A radiographic examination of constriction location for vowels. *Journal of Phonetics 7,* 25-43.

Zeman, G. (1976). Analysis of the interrelationship between image quality and radiation exposure in xeroradiography. Unpublished doctoral dissertation, Johns Hopkins University, Baltimore, MD.

Suggested Readings

Point-Tracking Measurements

Electromagnetic Midsagittal Articulometer (EMMA) System

Perkell, J. S., Cohen, M. H., Svirsky, M. A., Matthies, M. L., Garabieta, I., & Jackson, M.T.T. (1992). Electromagnetic midsagittal articulometer systems for transducing speech articulatory movements. *Journal of the Acoustical Society of America, 92,* 3078-3096.

X-Ray Microbeam

Westbury, J. (1991). The significance and measurement of head position during speech production experiments using the x-ray microbeam system. *Journal of the Acoustical Society of America, 89,* 1782-1791.

Westbury, J. (1994). On coordinate systems and the representation of articulatory movements. *Journal of the Acoustical Society of America, 95,* 2271-2273.

Strain Gauges

Barlow, S., & Abbs, J. (1983). Force transducers for the evaluation of labial, lingual, and mandibular motor impairments. *Journal of Speech and Hearing Research, 26,* 616-621.

Barlow, S., & Burton, M. (1990). Ramp-and-hold force control in the upper and lower lips: Developing new neuromotor assessment applications in traumatically brain injured adults. *Journal of Speech and Hearing Research, 33,* 660-675.

Kuehn, D. P., Reich, A. R., & Jordan, J. E. (1980). A cineradiographic study of chin marker positioning: Implications for the strain gauge transduction of jaw movement. *Journal of the Acoustical Society of America, 67*(5), 1825-1827.

Optoelectronic Measurement of Orofacial Motions

Vatikiotis-Bateson, E., & Ostry, D. J. (1992). Rigid body reconstruction of jaw motion in speech. *Journal of the Acoustical Society of Japan, 4*(10), 281-283.

Vatikiotis-Bateson, E., & Ostry, D. (1995). An analysis of the dimensionality of jaw motion in speech. *Journal of Phonetics, 23* (101-119).

Imaging Techniques

X-Ray

Fant, G. (1965). Formants and cavities. In *Proceedings of the Fifth International Congress of the Phonetic Sciences.* Basel: Karger (pp. 120-141).

Subtelny, J., Li, W., Whitehead, R., & Subtelny, J. D. (1989). Cephalometric and cineradiographic study of deviant resonance in hearing impaired speakers. *Journal of Speech and Hearing Disorders, 54,* 249-265.

Subtelny, J., Oya, N., & Subtelny, J. (1972). Cinera-diographic study of sibilants. *Folia Phoniatrica, 24,* 30-50.

Wood, S. (1979). A radiographic examination of constriction location for vowels. *Journal of Phonetics, 7,* 25-43.

Zawadski, P. (1981). Tongue apex activities during alveolar stops. *Phonetica 38,* 227-235.

Xeroradiography

Schertel, L., Puppe, D., Schnepper, E., Witt, H., & Winkel, K. (1976). *Atlas of Xeroradiography.* Philadelphia: W. B. Saunders.

Zeman, G. (1976). Analysis of the interrelationship between image quality and radiation exposure in xeroradiography. Unpublished doctoral dissertation, Johns Hopkins University, Baltimore, MD.

Tomography

Putnam, C.E., & Ravin, C.E. (1988). *Textbook of diagnostic imaging* (Vol. 2). Philadelphia: W.B. Saunders.

Computed Tomography

Kiritani, S., Kakita K., & Shibata, S. (1977). Dynamic palatography. In Sawashima, M., & Cooper, F. (Eds.), *Dynamic aspects of speech production,* Tokyo: Tokyo University Press (pp. 159-170).

Muraki, A, Mancuso, A., Harnsberger, H., Johnson, L., & Meads, G. (1983). CT of the oropharynx, tongue base and floor of the mouth: Normal anatomy and range of variations, and applications in staging carcinoma. *Radiology, 148,* 725-731.

Sundberg, J., Johansson, C., Wilbrand, H., & Ytterbergh, C. (1987). From sagittal distance to area: A study of transverse vocal tract cross sectional area. *Phonetica, 44,* 76-90.

Magnetic Resonance Imaging

Baer, T., Gore, J. C., Boyce, S., & Nye, P. W. (1987). Application of MRI to the analysis of speech production. *Journal of Magnetic Resonance Imaging, 5,* 1-7.

Baer, T., Gore, J. C., Gracco, L. C., & Nye, P. W. (1991). Analysis of vocal tract shape and dimensions using magnetic resonance imaging. *Journal of the Acoustical Society of America, 90,* 799-828.

Ultrasound

Miles, K. A. (1989). Ultrasound demonstration of vocal cord movements. *The British Journal of Radiology, 62,* 871-872.

Stone, M., Faber, A., Raphael, L., & Shawker, T. (1992). Cross-sectional tongue shape and linguopalatal contact patterns in [s], [ʃ], and [l]. *Journal of Phonetics, 20,* 253-270.

Watkin, K., & Rubin, J. (1989). Pseudo-three-dimensional reconstruction of ultrasound images of the tongue. *Journal of the Acoustical Society of America, 85,* 496-499.

Measurement of Complex Behaviors

Dynamic Electropalatography (EPG)

Hardcastle, W. J., Jones, W., Kright, C., Trudgeon, A., & Calder, G. (1989). New developments in electropalatography: A state-of-the-art report. *Clinical Linguistics and Phonetics, 3*(1), 1-38.

Electromyography

Basmajian, J. V., & Deluca, C. J. (1985). *Muscles Alive: Their Functions Revealed by Electromyography.* Baltimore: Williams & Wilkins.

Oshima, K., & Gracco, V. L. (1992). Mandibular contributions to speech production. In *Proceedings of the Second International Conference on Spoken Language Processing.* Banff, Canada (pp. 773-778).

Electroglottography (ECG)

Colton, R., & Conture, E. (1990). Problems and pitfalls of electroglottography. *Journal of Voice, 4,* 1, 10-24.

Rothenberg, M. (1992). A multichannel electroglottograph. *Journal of Voice, 6,* 36-43.

Rothenberg, M., & Mahshie, J. (1988). Monitoring vocal fold contact through vocal fold contact area. *Journal of Speech and Hearing Research, 31,* 338-351.

Inductance Plethysmography

Baken, R. (1987). *Clinical measurement of speech and voice.* Boston: College-Hill Press (pp. 468-470).

Chapter 15

Instrumentation and Methodology for the Study of Speech Perception

James R. Sawusch

INTRODUCTION

The study of speech perception is a behavioral science. The essential elements and assumptions of the methodology are the same as those in other behavioral sciences (Kintsch, Miller, and Polson, 1984). The key element of research in a behavioral science is to make repeatable observations. In speech perception this requires maintaining control over the details and conditions of stimulus presentation, the responses or task required of the listener, and any attributes of the listener relevant to the task, including instructions.

Without control over these aspects, observations are unique and unverifiable. Control over these aspects leads to the ability to map the relationship between attributes of the speech sound and the listener's perception of that sound as inferred from his response. If the experiment is designed to test a theory or model of speech perception, the results will either support or refute the ideas being tested. This is why experiments and methods are key elements in advancing our understanding of the mental operations involved in speech perception.

This chapter describes the basics of an experimental approach to speech perception. This approach is essential for understanding the mental operations of perception and the relation between attributes of the speech signal and recognition of the message intended by the talker. The impression of speech perception in any native language is a sequence of words heard in an apparently effortless, automatic fashion. However, perception is neither effortless nor automatic, and this subjective impression hides a complex process of mapping sound onto words (Nusbaum and Schwab, 1986; Pisoni and Luce, 1987).

This subjective experience raises two fundamental issues that methodology must address. The first is the impression that speech consists of a series of discrete sounds. This is most clearly seen in the experience of speech as a sequence of words. Perhaps because of this, in most speech perception experiments the listener is asked to identify sounds as words, syllables, or phonemes. The second aspect that methods must address is that human perception is an **on-line** process that occurs in **real time**. In this chapter *on-line* means that perception and interpretation of the speech signal take place as the signal is presented, and *real time* refers to the facts that speech is a rapidly changing signal and that

human perception keeps pace with it. If perception did not keep pace with the signal, the listener would quickly fall behind the talker and spoken communication would be impossible. Consequently, it is essential to evaluate whether or not experiments reflect the on-line quality of human perception.

This chapter has two goals. One is to present the essentials, distilled into a cookbook-like set of recipes for setting up and running experiments. The second is to explore the logic behind the recipe and how it relates to theories of perception. While it is tempting to focus on the cookbook approach, designing an experiment requires an understanding of the logic of experimental science. First the methodology of speech perception will be described, and then instrumentation for perceptual studies will be discussed.

A brief overview of the classic psychophysical methods will introduce recurring issues and ideas. The basic elements of theories of perception and judgment will be introduced and their effects on choices in methodology described. A discussion of some limits of the use of the methodology due to the nature of speech will complete the section. (For a more exhaustive discussion of psychophysical methods as they apply to research in perception, see Coren and Ward [1989]. For a treatment of experimental design in behavioral science, see Elmes, Kantowitz, and Roediger [1989].)

The second section considers **tasks** that investigate perception. This includes reaction time as a convergent measure, the relationship between discrimination and identification task performance (categorical perception) and variations in tasks such as selective adaptation, perceptual learning, and training procedures. The constraints on interpreting the data from these tasks and the nature of various control conditions that rule out alternative explanations of data will also be examined.

The section on methodology concludes with an examination of extensions to the basic methods used when perceptual experiments are conducted with infants, young children, and animals. The section on instrumentation covers the two elements required for studies in perception: reproduction of the stimulus and collection of responses. The nature of computer hardware and software for presenting speech sounds to human listeners and recording responses is outlined, with an emphasis on the capabilities of the system rather than on specific hardware and software.

PSYCHOPHYSICS

In 1860 Fechner (1966) described the three basic methods for presenting stimuli to observers and collecting responses. These methods are still the basis of experimental research, though with some elaboration. They are the methods of adjustment, limits, and constant stimuli. Some elements are common to all three procedures.

Human responses to sensory stimuli show variability. That is, the same listener will not always respond in the same way to a particular stimulus. This variability can arise from any of a number of factors, including the listener's attention to the task, experience with the task and the stimuli, memory of previous stimuli and responses to them, and interpretation of the instructions regarding the task. This variability in responding can pose a problem. Consider this simple experiment whose goal is to investigate how a listener's ability to recognize a word varies as a function of the intensity of the word. A single word is presented at a low intensity to the listener, who is asked to say "yes" if he recognizes the word or "no" if not. On this particular **trial** the listener responds "yes". Later the word is presented again at the same intensity and the listener responds "no". At this point it appears that the listener has about a 50% chance of recognizing the word. However, if we present the word again, the listener will respond either "yes" or "no" again. This will change the overall proportion of responses to either 67% yes or 33% yes.

Each additional response changes the overall proportions, but by an ever-decreasing amount. As the number of times the listener responds to each stimulus increases, the change caused by additional responses decreases. The data become a "better" (more stable) estimate of the listener's ability to perform the task. For this reason, in many experiments the listener must respond to the stimulus several times. In speech perception studies, 10 to 20 presentations of each sound are commonly used. If 10 responses to each stimulus have been collected, an additional response will produce less than a 10% change in the data. That is, the eleventh response can produce no more than a 1 in 11 (about 9%) change in the proportion of "yes" and "no" responses. If the changes in perception produced by different experimental conditions and stimuli are on the order of 20% to 30%, collecting a minimum of 10 responses assures that the variability in each listener's response to each stimulus is smaller than the effect of changes in experimental conditions.

If this experiment were conducted not just for one word intensity but for seven different intensities, tabulating the proportion of "yes" responses to each intensity would produce results like those shown in Figure 15-1. On the left and in the center are hypothetical data for two listeners showing the proportion of "yes" responses to each of the seven intensities. The points in each graph are connected, and the resulting curve is the **psychometric function** relating word intensity to recognition. Notice that the data for the two listeners are not identical, although the overall form of the two functions is similar. On the right-hand side of Figure 15-1 is the psychometric function that corresponds to the average (mean) of the two listeners.

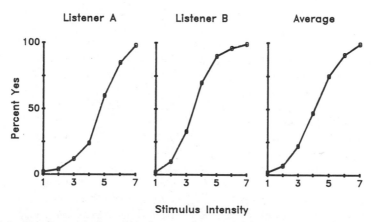

FIGURE 15-1   Psychometric functions for two listeners (left and center) and the average performance for the two listeners (right).

Three Basic Methods

Method of Adjustment

In the **method of adjustment,** the listener controls the stimulus and can vary some quality until it meets all the **criteria** set by the experimenter. Using the same example as in the previous section, the subject is given control over the stimulus intensity, perhaps by adjusting a potentiometer, or volume control, and asked to adjust the sound intensity until he or she can just recognize the word. This process is repeated a number of times. On each trial the initial setting of the stimulus intensity is at a different level, with some above and some below the threshold. The minimum intensity, or threshold, for word recognition is taken to be the mean for the intensities on the individual trials.

Another example of the use of this method comes from a study by Johnson, Wright, and Flemming (1992) in which the method of adjustment was used to examine vowel perception. The listeners were asked to pick the best example of a vowel category (e.g., the vowel in "beat") from among a set of stimuli. In the stimulus set, the first and second formants varied in frequency. The listeners were shown a two-dimensional grid on a screen along with the position on the grid of the first stimulus. One dimension of the grid corresponded to variation in the first formant frequency of the stimuli, and the other dimension corresponded to variation in second formant frequency. The listeners determined which stimulus was presented next by choosing different points in the grid. In this way, listeners were able to choose from among alternatives to select the stimulus that best exemplified a particular vowel category. Once listeners were satisfied with their choice of the best example of a category, a new trial was started.

The advantage of the method of adjustment is speed. Since the listener is allowed to choose which stimulus to listen to next and can set the pace, this method will rapidly produce an estimate of a threshold, the best example of a category, or any other criterion set by the experimenter. However, there are three disadvantages to this method. First, what if the researcher is interested in more than just the threshold? How well are stimuli recognized above and below the threshold? What is the listener's experience of the stimuli other than the one finally chosen? These questions cannot be answered with the method of adjustment because the listener does not respond to all of the stimuli. Second, how do we explain the difference between two listeners? Are their recognition abilities fundamentally different or does some other factor account for the difference? Finally, suppose the stimulus quality in question cannot be easily adjusted. Complex stimuli that vary on multiple dimensions are the norm in speech perception research, and providing listeners with control over stimulus qualities is not always feasible. In other experiments the stimuli form a discrete set (such as all consonant-vowel-consonant words) and adjustment is impossible. For all of these reasons, the method of adjustment is seldom used.

Method of Limits

The **method of limits** is similar to the method of adjustment. A set of discrete stimuli are presented to the listener one at a time, according to a predetermined algorithm. The two simplest algorithms are ascending and descending limits. Using the word recognition example, in ascending limits the first presentation is at a very low intensity. Presumably, the listener says the word was not recognizable. It is then presented at the next higher intensity. Every time the listener says "no", the word is unrecognizable, the next higher stimulus intensity is presented. Eventually the listener says "yes", the word is recognizable, and the task stops. The threshold is taken to be the intensity halfway between the last "no" and the first "yes". This task is repeated a number of times. The mean of the thresholds on individual trials is the estimate of the overall threshold. Descending limits are run similarly, with the first stimulus at an intensity above threshold. Each time the listener says "yes", the next lower intensity is presented until the listener eventually says "no". Again, the threshold is taken as the halfway point between the last "yes" and the first "no".

Often, both ascending and descending limits are used and their results averaged. A set of four trials using the method of limits is shown in Table 15-1. The first and third trials use ascending limits, and the second and fourth use descending limits. The threshold for each trial is shown at the bottom as the halfway point between the "yes" and "no" responses for that trial. The overall threshold as the mean of the results on the four trials appears at the bottom.

TABLE 15-1 Ascending and descending method of limits

Word Intensity	Trial 1 Ascending	Trial 2 Descending	Trial 3 Ascending	Trial 4 Descending
50		Y		Y
47		Y		Y
44		Y		Y
41		Y		Y
38		Y		Y
35		N	Y	Y
32	Y		N	Y
29	N		N	N
26	N		N	
23	N		N	
20	N		N	
Trial threshold	30.5	36.5	33.5	30.5
Overall threshold $(30.5 + 36.5 + 33.5 + 30.5) \div 4 = 32.75$				

The method of limits addresses one problem with the method of adjustment. Since responses are obtained for a range of values above and below the threshold, a psychometric function can show the listener's performance for these stimuli. Thus, the data shown in Figure 15-1 could have been obtained using this procedure by simply plotting the proportion of yes responses to each stimulus over trials. Many variants of the method of limits are designed to meet various special needs. The transformed up-down method (Levitt, 1970) and PEST (Taylor and Creelman, 1967) are designed to yield rapid, reliable estimates of the threshold.

In speech perception this method has two of the disadvantages of the method of adjustment. First, it can be used only with stimuli ordered along a continuum. With some sets of stimuli, such as consonant-vowel-consonant (CVC) words, there is no objective order of stimuli. Thus, if the question is whether words from a set are intelligible and easy to recognize, there is no way to order the words to present them with this method. Second, it does not account for the difference in performance between two listeners.

Method of Constant Stimuli

In the **method of constant stimuli,** the third of Fechner's basic methods, a set of stimuli is constructed. The stimuli from this set—for example, a set of stimulus intensities—are presented to the listener one at a time in random order. After each presentation the listener responds yes, the word was recognizable, or no, it was not. The set of stimuli is repeated in random order and the proportion of "yes" and "no" responses is determined for each stimulus to yield a psychometric function. Compared with the methods of adjustment and limits, constant stimuli has one distinct disadvantage: it is slow. Since each stimulus of the set must be presented several times in random order, it can take substantially longer than the other two methods. Conversely, it does collect data for all stimuli in the set, so the listener's response to stimuli both near and far from the threshold can be determined. This method is also the only one that can be used with sets of stimuli that have no objective order. For example, if the question is a listener's ability to recognize the words produced from a speech synthesis by rule system, only constant stimuli is suitable. The researcher presents the words one at a time in random order and asks the listener to identify each word.

These three methods can be used with both **identification** and **discrimination** tasks. The previous examples are all variations of an identification task, in which the listener is asked to label a stimulus (here, yes or no). In a discrimination task, two or more stimuli are presented to a listener, who is asked to discriminate, or tell apart, the stimuli. In the simplest form, two stimuli differ by a small amount. The listener is asked to indicate whether the two

TABLE 15-2 The four possible outcomes for trials using the method of constant stimuli

Trial	Listener's Response	
	Yes	No
Target present	Hit (correct)	Miss (error)
No target (catch or noise)	False alarm (error)	Correct rejection (correct)

stimuli sound the same or different. There are numerous variations on this basic procedure.

Discrimination does not require that listeners label the stimuli. Rather, they are free to use any and all information in the stimuli to perform the task. In this respect, the task is unlike the subjective experience of listening to speech. The utility of discrimination tasks lies in their ability to assess the limits of perception. That is, identification shows us how listeners categorize what they hear, and discrimination reveals how well listeners can use the fine details of sound. The primary emphasis in the sections that follow is on identification tasks, since the subjective experience of listening is that of labeling while generally ignoring fine details.

Of the three problems with the method of adjustment, only one remains: the differences in performance between two listeners. For the solution, consider the nature of information processing and the mental processes that the listener uses in experimental tasks.

Objective Psychophysics

A fundamental problem with all three methods is that they are **subjective methods.** The stimulus is presented on every trial, and the listener is asked to make a judgment about it. However, there is no way of verifying the judgment of the listener. That is, the correct answer is yes on every trial, and the listener "knows" it. The researchers asked the listeners to use their best judgment. If listeners interpret the instructions given by the experimenter differently, their judgments will reflect it. For example, listener A may have interpreted the instructions as "Be very sure you can recognize the word before responding 'yes'." This leads to a lot of "no" responses at low intensities. It also leads to a relatively high threshold. Listener B may have interpreted the instructions as "If you hear any hint of a recognizable word, respond 'yes'." This interpretation leads to more "yes" responses to low-intensity items and to a lower threshold. The point is that

listeners A and B differ only in their interpretation of the instructions. Their underlying perceptual processes are largely identical, but their responses differ because they have different decision rules for when to respond "yes".

Alternatively, if these two listeners have differences in their basic perceptual abilities, their judgments will reflect it. Listener B may have a lower threshold for hearing. These methods cannot distinguish whether listeners A and B differ in their underlying perceptual abilities, their decision rules, or both. Without an objective reference for what the response to the stimulus could (or should) be, there is no way to compare the performance of different listeners or to distinguish different mental processes in perception. We need an objective method.

Basic Signal Detection Theory

The use of an **objective method** can be seen most clearly in **signal detection theory** (SDT) (Green and Swets, 1974). The modification is to include trials with no stimulus (**catch trials**) as well as trials with the word varying in intensity. This provides an objective criterion for the listener's response. A "yes" response when no word was presented is an error. A "no" response when the word was presented is also an error. Correct responses are "yes" when a word was present and "no" when no word was present (Table 15-2).

The key to making a test objective is the **forced-choice** procedure where the listener must choose among a set of predefined alternatives on each trial, and the use of catch trials, in which different stimuli have different correct responses. The proportions of hits (responding yes to a target) and false alarms (responding yes to a nontarget or catch trial) can be used to evaluate the performance of each subject. The details of this evaluation depend on some assumptions about the perceptual processes used by the listener. The general version of SDT is the basis for more detailed theories of perception (Durlach and Braida, 1969; Braida and Durlach, 1972; Braida et al., 1984). Moreover, SDT has also been used in other domains of research such as memory and visual perception. A thorough treatment of SDT can be found in Macmillan and Creelman (1991).

SDT will be briefly described and then some aspects of the work of Braida and Durlach (1972) will be discussed. The basic idea of SDT is that a listener's performance is a result of two processes. One is a coding process that transforms the stimulus into an internal percept or sensation. The second is a decision process that maps the internal percept onto a response. This decision process compares the internal percept with a criterion. When the percept exceeds the criterion, one response is made, and when it is less than the criterion, the other response is made. Thus, a hit occurs when the target stimulus results in an internal percept that exceeds the criterion. A false alarm will occur whenever a nontarget stimulus produces an internal percept that exceeds the criterion. Using the example experiment previously presented, each listener's performance is a function of both the perceptual coding of each word and the decision rule about the certainty required for a yes response. Misses result from a stimulus intensity insufficient to produce an internal percept that exceeds the criterion. A false alarm occurs when noise in the perceptual system gives rise to an internal percept that does exceed the criterion, even though no stimulus was presented.

If two listeners have identical coding processes but place their criteria at different points along the internal perceptual dimension, they will produce different proportions of hits and false alarms. If listener A sets the criterion relatively high, nontarget stimuli will rarely produce an internal percept that exceeds the criterion, and a low false alarm rate will be found. However, this will also result in trials on which the internal percept of the target fails to exceed the criterion, and this will reduce the hit rate. Conversely, if listener B has a relatively low criterion, most target stimuli will produce an internal percept that exceeds the criterion, resulting in a high hit rate. However, a fair number of nontarget stimuli will also produce an internal percept that exceeds the criterion, leading to a relatively high false alarm rate. Thus, two listeners may have identical perceptual coding processes yet produce very different performances due to different decision rules

(criterion placement). When two listeners differ primarily in their criterion placement, they differ in both hit and false alarm rates, with the listener who has the higher hit rate also having a higher false alarm rate. Different criteria would explain the difference between the two listeners in Figure 15-1.

More detailed comparisons between two or more listeners require some assumptions about how likely each stimulus, target and nontarget, is to produce a particular value on the internal dimension. The standard assumption is that the internal dimension for each stimulus has a **normal (gaussian) distribution** and that the distributions all have the same variance (Green and Swets, 1974). Using these assumptions, the hit and false alarm rates can be used to determine both the placement of the criterion for a listener and a second quality, sensitivity of the underlying perceptual coding process.

These assumptions are embodied in Figure 15-2. The two distributions correspond to the probability of catch and signal trials resulting in particular values on the internal, perceptual dimension. The placement of the listener's criterion is shown by the vertical line. The means of the two distributions are also marked. Based on this diagram, a trial on which the signal is present would result in a hit whenever the value for the stimulus on the internal dimension exceeds (is to the right of) the criterion. Over trials, the probability of a hit corresponds to the proportion of the area of the signal distribution to the right of the criterion. Conversely, the cumulative probability of a false alarm is represented by the proportion of the area of the catch trial distribution to the right of the criterion. If the probabilities of a hit and false alarm are converted into z-scores, the distance along the perceptual dimension between the mean of the catch trial distribution and the mean of the signal distribution can be computed. This value is referred to as the listener's *sensitivity* (or d').

Using this generic version of SDT, we can compare the performance of two listeners. If the listeners have the same sensitivity but differ in criteria, in some sense their perceptual processing of the stimuli is identical. That is, if two listeners differ only in their criterion placement, the perceptual processes that code the stimulus and convert it to a value on the internal dimension for the two listeners are indistinguishable. Only their decision rules for converting an internal percept into an external response

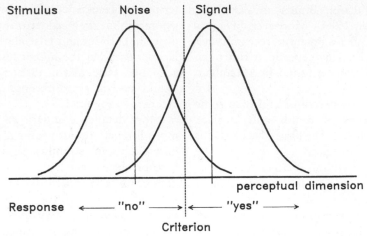

FIGURE 15-2　The general signal detection model with distributions showing the probability of stimuli (noise or catch trials and signal trials) yielding different values on the internal perceptual dimension and the placement of a decision criterion for mapping perceptual values onto responses.

differ. If the sensitivity of the two listeners is different, the perceptual coding processes must differ in some way. This makes SDT a powerful tool for evaluating the effects of changes in stimulus presentation or other experimental and task conditions upon the listener.

For example, models of vowel perception often include a normalization process that is supposed to alter perception to match the range of variation present in an individual talker's vowels. Some researchers have proposed that the point vowels /i/, /a/, and /u/ are critical to this adjustment process. SDT could be used, along with a suitable experimental task, to examine this hypothesis. To oversimplify, a listener's experience with the point vowels of a talker is expected to lead to changes in sensitivity between vowels, and experience with other vowels should lead to either no changes or changes in the criterion. In fact, this is what Sawusch, Nusbaum, and Schwab (1980) found. Thus, SDT can be useful in testing models of speech perception because of its ability to separate effects of perceptual coding (sensitivity) from effects of the decision process used to map internal, perceptual coding onto a response.

Advanced Signal Detection Theory

Braida and Durlach (1972) developed a theory of intensity perception that incorporates many of these aspects of SDT. In addition, their model includes a memory component and other elements (Macmillan, 1987). Part of the model is an

extension of SDT to deal with tasks involving more than two stimuli (Fig. 15-3). Assume the observer is listening to a series of vowels that vary from /i/ as in "beat" (stimulus 1) to /I/ as in "bit" (stimulus 7). Each of seven different stimuli gives rise to a distribution of internal perceptual coding along the internal dimension. These distributions are labeled 1 through 7 in Figure 15-3. The listener has a seven-point rating scale to use in identifying the vowels as they are presented (method of constant stimuli). To use this seven-point scale, the listener places six criteria along the perceptual dimension, dividing it into seven regions. A detailed description of how the data from the listener are used to determine the distances between adjacent stimulus distributions (sensitivity) and criterion placement can be found in Braida and Durlach (1972). This is the version of SDT used by Sawusch, Nusbaum, and Schwab (1980) in the experiment described earlier. In principle this version of SDT can be scaled to any number of stimuli and any number of responses.

Up to this point, I have focused on SDT and its advantages. It also has some limitations. First, the underlying distributions of the results of perceptual coding of the stimuli are assumed to be normal and to have the same variance. Second, the underlying perceptual coding process is presumed to be unidimensional. Macmillan (1987) describes these assumptions and the degree to which SDT is robust when they are violated. From the perspective of speech perception, the unidimensional nature of the stimuli

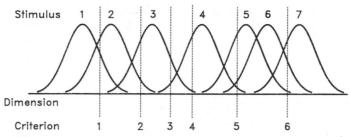

FIGURE 15-3 Generalization of the signal detection model to seven stimuli with their probability distributions along an internal perceptual dimension. Six criteria are shown yielding seven response categories.

can be a problem. The issue for SDT is not whether the stimuli are multidimensional but whether the perceptual processing by a human observer of a particular set of stimuli can be characterized as differing along a single dimension. For many stimuli, especially continua between two speech sounds that are highly confusable or similar, this assumption may be reasonable. Using the model of Braida and Durlach (1972), it is possible to check the degree to which the data obtained from listeners meets the unidimensional, equal variance, and normal assumptions (see Sawusch, Nusbaum, and Schwab [1980] for an example).

There is also another basic limit to SDT. It is fundamentally a two-stage model. All perceptual coding is lumped into a single stage that yields a value on the internal dimension. However, in a number of models the perceptual coding process is represented as a series of steps (e.g., Sawusch, 1986; Klatt, 1989). If speech perception is a sequence of processing steps, SDT cannot be used to distinguish the relative contribution of each to perception. Rather, some alternative approach is needed to allow researchers to pinpoint the nature of speech perception processes and test theories of perception.

Finally, a word of caution about objective methods. Consider a set of synthetic syllables varying the initial consonant from /ba/ to /wa/. Researchers present them to listeners for forced-choice labeling as /b/ or /w/, and the listeners consistently label the stimuli. Does this imply that the acoustic information in the stimuli cues the perception of /b/ and /w/? Not necessarily. If the listeners had a larger set of response alternatives such as /b/, /w/, /v/, and "other," some of the syllables might have been identified as /va/ (Shinn and Blumstein, 1984). If a limited set of alternatives is provided to listeners in a forced-choice task, listeners may comply with the

instructions of the experimenter even though the labels do not correspond to their subjective experience. The only way to deal with this possibility is to run a pilot experiment that assesses the labeling of the stimuli. This can be done either with an open-ended set of labels or with a set of reasonable alternatives plus an "other" category (Shinn and Blumstein, 1984). These data can be used to determine an appropriate set of labels for a forced-choice task or as a guide to modifying the stimuli. Without this type of pilot data, possible alternative explanations may render the data uninterpretable.

The Limits of Perception and On-line Processing

Because speech perception is an on-line, real-time process, the methods and tasks used in experiments are generally aimed at explicating the processes used in understanding fluent speech. However, sometimes the key question is not about the processes routinely used in perception. Rather, it may be in the limits of perception and processes that are not real-time.

Grosjean (1985) and Salasoo and Pisoni (1985) used a gating task to investigate word recognition. For example, a short portion of a target word, the first 100 ms of the word "blanket," is presented to the listener for identification. The listener is often incorrect in identifying this short segment of the target word. On subsequent trials, the portion of the target word presented to the listener is gradually lengthened (for example 50 ms at a time) until the word is correctly recognized. Using this task, Grosjean showed that monosyllabic words embedded in a sentence often are not correctly recognized until the end of the syllable following the target word.

Gating does not assess the on-line recognition of words. Since the target is repeated from trial to trial, the listener can accumulate information over successive trials in a fashion that does not occur in normal word recognition. The listener may also use active problem-solving strategies to deduce the word or systematically sample memory for candidate words in a fashion very unlike the rapid processing that takes place in on-line perception. Consequently, the processing strategies used by listeners in a gating task may be substantially different from those of normal word recognition. This limits the generality of conclusions drawn from this task. Put simply, performance in a task such as gating probably does not reflect the real-time, on-line processing of fluent speech.

This does not imply that such *off-line* tasks are not valuable sources of information. In the case of Grosjean (1985), the key issue was the isolation point for word recognition in continuous speech—that is, at what point in the utterance the listener could confidently identify the target word. Gating was appropriate for this question because it provides an estimate of the earliest point at which the target word can be recognized. However, in normal on-line processing the point at which a word is recognized may not correspond to the isolation point found in a gating task. An on-line task is needed to provide additional data that can be combined with that from the off-line task to yield a more complete picture of perception. This approach of combining data from different tasks, known as **converging operations**, is a central concept of experimental methodology and is part of the next topic.

EXPERIMENTAL TASKS AND CONVERGING OPERATIONS

The use of SDT and objective measurement in experimental tasks is an attempt to understand the internal processing or mental operations involved in perception. The work of Braida et al. (1984) shows how the SDT framework can be retained in a more elaborate model of perception. Most models of speech perception are less detailed than the model of intensity perception (Braida et al., 1984). However, the emphasis on multiple stages of processing or on processes that are specialized for dealing with speech has led to the use of a range of different tasks. The task and the particular measure of a listener's performance are often chosen to test one or more theories of speech perception. All are

variations on the method of constant stimuli. What distinguishes these tasks is the instructions to the listener, the conditions of stimulus presentation, and the response measurements.

The use of converging operations will also be emphasized throughout this section. The basic assumption of the use of converging operations is that the underlying nature of perception can be found by using various tasks that examine different aspects of perception or different predictions from theories. The pattern of results across tasks provides convergent evidence of the nature of perception. Rather than relying on a single result, the pattern of results across experiments is emphasized. Converging operations lie at the heart of most contemporary research in speech perception. Experimental studies of **selective adaptation, categorical perception,** priming, and speech versus nonspeech modes of perception all involve either multiple tasks or multiple measures of the listener's response. From the pattern of results, some explanations or theories can be eliminated. The use of these tasks and measures is the focus of this section.

Reaction Time as a Measure of Mental Processes

Up to this point, only one measure of a listener's response to speech stimuli has been used: percent categorization. Using just the proportion of trials on which the listener assigns each stimulus to each response category ignores an important aspect of the listener's performance: the time it takes the listener to respond. This *reaction time* (RT), or *latency,* is a powerful source of information. Other things being equal, a listener will take longer to respond when additional perceptual processing of the stimulus is required. This additional processing may be on the same or another level. Thus, two stimuli that yield equivalent performance in percent response may either have engaged different perceptual processes or have produced differences in the amount of processing at some point in perception. RT provides a means of assessing differences in the time course of perception and thus provides a window into speech perception processes.

In principle, RT can be used with any task if a few basic requirements are met. First, the task must have an interval to measure—reference points for when to start measuring time and when to stop. For example, in a simple categorization task, speech sounds are presented one at a time and the listener sorts each into one of two categories. The starting point for measuring RT is the onset of the speech sound. The stopping point is when the listener makes the response, typically by pushing one of two buttons to stop a timer.

In addition, the motor (response) component of the task must be held constant so that variations do not contaminate the measurements. Suppose the test stimuli represent a synthetic speech continuum from /ba/ to /da/ and the listener classifies the syllables by pushing a button under the right index finger for /b/ and the left index finger for /d/. A right-handed listener will probably respond faster to the /b/ syllables than to the /d/ syllables because of motor dominance. Consequently, any differences in perception of /b/ and /d/ can be masked by this motor contaminant in the RT.

Since the handedness of the listener cannot be changed, the general rule is to counterbalance the assignment of response labels to hands. For every listener run with the /b/ label on the right and /d/ on the left, another listener is run in the same task with the same stimuli and the labels reversed. Alternatively, the two response buttons can be placed under the index and middle fingers of one hand, so both responses are made by the dominant side. Half the listeners make response A with the index finger, and the other half make it with the middle finger. The mapping of response to hand or finger is **counterbalanced** to avoid differences in the ease of motor control producing a systematic difference in RT.

Finally, in using RT, consider the overall difficulty of the response and how it changes with practice. A two-alternative, forced-choice task does not pose serious difficulty, since it is fairly easy to remember a mapping of two categories to two responses. However, human memory is limited, and using more than two categories or more than two responses can lead to long RTs. Since the question is the perceptual processes that result in categorization and not in how categories are mapped onto button presses, it is essential to avoid unnecessary complication of the response task.

Consider a synthetic speech series that varies from /ba/ to /da/ to /ga/. The subject must choose among three responses. This requires mapping three categories onto three motor responses, and those responses must be easy to make and comparable in speed. Listeners are likely to find

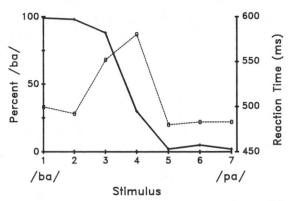

FIGURE 15-4   Percent categorization as /ba/ (solid line) and RT (dashed line) for a synthetic speech /ba/–/pa/ series. (Adapted from Pisoni, D. B., & Tash, J. B. [1974]. Reaction times to comparisons within and across phonetic categories. *Perception & Psychophysics, 15,* 285-290.)

this task a bit more difficult than the two-alternative case. Consequently, they may need more practice before they can perform the task reliably. In general, the more difficult the task, the more practice the subject will require to learn the category-to-response mapping. The upper limit for the number of response categories is established by the difficulty of remembering the category-to-response mapping and the motor requirements. Humans are limited to about seven categories in many tasks (Miller, 1956), and even this may be too many for button-press responses.

This does not mean that RT cannot be used with a large set of stimuli. Rather, the category-to-response mapping must be easy to remember and the motor response easy to execute. Thus, the subject may be asked to shadow or name the speech sound presented. This makes use of a highly skilled motor system and easy perception-to-response mapping. As long as the task meets these requirements, RT can provide valuable information about the nature of perceptual processes.

Consider a simple experiment. Pisoni and Tash (1974) used seven synthetic syllables varying in voice onset time from /ba/ to /pa/. The listeners were asked to classify the stimuli as either /b/ or /p/ as fast and accurately as possible (Fig. 15-4). RT was longest for the syllables near the category boundary. That is, the syllables that are ambiguous (sometimes classified as /b/ and other times as /p/) take longest to classify. This implies that stimuli near the category boundary require additional processing. These results and many others like them demonstrate that RT is a sensitive measure of perceptual processing.

The use of RT is not without problems. The most serious is the possibility of finding a speed for accuracy trade-off in the data. A speed-accuracy trade-off occurs when a listener is faster and less accurate in one condition than in another condition. The two conditions cannot be compared on the basis of speed or accuracy because both vary, and the faster speed of the one listener could have been bought at a cost of more errors. Pachella (1974) systematically explored the speed-accuracy trade-off. If it is present, differences in performance between groups of listeners in different conditions cannot be interpreted. Examining data for a speed-accuracy trade-off requires statistical tests of both the RT and percent correct data. A significant difference in RT going in one direction while percent correct differs significantly in the other direction indicates a speed-accuracy trade-off, and the data are uninterpretable.

The differences in accuracy need not be large to produce substantial differences in RT (Pachella, 1974). This does not imply, however, that listeners should not make errors. If listeners make no errors, they may not be performing the task as rapidly as possible. If they are not performing as rapidly as possible, the RTs are not an accurate indicator of perceptual processing, since extra time could be taken anywhere in processing. What is desired is a 5% to 10% error rate that does not vary across conditions. In this case any differences in RT reflect differences in perceptual processing and can be used as an indication of the difficulty of the conditions. The usual instructions are that listeners should respond as rapidly and accurately as possible. In addition, listeners get to practice the task so that initial unfamiliarity does not influence the results.

Fox (1984) was interested in how a listener's knowledge of which sequences of phonemes constitute words might **bias** perception of phonemes. Previous studies (e.g., Ganong, 1980) showed that ambiguous phonetic sequences that may be either a word (e.g., "bag") or a nonword (e.g., "dag") tend to be heard as words. Fox contrasted two models for this effect. One proposed that the effect happens relatively late in perception, after an auditory-to-phonetic-to-lexical coding process and was based on a lexical bias that items should be words. (Fig. 15-5, A,). If the listener waits until after the lexical coding

process to retrieve the initial phoneme, ambiguous stimuli will be treated as words and the initial phoneme will be identified as the one that makes a word.

The alternative model proposed that words are recognized directly from auditory cues and that the phonetic representation existed only after the word was recognized (Fig. 15-5, B). Fox reasoned that the second model, which we will call *postlexical only,* predicts that the lexical bias will be present in listeners' categorization data no matter how fast they respond. This is because the listener must finish lexical coding before a phonetic representation of the stimulus is available for the listener to respond.

However, the first, the pre- and postlexical model makes another prediction. Slow responses by listeners should show the lexical bias because a slow response is likely if the listener processes the stimulus all the way through the lexical coding, which produces a lexical bias. However, fast responses may be made on the basis of auditory-to-phonetic coding before consulting the lexicon. Thus, the pre- and postlexical model predicts that the lexical bias will disappear for listeners' fastest responses. (Figure 15-5, A). Fox partitioned his RT data for each subject into three sets: fast, intermediate, and slow. The lexical bias was present for the slow responses but disappeared for the fast responses. Thus, the partitioning of RT data offers a useful tool for the researcher to distinguish between competing theories based on their predictions regarding the internal stages of processing in perception (see also Wannemacher and Sawusch, 1989).

Experimental Tasks

The key element of converging operations is the use of multiple tasks, multiple sets of instructions to the listener, or multiple sets of stimuli to provide a pattern of data that fits only one theory. To illustrate this, we will examine three uses of this methodology in areas generally called categorical perception, speech versus auditory modes of processing, and selective adaptation.

Categorical Perception

The research on categorical perception grew out of some results reported by Liberman et al. (1957). Using a synthetic speech continuum, listeners performed two tasks, identification

Pre- and Post-Lexical Phonemes

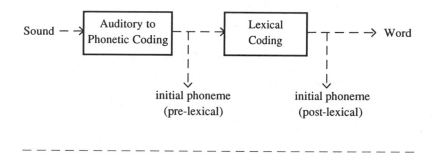

Post-Lexical Phonemes Only

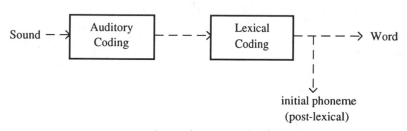

FIGURE 15-5   **Outlines of two models of word recognition.**

and discrimination. Consider again the seven-element /ba/–/pa/ continuum. In the identification task, syllables are presented one at a time and listeners classify each as /b/ or /p/. The results are shown as the solid line in Figure 15-6. A number of different discrimination tasks have been used, but the most common is ABX, or odd-ball discrimination. In the ABX task, the listener hears three stimuli from the series in sequence. The first two, A and B, are always different. The third, X, always matches either A or B. The listener's task is to indicate whether the third matches the first or second. These trials are chosen so that A and B are always two steps apart in the series. That is, they are stimuli 1 and 3, 2 and 4, 3 and 5, 4 and 6, and 5 and 7.

Figure 15-7 shows two ABX trials. At the top is a trial in which stimulus 3 is presented first (A), followed by stimulus 1 (B) and then stimulus 1 again (X). The correct response is that the third item matches the second. The bottom panel of Figure 15-7 shows a trial of the same stimuli, only in this case the third stimulus matches the first. In an ABX discrimination task, all of the different pairings of stimuli are presented in

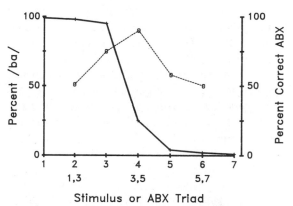

FIGURE 15-6   **Percent categorization as /ba/ (solid line) and percent correct ABX discrimination (dashed line) for a synthetic speech /ba/ – /pa/ series.**

random order, as in all constant stimuli tasks, with the subject simply indicating which pair is identical.

The percent correct ABX discrimination for each A-B pairing is shown by the broken line in Figure 15-6. The performance for each pair is plotted over the stimulus in between the two in the pair (e.g., the data for the stimulus 1-3 pairs

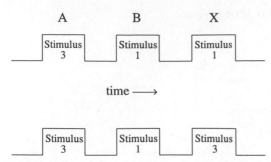

FIGURE 15-7 Schematic representation of the order of stimuli within an ABX discrimination trial.

is plotted over stimulus 2). The prototypical finding was that listeners could discriminate between stimuli only to the extent that they classified the two stimuli as different. For example, stimuli 1 and 3 in Figure 15-6 are both identified as /b/, and the listener's discrimination performance is near chance (50%). Stimuli with different labels, such as 3 and 5 in Figure 15-6, are well discriminated.

There are a number of interpretations of categorical perception, and examining them in any detail is beyond the scope of this chapter. Harnad (1987) and Watson (1987) offer alternative explanations. The importance of categorical perception here is that the basic phenomenon can be demonstrated and explored only through the use of converging operations. Both identification and discrimination tasks are needed to examine categorical perception.

The more recent research on categorical perception has investigated explanations of the phenomenon involving attention (Watson, 1987), the use of multiple memory codes for the stimuli (Pisoni, 1975; Cowan, 1984; Macmillan, 1987), and psychophysical boundaries (or discontinuities) that may underlie phonetic categories (Miller et al., 1976; Pisoni, 1977; Pastore, 1987). Testing of these alternatives generally involves modifications to the discrimination task to alter the memory (Pisoni, 1975) or attentional demands of the task (Watson, 1987; Kewley-Port, Watson, and Foyle, 1988), the use of signal detection methodology (Macmillan, 1987), or comparisons of performance across multiple sets of stimuli including nonspeech stimuli (Miller et al., 1976; Pisoni, 1977). In all these cases, convergent operations are used in the attempt to establish a pattern of data that can be explained by only one theory.

Speech Mode

Research into the speech mode of processing has taken a somewhat different approach to the use of convergent operations. The issue is whether the processing of speech makes use of specialized capabilities (Liberman, 1982; Liberman and Mattingly, 1985) or speech coding is layered on a distinctive complex auditory coding of the speech signal (Sawusch, 1986). To answer such a question two requirements must be met. The first is the use of a task that can show differences between speech coding processes and nonspeech (auditory) coding processes. The second is a set of stimuli that are ambiguous, that is, can be perceived as speech or nonspeech.

Virtually any experimental task will meet the first requirement. However, interest has focused on identification and discrimination tasks (Best, Morrongiello, and Robson, 1981; Tomiak, Mullennix, and Sawusch, 1987; Best et al., 1989; Pastore, Li, and Layer, 1990) and Pastore, Li, and Layer (1990) compared the identification and discrimination performance of groups of listeners. Best et al. (1989) gave one group of listeners instructions about the phonetic labels to use in categorizing the stimuli; another group was not told about the speech basis for the stimuli. This is the second requirement described above.

Early studies of the speech mode used synthetic speech stimuli and complex nonspeech control stimuli. These studies often reported categorical perception based on identification and discrimination data for the speech stimuli but no evidence of categorical perception for the nonspeech stimuli (Mattingly et al., 1971). Drawing any conclusion that there is a speech mode of processing from these early experiments is problematic for two reasons. Any failure to classify nonspeech stimuli consistently may simply reflect uncertainty about what aspect of the stimuli to listen to. Many nonspeech stimuli that are comparable to speech contain rapid spectral or temporal changes. If listeners do not attend to the relevant changes and ignore irrelevant information, they will not be able to categorize the stimuli consistently. Conversely, listeners given speech stimuli (or instructions) are told precisely which aspects of the stimulus are salient. Thus, listeners to speech do not have the same problems in categorizing the stimuli. A suitable task will minimize uncertainty or train the listener to the relevant information in the stimuli.

The second problem with early research was that since the speech and nonspeech stimuli were not identical, there is little reason to suppose that coding processes used on the stimuli were the same. That is, using synthetic speech for one group and different nonspeech stimuli for the other group makes for two differences between the groups. They differ in their instructions and expectations, and the stimuli presented to the two groups are not parallel. Either of these differences can explain any differences in performance, so no conclusion about the hypothetical speech mode was justified.

The resolution to this problem resides in stimuli that can be identified either as speech or nonspeech. Cutting (1974) described such a set of stimuli. Sine wave tones that follow the center frequencies of the formants of speech are ambiguous. If listeners are told that the stimuli are synthetic speech, they are likely to be consistent in using phonetic labels (Remez et al., 1981). Alternatively, the stimuli can be presented as complex tones. If two groups of listeners hear such a set of stimuli, with one group given speech labels and the other given nonspeech labels, any differences observed must be due to the difference between speech and nonspeech modes. This still leaves open the question of an appropriate task to minimize uncertainty or train the subjects listening to nonspeech stimuli as to the relevant stimulus information and the corresponding response. Discussion of these issues is a topic of current research, and new training procedures have been described (Gagnon and Sawusch, 1990; Pastore, Li, and Layer, 1990). Using speech and nonspeech instructions with an ambiguous set of stimuli and comparing performance of the two groups across tasks are converging operations used to explore the presence and nature of a speech mode of processing.

Selective Adaptation

The third area of research that has used converging operations is selective adaptation. The basic task is deceptively simple: collect labeling data for a set of stimuli. This is the baseline condition. Next is an adaptation condition wherein the listener hears a stimulus (the adaptor) repeated and is asked to label the original stimuli. The repeated presentation of the adaptor and labeling of the stimulus set by the listener is itself repeated to collect sufficient adapted responses to

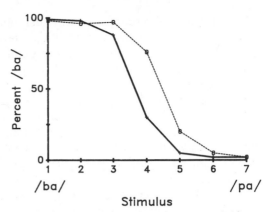

FIGURE 15-8 Baseline identification (solid line) and /pa/ adapted identification (dashed line) of a synthetic speech /ba/ – /pa/ series.

the stimuli. Typical data for the synthetic /ba/–/pa/ continuum are shown in Figure 15-8. The solid line represents listeners' labeling of this voice onset time (VOT) series in the baseline condition. The broken line represents the listeners' labeling of the same stimuli after repeated presentation (adaptation) with /pa/ (the + 60 ms VOT end of the series). The adaptor has altered the listeners' labeling of the series so that ambiguous syllables are labeled as /b/. That is, the category boundary has moved toward the end of the series from which the adaptor (/pa/) was drawn.

Early work on selective adaptation (Eimas and Corbit, 1973; Ades, 1974) focused on issues such as whether this adaptation effect reflected the operation of phonetic feature detectors. Later work suggests that the effects of adaptation are auditory, not phonetic (Samuel, 1986; Sawusch, 1986), and that mechanisms other than feature detectors are involved (Remez, 1987). These issues were addressed through the use of converging operations. Basically, the work on selective adaptation has proceeded along two lines. One involves systematically modifying the acoustic-phonetic relationship between the adaptor and the test series. In doing this, the researchers have sought to discover the information or acoustic elements that the adaptor and test series must have in common for the change in the category boundary to occur. This in turn allows the researcher to infer something about the nature of the acoustic information a listener uses to recover phonetic labels. For example, an adaptor could be phonetically similar to the /pa/ end of the test series but different in its precise acoustic structure or phonetic identity. A /ta/ adaptor would share the voiceless feature with the /pa/ but have a different place of articulation. A /pi/ adaptor would share the same initial phoneme but differ in the detailed spectral structure of the /p/ and the following vowel. Many other adaptors could be used. This approach was present in the early work (Eimas, Cooper and Corbit, 1973; Ades, 1974) and has continued as an underlying theme in this research (see Samuel [1986] and Sawusch [1986] for partial reviews).

The second use of converging operations has been in additional tasks. If these tasks produce results similar to selective adaptation, common underlying mechanisms or processes may be responsible for both. For example, Diehl, Elman, and McCusker (1978) and Diehl, Kluender, and Parker (1985) evaluated the feature detector fatigue explanation of selective adaptation. They used an experimental task in which the adaptor was presented only once yet still produced a shift in phonetic categorization of the test stimuli. This led to further studies that compared various tasks with adaptors that shared with the test series the acoustic structure, phonetic identity, or both. That is, both the experimental tasks and the stimuli used as adaptors were modified to provide convergent evidence of the nature of selective adaptation effects (Roberts and Summerfield, 1981; Sawusch and Jusczyk, 1981; Garrison and Sawusch, 1986; Samuel, 1986). The pattern of data reveals that multiple representations or stages of processing are involved in the auditory to phonetic coding of speech. That is, the effects observed with selective adaptation consistently follow the acoustic and auditory similarity of the adaptor to the test series. Other tasks (Diehl, Elman, and McCusker, 1978) seem to show effects based on the phonetic similarity of the adaptor to the test items. Only with multiple tasks and adaptors (converging operations) could this be demonstrated.

In essence, the theories and models of speech perception are complex enough that a single experiment is seldom sufficient to distinguish among them. Converging operations, involving the systematic modification of the stimuli, tasks, and instructions to the listeners, provide a pattern of data that can be used to evaluate competing explanations.

METHODS FOR NON-ADULT LISTENERS

When the listener in an experiment is not an adult human, additional issues must be ad-

dressed. First, how are instructions to be given? With adults, this is relatively simple: they are told or given written instructions. With young children, verbal instruction is feasible, although careful attention must be given to making sure the child understands the task. With infants and nonhuman listeners, verbal instructions are useless and an alternative is needed. Second, the task must be within the cognitive capabilities of the listener. For example, an infant is unlikely to have the memory capacity, motor skills, or ability to sustain attention to a task that an adult has. With young children, the cognitive abilities may be further developed, but the task must still engage the child and sustain his or her attention.

The primary concern with young children is structuring the experiment to keep the child interested. If the child attends to the task, then virtually any of the tasks used with adults can be used with children. Adults will attend to a boring task (selective adaptation comes to mind), but children generally need something more interesting to keep them engaged and attentive. In addition, the duration of the experiment must be kept short by reducing either the number of trials or the number of conditions. Having the listener respond only a few times to each stimulus has its own disadvantage, but it may be the only way to collect data from young children.

Making the task interesting for a child generally involves either turning it into a game or constructing a story around the task. Treiman (1985) used a rhyming task to investigate whether children perceive the internal structure of syllables, and Sussman and Carney (1989) modified the selective adaptation task for use with children.

Adult tasks cannot be used with infants or nonhuman subjects. Since verbal instructions are useless with infants, an operant conditioning procedure such as high-amplitude sucking (Jusczyk, 1985) or head turning (Kuhl, 1985) is typically used. These techniques and others used with nonhumans are treated in detail in Gottleib and Krasnegor (1985). However, it is useful to point out certain similarities between the tasks used with infants and tasks used to train adults with nonspeech contrasts or speech contrasts that are not part of their native language. In both cases the listener is trained to make an appropriate response. In both cases the memory load must be carefully considered (see Jusczyk, Pisoni, and Mullennix [1992] regarding mem-

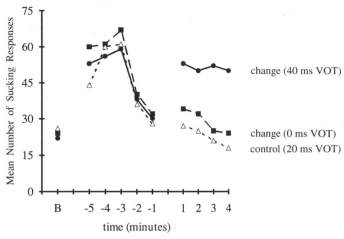

FIGURE 15-9 Average sucking rate for three groups of infants in a high amplitude sucking experiment listening to /ba/ and /pa/ stimuli (adapted from Eimas et al., 1971).

ory limits in infants). Finally, in both cases verbal description of the stimuli is useless.

The solutions to these problems come from work in animal psychophysics. A response within the capabilities of the infant is chosen. With infants up to 6 to 8 months of age, high-amplitude sucking (HAS) is typically used. Somewhat older infants (6 months and up) can be run in the head-turning task. In both cases, the infant is reinforced for responding to the stimuli appropriately.

For a review of the HAS procedure, see Chapter 9 of this volume. The prototype for this experiment is the study by Eimas et al. (1971) on infants' perception of the voicing contrast between /ba/ and /pa/. Figure 15-9 shows the base sucking rate for three groups of infants at the start of an experiment on the far left (B). The higher rates at 5, 4, and 3 minutes before the change (or control) trials show that the infants have learned the contingency between sucking on the pacifier and the presentation of the sound.

After a few minutes the infant's sucking rate declines, apparently because the infant loses interest in the sound. The middle part of Figure 15-9 shows this decline at 2 and 1 minutes before the change (control) trials. When the sucking rate has dropped to 75% of the highest rate, either a new stimulus is presented to the infant (a change trial) or the same stimulus is repeated (a control trial). If the infant notices the change in the stimulus on a change trial, the sucking rate increases. If the infant does not notice the change in the stimulus, the rate of sucking should stay low and be indistinguishable from that of infants who listened to control trials.

Two types of change trials as well as control trial results are shown on the right side of Figure 15-9. The infants' sucking rate on the control trials has remained low. The sucking rate for the change trial from the 20-ms VOT stimulus to a 40-ms VOT stimulus shows a marked increase. This indicates that the infants noticed the change and can distinguish between 20- and 40-ms VOT stimuli. Finally, the sucking rate for the infants who received a change from 20-ms VOT to 0-ms VOT shows no increase. This indicates that the infants in this condition did not discriminate the 0-ms VOT stimulus from the 20-ms VOT stimulus.

The HAS procedure assesses the infant's ability to discriminate between different sounds, but it does not assess categorization or labeling. The head-turning task, in contrast, is a categorization task. Here the infant is conditioned to make different responses to two different stimuli, for example, to turn to the right on hearing a /pa/ and turn to the left on hearing a /ba/. Once the infant has been trained to make the two responses consistently, new stimuli can be presented. The direction in which the infant turns to each stimulus then represents the categorization of each sound.

The head-turning task cannot be used with very young infants for two reasons. First, they do not have the muscle control to turn their heads reliably. Second, they do not seem to make the left-right distinction, which is critical for indicating categorization.

Because issues in methodology are really issues in interpreting results, as our understanding of perception and the mind advances, the methodology and tasks are adapted to distinguish among competing theories. Much early research on speech perception focused on the correspondence between the acoustic structure of speech and perception of phonemes, syllables, and words. Some issues such as comparisons between speech and nonspeech modes are topics of debate (Fowler, 1990). In addition, speech perception research seems to be moving to understand the perception of fluent speech, including the use of intonation. There is an increasing emphasis on tasks that measure on-line processing when the listener is performing a task relevant to normal language use. Pisoni and Luce (1987) described some of these issues as they relate to spoken word recognition. Eimas, Marcovitz Hornstein, and Payton (1990) addressed methodological and theoretical issues of the phoneme-monitoring task. In both cases the methods and tasks used are refinements and elaborations of the basic elements described here.

INSTRUMENTATION

The issue in this section is the technological implementation of the methodology and tasks described previously. In the late 1960s and early 1970s minicomputers such as the PDP-11 began to be used for speech analysis and synthesis and to run listeners on line in experimental tasks. However, because of the expense, typically in excess of $30,000, many laboratories continued to use tape recorders to present stimuli to listeners, who wrote their responses on an answer sheet. More recently computers have become widely available at a low cost. With an analog subsystem and appropriate software, a computer system can both present speech stimuli to a listener and record the listener's responses. That is, experiments can be run on line.

The next sections discuss the basic requirements of hardware and software for running speech perception experiments. The first considers the requirements for reproducing and recording sound. The second compares on-line and off-line methods for experiments with human listeners. Finally some basic requirements and guidelines for an on-line system are presented. In each section the emphasis will be on what is expected of the hardware and software and why, rather than on particular products because products change rapidly and manufacturers constantly introduce new models.

Audio Reproduction

The basic issue of sound reproduction is fidelity. The signal that is reproduced for the listener should be as close to the original as possible. When using an analog tape recorder, this means a high signal-to-noise ratio and low wow and flutter. For digital (digital-to-analog) reproduction, this means a high signal-to-noise ratio and a sufficiently high sampling rate.

The signal-to-noise (S/N) ratio represents the intensity of the signal relative to any noise inherent in the system. In essence, a high S/N ratio means that the signal will be clear and background noise will be low or inaudible. This S/N ratio should exceed the dynamic range of the signal being reproduced. If it does not, the weak, or low-intensity, portions of the target signal will be masked by the background noise of the system. The dynamic range of speech is about 55 dB. That is, the intensity difference between the highest intensity in the speech signal (such as that of a vowel in a stressed syllable) and the lowest intensity (such as a soft fricative in an unstressed syllable) can be as great as 55 dB. Figure 15-10 shows the waveform for the word "first" excised from fluent speech. The /f/, on the left of the top panel, is substantially less intense than the vowel in the center of the top panel. If the weakest portions of the speech signal are to be more intense than the background noise, the S/N ratio must be 60 to 70 dB for speech experiments. If the system is also to be used for psychophysical experiments on hearing, a somewhat greater dynamic range is needed. In this case, the entire range of hearing to be tested (generally about 80 to 90 dB) has to be represented and an S/N ratio of 100 to 110 dB is necessary.

Analog tape recorders with a 60- to 70- dB S/N ratio without using noise reduction are readily available. Both reel-to-reel decks and cassette decks are suitable. The cassette decks are easier to use and cassette tapes are easier to handle. However, it is easier to edit reel-to-reel tapes. In either case, stimuli should be recorded without noise reduction. Noise reduction circuits can alter the attack (amplitude rise from silence) of a sound, especially a sound with a rapid attack such as a stop consonant. Since speech perception experiments are often concerned with the effect of various acoustic qualities on a listener's perception, the tape reproduction system should not be adding or modifying stimulus information. Finally, low

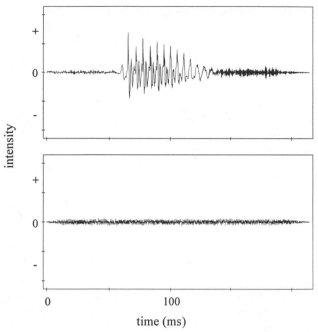

FIGURE 15-10   Waveforms for the word "first" (top) and noise (bottom).

wow and flutter require that the tape move at a constant speed. Variation in speed shifts the pitch (wow) of the speech signal or otherwise distorts it (flutter).

The alternative to an analog tape recorder is digital audio. Digital recording can be done either with a digital audio tape (DAT) or an analog-to-digital conversion system attached to a computer. With digital audio, a higher S/N ratio is achieved by using more bits (binary digits) to represent each point in the waveform. The analog waveform is represented as voltage (the electrical equivalent of intensity). In the digital domain, each voltage is represented by a number. The larger the range of numbers used, the more accurately the analog waveform is represented (greater fidelity). Since adding a bit to a binary number doubles the range of numbers that can be represented, and a doubling of intensity corresponds (approximately) to a 6 dB change, the rule of thumb is that the S/N ratio of a digital audio system is approximately the number of bits times 6 dB per bit.

DAT decks typically use 16-bit converters and thus have an S/N ratio of about 100 dB. Audio systems available for computers typically have 8-, 12-, or 16-bit converters yielding S/N ratios of 48, 72, and 96 dB, respectively. The 8-bit systems do not have adequate fidelity and should not be used for experimental studies. However, the 12-bit systems are quite adequate

for most speech studies. The lower panel of Figure 15-10 shows noise from an 8-bit system on the same intensity scale as the waveform in the upper pannel, which was recorded with a 12-bit system. The initial /f/ of the waveform is less intense than the noise in the 8-bit system. If the word had been recorded on an 8-bit system, the /f/ would have been inaudible. A system designed to handle both psychophysical and speech studies should use a 16-bit digital audio system, since analog systems do not have an adequate S/N ratio.

The second factor in choosing a digital audio system is the sampling rate, which corresponds to the number of times per second that a digital value (representing a point in the analog waveform) is reproduced. The rule of thumb is that the sampling rate must be at least twice as high as the highest frequency to be reproduced. The rationale for this is simple: to reproduce a particular frequency requires a minimum of two values. One corresponds to the positive part of the waveform, the other to the negative part. Accurate reproduction of a frequency requires more samples for each cycle. The frequency range for speech is approximately 40 to 8000 Hz. Thus, a sampling rate in the range of 16,000 to 20,000 samples per second (16 to 20 kHz) captures the speech range. However, the frequency range of 5 to 8 kHz contains very little speech information, so in practice, systems with a 10 kHz sampling rate are adequate.

A system for psychophysical experiments again imposes somewhat higher requirements. Since the upper limit for human hearing is about 20 kHz, a higher sampling rate is needed. A sampling rate in the range of 40 to 50 kHz is adequate here. The sampling rate typically used in a DAT deck is 48 kHz. For comparison, the digital audio on a compact disk is recorded at 44.1 kHz.

The next step in reproducing sound from the tape deck is to amplify the sound to the desired intensity and reproduce it over a loudspeaker or headphones. For a digital audio system, the analog signal is first filtered to remove high-frequency components that result from the digital-to-analog conversion process and then amplified and presented to the listener. The filters used in a digital system are generally low-pass filters that eliminate all frequencies above half of the sampling rate. The amplifier should be stereo for dichotic presentation. Separate stepped volume controls for the two channels allow the experimenter to vary the intensity on the two channels independently and to reproduce previous settings accurately. In a computerized system, programmable attenuators are often used so that stimulus intensity can be controlled by the computer during an experiment. The response of any loudspeakers used should be as flat over the target frequency range as possible. Similarly, for headphones, the response should be flat. The term *flat* means that all frequencies should be reproduced as accurately as possible and without amplification or attenuation by the speakers or headphones. The two headphone channels should also be matched so that no localization or lateralization cues are introduced when sound is reproduced. Most speech laboratories, even if they use loudspeakers for some experiments, have headphones for use in dichotic studies. Further discussion of the issues in audio reproduction and recording can be found in Cudahy (1988).

Listener Participation in Experiments

Having listeners participate in an off-line experiment involves using the audio equipment to reproduce the stimuli as required by the task. The listeners record their response, often by writing it on an answer sheet. A tape deck, amplifier and headphones, or loudspeaker are all that is required for the off-line approach. This approach is relatively inexpensive but very limited. For example, to measure RT, additional hardware is needed to time the interval from the onset of the stimulus to the listener's response, and then the RT must be recorded. In tasks that use training, feedback about the correct response must be given. Finally, for each new experiment or variation, new tapes of the stimulus sequence must be constructed. The answer to all of these problems is to automate the process of running listeners: to run them on-line.

When a listener participates in an on-line experiment, the computer controls the presentation of stimuli, times intervals, collects the responses from the listener, and provides feedback. At a minimum, this requires having a single listener seated at the keyboard. Responses can be entered either by typing or by pushing a button on the mouse, and feedback can be provided on the screen. This on-line approach uses software to control all the elements of a particular task. Setting up a new experiment using a task that has been previously programmed involves substituting one set of stimuli for another. Setting up a new task depends on the software. If the program already can run the new task, configuring the program (often simply by answering a few questions) is sufficient. Alternatively, a new control program to coordinate the events and timing in the new task may have to be written.

On-line listener participation also makes collecting RTs easier. Finally, certain adaptive tasks in psychophysical experiments are impossible without computer control. In an adaptive task the computer monitors the listener's response on each trial and determines which stimulus to present on the next trial based on how the listener has responded on previous trials. These adaptive tasks are useful for quickly determining a category boundary in a synthetic speech series (Penner, 1978). The experiment of Johnson, Wright, and Flemming (1992), described in the section on the method of adjustment, is a task in which a computer is necessary to determine which stimulus to present based on the listener's actions.

There is one additional advantage to running listeners on line. Since the responses are collected by the computer, they are available for analysis by other programs, including statistical packages. Either these statistical packages can be run on the laboratory computer or the data can be transferred to another computer for analysis. The computer used to run the experiments can

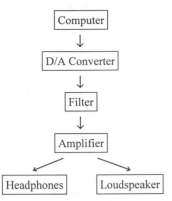

FIGURE 15-11 Components for a computer system to reproduce audio and present it to listeners.

also be used for recording audio signals such as natural speech, waveform measurement and editing, spectral analysis, and synthesis. The hardware required for these tasks is also used for the running of experiments. Thus, the use of an on-line system provides flexibility and ease of use and eliminates tedious work.

An On-line System

There are three elements for a basic on-line system: the computer, the analog input-output (I/O) system, and the software. The choices for these elements are interrelated. However, a good rule of thumb is to choose the software first, then choose the computer and analog systems to work with the software. Since the hardware must also have certain basic capabilities, we will briefly consider the specifications for the computer and analog I/O system first.

A block diagram of the computer and analog input/output system is shown in Figure 15-11. The computer system can be virtually any micro- or minicomputer with sufficient memory, disk space, and speed. The speed should be sufficient to match the requirements of the analog I/O system and support the sampling rates to be used, furthermore, the memory must be large enough for the operating system, programs to run on-line experiments, and any buffer areas needed for speech input and output. The disk space is needed for software and speech stimuli. Speech stimuli can use huge amounts of disk storage. A typical sentence may be about 2 seconds in duration. At a 20 kHz sampling rate, this is 80,000 bytes of storage (uncompressed). If several sentences are being presented, they will use substantial space on the disk. As another point of comparison, a compact disk holds about

70 to 75 minutes of stereo (two-channel) sound at a 44.1 kHz sampling rate. This corresponds to over 600 million bytes, or 600 megabytes (MB) of storage. Finally, an experiment using monosyllabic words might involve 200 items spoken by each of four talkers. With a 10 kHz sampling rate and an average duration of 500 ms, this corresponds to about 16 MB of storage. Examine the type of stimulus materials to be used and scale the disk space accordingly.

For the analog I/O system, the basic requirements are as follows. First, the system should have analog input and at least two channels of analog output. The converters can be 12-, 14-, or 16-bit but should run at a sustained rate of 44.1 kHz or higher. *Sustained* means that the analog I/O system together with the computer and software should be capable of handling utterances of arbitrary duration with the only limit being the available disk space. The two channels of analog output are used for dichotic presentation, and the analog system should be capable of dichotic (stereo) output. Whalen et al. (1990) describe these requirements and how they were implemented at Haskins Laboratories. Finally, a programmable clock that can be used to time intervals and RTs is needed. This may either be part of the analog system or a separate device. It should be capable of timing with millisecond resolution. Yaphe, Raftery, and Jamieson (1989) describe a microcomputer-based system for running listeners in adaptive procedures that meets these criteria.

The software component and choices are perhaps the most difficult. Some off-the-shelf packages are designed to run basic experimental tasks. Their users need not know how to program the computer. An alternative is to clone an existing laboratory facility. Software is often shared across laboratories, and at least one journal, *Behavioral Research Methods, Instruments and Computers,* publishes descriptions of software, hardware, and algorithms. Cohen et al. (1993) describe a general-purpose experimental package for the Macintosh that includes audio output. A third alternative for those who can do programming is to buy a computer and compatible analog I/O system and write experimental control programs for the hardware.

Table 15-3 describes some alternative systems. They illustrate systems using two popular microcomputers (IBM PC/AT or compatible and Apple Macintosh). Systems similar to these are in use in speech perception laboratories (Yaphe, Raftery, and Jamieson, 1989; Blount

TABLE 15-3 Microcomputer systems for running listeners on-line in speech perception experiments

	System	
	PC-compatible	Macintosh
Computer	386-based PC/AT compatible with ISA bus (at least two free slots)	Model with NuBus (at least two free slots)
Analog I/O	Data translation DT2821 series Ariel DSP-16	Data translation Topflight series Digidesign Audiomedia
	National Instruments AT-MIO-16 series	National Instruments NB-MIO-16 series GW Instruments MacAdios
Other	Filters such as TTE model 411AFS, microphone, speakers and headphones	
Software	Laboratory microsystems APRLS CSRE User written	PsyScope User written

Vendors:
  Ariel—433 River Road, Highland Park, NJ 08904
  CSRE—Dr. Donald G. Jamieson, Department of Communicative Disorders, University of Western Ontario, London, Ontario, Canada N6G 1H1
  Data Translation—100 Locke Drive, Marlboro, MA 01752
  Digidesign—1360 Willow Road, Suite 101, Menlo Park, CA 94025
  GW Instruments—PO Box 2145, Cambridge, MA 02141
  Laboratory Microsystems—450 Cloud Drive #11, Baton Rouge, LA 70806
  National Instruments—6504 Bridge Point Parkway, Austin, TX 78730
  PsyScope—Jonathan Cohen, Department of Psychology, Carnegie Mellon University, Pittsburgh, PA 15213
  TTE—11652 W. Olympic Blvd, Los Angeles, CA 90064

and Blount, 1990). It is also possible to assemble a system for running multiple listeners simultaneously. However, additional hardware is required for each subject. These types of systems are beyond the scope of this chapter. The systems illustrated in Table 15-3 can also be used for speech recording, editing, analysis, and synthesis to provide a flexible laboratory computer system. The list is not exhaustive, and many laboratories have developed their own software for on-line experiments.

SUMMARY

The basis of research in speech perception is measurement of a listener's response to a speech stimulus under controlled circumstances. The method of constant stimuli, one of the classic methods of psychophysics, underlies most contemporary work using identification, discrimination, adaptation, and other tasks. With the emergence of signal detection theory and the emphasis in cognitive psychology on converging operations (using multiple tasks or dependent measures), a powerful set of tools is available to the researcher to investigate the mental processes that underlie speech perception.

Instrumentation for speech perception experiments emphasizes the use of computers for gathering data from listeners on-line. This automated data collection allows new experimental tasks and modifications to existing tasks to be easily and quickly programmed and speeds collecting and analyzing of data.

The development of new tasks and new uses or variations of current tasks is largely a result of new questions raised by theory and research. Thus, methodology is a product of our understanding of perception and can be expected to change to answer new questions.

Review Questions

1. What is the importance of catch trials or their equivalent of trials with different correct answers in studies of speech perception?

2. What is a speed-accuracy trade-off and how does it affect the interpretation of reaction-time data?

3. Illustrate the use of converging operations in speech perception research.

4. When is it appropriate to use open categorization in collecting perceptual data and when is it appropriate to use forced choice?

5. Speech perception is a real-time process in humans. How does this affect our choice of experimental tasks in designing perceptual experiments?

6. Why should trials in an experiment be presented in random order? Why are stimuli presented more than once to the listener for response?

References

Ades, A. E. (1974). How phonetic is selective adaptation? Experiments on syllable position and vowel environment. *Perception & Psychophysics, 16*, 61-67.

Best, C. T., Morrongiello, B., & Robson, R. (1981). Perceptual equivalence of acoustic cues in speech and nonspeech perception. *Perception & Psychophysics, 29*, 191-211.

Best, C. T., Studdert-Kennedy, M., Manuel, S., & Rubin-Spitz, J. (1989). Discovering phonetic coherence in acoustic patterns. *Perception & Psychophysics, 45*, 237-250.

Blount, J. P., & Blount, M. A. (1990). Teaching about speech perception and production inexpensively on microcomputers. *Behavior Research Methods, Instruments, & Computers, 22*, 219-222.

Braida, L. D., & Durlach, N. I. (1972). Intensity perception: 2. Resolution in one-interval paradigms. *Journal of the Acoustical Society of America, 51*, 483-502.

Braida, L. D., Lim, J. S., Berliner, J. E., Durlach, N. I., Rabinowitz, W. M., & Purks, S. R. (1984). Intensity perception: 13. Perceptual anchor model of context-coding. *Journal of the Acoustical Society of America, 76*, 722-731.

Cohen, J., MacWhinney, B., Flatt, M., & Provost, J. (1993). PsyScope: An interactive graphic system for designing and controlling experiments in the psychology laboratory using Macintosh computers. *Behavior Research Methods, Instruments, and Computers, 25*, 257-271.

Coren, S., & Ward, L. M. (1989). *Sensation & Perception*. San Diego: Harcourt Brace Jovanovich.

Cowan, N. (1984). On short and long auditory stores. *Psychological Bulletin, 96*, 341-370.

Cudahy, E. (1988). *Introduction to instrumentation in Speech and Hearing*. Baltimore: Williams & Wilkins.

Cutting, J. E. (1974). Two left-hemisphere mechanisms in speech perception. *Perception & Psychophysics, 16*, 601-612.

Diehl, R. L., Elman, J. L., & McCusker, S. B. (1978). Contrast effects on stop consonant identification. *Journal of Experimental Psychology: Human Perception and Performance, 4*, 599-609.

Diehl, R. L., Kluender, K. R., & Parker, E. M. (1985). Are selective adaptation and contrast effects really distinct? *Journal of Experimental Psychology: Human Perception and Performance, 11*, 209-220.

Durlach, N. I., & Braida, L. D. (1969). Intensity perception: 1. Preliminary theory of intensity resolution. *Journal of the Acoustical Society of America, 46*, 372-383.

Eimas, P. D., Cooper, W. E., & Corbit, J. D. (1973). Some properties of linguistic feature detectors. *Perception & Psychophysics, 13*, 247-252.

Eimas, P. D., & Corbit, J. D. (1973). Selective adaptation of linguistic feature detectors. *Cognitive Psychology, 4*, 99-109.

Eimas, P. D., Marcovitz Hornstein, S. B., & Payton, P. (1990). Attention and the role of dual codes in phoneme monitoring. *Journal of Memory and Language, 29*, 133-159.

Eimas, P. D., Siquiland, E. R., Jusczyk, P., & Vigorito J. (1971). Speech perception in infants. *Science, 1971*, 303-306.

Elmes, D. G., Kantowitz, B. H., & Roediger III, H. L. (1989). *Research methods in Psychology*. St. Paul: West.

Fechner, G. T. (1966). *Elements of psychophysics* (Adler, H. E., Trans.). Howes, D. H., & Boring, E. G. (Eds.), New York: Holt Rinehart and Winston. (Original work published in 1860)

Fowler, C. A. (1990). Sound-producing sources as objects of perception: Rate normalization and nonspeech perception. *Journal of the Acoustical Society of America, 88,* 1236-1249.

Fox, R. A. (1984). Effect of lexical status on phonetic categorization. *Journal of Experimental Psychology: Human Perception and Performance, 10,* 526-540.

Gagnon, D. A., & Sawusch, J. R. (1990). Rediscovering auditory coherence in phonetic patterns. *Journal of the Acoustical Society of America, 88,* (Suppl. 1), S177 (Abstract).

Ganong, W. F. (1980). Phonetic categorization in auditory word perception. *Journal of Experimental Psychology: Human Perception and Performance, 6,* 110-125.

Garrison, L. F., & Sawusch, J. R. (1986). Adaptation of place perception for stops: Effects of spectral match between adaptor and test series. *Perception & Psychophysics, 40,* 419-430.

Gottleib, G., & Krasnegor, N. A. (Eds.) (1985). *Measurement of audition and vision in the first year of postnatal life: A methodological overview.* Norwood, NJ: Ablex.

Green, D. M., & Swets, J. A. (1974). *Signal detection theory and psychophysics.* Huntington, NY: Krieger.

Grosjean, F. (1985). The recognition of words after their acoustic offset: Evidence and implications. *Perception & Psychophysics, 38,* 299-310.

Harnad, S. (Ed.) (1987). *Categorical perception.* Cambridge, UK: Cambridge University Press.

Johnson, K., Wright, R., & Flemming, E. (1992). Using the method of adjustment to study vowel spaces. *Journal of the Acoustical Society of America, 91,* 2387 (Abstract).

Jusczyk, P. W. (1985). The high-amplitude sucking technique as a methodological tool in speech perception research. In Gottleib, G., & Krasnegor, N. A. (Eds.), *Measurement of audition and vision in the first year of postnatal life: A methodological overview.* Norwood, NJ: Ablex (pp. 195-222).

Jusczyk, P. W., Pisoni, D. B., & Mullennix, J. (1992). Some consequences of stimulus variability on speech processing by 2-month-old infants. *Cognition, 43,* 253-291.

Kewley-Port, D., Watson, C. S., & Foyle, D. C. (1988). Auditory temporal acuity in relation to category boundaries: Speech and nonspeech stimuli. *Journal of the Acoustical Society of America, 83,* 1133-1145.

Kintsch, W., Miller, J. R., & Polson, P. G. (Eds.) (1984). *Method and tactics in cognitive science.* Hillsdale, NJ: Erlbaum.

Klatt, D. H. (1989). Review of selected models of speech perception. In Marslen-Wilson, W. (Ed.), *Lexical representation and process.* Cambridge, MA: MIT Press (pp. 169-226).

Kuhl, P. K. (1985). Methods in the study of infant speech perception. In Gottleib, G., & Krasnegor,

N. A. (Eds.), *Measurement of audition and vision in the first year of postnatal life: A methodological overview.* Norwood, NJ: Ablex (pp. 223-251).

Levitt, H. (1970). Transformed up-down methods in psychoacoustics. *Journal of the Acoustical Society of America, 49,* 467-477.

Liberman, A. M. (1982). On finding that speech is special. *American Psychologist, 37,* 148-167.

Liberman, A. M., Harris, K. S., Hoffman, H. S., & Griffith, B. C. (1957). The discrimination of speech sounds within and across phoneme boundaries. *Journal of Experimental Psychology, 54,* 358-368.

Liberman, A. M., & Mattingly, I. G. (1985). The motor theory of speech perception revised. *Cognition, 21,* 1-36.

Macmillan, N. A. (1987). Beyond the categorical/continuous distinction: A psychophysical approach to processing modes. In S. Harnad (Ed.), *Categorical perception.* Cambridge, UK: Cambridge University Press (pp. 53-85).

Macmillan, N. A., & Creelman, C. D. (1991). *Detection theory: A user's guide.* Cambridge, UK: Cambridge University Press.

Mattingly, I. G., Liberman, A. M., Syrdal, A. K., & Halwes, T. (1971). Discrimination in speech and nonspeech modes. *Cognitive Psychology, 2,* 131-157.

Mayzner, M. S., & Dolan, T. R. (Eds.) (1978). *Minicomputers in sensory and information-processing research.* Hillsdale, NJ: Erlbaum.

Miller, G. A. (1956). The magic number seven, plus or minus two: Some limits on our capacity for processing information. *Psychological Review, 63,* 81-96.

Miller, J. D., Wier, C. C., Pastore, R. E., Kelly, W. J., & Dooling, R. J. (1976). Discrimination and labeling of noise—buzz sequences with varying noise—lead times: An example of categorical perception. *Journal of the Acoustical Society of America, 60,* 410-417.

Nusbaum, H. C., & Schwab, E. C. (1986). The role of attention and active processing in speech perception. In Schwab, E. C., & Nusbaum, H. C. (Eds.), *Pattern Recognition by Humans and Machines,* Vol. 1. New York: Academic Press (pp. 113-157).

Pachella, R. G. (1974). The interpretation of reaction time in information-processing research. In Kantowitz, B. (Ed.), *Human information processing: Tutorials in performance and cognition.* Hillsdale, NJ: Erlbaum (pp. 41-82).

Pastore, R. E. (1987). Categorical perception: Some psychophysical models. In Harnad, S. (Ed.), *Categorical perception.* Cambridge, UK: Cambridge University Press (pp. 29-52).

Pastore, R. E., Li, X. F., & Layer, J. K. (1990). Categorical perception of nonspeech chirps and bleats. *Perception & Psychophysics, 48,* 151-156.

Penner, M. J. (1978). Psychophysical methods and the minicomputer. In Mayzner, M. S., & Dolan, T. R. (Eds.), *Minicomputers in sensory and information-processing research*. Hillsdale, NJ: Erlbaum (pp. 91-122).

Pisoni, D. B. (1975). Auditory short-term memory and vowel perception. *Memory & Cognition, 3*, 7-18.

Pisoni, D. B. (1977). Identification and discrimination of the relative onset time of two component tones: Implications for voicing perception in stops. *Journal of the Acoustical Society of America, 61*, 1351-1361.

Pisoni, D. B., & Luce, P. A. (1987). Acoustic-phonetic representation in word recognition. In Frauenfelder, U. H., & Tyler, L. D. (Eds.), *Spoken word recognition*. Cambridge, MA: MIT Press (pp. 21-52).

Pisoni, D. B., & Tash, J. B. (1974). Reaction times to comparisons within and across phonetic categories. *Perception & Psychophysics, 15*, 285-290.

Remez, R. E. (1987). Neural models of speech perception: A case history. In Harnad, S. (Ed.), *Categorical perception*. Cambridge, UK: Cambridge University Press (pp. 199-225).

Remez, R. E., Rubin, P. E., Pisoni, D. B., & Carrell, T. D. (1981). Speech perception without traditional speech cues. *Science, 212*, 947-949.

Roberts, M., & Summerfield, Q. (1981). Audiovisual presentation demonstrates that selective adaptation in speech perception is purely auditory. *Perception & Psychophysics, 30*, 309-314.

Salasoo, A., & Pisoni, D. B. (1985). Interaction of knowledge sources in spoken word identification. *Journal of Memory and Cognition, 2*, 210-231.

Samuel, A. G. (1986). Red herring detectors and speech perception: In defense of selective adaptation. *Cognitive Psychology, 18*, 452-499.

Sawusch, J. R. (1986). Auditory and phonetic coding of speech. In Schwab, E. C., & Nusbaum, H. C. (Eds.), *Pattern recognition by humans and machines*, Vol. 1. New York: Academic Press (pp. 51-88).

Sawusch, J. R., & Jusczyk, P. (1981). Adaptation and contrast in the perception of voicing. *Journal of Experimental Psychology: Human Perception and Performance, 7*, 408-421.

Sawusch, J. R., Nusbaum, H. C., & Schwab, E. C. (1980). Contextual effects in vowel perception: 2. Evidence for two processing mechanisms. *Perception & Psychophysics, 27*, 421-434.

Shinn, P., & Blumstein, S. E. (1984). On the role of the amplitude envelope for the perception of [b] and [w]. *Journal of the Acoustical Society of America, 75*, 1243-1252.

Sussman, J. E., & Carney, A. E. (1989). Effects of transition length on the perception of stop consonants by children and adults. *Journal of Speech and Hearing Research, 32*, 151-160.

Taylor, M. M., & Creelman, C. D. (1967). PEST: Efficient estimates on probability functions. *Journal of the Acoustical Society of America, 41*, 782-787.

Tomiak, G. R., Mullennix, J. W., & Sawusch, J. R. (1987). Integral processing of phonemes: Evidence for a phonetic mode of perception. *Journal of the Acoustical Society of America, 81*, 755-764.

Treiman, R. (1985). Onsets and rimes as units of spoken syllables: Evidence from children. *Journal of Experimental Child Psychology, 39*, 161-181.

Wannemacher, C. A., & Sawusch, J. R. (1989). The role of phonological permissibility in the phonetic coding of speech. *Journal of the Acoustical Society of America, 86*, S100 (Abstract).

Watson, C. S. (1987). Uncertainty, informational masking, and the capacity of immediate auditory memory. In Yost, W. A., & Watson, C. S. (Eds.), *Auditory processing of complex sounds*. Hillsdale, NJ: Erlbaum (pp. 267-277).

Whalen, D. H., Wiley, E. R., Rubin, P. E., & Cooper, F. S. (1990). The Haskins Laboratories' pulse code modulation system. *Behavior Research Methods, Instruments, & Computers, 22*, 550-559.

Yaphe, M., Raftery, E., & Jamieson, D. G. (1989). A general-purpose facility for adaptive testing in psychoacoustics. *Behavior Research Methods, Instruments, & Computers, 21*, 275-280.

Suggested Readings

Basic Methodology

Elmes, D. G., Kantowitz, B. H., & Roediger, H. L. (1989). *Research methods in Psychology*. St. Paul: West.

Kintsch, W., Miller, J. R., & Polson, P. G. (Eds.) (1984). *Method and tactics in cognitive science*. Hillsdale, NJ: Erlbaum.

Psychophysical Methods in Perception

Coren, S., & Ward, L. M. (1989). *Sensation and perception*. San Diego: Harcourt Brace Jovanovich.

Signal Detection

Macmillan, N. A., & Creelman, C. D. (1991). *Detection theory: A user's guide*. Cambridge, UK: Cambridge University Press.

Converging Operations

Reaction Time

Pachella, R. G. (1974). The interpretation of reaction time in information-processing research. In Kantowitz, B. (Ed.), *Human information processing: Tutorials in performance and cognition.* Hillsdale, NJ: Erlbaum (pp. 41-82).

Categorical Perception

Harnad, S. (Ed.). (1987). *Categorical perception.* Cambridge, UK: Cambridge University Press.

Speech and Nonspeech Mode

Fowler, C. A. (1990). Sound-producing sources as objects of perception: Rate normalization and nonspeech perception. *Journal of the Acoustical Society of America, 88,* 1236-1249.

Liberman, A. M., & Mattingly, I. G. (1985). The motor theory of speech perception revised. *Cognition, 21,* 1-36.

Tomiak, G. R., Mullennix, J. W., & Sawusch, J. R. (1987). Integral processing of phonemes: Evidence for a phonetic mode of perception. *Journal of the Acoustical Society of America, 81,* 755-764.

Selective Adaptation

Samuel, A. G. (1986). Red herring detectors and speech perception: In defense of selective adaptation. *Cognitive Psychology, 18,* 452-499.

Sawusch, J. R. (1986). Auditory and phonetic coding of speech. In Schwab, E. C., & Nusbaum, H. C. (Eds.), *Pattern recognition by humans and machines,* Vol. 1. New York: Academic Press (pp. 51-88).

Other

Pisoni, D. B., & Luce, P. A. (1987). Acoustic-phonetic representation in word recognition. In Frauenfelder, U. H., & Tyler, L. D. (Eds.), *Spoken word recognition.* Cambridge, MA: MIT Press (pp. 21-52).

Infant and Nonhuman Subjects

Gottleib, G., & Krasnegor, N. A. (Eds.) (1985). *Measurement of audition and vision in the first year of postnatal life: A methodological overview.* Norwood, NJ: Ablex.

Instrumentation

Sound Reproduction

Cudahy, E. (1988). *Introduction to instrumentation in speech and hearing.* Baltimore: Williams & Wilkins.

Computerized Experiments

Mayzner, M. S., & Dolan, T. R. (Eds.) (1978). *Minicomputers in sensory and information-processing research.* Hillsdale, NJ: Erlbaum.

Schwartz, A. H. (Ed.) (1984). *The handbook of microcomputer applications in communicative disorders.* San Diego: College-Hill Press.

Glossary

accent—Prosodic prominence involving more than one of the three prosodic features of duration, pitch, and stress.

acoustic-phonetic invariance—The central "problem" of speech perception; the physical manifestations of phonetic contrasts vary widely across different talkers, phonetic environments, and speaking rates.

acoustic-regulation hypothesis—Hypothesis that speech pressures are maintained at certain levels primarily for acoustic purposes rather than for aerodynamic needs.

active mechanical properties—Properties of muscles that are manipulated by variations in muscle contraction, viz., the stiffness of the lips, tongue tip, and vocal folds that is changed as facial, tongue and vocal muscles contract, respectively.

adaptation—The decline in probability of a neuron firing as a function of time. At the beginning of a stimulus the probability of discharge is high. It declines rapidly over the first 15 ms (rapid adaptation). A slower but significant decrease in firing probability occurs over the following 40 ms. A much longer, more gradual decrease in firing occurs over a time span of about 1 second (slow adaptation).

afferent—When used in relation to the nervous system, referring to nerves that carry information to the central nervous system, including the spinal cord and brain stem; most often associated with sensory functions.

affricate—A speech sound that involves the two articulatory phases of a stop (vocal tract obstruction) and a fricative (release of air through a constriction). These two phases relate to the acoustic events of a stop gap and a noise segment.

airway resistance—Opposition to motion produced by the forces of friction, which dissipate energy as heat.

aliasing—A process by which artifacts or errors arise during digitization of a signal; the loss of information resulting from sampling an analog signal that has energy above half of the sampling frequency used in digitizing the analog signal. Spurious energy appears in the analysis. See **Nyquist sampling theorem**.

allophone—Phone that is treated as a variant or instance of the same phoneme within a particular language.

alternating magnetic field—A magnetic field caused by an alternating current passing through a wire. The poles reverse as the current reverses.

amplitude—The magnitude of displacement for a sound wave. The waveform of a sound is represented on a two-dimensional graph in which amplitude is plotted as a function of time. The amplitude of sound largely determines the perceived loudness of the sound.

amplitude modulation (AM)—The periodic or quasi-periodic oscillation of the magnitude of a mathematically defined signal, such as a sinusoid or spectrally more complex sound such as Gaussian noise. The consequence of amplitude modulation is to increase the complexity of the spectrum in a systematic way. Thus, a sinusoid signal of frequency f_c, modulated by a second sinusoid of frequency f_m, will generate a spectrum consisting of three components, $f_c - f_m$, f_c, and $f_c + f_m$. Amplitude modulation is observed in many speech sounds (voiced segments).

analog signal—A continuous function of time that can take any real value. An analog signal can represent the value of a physical measurement like the sound pressure captured by a microphone.

antiformant—A property of the vocal tract transfer function in which energy is not passed effectively through the system; it is opposite in effect to a formant. Antiformants, or zeros, arise because of divided passages or constrictions in the vocal tract. The antiformant acts like a short circuit, trapping energy in the system so it is not radiated into space.

antinode—A region in the resonating vocal tract where particle vibration is minimized (i.e., a region of volume velocity minimum) and pressure is maximized. Antinodes alternate with nodes in accounting for the standing wave distribution of volume velocity for its inverse, pressure) in the resonating tube.

aperiodic—The characterization of a signal that does not repeat itself.

apparent viscosity—The inherent characteristic of muscle contraction that limits the rate at which actin/myosin cross-bridges can be made and broken, leading to a limitation in rate of muscle shortening.

articulation—Movement; in speech production, the movement of a speech organ.

articulatory model—A model that accounts for the movements of speech.

articulatory undershooting—The phenomenon whereby an articulator does not reach its target position for the production of a particular sound, thereby decreasing the acoustic distinctiveness for that sound.

artifact—An apparent object or surface that appears in an image but is not really there.

attractors—A concept used in dynamic systems perspectives to account for transitions and stabilities in motor behaviors; three major types are point attractors, limit cycle attractors, and strange attractors.

auditory induction—The perceptual reconstruction of sounds obliterated by louder sounds. This process reverses the effects of masking on the basis of collateral information concerning the nature of the missing segments. There are two types of auditory induction: (1) *temporal induction,* which restores missing fragments based on prior and/or subsequent information concerning its identity; (2) *contralateral induction,* which restores sounds masked at one ear on the basis of information reaching the other ear.

autocorrelation (AC)—A mathematical procedure for estimating the periodicity of a given signal. A copy of the signal is multiplied (correlated) with the original and the product stored in a buffer. The copy is shifted by a small amount of time and the correlation recomputed and the product appended to the buffer. This procedure is repeated a sufficient number of times to obtain a reliable estimate of the periodicity, which is reflected in the interval over which the correlation function achieves its maximum amplitude at least twice.

automatic gain control (AGC)—The processes by which the auditory system compensates for large changes in sound pressure level. Faint sounds produce a larger response than otherwise, while very intense sounds evoke a smaller response that would normally occur. The result is to compress a very large dynamic range of signal intensities within a manageable scale of neural firing rates.

bandwidth—A measure of the extent to which a sound component is dispersed among a group of adjacent frequencies. Resonances and formants are defined as having a center frequency and a bandwidth, which is the difference in hertz between the center frequency and the frequency at which the power is half of the power at the center frequency. That is, both the lower and higher frequencies that define the bandwidth are 3 dB less intense than the peak energy in the band.

Bark scale—A nonlinear transformation of frequency that corresponds to the analysis accomplished by the ear. The Bark scale is closely related to the concept of critical band in auditory perception.

Bernoulli force or effect—A decrease in pressure at a constriction due to an increase in air or fluid velocity in the face of a constant volume flow. It is based on Bernoulli's principle that states that when fluid velocity is high, the pressure will be low. The low pressure caused by the Bernoulli force as a result of airflow through the vocal folds is part of the effect causing the vocal folds to come together during voicing.

bias—The decision rule used by a listener to map internal perception of a stimulus onto a response. Synonym of **criterion**.

bite block—A device for changing the vertical space between the upper and lower jaws.

bleed valve—Tube offering different diameters used to create an oral air leak during speech production.

burst—The brief noise created during the release of a stop consonant, typically about 10-30 msec.

cascade—An arrangement of a group of filters in which a signal first passes through one filter, then the next, and so on, until it has passed through all the filters. It contrasts with parallel designs.

catch trial—A trial on which no stimulus is present or on which a different stimulus, requiring a different response by the listener, is presented.

categorical perception—The relationship between identification and discrimination task performance where a listener can only discriminate between stimuli to the extent that he can label them differently; i.e., the ability to discriminate between two stimuli is no better than one's ability to identify them as belonging to different categories.

central spectrum—A term used originally by Srulovicz and Goldstein (1983) to describe the neural representation of spectral information in the central auditory pathway. It is important for understanding the theoretical basis of certain place models of pitch perception.

cepstrum—A Fourier transform of the power spectrum of a signal. The transform is described in terms of quefrency (note the transposition from frequency), which has timelike properties. The cepstrum is used to determine the fundamental frequency of a speech signal. Voiced speech tends to have a strong cepstral peak, at the first rahmonic (note the transposition from harmonic).

channels (frequency) — A population of tonotopically organized neurons whose characteristic frequencies span a specified range. For conceptual and modeling simplicity the response of a large number of neural elements is often analyzed as a smaller series of frequency channel, in which the constituent neural elements are considered relatively homogeneous in response properties.

characteristic frequency (CF) — The frequency to which an auditory neuron is most sensitive. This is the frequency (or center of a frequency range) to which it is possible to evoke a significant increase in firing rate above the background level at the lowest possible sound pressure level.

child-directed speech — The manner of speaking that one uses when talking to an infant or young child. Typically it has short sentences and is slow, with high pitch and great fluctuations in pitch.

chopper — The predominant physiological response pattern observed in the ventral cochlear nucleus and found in more centrally located nuclei such as the inferior colliculus. Its name derives from the fact that the discharge level oscillates at a relatively regular interval (typically ranging between 2 and 10 ms). The function of these cells is not entirely clear, though they seem to be important for encoding spectral information.

click — A type of speech sound produced by placing some portion of the tongue in contact with a location on the palate. A vacuum is created behind the point of contact and the resulting sound produced as the tongue is pulled away from the palate is referred to as a click.

clipping — The cutting off of a signal past a given amplitude threshold, frequently the effect of introducing a signal with a greater dynamic range than the amplifier or computer program can handle.

coarticulation — A phenomenon of speech production in which simultaneous adjustments are made to two or more speech segments; i.e., articulation of more than one phoneme at a time: the reciprocal influence of neighboring phonemes upon the production and acoustic nature of each other; the effect of speech sounds on the articulation of adjacent speech sounds. One feature of a speech unit may be anticipated during production of an earlier unit in the string (anticipatory or forward coarticulation) or retained during production of a unit that comes later (retentive, or backward, coarticulation).

coherent modulation — The condition in which two or more elements of an acoustic signal (such as the spectral peaks) covary in time; indicative of being produced by a common source (e.g., a human vocal tract).

cohort — A collection of words in the mental lexicon that all begin with the same sound sequence.

coincidence detection — A property of certain auditory neurons such that a cell will discharge when and only when two or more neural inputs arrive approximately simultaneously (i.e., within about 100 μs). The consequence of such triggered correlation is to focus the auditory system's response on common elements of the acoustic signal and to provide a means of filtering out background noise.

complex signal — A signal whose spectrum contains more than a single frequency. Technically, any signal that is not a sinusoid is complex. However, the term is usually reserved for signals with periodic or quasi-periodic properties and with a well-defined harmonic structure.

composite model — An integration of various subsystem models into a single overall model of speech production.

concatenation — In speech, the joining together of speech segments one after the other.

connectionist model — The proposition that speech production involves parallel patterns of activation in networks of densely interconnected units; some connectionist systems may take the form of neural networks.

consonant transitions — The portion of speech just before the onset or just after the offset of contact for a consonant.

context-sensitivity problem — The issue of how the speech control system regulates action while permitting extensive adjustments to context.

continuant — A speech sound that does not stop the flow of air in the mouth.

continuous speech — A modality of input to a speech recognition system in which words are spoken without pauses between them. This type of speech contrasts with the isolated speech mode required by earlier, simpler systems.

control — The process of management and the means by which a parameter is kept fairly constant or is regulated.

converging operations — The use of two or more tasks, sets of stimuli, or sets of instructions to listeners designed to provide a pattern of data to test a theory or theories.

coordinative structure — A synergy or linkage among a group of muscles to accomplish a particular task.

coproduction — A proposition that vowels and consonants can be produced in parallel to yield combined and simultaneous effects in articulation.

correlation — The degree of similarity between data patterns. Typically, the magnitude of correlation is computed through a multiplicative operation. Large products result from high degrees of correlation, and low products are associated with little correlation. The sign of the magnitude indicates whether the correlation is positive (+) or negative (−).

counterbalance—The process of altering or varying the order of events so that the effects observed in an experiment are not due to the qualities of one particular order.

coupling—Interaction between two or more systems; e.g., oral-nasal coupling is interaction between the two resonating cavities. No coupling means no interaction; strong coupling means substantial interaction.

criterion—See **bias**.

criterion shift rule—A general perceptual principle that the criteria serving as the bases for evaluation and categorization of stimuli are displaced in the direction of recently experienced values.

critical band—A range of frequencies surrounding a given frequency that are most effective in masking, or preventing the hearing, of that frequency.

crossed olivocochlear bundle (COCB)—A small population of fibers originating in the olivary complex of the auditory brain stem, which projects to the cochlea of the opposite ear. It is thought to be important for providing recurrent short-term (50 to 100 ms) feedback for spectral and intensity processing and is believed to act as an automatic gain control at the level of the cochlea. The COCB is the major component of the efferent system.

damping—The rate of absorption of sound energy. Damping is related to bandwidth: the greater the damping of a sound in a system, the larger is the bandwidth.

decibel (dB)—A logarithmic scaling of sound intensity (or sound pressure) relative to a reference intensity (or sound pressure).

declination—The overall slope of the fundamental frequency of an utterance; an intonational phenomenon manifested as lowering of the fundamental frequency of successive peaks in declarative sentences.

degrees of freedom problem—The issue of how the large number of muscles and structures are controlled and coordinated during speech production.

delta spectrum—A function formed by computing the (smoothed) difference of the values of consecutive spectra (see **spectrum**) for each frequency. The delta spectrum gives a measure of the instantaneous rate of change of the spectrum at each frequency. It provides a way to represent dynamic information about a speech signal.

demisyllables—The portion of a syllable including part of a consonant and half of the following vowel portion, or half of the vowel and part of the following consonant. Demisyllables are sometimes used as the basic unit in speech synthesis.

dendritic arborization—The anatomical pattern of connections that a cell receives from other neurons. A dendrite collects information from other neurons and transmits some form of weighted average to the neuronal soma (cell body).

depolarization—The process by which the electrical potential of a cell changes from its resting level (typically −50 to −70 mV) to a level close to or greater than 0 volts DC. That is, the electrical potential at a given location of the cell changes sign from negative to positive, an indication that the neuron has discharged.

dicrotic pulse phonation—A low-frequency phonation associated with a double opening and closing of the vocal folds for each vocal cycle.

difference limen (DL)—A behavioral measure of the smallest difference reliably discriminated along a designated perceptual parameter, such as frequency or intensity. The just noticeable difference between two sounds, the value at which half of listeners' judgments are that two sounds are different.

differentiation—A mathematical function whose acoustic effect, applied to a signal, is to produce a relative increase in the amplitude of the higher frequencies.

digital signal—A function that usually corresponds to a sequence of samples taken periodically from an analog signal. In a digital signal each sample is represented by an integer. The larger the number of bits used to represent each integer, the better will be the approximation to the true value of the original analog signal. In addition, the samples have to be taken close enough together in time so that the digital signal is a good representation of the original analog signal. In general, an accurate rendering of an analog requires a digital sampling rate of more than twice the frequency of the highest frequency component of the original signal.

diphthong—A vowel-like sound involving a gradual change in articulatory configuration from an onglide to offglide position. The usual phonetic symbol is a digraph, or combination of two symbols, to represent the onglide and offglide portions.

discrete Fourier transform—An algorithm that may be used to generate a spectrum on a digital computer. The value of the spectrum is computed only for a discrete number of frequencies, but there is no loss of information if the frequency values are close enough. The fast Fourier transform (FFT) is a very efficient procedure to compute discrete Fourier transforms.

discrimination—A task in which the listener tries to distinguish two or more stimuli, such as indicating whether two stimuli are the same or different.

distributed representation—The spatial dispersion of perceptually related information across an array of frequency channels. This often occurs at moderate to high sound pressure levels for information pertaining to low-frequency spectral peaks.

dominant frequency—The observation that many frequency channels often synchronize to the same spectral information, such as a speech formant or some other spectral peak.

downdrift—See **declination**.

downsampling—The sampling at a relatively low rate from a signal that has already been sampled at a higher rate.

dynamic range—The range over which an element (in this instance a neuron's firing rate) responds to changes in the magnitude of a specified stimulus parameter. For example, auditory-nerve fibers typically increase their firing rate in response to intensity increments as long as the sound pressure level is approximately 20 to 30 dB above the cell's rate-defined threshold. Above or below this intensity range no significant changes in firing level occur.

dynamic systems—An explanation of motor control in which behavior is viewed in terms of the interactions between biomechanical and environmental variables.

efferent—When used in relation to the nervous system, referring to nerves or bundles of nerves that transmit signals or commands from the central nervous system (including the spinal cord or brain stem) to peripheral nuclei and to muscles.

efferent system—A series of fiber tracts originating in the olivary complex that project to the outer hair cells and auditory-nerve fibers in the cochlea. The efferent system is thought to be involved in some form of feedback pertaining to automatic gain control.

electrostatically charged—Containing a stationary electric charge.

emphasis—High degree of sentence-level stress, used to assign particular prominence to a constituent of the utterance.

entrainment—The ability of certain auditory neurons, principally located in the posteroventral cochlear nucleus, to discharge on each modulation cycle in a manner highly synchronized to the waveform. Each cycle of the signal evokes a discharge that is locked to a specific phase of the stimulus. Thus, there is a one-to-one relationship between stimulus cycle and neural event.

error rate—An overall measure of performance of a speech recognition system. The most common characterization in a given task is word error rate, which is computed as the number of total word errors divided by the total number of words in a given test set. The counted errors are the number of substitutions plus deletions plus insertions.

event detectors—The capability of neurons to respond to significant changes in the acoustic signal, such as a rapid increase in amplitude, or a sudden shift in the spectrum. These abrupt changes indicative transitions in the state of the source producing the signal, such as when the vocal tract changes shape.

event stream—A series of acoustic events such as occurs in continuous speech. Each phonemelike segment is considered a separate event joined by spectral and amplitude transitions.

fast Fourier transform (FFT)—An algorithm commonly used in microcomputer programs to calculate a Fourier spectrum. The FFT is a special type of discrete Fourier transform in which the number of points transformed is a power of 2. The number of points expresses the bandwidth of analysis; the higher the value, the narrower the bandwidth.

feedback system—A controlled system in which information regarding the output of the system is used to modify the system's performance.

feedforward system—A controlled system in which planning and predicting mechanisms make ongoing changes in the system's output.

filter—A hardware device or software program that provides a frequency-dependent transmission of energy. Commonly, a filter is used to reject energy at certain frequencies while passing the energy at other frequencies. A *low-pass filter* passes energy at frequencies below a certain cutoff frequency; a *high-pass filter* passes energy at frequencies above a certain cutoff frequency; and a *band-pass filter* passes energy between a lower and an upper cutoff frequency.

filtering—One of the most important properties of auditory neurons, namely the capability of responding selectively to different frequencies in a systematic fashion. Most neurons act as bandpass filters in that they respond well to a continuous range of frequencies and respond poorly to frequencies lying outside this specified range. Cells can also act as low-pass filters in that they respond to all frequencies below some cutoff and poorly above this limit.

fine-temporal structure—The detailed modulation of an acoustic waveform or neural firing pattern. Specifically, the fine structure refers to the time intervals between peaks (or modes) in the waveform.

finite state machine—A general abstraction consisting of a finite set of states and the transitions among them. It is usually represented by a graph in which the nodes represent the states and the arrows represent the transitions.

first spike latency—The point in time relative to stimulus onset when a neuron reliably responds to a signal; important for coincidence detection and phase-place models of frequency coding.

flap—An articulation in which one articulator strikes another in passing while on its way back to its rest position.

fleshpoint—A specific point on an articulatory structure, usually marked by a pellet affixed to it.

forced choice—A task in which the listener must choose the response to each trial from a limited, predetermined set.

formant—A resonance of the vocal tract; the concentration of energy at certain frequencies in speech resulting from the time-varying resonances of the vocal tract. A formant is specified by its center frequency (commonly called formant frequency) and bandwidth. Formants are identified by integers that increase with the relative frequency location of the formants. F_1 is the lowest-frequency formant, F_2 is the next highest, and so on.

formant transition—A change in formant pattern, typically associated with a phonetic boundary; for example, the CV formant transition refers to formant pattern changes associated with the consonant-vowel transition.

Fourier theory—Named after the early nineteenth-century physicist, Jean-Baptiste Fourier, who was the first to conceive of how a complex waveform could be mathematically described using sinusoidal functions. Fourier's technique was originally applied to heat transfer but was used by Ohm in the mid-nineteenth century to describe the process by which the auditory system analyzes and encodes spectral information. The basic concept underlying Fourier theory is that any waveform can be uniquely described as a series of sinusoidal functions of specified frequency, amplitude, and starting phase. One could then substitute this frequency-domain representation for the much less mathematically tractable time-domain description.

Fourier transform—A mathematical procedure that converts a series of values in the time domain (waveform) to a set of values in the frequency domain (spectrum). The spectrum is the Fourier transform of a waveform; the waveform is the inverse Fourier transform of the spectrum. It is frequently used to obtain the frequency spectrum of a given signal.

frame—A segment of the speech signal short enough so that the signal within can be considered stationary. Normally, the length of a frame is around 20 ms. Usually, speech frames are tapered by a window function that smooths the discontinuities arising from the cutting of the speech signal.

free stress—Stress whose placement on a syllable within a word is not predictable by distributional, morphological, or lexical criteria.

frequency—The rate of vibration of a periodic event; e.g., a periodic sound has a frequency measured as the number of cycles of vibration per second expressed in hertz.

frequency declination—See **declination**.

frequency-domain operation—An operation that is performed in the frequency domain, e.g., with a fast fourier transform or linear predictive coding spectrum.

frequency modulation (FM)—A systematic change in the spectrum. For example, a sinusoidal signal can be modulated so that its instantaneous frequency continuously changes as a function of time. If the change is unidirectional, the resultant signal is an FM *sweep*, similar to certain forms of police sirens and alarms. The formant transitions of speech are often considered to represent a form of FM, although in this instance the modulation is imposed only on the peaks of the spectrum.

frequency spectrum—A distribution of sinusoidal wave components of a given segment of a signal. Normally a frequency versus amplitude diagram is used to display the frequency spectrum.

frequency-threshold curve (FTC)—The most commonly used characterization of an auditory neuron's filtering properties. The FTC is generated by presenting a sinusoidal stimulus over a range of sound pressure levels and frequencies in such a manner as to trace out a contour delineating the stimulus parameters effective in evoking a discharge rate just greater than a cell's background firing level. The FTC is useful only for characterizing filter properties close to threshold, where the unit's response properties behave in a quasi-linear fashion. FTCs are also called *tuning curves*.

frication—The creation of noise through the turbulent flow of air through a relatively small area.

fricative—A speech sound produced by maintaining a narrow airflow path, resulting in turbulence and causing frication. Fricatives are often classified as stridents or nonstridents, depending on the degree of noise energy.

front end—The stage of an automatic speech recognition system concerned with transforming the acoustic waveform into a representational format that facilitates the extraction of phonetic features by the higher-level components of a recognition system. Front ends typically will transform the acoustic waveform into some form of spectral representation, often with nonlinear operations, to simulate some of the preconditioning imposed by the auditory pathway.

fundamental frequency (f_o)—The lowest frequency component of a periodic signal. A periodic signal consists of a fundamental frequency and its harmonics. The voiced portion of a speech signal is pseudo-periodic and its fundamental frequency corresponds to the perceived pitch of the signal. In music f_o is associated with the musical pitch of a tone (e.g., middle C), and in speech it is associated with voice pitch (e.g., male versus female pitch) or linguistic tone (as in Chinese and many Bantu languages).

fundamental frequency perturbation—The average absolute difference between the successful vocal periods of a sustained phonation; may be expressed as a percent of the mean phonatory frequency.

genioglossus—An extrinsic tongue muscle that originates on the interior surface of the jaw at midline, fans out as it passes through the tongue, and inserts along the entire lengthwise upper surface of the tongue at midline.

gestural patterning model—A proposal that bundles

of gestures or functionally equivalent movement patterns are actively regulated to achieve speech goals.

glide — A consonant sound that has a gradual (gliding) change in articulation reflected by a relatively long interval of formant-frequency shift.

glossometry — A light emitting and sensing device embedded on a pseudopalate, which measures the distance of the tongue from the palate.

glottal attack — The initiation of vocal fold vibration, phonatory airflow, and/or voice production.

glottal volume velocity — The flow of air through the glottis during phonation. Also called the *glottal flow;* may be represented by a flow glottogram.

glottis — The space between the vocal folds, usually measured as a width or area.

harmonic — An integer multiple of the fundamental frequency in voiced sounds. Ideally, the voice source can be conceptualized as a line spectrum in which energy appears as a series of harmonics.

headroom — An informal term for a safety margin between the maximum signal strength expected and the maximum level that can be handled by an amplifier or computer algorithm.

Hebbian learning — A cell modifies its responsiveness based on previous exposure to excitatory inputs from other neurons. This history of neural excitation also influences the connections of that cell, such that neurons that send excitatory signals to it will have their synaptic connections strengthened, while those that rarely send impulses will show a weakening of synaptic connectivity (illustrating the "use it or lose it" principle). Named after the psychologist Donald Hebb, who first proposed such a mechanism for the neural basis of learning.

hertz (Hz) — A measure of frequency, the number of cycles (i.e., periods) per second.

hidden Markov model — A mathematical model in which there is (1) a finite set of states, (2) transition probabilities among them, (3) a finite set of possible observations or outcomes, and (4) a different probability distribution over the set of observations or outcomes associated with each state. The probability of being in a state depends only upon the previous state. Unlike a regular Markov model, in a hidden Markov model the states themselves are not directly associated with outcomes or observations; instead, the states control the probability of the outcomes or observations.

homeostasis — A tendency toward stability of the internal environment of the body.

hybrid — Combination of two or more distinct entities. In synthetic speech, this most frequently refers to two filter arrangements.

hypernasality — Quality of speech characterized by excess nasal resonance.

identification — A task in which the listener categorizes or labels the stimuli presented on a trial.

imaging techniques — Instruments that produce pictures of structures internal to the body, usually without entering the body.

indexical information — Information regarding a speaker's gender, age, mood, and so on, that can be inferred from vocal characteristics.

inertia — The property of a mechanical body (element) to maintain its state of motion or conversely to resist changes in motion; a body at rest tends to stay at rest, and a body in motion tends to stay in motion. The amount of inertia is related to the mass (roughly weight) of a body, and the force (muscle force) needed to overcome inertia is related to the amount of change in motion.

info-elements — Portions of the acoustic signal that contain significant phonetic information. For voiced speech sounds info-elements are typically the formant transitions near phonetic segment boundaries.

inhibition — The ability of a nerve cell to reduce the discharge activity of another neuron through transmission of an inhibitory neurotransmitter that hyperpolarizes (increases the negative electrical potential) of the target cell. Inhibition is an important means of providing negative feedback for stabilization and fine-tuning of the neural representation.

inner hair cell (IHC) — The motion of the basilar membrane is transmitted to higher auditory centers through the inner cells, of which there are about 9000 in the human ear. Approximately 95% of the auditory-nerve fibers innervate IHCs. The cilia on top of the cell (the hair bundle) sense the motion of the tectorial membrane, which passively follows basilar membrane motion. Deflection of the cilia in one direction results in depolarization of the cell, which in turn releases a neurotransmitter that depolarizes innervating auditory-nerve fibers.

input-to-the-system problem — The issue of what are the basic elements of speech production and how these are input to the system; some possible input units are features, gesture bundles, phonemes, allophones, and syllables.

integration — A mathematical function whose acoustic effect, when it is applied to a signal, is to produce a relative increase in the amplitude of the lower frequencies.

integrator — A circuit or algorithm that performs integration on a signal.

intensity — The sound energy per unit of time (i.e., sound power) distributed over a given surface area.

interface — A surface causing a common boundary between adjacent regions.

interval histogram — A measure of the periodicity-encoding properties of a neuron. The interval between each pair of successive discharges is plotted as a frequency histogram. If a neuron is synchronized to a particular frequency, the modes in the histogram will cluster around the period of the frequency and integral multiples thereof, reflecting the fact that the cell may not be able to fire on every stimulus cycle.

intonation—Fundamental frequency pattern associated with a sentence.

intrinsic duration, pitch, intensity—Duration, fundamental frequency, and intensity associated with the phonetic nature of the segment.

intrinsic oscillators—Cells that fire at a relatively constant rate, acting as internal clocks for precise periodicity measurement. They can also serve as synch pulses for resetting a neural process. Intrinsic oscillators are used in certain models of periodicity coding to account for the extraordinary precision with which human listeners can discriminate between signals of very similar fundamental frequency.

invariant representation—The observation that a large variety of sensory stimuli are categorized as the same perceptual entity. In speech this means that a phonetic segment spoken by many different speakers spanning a wide range of regional dialects, speaker rate, age, and voice characteristics are all classifiable as the same phoneme. Despite the variation in acoustic detail, common properties of the spectrotemporal patterns lead to a similar percept.

inverse filter—Filter that cancels the characteristics of another filter. Since the vocal tract acts as a filter on the signal from the vocal folds, a filter with an inverse response can remove the effect of the vocal tract and permit the measurement of the vocal fold signal.

isofrequency representation and contour—The pattern of tonotopic organization of certain nuclei in the auditory pathway, such that all of the neurons along a plane of intersection are most sensitive to the same range of frequencies.

isolation point—The point in a word at which it resembles no other members of its cohort.

laminar flow—A type of air flow in which the air moves in smooth layers; streamline flow, wherein the fluid moves in parallel layers, in contrast to turbulence.

lateral inhibitory network (LIN)—Ability of a neural system to enhance its stimulus representation through the coordinated interaction of excitatory and inhibitory projections. It sharpens the representation by etching the boundaries of the population response to a given signal in such a fashion that the spatial distribution of activity is more clearly defined than would otherwise be the case. At the skirts of the excitation region, inhibitory inputs predominate, restricting the neural activity to a smaller population of nerve cells than would otherwise occur without inhibitory interaction. This mechanism is important for place coding of spectral information.

lateral suppression—Similar to lateral inhibition in appearance but mediated by mechanical properties of the basilar membrane rather than through active neural inhibition.

linear predictive coding (LPC)—A class of methods, used to obtain a spectrum, that employs a weighted linear sum of samples to predict an upcoming value.

linear prediction method—A mathematical method for estimating the vocal tract characteristics by computing the linear regression coefficients from a given segment of speech signal. The regression coefficients correspond to the impulse response of the inverse vocal tract characteristics.

linear regression—The relationship between the mean value of a random variable and the corresponding values of one or more independent variables, approximated by a straight line. The slope of the straight line is called the *regression coefficient*.

linear system—A mathematical representation of a system in which subelements are assumed to be independent of each other. When a linear system is presented by a serial concatenation of subelements, the order can be interchanged freely.

linear, time-invariant (LTI) system—A system in which known inputs yield quantitatively predictable outputs. For example, given two signals of frequency f_1 and f_2, passed through an LTI system, the output should contain those frequencies and no other. However, their amplitude and phase characteristics may change, depending on the nature of the filter.

liquid—A cover term for the phonemes /l/ and /r/.

localization (sound)—The ability of the auditory system to pinpoint the location of a sound source through analysis of binaural time and intensity cues, as well as using spectral cues for elevation localization.

loft register voice—Also called falsetto; the speaking voice register comprising the highest fundamental frequencies, associated with a relatively high open quotient.

logogen—A theoretical device that stands for a word in the mental lexicon. Logogens become activated if a perceptual input resembles their respective word, eventually crossing a threshold and allowing word recognition to occur.

loudness—The perception of intensity, influenced by the frequency and spectral composition of the sound.

low pitch—The perceptual attribute associated with the fundamental frequency of complex signals such as speech and musical tones. It is often correlated with the envelope periodicity of the waveform.

magnitude spectrum—A graph displaying the relative magnitudes of the frequency components of a sound.

manometer—Device for measuring pressure in terms of displacement of water.

Markov model—A mathematical model in which there is a finite set of possible events or outcomes that are observed sequentially. At each time the probability of seeing an event depends only upon the previous event (or in general, for Markov models of order N, the set of N previous events). Usually a Markov model is represented by a graph or a finite state machine consisting of a set of states (representing the events or outcomes) connected with a set of arrows, representing the probabilities of transitions among states.

masking—The perceptual obliteration of a signal by a louder sound.

mass-spring model—A model in which the properties of movement are likened to those of a mass attached to a spring; in some models the speed of movement is linked to the explicit control of articulatory stiffness.

matched filter—A specific form of filter in which the filter output is highly correlated with the central portion of its bandpass characteristic.

mechanoreceptors—Sensory receptors found in the skin and in joints that are sensitive to mechanical stimuli such as skin stretch, joint rotation, and skin indentation.

mel—An auditory unit for the measurement of frequency. It follows certain nonlinear properties of the human perception of frequency.

mental lexicon—Knowledge accumulated about words, their sounds and meanings, and their grammatical uses.

method of adjustment—A basic experimental method in which the observer is given control over the stimulus and allowed to vary it to meet some criterion.

method of constant stimuli—A basic experimental method where the stimuli are presented to the observer in random order.

method of limits—A basic experimental method in which the stimuli are presented to the observer in a fixed order.

modal register voice—The most commonly used voice register, a series of sequential fundamental frequencies between the pulse and loft registers.

model—A simplification of a complex system or process that identifies major components or principles of regulation or action.

modulation—The altering of a signal by a filter or by another signal.

modulation frequency—The most basic (i.e., lowest) periodicity of a complex waveform.

morphological decomposition—The analysis of a word into its morphemes.

motor control model—A model that is concerned with the activation patterns and motoric processes of action.

motor program—A ready-made plan or prescription for a movement or movement sequence.

motor theory—A theory of speech perception described by Liberman and colleagues at Haskins Laboratories proposing that speech perception is mediated by reference to articulatory knowledge so that listeners perceive speech by using information about the sequence of articulatory gestures used to produce the utterance. That is, speech is perceived by translating the acoustic signal into the underlying articulatory gestures that produced it. It is an attempt to account for the perceptual invariance of speech segments. To date, there is little objective experimental evidence to support it.

mucosal wave—The passive undulation of the vocal fold mucosa during phonation.

murmur—A mode of voicing in which the opening and closing of the vocal folds is less abrupt than in other modes and in which the closure may be incomplete.

narrowband analysis—An analysis in which the analyzing bandwidth is relatively narrow (such as 45 Hz in speech analysis). A narrowband analysis is preferred when the interest is to increase frequency resolution, as in the analysis of harmonics for a man's voice.

nasal—A speech sound containing radiation of sound energy from the nose, either with or without accompanying oral radiation.

nasal emission—Flow of air through the nose, usually indicative of an incomplete velopharyngeal seal.

nasal formant—The low-frequency resonance associated with the nose. For men's speech, the nasal formant has a frequency of less than 400 Hz.

nasal grimace—Constriction of the nasal valve to increase resistance and diminish emission from the nose when the velopharyngeal mechanism is inadequate.

neighborhood density—A measure of the absolute number of words in a similarity neighborhood.

neighborhood frequency—A measure of the average or summed frequency of the words in a similarity neighborhood.

neural delay lines—The hypothesized neural implementation of auto- and cross-correlational mechanisms in the auditory system. A delay line is imposed to provide a means for the nervous system to compare the neural activity to the same signal through two different paths. One path projects directly to the neural comparator; the other path takes a more circuitous route of known excursion. The comparator neurons are spatially organized according to the amount of delay imposed. The delay line is an efficient means of computing periodicity because it translates a temporal parameter into an explicitly spatial (place) one. To date there is physiological and anatomical evidence for a neural delay line only in the barn owl.

neural model — A model that relates the various phases of speech motor control to specific brain structures and neural pathways.

node — A region in the resonating vocal tract where particles vibrate with maximum amplitude (i.e., a region of volume velocity maximum) and pressure is at a minimum. Nodes alternate with *antinodes* in accounting for the standing wave distribution of volume velocity (or its inverse, pressure) in the resonating tube.

noise — Essentially any sound (or time series data) without a deterministic structure; in practice, one of two types of sound. The first is acoustic signals that fulfill certain statistical and spectral criteria (e.g., white noise, or equal energy per Hz band over the bandwidth of the signal). The second is extraneous background sounds, regardless of their statistical and spectral properties.

noise-rejection filter — The means by which the auditory system reduces the effect of noise or background sounds by enhancing the response to a more intense (foreground) signal, effectively suppressing activity to the noise through some form of lateral inhibition or neural suppression.

nonlinear system — One in which the output disobeys the rules of a linear, time-invariant system. For example, in response to the input of two signals, f_1 and f_2, a nonlinear system will produce an output that contains not only these frequencies but others as well, such as $f_1 + f_2$ (even-order distortion). Threshold (a point below which there is no effective response) and saturation (a point above which there is no increase in response activity) are inherent properties of a nonlinear system.

nonmonotonic — The change in direction of a function describing the behavior of a system. Its usage is most clearly illustrated by defining its antithesis, the monotonic function. The latter is one in which the function (a straight line) always goes up or down, but not both. When the function goes up over a portion of its dynamic range and down over the remainder, that function is termed nonmonotonic. In this context, nonmonotonic refers to the fact that the discharge rate of certain neurons in the central auditory pathway increases in response to a gain in sound pressure level and then decreases when the amplitude reaches a certain limit.

normal (gaussian) distribution — The bell-shaped curve of probability density for a variable.

normalization — A correction for variance. Speaker normalization is the correction or scaling that reduces variability in acoustic measures such as formant frequencies; time normalization is the correction or scaling that reduces variability in the durations of sound sequences. In synthetic speech, the regularizing of input so that a text-to-speech system receives only text that it is able to turn into speech. For example, the expression ⁵/₁₆ is turned into five-sixteenths, and data that do not translate into text are discarded.

normalizer — A component in a text-to-speech system for normalizing input.

Nyquist sampling theorem — The theorem that a digital representation requires at least two sampling points for every periodic cycle in the signal of interest. Therefore, the sampling rate of digitization should be at least twice the highest frequency of interest in the signal to be analyzed. Unfortunately, the Nyquist frequency is inconsistently used. Some use it to indicate the highest frequency of interest in an analysis; others use it to refer to twice the highest frequency of interest, i.e. to the sampling rate needed to prevent aliasing.

objective method — Any method with trials that have only a limited number of response alternatives and a predetermined correct answer for trials.

obstruent — A consonant sound made with a radical constriction of the vocal tract; it includes stops, fricatives, and affricates.

obturator — An appliance used to occlude an opening between the nasal and oral cavities.

on-line — A process or task run by a real-time device that coordinates actions or other processes.

onset choppers — Physiological response class of the posteroventral cochlear nucleus. They differ from onset lockers in that their response pattern to high-frequency signals looks like a chopper unit and the bandwidth of their filtering is about twice as broad. These cells may form the basis of intensity and pitch coding in the auditory periphery.

onset lockers — Physiological response class of neurons in the posteroventral cochlear nucleus. Onset lockers synchronize to low-frequency signals with a high degree of precision and are so named because of their tendency to concentrate their discharge at the beginning of the stimulus.

open categorization — A task in which the listener is given a large set of response alternatives to allow him or her to choose the one closest to the subjective impression of the stimulus.

open quotient (OQ) — The percent of an entire vocal cycle during which the glottis is open.

orbicularis oris — Muscle that rounds the lips.

orchestration — The coordination of vocal tract gestures in natural speech or in articulatory synthetic speech.

orifice flow — Flow through a narrow opening where the actual flow varies from the theoretical flow depending upon the geometry of the orifice and on Reynolds number.

parallel — An arrangement of a group of filters in which a signal is simultaneously passed to all the filters. The output of all the filters is summed.

parietal pleura — Inner surface of the thoracic cavity.

parsing — The ability of the auditory system and higher cortical centers to distinguish separate sound sources concurrently presented.

partial correlation (PARCOR) — Correlation (sometimes called total correlation) that includes the contribution from various factors. Correlation computed after the contribution from certain factors is eliminated is called partial correlation. The partial correlation coefficients in linear prediction analysis correspond to the reflection coefficients in the discrete cylindrical model of the vocal tract.

Passavant's pad — The anterior movement of the posterior pharyngeal wall produced by the contraction of the overlapping superior and middle constrictors of the pharynx; possibly an airway response to a decrease in velar resistance.

passive mechanical properties — Elastic, frictional, and inertial characteristics of bones, skin, tendons, ligaments, and other nonactive (noncontracting) tissue.

pauser buildup — A physiological response class of neurons in the dorsal cochlear nucleus. They exhibit a complex response pattern such that the cell typically requires between 50 and 200 ms to attain its maximum response level. The pauser variety discharges at stimulus onset and then shuts off for approximately 20 to 50 ms. The buildup pattern does not fire during the first 50 ms and then gradually increases its firing rate until reaching its asymptotic firing level.

perceptual module — A perceptual device described by Fodor as an autonomous, cognitively impenetrable system.

period (t) — The amount of time in seconds required to complete one cycle of oscillation.

periodic or periodicity — The temporal interval over which a waveform (or any time series) repeats itself (either in exact or approximate fashion). Thus, a sinusiodal signal repeats at an interval equal to the reciprocal of its frequency (for a 1 kHz signal the period is 1 ms). Periodicity can also refer to the envelope of the waveform. For a sinusoidal signal the periodicity of the waveform envelope and that of the temporal fine structure are identical. For an amplitude-modulated tone consisting of three harmonics of a common fundamental component, the waveform envelope periodicity is the reciprocal of the fundamental frequency, while the fine structure periodicity is equal to the reciprocal of the average frequency, which in this instance is the same as the middle harmonic.

peripheral representation — The pattern of neural excitation in the auditory nerve or cochlea across the tonotopic axis and through time associated with a particular event or segment.

perplexity — The average number of words that may follow any word at each decision point, using a given grammar. The perplexity of a grammar gives an idea of the degree to which the grammar limits the number of allowable sequences of words. Normally, for a given system a larger task perplexity leads to a larger error rate.

perturbation — A local constriction of the vocal tract. In the perturbation theory of resonance, the effects of a local constriction on resonant frequencies depend on whether the site of constriction is proximal to node or antinode.

phase characteristic — The portion of the Fourier spectrum that pertains to the temporal registration of a frequency component. Phase is computed relative to a cycle of the signal. A full cycle is 360 degrees. A sinusoid by convention begins at 0 degrees. A cosine wave begins at 90 degrees. Although phase is measured in degrees relative to the signal period, it really is a measure of time delay.

phase–locking — The capability of cells to distribute their firing temporally so as to be in registration with the temporal fine structure or envelope of the stimulus waveform. The term derives from the fact that the discharges tend to occur over a restricted phase range of the stimulus cycle. Also called *synchrony.*

phase transition — A qualitative change in a system's behavior.

phonation — The act of producing voice; the generation of acoustic energy by vocal fold vibration.

phone — An elementary sound unit that can be combined to form syllables and words. Phones are the basic building blocks of words. Substituting one phone for another may produce meaning distinction between two words in a particular language.

phonemic restoration — A linguistic form of temporal induction in which listeners restore masked segments of speech on the basis of context.

phonemic transformation — Illusory organization of repeated sequences of brief steady-state vowels into syllables and words.

phonotactics — Constraints on the possible orders of phonetic sequences that can occur within the words of a particular language.

piezoelectric crystal — A dielectric crystal transducer that emits a pressure wave (high-frequency sound wave) when subjected to an applied voltage. It also emits a voltage when subjected to pressure. Thus, it sends and receives ultrasound waves.

pitch — The perception of frequency, influenced by the intensity and spectral composition of the sound; perceptual correlate of fundamental frequency.

pitch period — The interval of speech correlated with a single pulsation cycle of the glottis. For male adult speech this interval ranges from 6 to 12 ms, and for adult female speech the interval is between 3 and 6 ms.

pitch sigma — The standard deviation of fundamental frequencies used in a spoken utterance or series of utterances.

pitch-synchronous analysis (PSA) — A form of spectral analysis in which the estimation of the resonance patterns is based on a single glottal cycle. The estimation of the vocal tract transfer function tends to be most accurate when the analysis window corresponds to the glottal vibration pattern.

place theory — Based on the observations that at low sound pressure levels only a small proportion of nerve cells respond to a given frequency and that this active group of neurons changes in a systematic fashion with corresponding changes in signal frequency (tonotopic organization). The place theory posits that frequency information is encoded entirely or primarily by spatial location of neural activity in auditory nuclei. It is often invoked as an alternative to temporal-based models, in which the frequency information is thought to be encoded in the timing intervals between neural discharges.

PLP method—Perceptually based linear prediction method in which speech spectrum is represented by a perceptual model instead of based on a production model.

pneumotachograph—A device used for measuring volume rate of airflow.

point-tracking techniques—Instruments that track fleshpoints on the surface of an articulator, usually by tracking markers attached to the structure.

preboundary lengthening—Decrease in tempo in anticipation of a linguistic boundary.

preemphasis—In speech analysis, a filtering that boosts high-frequency energy relative to low-frequency energy. Because speech normally contains its strongest energy in the low frequencies, these frequencies would dominate analysis results if preemphasis were not performed.

pressure head—The height of a column of homogeneous fluid that will produce a given intensity of pressure.

pressure transducer—The property of certain structures in the auditory system, such as the tympanic membrane, ossicular chain, and organ of Corti, that systematically respond to pressure variations within the sonic range (0.05 to 30 kHz for human listeners). Nonbiological pressure transducers include microphones, headphones, tweeters, and woofers.

prevoicing—The onset of voicing before the appearance of a supraglottal articulatory event; for stops, prevoicing means that voicing precedes the stop release. Also called *voicing lead*.

primary-like—A physiological response class of neurons in the anteroventral cochlear nucleus. They exhibit a response pattern similar to that of auditory nerve fibers in many respects. These cells send their axonal projections to the olivary complex via the trapezoid body and are thought to be important for binaural analysis of sound for spatial localization.

primary-like with notch—Yet another physiological response class in the anteroventral cochlear nucleus. These neural elements are similar to primary-like units but exhibit a brief (about 5 ms) but pronounced reduction in activity a few milliseconds after firing. These cells exhibit temporal phase-locking capability superior to that of primary-like units.

probability of firing—The likelihood that a cell will fire during a specified interval of time. For certain cells the probability of firing is virtually certain within a few milliseconds of stimulus onset (such as the onset units of the cochlear nuclei or auditory cortical units). Because of the restricted rate of discharge for many auditory neurons, the characterization of a cell's firing pattern in terms of probability is a more accurate gauge of its encoding properties than purely numerical indices of firing behavior.

projection x-ray—Creates an x-ray image by projecting an x-ray beam through the structure of interest onto a sheet of film. A projected image records everything in the path of the beam.

prominence—The condition or quality of being immediately noticeable, eminent, standing out from the environment.

prosodeme—Prosodic distinctive feature.

prosodic bootstrapping—The notion that attention to important changes in the prosody of utterances may provide the language learner with clues to portions of speech that correspond to important grammatical units.

prosodic markers—Changes in prosody such as the introduction of pauses, the lowering of pitch and increases in duration of syllables that occur at points in an utterance where important grammatical changes (such as the end of a phrase or clause) also occur.

prosody—The characteristics of speech sounds having to do with rhythm and intonation. These properties are sometimes called **suprasegmental features** because they apply to stretches of speech longer than a single segment.

prototype—An ideal instance or example from a category that includes most properties typically associated with members of the category and very few properties associated with members from other similar categories.

psychometric function—The relation (function) between the variation in the stimulus and the listener's performance in the experiment.

pulse register voice—Also called *vocal* or *glottal fry*; the speaking voice register comprising the lowest fundamental frequencies, associated with a relatively low open quotient and a perceived rough and bubbly quality.

pulse-ribbon model—Proposed by Patterson to account for many properties of musical pitch and other periodicity pitch phenomena. The basic idea is that patterns of temporally organized neural impulses are sent via the auditory nerve to the central auditory nuclei, where an autocorrelation-like operation is performed based on the spiral shape of the tonotopic axis. Because the spiral has its own spatial periodicity, the effect is to perform a spatial autocorrelation. It is similar in its mathematical properties to several other space-time models of pitch.

pyramidal cell—Relatively large nerve cell found in the motor fields of the cerebral neocortex. These cells are thought primarily to be responsible for outgoing motor command signals going to the spinal cord or brain stem motor nuclei.

quantal theory—A theory that proposes a highly nonlinear relationship between articulatory configurations and acoustic output of the vocal tract, such that the acoustic product for some articulatory constrictions is highly sensitive to slight variations in articulatory positioning.

quantity—Contrastive duration within a phonological system.

radiation characteristic—The term in source-filter theory associated with the radiation (dispersion) of sound from the lips to the atmosphere. Radiation from the mouth has the effect of raising the amplitude of the higher frequencies. It is typically expressed as a 6 dB per octave increase in sound energy (hence, a high-pass filter).

radio waves—Radio frequency electromagnetic waves.

rate-intensity curve—The relationship between sound pressure level and firing rate. Typically, the curve will be flat at low sound pressure levels. Above rate threshold, it will then increase proportional to sound pressure level for 20 to 40 dB and then level off at a rate equal to saturation level.

rate-place—A form of encoding frequency information in terms of the spatial distribution of the magnitude of neural activity. This encoding scheme works best at very low sound pressure levels, where most neurons are not saturated, or with cells that exhibit extended dynamic ranges of response.

rate saturation—Over a certain range of intensities, nerve cells will fire at a rate roughly in proportion to sound pressure level. Above a certain level, however, the cell will no longer respond with an increase in firing. This property, referred to as *saturation*, refers to the fact that neurons have limitations on their discharge activity.

real time—A process that proceeds rapidly enough to keep pace with other events such as changes in an external stimulus.

receptor potential—The electrical potential inside a sensory cell, frequently applied to the characterization of inner and outer hair cell responses. The receptor potential of both types of hair cells is modulated at a rate equal to the driving stimulus over much of the audible hearing range. This is the basis for neural phase locking and temporal coding of frequency.

regulation—A system is said to be regulated if structures respond to change and by their activity preserve or attempt to preserve some level of constancy. An example is the maintenance of a fairly constant pH.

representation—The systematic organization of information in terms of the spatial and temporal distribution of neural activity that underlies the behavioral ability to recognize and categorize based on distinctive neural patterns.

residue—A term originally used by Jan Schouten in the late 1930s to describe the high-order harmonics of a complex tone, which he believed were responsible for generating the low pitch of such signals. The term *residue pitch,* often used as a synonym for low pitch, derives from his work. It is known that low pitch stems principally from lower-order harmonics outside the residue region. In linear predictive coding (LPC), the term residue (or error) is the difference between the actual signal and the signal predicted by the LPC algorithm.

resolution—The fineness of detail of a measurement. In speech this typically refers to the duration of the time intervals or the frequency spacing used in measurement.

resonance—The characteristic of resonators, enclosed bodies of air or other elastic objects, such as metal springs, to vibrate at certain frequencies. In speech, the amplification of a restricted portion of the spectrum, as occurs for sounds emitted through the human vocal tract. At the point of resonance the medium (in this instance, air) responds so that energy associated with resonant frequencies is increased due to reinforcement.

respiratory effort—Increased energy expenditure of the respiratory muscles resulting in increased airflow rate and volume.

resynthesis—The synthesis of speech from parameters extracted from spoken speech.

Reynolds number—A dimensionless number in excess of 2000; an index of the development of turbulence.

rhythm—The temporal pattern or stress pattern of a syllable sequence.

rounding—Constriction and protrusion of the lips. Rounding is associated with a lowering of the frequencies of all vowel formants. In English, only certain back and central vowels are rounded.

sampling—The process of making a series of measurements from a continuous signal. In the computer processing of speech, these measurements are used to represent the signal.

sampling theorem—Nyquist's theorem that S samples per second are needed to represent a waveform with a bandwidth of S/2 Hz.

schema theory—A generalized motor program theory that includes mechanisms for correcting ongoing movements and offers an explanation of motor learning.

segmental features—The phonetic features of phonemes.

segmentation—The delineation of successive sound segments in a speech signal. Typically, segmentation yields units such as phonemes, allophones, or some other phonetic segment.

selective adaptation — An experimental task in which the observer responds to a set of stimuli before and after exposure to a repeated stimulus (the adaptor).

semitone (ST) — A logarithmic scaling of one frequency relative to another.

sensation level (SL) — The decibels above an individual's threshold level for a particular sound (the threshold for that sound by an individual is rated as 0 dB SL).

servosystem model — A model that proposes specific feedback mechanisms in the control of speech production.

signal detection theory (SDT) — A theory of decision making in psychophysical tasks.

signal-to-noise (S/N) ratio — The quantitative relationship between the energy associated with a signal (e.g., a sinusoid or speech sound) and the background noise. The procedures for computing the S/N ratio are complicated and controversial. Human listeners can detect and process sound under extraordinarily low S/N ratios (-10 to 0 dB), probably as a consequence of neural phase locking.

similarity neighborhood — A collection of words in the mental lexicon that share phonetic similarity.

sine wave speech — Nonspeech signals created by tracing natural speech formants with simple sinusoidal waves. Sine wave speech is readily perceived as speech, although it preserves little of the information typically considered as vital speech cues.

sinusoids — The most basic acoustic (and one of the most basic mathematical) functions. The concept of frequency is based on sinusoidal functions (see Fourier theory). The basic mathematical form is:

$$s(t) = A \sin (wt + f)$$

where s(t) is the resultant sine wave; A is a scaling parameter equivalent to amplitude; w is the frequency parameter expressed in radians per unit time (sec.); t is the sampling frequency; f is the phase; 1 cycle is equivalent to 2π radians or 360°. The higher the frequency parameter, the more signal cycles per unit time will result. The greater the value of A, the larger (more intense) the sinusoidal waveform will be.

sound pressure level (SPL) — The decibels above a physical reference standard (0 dB SPL) for a particular sound. SPL is measured by a sound level meter.

source-filter theory — A theory of the acoustic production of speech; that the energy from a sound source is modified by a filter or set of filters. For vowels the vibrating vocal folds usually are the source of sound energy, and the vocal tract resonances (formants) are the filters. The source-filter theory makes possible a description of speech sound production in terms of two fundamental processes or stages: generation of energy and modification of that energy.

speaker adaptation — The process by which a speech recognition system learns characteristics of a new speaker and modifies its internal speech models to improve performance for that speaker. The goal is to approach speaker-dependent performance using the smallest possible amount of speaker-dependent speech data.

speaker dependent system — A speech recognition system in which the acoustic models represent the speech of a particular individual. Such a system is intended to be used only for that person. Normally speaker dependent systems have to be trained for each new user. For speech from the modeled speaker, speaker dependent systems can outperform **speaker independent systems**.

speaker independent system — A speech recognition system in which the models of the speech signal have been trained using many speakers, so that they will cover most of the possible acoustic variations of each sound. This characteristic allows the system to be used by any new user without any prior training for that user. Speaker independent systems usually do not perform as well as **speaker dependent systems**.

spectrogram — A graphic representation of sound; a pattern for sound analysis containing information on intensity, frequency, and time. The typical spectrogram provides a three-dimensional display of time on the horizontal axis, frequency on the vertical axis, and intensity at a particular time and frequency by the darkness of a gray-scale display. A spectrogram can be printed as hard copy or displayed on a video monitor.

spectrograph — A device for producing spectrograms.

spectrum — A signal's energy as a function of frequency. The spectrum is usually represented in a graph in which the x-axis is the frequency and the y-axis is the logarithm of the energy. Spectra are defined only for stationary signals (signals whose statistical properties do not change with time). For nonstationary signals like speech, the spectrum is computed over short enough frames so that the signal within can be considered stationary; a sequence of spectra is used to characterize the nonstationary signals.

speech mode of perception — A hypothetical mode of perception involving listening to potentially ambiguous sounds such that they are perceived as speech.

speech sine wave — The speech spectrum can be pared down to a minimal representation based on sinusoidal components in place of formant patterns. Such a minimalist representation is effective under certain conditions in communicating the phonetic and semantic information in the original speech waveform.

spike—A term for the discharge of a neuron. Typically the electrical potential recorded from nerve cells is amplified and routed to the trigger port of an oscilloscope. Although the cell's action potential is not in the shape of a pulse, the circuit used to trigger the display of the oscilloscope converts the potential into a pulse or spikelike signal, accounting for the use of this term.

spindles—Specialized mechanoreceptors found within muscles containing fibers that are classically thought to be sensitive to changes in muscle length. Muscle spindles' sensitivity is unique in that it can be changed by special small fiber motoneurons (gamma motoneurons).

stiffness—The property of a mechanical body (or element) to maintain its position or shape; roughly equivalent to elasticity. The muscle force needed to overcome stiffness is related to how far the body is moved to change in shape.

stop—A speech sound characterized by a complete obstruction of the vocal tract, usually followed by an abrupt release of air that produces a burst noise.

stop gap—The acoustic interval corresponding to articulatory closure for a stop or affricate consonant; it is identified on a spectrogram as an interval of relatively low energy, conspicuously lacking in formant pattern or noise.

strain gauge—A coiled wire transducer placed on a beam. When the beam bends, the wire emits a voltage proportional to the degree of bend.

strain gauge transducer—A device to measure pressure.

stress—Prominence of a syllable in a spoken chain, usually achieved by greater articulatory effort.

strident—A fricative with an intense noise energy; also called a sibilant; /s/ and /ʃ/ are examples. The nonstrident fricatives have less energy; /θ/ is an example.

subjective method—Any method that asks the listener to introspect about his perception of a stimulus without providing a basis for determining whether the response by the listener is correct.

suppressor—A signal effective in reducing the magnitude of discharge to a second excitatory stimulus. Often a suppressor signal is ineffective in exciting a neuron by itself, and its suppressive potential is only revealed when presented in tandem with another sound.

suprasegmental information—Features whose domain extends over more than one segment, including intonation, stress, and quantity.

syllable stress—Accent or emphasis on a particular syllable relative to surrounding syllables. Stressed syllables are typically loud and long and may have a different pitch relative to immediately adjacent syllables.

synchronous activity—The fact that large numbers of neurons tend to fire at the same time in response to a high-intensity, low-frequency signal. This synchronous activity of neurons associated with different frequency channels can be an important cue for event detection and sound source segregation.

synchrony capture—The ability of a high-intensity signal to recruit neurons of distant characteristic frequency to its timing pattern. For example, it is possible for a 500 Hz signal to have auditory nerve fibers responding to its temporal pattern whose characteristic frequencies are several octaves distant, particularly higher in frequency.

synchrony-place—Similar to the rate-place model of frequency coding in that it relies on the tonotopic organization of the auditory pathway to represent the frequency dimension. However, the magnitude parameter is encoded in terms of neural synchrony to frequencies close to the fibers' characteristic frequencies rather than in terms of discharge rate.

synchrony suppression—A phenomenon related to synchrony capture. In the absence of a suppressor signal a population of neurons may synchronize its discharge to a signal close in frequency to their characteristic frequencies. When a second, more intense signal is introduced, the same neurons respond to this stronger sound. In this sense it acts to suppress the synchrony of the cells' response to the original signal.

synergies—See **coordinative structure.**

syntactic parser—A computer program that analyzes, or parses, a sentence by breaking it into its syntactic components. The parser imposes a structure, as defined by the syntactic rules of a language, upon a given sentence. For instance, a sentence may be defined as a sequence of "noun phrase, verb, noun phrase," and a noun phrase may be defined as any one of a list of possible sequences, such as "word determiner, noun" or "pronoun."

syntagma—A rhythmic grouping of syllables.

synthesis—The creation of speech by computer, circuits, or physical resonators.

tail—The portion of the auditory nerve fiber frequency threshold curve that is responsive only to high-intensity signals distant from the unit's characteristic frequency. This tail component indicates a low-pass filter–like process in peripheral transduction that enables low-frequency signals to drive high–characteristic frequency neurons.

tap—A very rapid articulation of a stop closure.

task—The format of presentation of stimuli to a listener and the responses.

tectorial membrane—Overlies the hair cells in the organ of Corti. This membrane's articulation with the cilia of the outer hair cells and its consequent interaction through fluid coupling with the cilia of the inner hair cells depolarizes the inner hair cells and thus transmits acoustic information from inner ear into the neural portion of the auditory pathway.

temporal integration—The perceptual property sensitive to signal duration. For example, the detection threshold in units of sound pressure level of a sinusoidal signal depends on signal duration such that the threshold lowers as a function of duration up to a certain limit, typically around 200 ms. Beyond this duration the threshold is relatively insensitive to stimulus duration. Similar phenomena have been demonstrated for other types of acoustic signals and sensory modalities. In each instance, the system appears to integrate energy over time up to a certain limit; hence the reduction in threshold proportional to stimulus duration. For durations greater than this limit no further increase in sensitivity (i.e., energy integration) occurs.

tendon organs — Specialized mechanoreceptors within muscle tendons and muscle-related connective tissue that are sensitive to changes in muscle tension.

timbre — Attribute of auditory sensation distinct from pitch and loudness and commonly associated with vowel quality and musical instrument identity. Helmholtz proposed that timbre is based on the distribution of energy across the spectrum. It is now known that timbre is also based on the attack characteristics of the initial 50 to 80 ms of the signal.

time-domain operation — An operation governed by duration; e.g., calculations performed with respect to the waveform of a sound.

time-intensity trading — The ability to compensate for changes in interaural time disparities with commensurate alterations to interaural disparities in sound pressure level in keeping the apparent location of a sound object the same.

tissue viscous resistance — Resistance due to friction from the peribronchial tissues, lung parenchyma, and vascular structures sliding over one another during movement of the lung.

tomograph — An image, not a projection, of a thin slice of tissue.

tone — Distinctive fundamental frequency associated with syllables or words.

tone sandhi — Influence of the tone on one syllable or word on the tone of an adjacent syllable or word.

tongue advancement — The relative position of the tongue in the anteroposterior dimension of the vocal tract. Front vowels tend to have relatively high F_2 values, relatively large values of the F_2-F_1 difference, and relatively small value of the F_3-F_2 difference. Back vowels tend to have relatively low F_2 values, relatively small values of the F_2-F_1 difference, and a relatively large value of the F_3-F_2 difference.

tongue height — The relative position of the tongue in the inferosuperior dimension of the vocal tract. As applied to vowels, tongue height relates primarily to the relative frequency of F_1; the higher the vowel, the lower F_1 tends to be. Tongue height also varies with jaw position such that high vowels tend

to have a nearly closed jaw position.

tonotopoic organization — The fact that there is a systematic relationship between the frequency to which a neuron is most sensitive and the spatial location of the cell relative to others. Thus, in most nuclei of the auditory pathway there is strict segregation of frequency sensitivity, such that units most sensitive to low frequencies will cluster together and those most sensitive to higher frequencies will be located a certain distance away, proportional to their characteristic frequencies. This anatomical-physiological correlation forms the basis of the place theory of frequency coding.

topographic representation — Similar to **tonotopic organization** but can apply to parameters of sensory coding other than frequency (e.g., intensity, sound location).

total lung capacity — The maximum amount of air that the lungs can contain when fully expanded.

training data — A set of recorded utterances used to estimate the model parameters in a speech recognition system. A training database is often comprised of thousands of sentences spoken by many different speakers in an effort to represent the variety of phonetic, phonological, lexical, syntactic, and indexical (personal) characteristics of the speech that a system is expected to recognize.

transducer — A device that converts energy from one form to another. For example, a microphone converts acoustical to electrical energy.

transform — A representation converted from a different domain. See **transformation**.

transformation — The conversion of data from one domain into another, as in the conversion of a speech signal (which indicates air pressures in the time domain) into a magnitude spectrum (which indicates the relative magnitudes of different components in the frequency domain).

transglottal pressure — The differential pressure across the glottis; the pressure difference between the intraoral and subglottal pressures.

transliteration — The representation of the sounds of one language using the writing system of another.

traveling wave — The form of wave pattern propagating across the basilar membrane. In contrast to standing waves, which pertain to airborne sound propagation, traveling waves are asymmetrical, with relatively little back propagation. This is the primary reason the filter characteristics of the cochlea are asymmetrical, with much sharper tuning on the high-frequency slope of the tuning function than on the low side.

trial — The cycle of presenting one stimulus or set of stimuli and collecting the response from the listener.

turbulence (turbulent flow) — A condition characterizing gases and liquids in which the velocity, and to an extent, the direction of flow of the particles fluctuate irregularly; a condition of air flow in which eddies (rotating volume elements of air) are generated. This condition is associated with the generation of noise energy. Turbulence contrasts with **laminar flow.**

user interface—The part of a computer system that facilitates interaction between the user and the computer. The user interface may consist of text or pictures displayed on a screen, sounds either generated or accepted by the computer, and keyboard or mouse input from the user.

vector codebook—The collection of vector prototypes representing the different spectrum (and delta spectrum) shapes used to represent the input speech.

velopharyngeal adequacy—Ability to maintain velopharyngeal closure sufficiently for normal speech.

velopharyngeal closure—Occurs when the velum is physically capable of forming a tight seal between the nasal and oral cavities.

velopharyngeal inadequacy—Failure to effect velopharyngeal closure, resulting in compromised speech.

velopharyngeal orifice—The space existing between the velum and the lateral and posterior pharyngeal walls.

verbal satiation—The loss of meaning that occurs when one repeats a word over and over to oneself.

verbal transformation—The illusory changes heard when a recorded word or phrase is played over and over.

visceral pleura—The outer surface of the lung.

viscosity—The property of a mechanical body (or element) to resist motion, approximately equivalent to friction or reflected on the resistance felt when pulling an oar through the water. The muscle force needed to overcome viscous resistance is related to the velocity of motion.

vital lung capacity—The volume of air that can be expelled by the most forcible expiration after the deepest inspiration.

vocalization—The production of voice for nonspeech purposes such as crying, laughing, grunting, sighing, and moaning.

vocal jitter—See **fundamental frequency perturbation.**

vocal shimmer—Also called *amplitude perturbation*; the average absolute decibel difference of the acoustic amplitude between successive vocal cycles of a sustained phonation; may be expressed as a percent of the mean sound pressure level.

vocal tract area function—A mathematical representation of the vocal tract in which its cross-sectional areas are specified as a function of the distance from the glottis.

vocal tract model—A model that focuses on the shaping of the vocal tract for speech production.

voice bar—A band of energy, typically reflecting the first harmonic of the voice source, that appears on a spectrogram; indicates voicing.

voice onset time (VOT)—A measure of the time between a supraglottal event and the onset of voicing; for stops, VOT is the interval between release of the stop (usually determined acoustically as the stop burst) and the appearance of periodic modulation (voicing) for a following sound.

voice register—A range of consecutive fundamental frequencies that can be produced with a perceptually distinct voice quality; a physiologically distinct mode of phonation.

volume velocity—A measure of the flow of air that takes into account both amount and speed of air.

waveform—A graph showing the amplitude versus time function for a continuous signal such as the acoustic signal of speech.

wavelength—The distance that a periodic sound travels in one complete cycle. Wavelength equals velocity (speed of sound) divided by frequency.

wideband analysis—An analysis in which a relatively large analyzing bandwidth is used (such as 300 Hz in speech analysis); preferred when the primary concern is to reveal formant pattern or to increase time resolution.

word frequency—An estimate of how commonly a word is used in conversation or text.

Index

Page numbers in *italics* indicate illustrations.
Page numbers followed by a *t* indicate tables.

Time waveform, visual analysis of, 250-251
Timing; *see* Prosody
Timing models, 22
Tissue resistance, 50
Tomographic images, 517
Tomography, 502-503
Tonal features, 234
Tonal tier, 236
Tone, 232-236
Tone-group, 264
Tone sandhi, 234
Tone-unit, 264
Tongue height, 200, 228
Tonotopic organization, 363, *369, 374, 375*
Tonotopic range, *373*
Topographic representation of waveform periodicity, 391
Total correlation, 479
TRACE model of speech perception, 301, 312, 313-315
Tracking points, 517
Trading relations, 282, 287-289
Training data, speech recognition systems, 423-424
Transducer, intraoral, 496
Transduction, auditory, 354
Transfer function, *187,* 187
  fricatives, 194
  linear prediction method, 480, 481
  nasal vowels, 196
  vocal tract area function, 486-487
Transformation, 247
Transglottal pressure, 129, 161
Transition cues, 211
Transitions, 209
  augmented transition network (ATN), 263
  speech signal, 204-206
Transition to turbulence, 193
Translation theories, 21
Transmission, speech production modeling, 470
Transmission line analog, 472
Traveling wave, 367, *369*
Trial, 527
Trigeminal nerve, 103
Tuning, 385
Turbulent flow, 50, 193
Turbulent (fricative) articulatory sound sources, 160
Turbulent (noise) source, 187
Two degrees of freedom model of vocal fold mechanics, 136
Two-mass models of vocal fold mechanics, 29, 135-136, 137

U

Ultrasound, *507-510, 515, 517*
Uncoupled cavities, 193
Units of analysis in speech perception, 280-281
User interface of speech recognition system, 412

V

Vagus nerve, 121, 123
Variability; *see also* Normalization, perceptual
  in memory and attention, 297-299
  speaker
    perceptual normalization, 330
    and speech signal, 264
  in speech perception and word recognition, 296-297
Vector codebook, 417, 423
Vector quantization
  simple-HMM signal analysis, 416-417
  speech recognition system, 415, 416
Vegetative laryngeal function, 113-114
Velar burst spectra, 204, *206*
Velar stop, *206*
Velopalatography, 511
Velopharyngeal closure, 68
Velopharyngeal inadequacy, 68-73, 79
  acquired, 72-73
  simulation of, 73-77
  structural adjustments with, 64
Velopharyngeal orfice measurement of, 82
Velopharyngeal orfice resistance, *58*
Velopharyngeal sphincter resistance, *56, 58*
Verbal satiation, 452, 459, 460
Verbal transformation (VT), 452
Verbal transformation effect, 451-461
  age and, 454-457, *458*
  interaurally asynchronous stimuli, 460-461
  phonemic restoration effect and, 458-459
  phonetic analysis of, 453
  verbal satiation, 452
  visual effects analogous to, 452-453
Veridical perception, 440
Vertical phase difference, 135
Viscoelastic components of muscle contraction, 97
Viscoelasticity
  aerodynamic coupling and, 138
  vocal fold mucosal wave, 135
Viscosity, 97
  active, 98
  and airway resistance, 48, 50
  vocal fold mucosal wave, 135